Psychiatric Disease: Metabolic and Immune Abnormalities

Psychiatric Disease: Metabolic and Immune Abnormalities

Editor: Brendan Tucker

AMERICAN
MEDICAL PUBLISHERS
www.americanmedicalpublishers.com

AMERICAN
MEDICAL PUBLISHERS
www.americanmedicalpublishers.com

Cataloging-in-Publication Data

Psychiatric disease : metabolic and immune abnormalities / edited by Brendan Tucker.
p. cm.
Includes bibliographical references and index.
ISBN 979-8-88740-404-2
1. Psychology, Pathological. 2. Mental illness. 3. Psychiatry. 4. Mental illness--Metabolism.
5. Psychology, Pathological--Immunological aspects. 6. Psychobiology. I. Tucker, Brendan.
RC435 .P79 2023
616.89--dc23

American Medical Publishers,
41 Flatbush Avenue,
1st Floor, New York,
NY 11217, USA

ISBN 979-8-88740-404-2 (Hardback)

Contents

Preface

This book has been an outcome of determined endeavour from a group of educationists in the field. The primary objective was to involve a broad spectrum of professionals from diverse cultural background involved in the field for developing new researches. The book not only targets students but also scholars pursuing higher research for further enhancement of the theoretical and practical applications of the subject.

A psychiatric disease is a mental illness which significantly disrupts the thinking, behavior and mood of an individual and severely increases the risk of pain, death, disability or loss of freedom. There are various categories of psychiatric diseases including anxiety disorders, depression, addictive behaviors, schizophrenia, personality disorders and eating disorders. Symptoms of psychiatric diseases comprise drug or alcohol abuse, suicidal thinking, confused thinking, inability to handle daily problems and stress, extreme tiredness, sleeping problems and more. Schizophrenia is a serious psychiatric disease. It results in detachment from reality and people having this disease experience disorganized speech and thinking, delusions, and hallucinations. Anxiety involves focusing on dangerous and bad things, which can happen and worrying about them excessively. It also comprises phobias such as irrational fears in regards to particular things like height. This book explores all the important aspects of psychiatry in the present day scenario. It presents researches and studies performed by experts across the globe. This book is appropriate for students seeking detailed information in this area as well as for experts.

It was an honour to edit such a profound book and also a challenging task to compile and examine all the relevant data for accuracy and originality. I wish to acknowledge the efforts of the contributors for submitting such brilliant and diverse chapters in the field and for endlessly working for the completion of the book. Last, but not the least; I thank my family for being a constant source of support in all my research endeavours.

Editor

1

Dynamic Patterns of Threat-Associated Gene Expression in the Amygdala and Blood

Adriana Lori[1†], *Stephanie A. Maddox*[2,3†], *Sumeet Sharma*[1,2], *Raül Andero*[4,5,6], *Kerry J. Ressler*[1,2,3] and *Alicia K. Smith*[1,7*]

[1] Department of Psychiatry and Behavioral Sciences, Emory University School of Medicine, Atlanta, GA, United States, [2] Neurobiology of Fear Laboratory, Division of Depression and Anxiety Disorders, McLean Hospital, Belmont, MA, United States, [3] Department of Psychiatry, Harvard Medical School, Boston, MA, United States, [4] Institut de Neurociències, Universitat Autònoma de Barcelona, Bellaterra, Spain, [5] CIBERSAM, Corporació Sanitaria Parc Taulí, Sabadell, Spain, [6] Department of Psychobiology and Methodology in Health Sciences, Universitat Autònoma de Barcelona, Bellaterra, Spain, [7] Department of Gynecology and Obstetrics, Emory University School of Medicine, Atlanta, GA, United States

***Correspondence:**
Alicia K. Smith
alicia.smith@emory.edu

† These authors have contributed equally to this work

Stress and trauma profoundly influence psychiatric biobehavioral outcomes. The identification of treatment and biomarker targets would be accelerated by a broad understanding of the biological responses to these events. The goal of this study was to determine genes responsive to auditory fear conditioning (FC), a well-characterized amygdala-dependent rodent model of threat-exposure, in the presence or absence of prior stress history, providing insight into the physiological processes underlying response to trauma. RNA-sequencing was performed in blood and amygdala from mice that underwent fear conditioning with (Immo+FC) and without (FC) prior immobilization stress, a paradigm that induces HPA axis, and behavioral stress sensitization. In the amygdala, 607 genes were regulated by FC vs. home-cage (HC) controls, and 516 genes differed in stress-sensitized mice (Immo+FC vs. FC). In the former, we observed an enhancement of specific biological processes involved in learning and synaptic transmission, and in the latter processes associated with cell proliferation and the cellular response to drugs. In the blood of stress-sensitized animals, 468 genes were dynamically regulated when compared to FC, and were enriched for the biological pathways of inflammation and cytokine signaling. This study identified genes and pathways that respond to threat in the amygdala and blood of mice with and without a prior stress history and reveals the impact of stress history on subsequent inflammation. Future studies will be needed to examine the role of these dynamically regulated genes may play in human clinical stress and trauma-related disorders.

Keywords: threat, fear, PTSD (post-traumatic stress disorder), amygadala, stress

INTRODUCTION

Post-traumatic stress disorder (PTSD) is a pervasive and debilitating psychiatric disorder that develops in vulnerable individuals after exposure to variable levels of trauma. A prior stress event, particularly early life trauma or abuse, has also been shown to cause poor psychiatric outcomes in adults, increasing risk for and the severity of PTSD (1, 2). The characteristic features of PTSD, such as hypervigilance and heightened startle reactions (DMS-V), associate with a patient's inability to regulate their fear response in the presence of a non-threatening situation (3, 4). Human neuroimaging studies and animal models have well established that the amygdala plays a central role in the processing of fearful and threatening stimuli and in mediating the constellation of responses that are associated with fear and threat-related behaviors (5, 6). Accumulating and compelling evidence now suggests that PTSD is associated with dysregulation of the amygdala, generally hyperactivity, in response to trauma-relevant or emotionally salient cues (7, 8).

Recent studies have identified differential gene expression patterns in blood between PTSD cases and trauma-exposed controls, reporting possible genes, and pathways associated with PTSD, several of which show dysregulation of the immune system and glucocorticoid pathways (9). However, there is limited knowledge of the degree of correlation between gene expression changes, accompanying trauma, and psychiatric conditions (e.g., PTSD) in the blood and those in the brain. Additionally, because of the obvious limitations of availability of human brain tissues, there had been paucity of brain-based transcriptomic studies. While transcriptomic studies from human post-mortem issues can aide in examining persistent, long-lasting changes in gene expression relevant to specific disease states, they do not permit examination of the transcriptional changes which occur in brain regions relevant for stress and trauma-related disorders at times proximal to trauma.

In this regard, traumatic memory formation in animal models can facilitate identification of genes whose expression is comparable between the amygdala and blood. As such, studies employing rodent models of stress and threat exposure may present a powerful approach toward bridging this gap. Moreover, studies examining the molecular mechanisms associated with the formation and persistence of threat-relevant memories have largely utilized Pavlovian fear-conditioning (FC), employing as conditioned stimulus either novel auditory cues to result in a largely amygdala dependent memory, or spatial, and contextual cues that integrate hippocampal and amygdala regions to regulate learning (5, 10). As much work has shown in human clinical studies has noted the importance of the amygdala in the pathophysiology of trauma-relevant disorders (11–13) and the impact of prior stress history on later risk for the development of PTSD accompanying trauma (14), we were most interested in examining the molecular changes occurring within the amygdala in the time period proximal to trauma. To meet this objective we used paradigm previously utilized by our group which has confirmed that mice immobilized for one 2 h session, 1 week prior to auditory FC have impaired fear extinction and retention, phenotypes that are seen in human clinical PTSD (15, 16). In addition to the observed behavioral phenotype, mice exposed to the immobilization paradigm had hypothalamic-pituitary-adrenal (HPA) axis hypersensitivity, and transient changes in plasma corticosterone levels (4, 17). HPA axis abnormalities, such as low levels of cortisol in urine and plasma or higher suppression of cortisol in response to dexamethasone have been also reported in PTSD patients (18, 19). As the prior (immobilization) stress history model replicates many of the behavioral and hormonal alterations that are observed with human clinical trauma-relevant disorders (20, 21), we utilized a robust mouse model of stress exposure and auditory fear conditioning to identify changes in gene expression in the amygdala response to fear conditioning with and without prior stress.

Ultimately, our goal was to identify correlated patterns of gene expression between blood and brain under these conditions to facilitate interpretation of blood-based studies of PTSD and to provide new insight into the pathophysiology stress-related disorders.

METHODS

Animals

All experiments were performed on adult male wild-type C57BL/6J mice aged 2–3 months obtained from The Jackson Laboratory. Male mice were group-housed in a temperature-controlled vivarium with set-point maintained at 72° F (±1°) and relative humidity controlled at 40–50%, with *ad libitum* access to food and water. Each experimental group consisted of 12 mice maintained on a 12-h light/dark cycle, with all behavioral procedures being performed during the light cycle. All procedures used were approved by the Emory University Institutional Animal Care and Use Committee (IACUC) and in compliance with National Institutes of Health Guide for the Care and Use of Laboratory Animals.

Mouse Immobilization Stress (Immo) and Fear Conditioning (FC)

Immobilization stress (Immo) and fear conditioning (FC) were conducted following the protocol from Andero et al. (4). Briefly, immobilization procedures were conducted in a room separate from housing and behavioral paradigms. Each animal was immobilized by restraining their four limbs with tape in a prone position to metal arms attached to a wooden board for 2 h. All cage-mate animals received the same treatment—either Immo or handling. Handling lasted ~1 min per mouse and consisted of letting the animal walk on top of their home cage and in the hands of the experimenter. After Immo, animals were returned to their home cage (HC) where they remained undisturbed for a week prior to fear conditioning (FC), which was performed in Immo animals and a subset of naïve animals. For auditory fear conditioning mice were habituated to white-light illuminated, standard rodent modular test chambers (ENV-008-VP; Med Associates Inc., St. Albans, VT) with an inside area of 30.5 cm (L) × 24.1 cm (W) × 21.0 cm (H) for 10 min on 2 consecutive days prior to fear conditioning. Fear conditioning consisted of five trials of a novel tone conditioned stimulus (CS; 30 s tone, 6 kHz, 70 dB), which co-terminated with a foot-shock (500 ms, 0.6 mA) unconditioned stimulus (US). The tone conditioned stimulus was generated by a Tektronix function generator audio oscillator delivered through a high-frequency speaker (Motorola, Model 948) attached to the side of each chamber. The Pre-CS period lasted 180 s and a variable inter-trial interval (ITI) was used between each CS-US pairing to result in a total conditioning session which lasted 840 s. The apparatus was cleaned with Quatricide® after each mouse.

Mice were sacrificed under basal conditions (HC group) or 2 h following auditory fear conditioning (Immo+FC and FC alone groups)—a time point that our group has consistently utilized for looking at changes in transcriptional processes in the amygdala following auditory fear conditioning—with a brief exposure to isoflurane anesthesia, <30 s, followed by decapitation and trunk blood collection. Trunk blood from two mice of the same behavioral group was collected into a single 3 ml EDTA BD-Vacutainer tubes. A 250 μL aliquot of each blood sample was allocated for complete blood count, and the remaining sample was stored at −80°C. Brains were immediately frozen on dry ice and stored at −80°C, and 1 week later brains were mounted on a sliding, freezing microtome using Tissue-Tek OTC, and sectioned slowly to approximately Bregma −1.34 mm (22) to reveal the amygdala. One millimeter of bilateral amygdala punches, centered on the basolateral nucleus were taken and immediately frozen in microcentrifuge tubes on dry ice and stored at −80 degrees for later RNA extraction. The bilateral amygdala punches (and the blood) from 2 mice of the same behavioral group were pooled together, thus resulting in a total of 6 pooled samples for each behavioral condition that were sequenced. As the murine basolateral amygdala is slightly larger than 1 mm, we cannot exclude the possibility that other amygdala subregions were including in these tissue samples.

RNA Extraction and Sequencing

RNA extraction, QC, library preparation, and sequencing were conducted by the Yerkes Non-Human Primate Genomics Core (Atlanta, GA). Amygdala punches were homogenized with a bead milling homogenizer, and total RNA was isolated and purified from each sample with the RNeasy Mini Kit (Qiagen, CA) following the manufacturer's instructions. RNA quality and quantity were verified with the 2100 BioAnalyzer PicoChip (Agilent Technologies, Santa Clara, CA) before sequencing, and all samples had an RNA Integrity Number (RIN) score of nine or higher. For blood samples, globin mRNA transcripts were depleted using the GLOBINclear^{TM}-Mouse kit (Ambion, Austin, TX) according to the manufacturer's instructions. Briefly, 1 μg of total RNA was treated with biotinylated oligonucleotides to selectively deplete the α- and β-globin sequences. Subsequently, streptavidin paramagnetic beads were added, to capture the hybridized globin mRNA biotinylated probes, resulting in an average 25% loss of total RNA. Further purification of the globin depleted RNA was performed with SPRI magnetic beads as per manufacturer's recommendation.

Libraries were prepared using the Illumina (Illumina Inc. San Diego, CA) TruSeq^{TM} RNA kit as per manufacturer's instructions. Briefly, 250 ng of total RNA was used for library preparation.

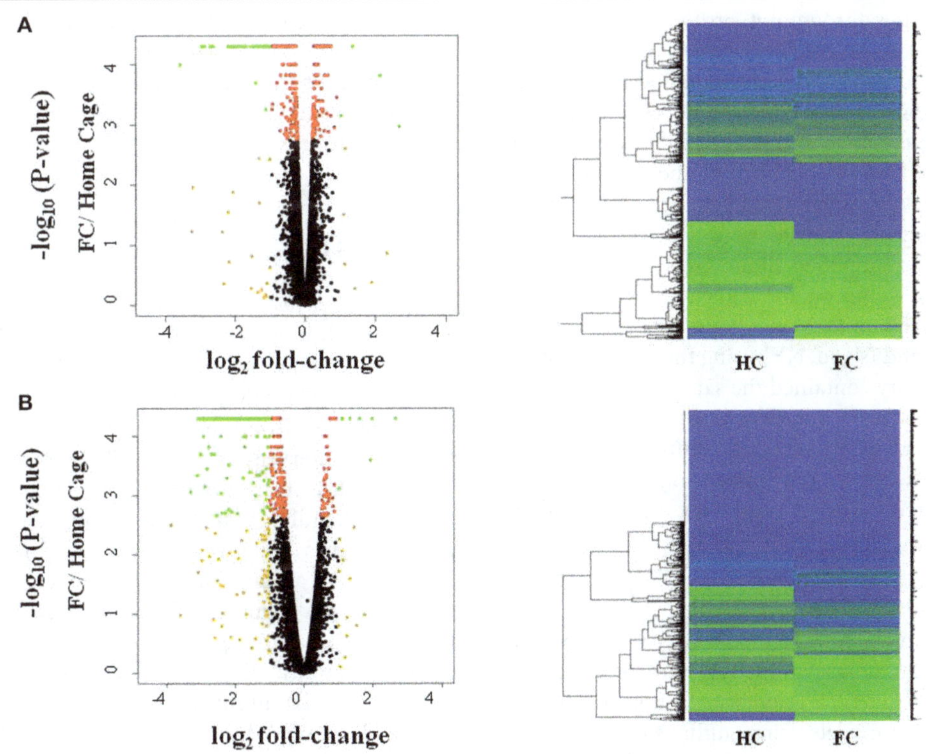

FIGURE 1 | Fear conditioning induces gene expression differences in amygdala and blood. Volcano plots and heatmaps show changes in gene expression in the amygdala **(A)** and blood **(B)** after fear conditioning compared to Home Cage (HC vs. FC). The horizontal axis of the Volcano plot is $\log_2$ fold change for differently expressed genes, and the vertical axis is the negative-$\log_{10}$ of the p-values are plotted. Each dot represents a gene, with red dots showing genes reaching an FDR corrected p-value of 0.05, and green dots representing genes with FDR < 0.05 and absolute fold change >1; orange dots have an absolute fold change>1 but do not reach experiment-wide significance; black dots are genes whose expression is similar between the two groups.

TABLE 1 | Enrichment biological process analyses for differential express genes in fear conditioning mice compared to control (FC vs. HC).

GO number	Description	FE[a]	*p*-value[b]
AMYGDALA			
GO:0007611	Learning or memory	8.20	4.18×10^{-4}
GO:0008306	Associative learning	8.47	0.010
GO:0007268	Chemical synaptic transmission	3.65	0.008
GO:0003007	Heart morphogenesis	5.99	0.008
GO:0035556	Intracellular signal transduction	2.44	0.012
GO:0055085	Transmembrane transport	2.49	0.023
GO:0007507	Heart development	2.80	0.025
GO:0048511	Rhythmic process	3.81	0.025
GO:0007612	Learning	5.28	0.030
GO:0007157	Heterophilic cell-cell adhesion via plasma membrane cell adhesion molecules	6.03	0.027
GO:0045944	Positive regulation of transcription from RNA polymerase II promoter	1.75	0.036
GO:0006811	Ion transport	2.03	0.036
GO:0006351	Transcription, DNA-templated	1.50	0.041
GO:0045053	Protein retention in Golgi apparatus	27.87	0.040
GO:0007626	Locomotory behavior	3.87	0.045
BLOOD			
GO:0007156	Homophilic cell adhesion via plasma membrane adhesion molecules	12.4	1.63×10^{-26}
GO:0002376	Immune system process	3.07	0.009

[a]*FE, Fold Enrichment.*
[b]*p-value following Benjamini-Hochberg correction for multiple testing.*

The TruSeq method (low-throughput protocol) employs two rounds of poly-A based mRNA enrichment using oligo-dT magnetic beads followed by mRNA fragmentation using cations at high temperature. First and second strand cDNA synthesis was performed followed by end repair of the blunt cDNA ends. One single "A" base was added at the 3′ end of the cDNA followed by ligation of barcoded adapter unique to each sample. The adapter-ligated libraries were then enriched using PCR amplification. The amplified library was validated using a High Sensitivity DNA chip on the Agilent Bioanalyzer. The libraries were further quantified on Qubit® 2.0 Fluorometer (Life Technologies, Grand Island, NY) using the High Sensitivity dsDNA assay. Each library contained the same amount of RNA, and eight sample pools were multiplexed in each lane of the flowcell. PhiX was used as an internal control on each lane to monitor the error statistics, and sequencing was performed on the Illumina HiSeq1000 system employing a paired-end 101 cycles run.

Statistical Analysis

Alignment to the 10 mm UCSC Mouse Assembly was performed using STAR version 2.3 (23); parameters were set using the annotation as a splice junction reference. Sample reads were assembled into transcript models using cufflinks (v2.1.1), which were then merged and processed with cuffdiff v2.1.1 (24) to produce per sample FPKM expression levels and estimate differential expression between the sample groups. Each tissue (amygdala and blood) was processed separately to allow for identification of tissue-specific differences for each behavioral condition. The false discovery rate (FDR) was controlled at 5% to account for multiple testing in all analyses ($q < 0.05$). Volcano plots were generated in R. Differentially expressed genes were further evaluated for the enrichment of biological processes using DAVID 6.8 (25). Differences in cell counts between groups were evaluated using an independent *t*-test.

RESULTS

In this study, two groups of mice (with and without a history of immobilization stress; Immo), were trained in an auditory fear conditioning paradigm (Immo+FC and FC, respectively); a third group of naïve, home-cage control animals was handled and removed from the vivarium but not exposed to any behavioral intervention (HC). All mice were sacrificed together 2 h after last fear conditioning (or an equivalent time of day after handling), and gene expression patterns from blood and amygdala were compared. Examination of the freezing behaviors of animals in the Immo-FC and FC groups did not reveal any significant differences in baseline, pre-tone CS freezing ($t = -0.39$, $p > 0.05$) or tone CS freezing across the auditory conditioning session ($t = 0.43$, $p > 0.05$). **Table S1** shows the total number of expressed genes in both tissues across the three different groups (HC, FC or Immo+FC). We observed tissue-specific gene expression, with an overall higher number of genes expressed in the amygdala relative to the blood in all three groups (HC, FC, Immo+FC). Overall 11,353 genes were expressed in both tissues, with 580 uniquely expressed in blood and 4,271 uniquely expressed in the amygdala.

TABLE 2 | Genes differentially expressed in FC compared to HC in amygdala and blood.

Gene	Amygdala			Blood		
	Fold change	*p*-value	*q*-value	Fold change	*p*-value	*q*-value
Nxpe4	−0.39	0.0003	0.010	−1.27	5.00*E*−05	0.002
Plxnd1	−0.22	0.0017	0.047	−0.82	5.00*E*−05	0.002
C1ql3	0.24	0.0012	0.037	−2.41	0.0001	0.004
Zhx2	0.29	0.0012	0.037	0.68	0.0001	0.006
Pbrm1	−0.26	0.0001	0.005	−0.68	0.0005	0.015
Adam8	0.47	0.0006	0.020	0.62	0.0008	0.022
Zbtb40	0.37	0.0002	0.007	0.67	0.0009	0.026
Myo5a	−0.30	0.0001	0.003	−0.53	0.001	0.030
Dmxl2	−0.42	0.0001	0.003	−0.66	0.002	0.045
Kif1b	−0.25	0.0012	0.036	−0.53	0.003	0.054
Sorl1	−0.37	0.0001	0.003	0.51	0.004	0.078
Sdc4	0.26	0.0008	0.025	0.46	0.005	0.088
Thada	−0.33	0.0010	0.032	0.49	0.006	0.098
Tra2a	0.32	0.0001	0.003	−0.45	0.006	0.106
Insr	−0.22	0.0015	0.044	−0.49	0.008	0.120
Galnt9	0.38	0.0001	0.003	−0.58	0.009	0.137
Myadm	0.22	0.0013	0.039	−0.48	0.011	0.152
Abhd2	−0.25	0.0007	0.023	0.50	0.013	0.172
Klf11	−0.41	0.0009	0.028	−0.48	0.016	0.195
Zfp280c	−0.31	0.0001	0.005	−0.50	0.020	0.225
Bptf	−0.25	0.0001	0.003	0.38	0.020	0.229
Numb	0.26	0.0005	0.017	0.39	0.022	0.241
Pds5a	−0.29	0.0001	0.005	0.39	0.023	0.248
Sdf2l1	0.58	0.0001	0.003	0.44	0.023	0.248
Egr3	0.33	0.0001	0.003	0.89	0.024	0.251
Arhgef12	−0.24	0.0004	0.015	−0.40	0.025	0.260
Kat6a	−0.28	0.0001	0.003	0.36	0.030	0.288
Guf1	−0.27	0.0006	0.021	−0.45	0.036	0.320
Phka2	−0.47	0.0001	0.003	−0.42	0.040	0.344
Zfp445	−0.21	0.0016	0.046	−0.33	0.044	0.362
Dusp1	−0.54	0.0001	0.003	0.37	0.045	0.364
Fkbp5	0.24	0.0007	0.024	0.35	0.048	0.377

Bold Gene Names: Adam8, a disintegrin and metallopeptidase domain 8; C1ql3, C1q-like 3; Dmxl2, Dmx-like 2; Myo5a, myosin VA; Nxpe4, Neurexophilin and PC-Esterase Domain Family, Member 4; Pbrm1, Polybromo 1; Plxnd1, Plexin D1; Zbtb40, Zinc finger and BTB domain containing 40; Zhx2, Zinc fingers and homeoboxes 2. [b]C1ql3 (C1q-like 3) changes in different direction in brain and blood.

Fear Conditioning Induces Robust Gene Expression Differences in Amygdala and Blood

We first investigated differences in response to fear conditioning (FC vs. HC). **Figure 1A** shows that FC induced gene expression changes in the amygdala, with 607 genes differentially expressed when compared to HC (**Table S2**; FDR < 0.05). FC resulted in a down-regulation of gene expression in the majority of these genes (76.6%). We then evaluated differentially expressed genes for enrichment of biological process and identified 15 processes that were enriched after multiple test correction (**Table 1**, **Table S3**). Among these processes, there was an enrichment of specific biological processes including memory formation and consolidation, and neurotransmission, with learning or memory ($p = 4.18 \times 10^{-4}$), and associative learning ($p = 0.01$).

In blood, FC results in expression differences of 352 genes in blood relative to HC (**Table S4**; FDR < 0.05; **Figure 1B**), with the majority of genes identified (84.3%) having lower expression levels in FC when compared to HC. Only two biological processes were enriched among these differentially expressed genes (**Table 1**; **Table S3**), homophilic cell adhesion of plasma membranes of adjacent cells ($p = 1.6 \times 10^{-26}$), and immune system processes ($p = 0.009$). Comparison of genes regulated in amygdala (FDR < 0.05) with those regulated in blood ($p < 0.05$) revealed 32 genes differentially expressed in FC vs. HC, 9 of which reached FDR significance in both tissues (**Table 2**).

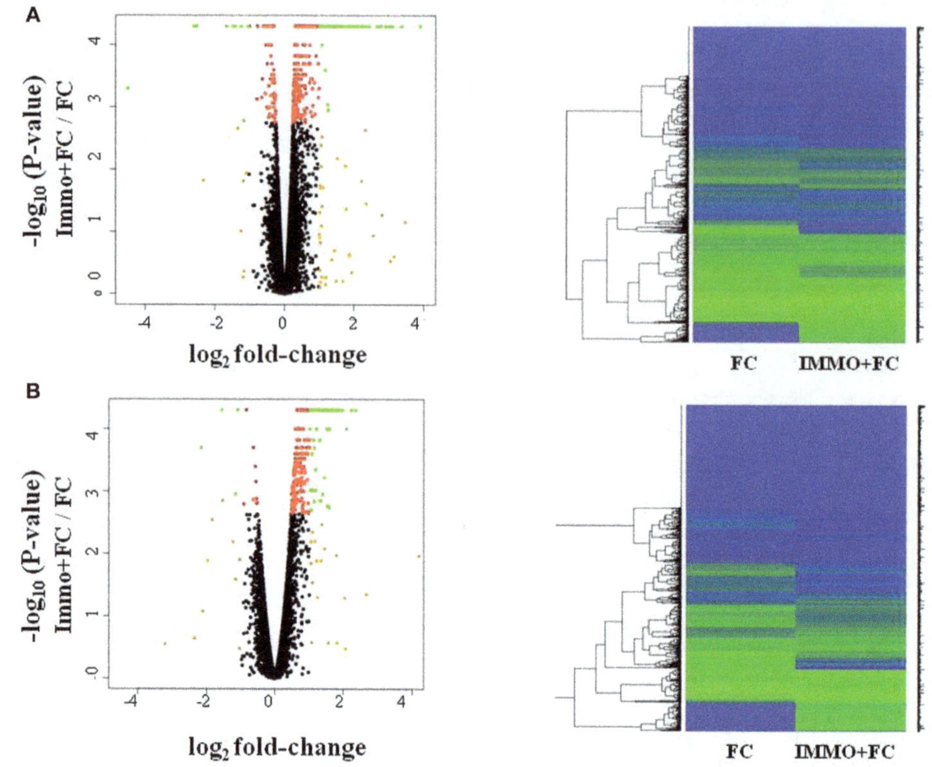

FIGURE 2 | Fear conditioning and prior immunization induce gene expression differences in amygdala and blood. Volcano plots and heatmaps show changes in gene expression in the amygdala **(A)** and blood **(B)** of animals that experienced immobilization (Immo+FC) prior to fear conditioning (FC). The horizontal axis of the Volcano plot is $\log_2$ fold change for differently expressed genes, and the vertical axis is the negative-$\log_{10}$ of the p-values are plotted. Each dot represents a gene, with red dots showing genes reaching an FDR corrected p-value of 0.05, and green dots representing genes with FDR < 0.05 and absolute fold change >1; orange dots have an absolute fold change>1 but do not reach experiment-wide significance; black dots are genes whose expression is similar between the two groups.

Prior Stress Sensitization Induces Gene Expression Changes in Response to Fear Conditioning

To evaluate how prior stress exposure may alter the transcriptional processes that accompany fear conditioning, we compared amygdala expression in the Immo+FC to the FC group (**Figure 2A**). We identified 516 genes that had differences in expression levels (FDR < 0.05; **Table S5, Figure 2A**), 84.3% of which were higher in FC. Among those, we observed genes that have been associated with PTSD in previous human studies (e.g., *DRD2* and *HTR2a*) (26–29) or linked to anxiety or PTSD-like behaviors in humans or animal models (*Igf2, Grm2, Clock, Trhr*) (30–32) (**Table S5**; **Figure 3**). Enrichment analyses of the 516 differentially expressed genes revealed four biological pathways, including cell proliferation and cellular response to drugs (**Table 3; Table S6**).

In blood, prior stress history (Immo+FC) associates with expression differences in 468 genes relative to FC (**Figure 2B**), the majority of which (97%) increased in expression compared to FC (FDR < 0.05; **Table S7**). Enrichment analysis revealed 39 pathways including immune response, inflammation, and cytokine signaling pathways (**Table 3**). To contextualize these differences, we compared the proportion of blood cell types (monocytes, neutrophils, and lymphocytes) between each group. Although there were no differences in blood cell composition between the HC and FC groups, Immo+FC had a higher proportion of neutrophils and a lower proportion of lymphocytes relative to both FC ($p = 0.013$) and HC ($p = 0.007$; **Figure 4**).

We then compared the genes whose expression differed in the amygdala (FDR < 0.05) with those that differed in blood. We identified 27 genes (**Table 4**) that change in Immo+FC vs. FC in both tissues, 20 (74%) of which occurred in the same direction in both tissues. Among the 10 genes that remained significant after multiple test correction in both tissues, *Dmxl2, Trps1, Fgd4,* and *Thbd* have similar expression patterns in Immo+FC and HC. Interestingly, the remaining genes in which immobilization (Immo+FC) had induced changes in expression seem to be involved in immune response (*Lbp* and *Lnc2*), anxiety behavior and schizophrenia (*Pde7b*), corticosterone homeostasis, and steroid transportation (*Lcn2* and *Soat1*; **Figure 5**). While we cannot state whether or not these genes are also regulated by immobilization alone, the observation of regulation in both stress exposed and non exposed animals following fear conditioning suggests that these genes are similarly transcribed in the amygdala following fear conditioning.

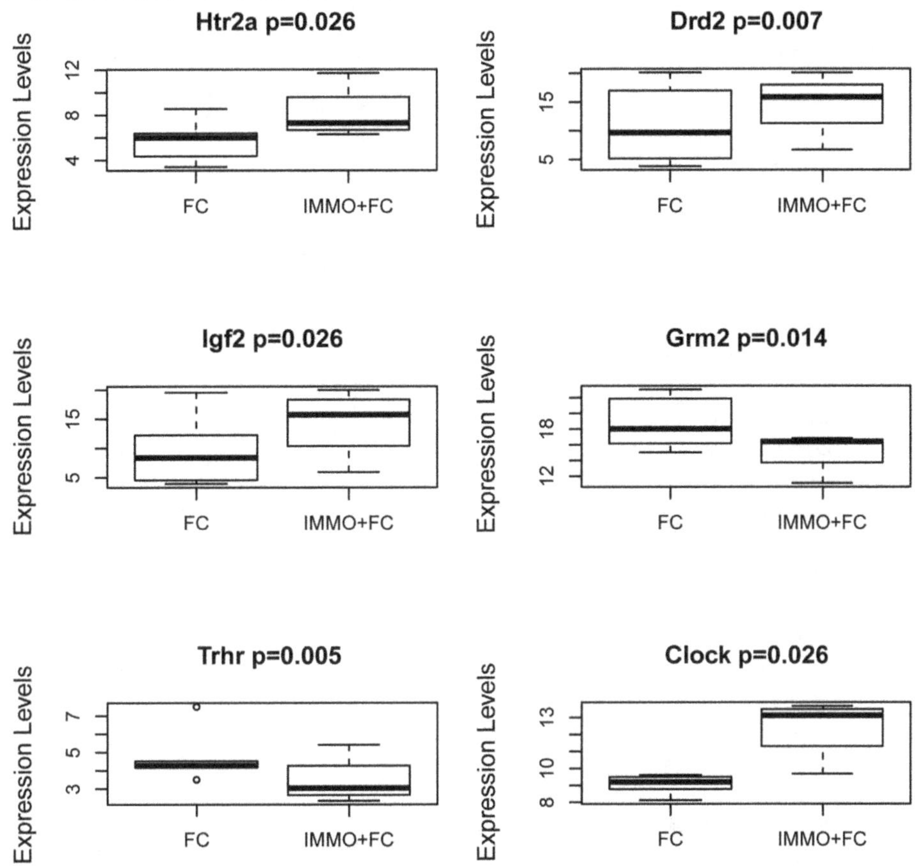

FIGURE 3 | Genes in the Amygdala traditionally associated with PTSD or psychiatric stress phenotypes. Box and Whiskers plots of gene expression in FC and Immo+FC animals for (a) 2 genes traditionally associated with PTSD (*Htr2a* and *Drd2*), and (b) 4 genes associated with stress phenotypes (*Igf2*, *Grm2*, *Trhr*, and *Clock*). On the y-axis, gene expression values from the different animal groups. The box represents their quartiles; whiskers the variability outside the upper and lower quartiles; the horizontal line represents the median.

DISCUSSION

This study utilized a translational animal model to examine molecular alterations associated with threat exposure in both the blood and amygdala of mice with and without a prior stress history. As much work has noted that, while trauma-related disorders can occur in individuals following exposure to a single trauma, individuals with a history of early stress and trauma are more likely to develop PTSD following subsequent trauma exposure (2, 33). We examined RNA expression changes in two different tissues: (1) the amygdala, often considered the "hub" of the fear and threat response in humans and animals (34, 35) and (2) the blood, the most common tissue used in human PTSD studies. Identification of a common gene expression response pattern presents a valuable step in translational biology, toward bridging the disconnect between how peripheral gene expression changes are relevant to PTSD-related behavioral alterations in humans.

In this study, fear conditioning resulted in differences in enrichment of genes implicated in learning and memory as well as general cellular processes in the amygdala (**Table 1**). These results provide confidence in our approach, as they are consistent with established pathways relevant to amygdala-mediated fear learning. However, our observation of fear conditioning induced down-regulation of gene transcription in the amygdala is noteworthy as one might expect that associative learning would increase transcription to support plasticity necessary for memory formation. As fear conditioning has been found to result in multiple waves of transcriptional processes occurring across the minutes to hours that follow (36), these data should be viewed as a static snapshot of the dynamic transcriptional processes that accompany fear conditioning, i.e., 2 h for the current study. Other recent studies have utilized time-points more proximal (30 min or 1 h) to fear conditioning and more distant (6 h and 24 h) to examine transcriptional changes, and have also demonstrated conditioning related down-regulation and up-regulation of gene targets (10, 37–39). Therefore, while 2 h has traditionally been used by our group for examining transcriptional processes following fear conditioning in the amygdala, these data must indeed be considered as only a subset of the dynamic and highly interwoven molecular processes, including translational and epigenetic processes, which also accompany fear conditioning.

TABLE 3 | Enrichment of biological process among genes associated with prior stress immobilization.

GO number	Description	FE[a]	p-value[b]
AMYGDALA			
GO:0008285	Negative regulation of cell proliferation	3.43	0.004
GO:0006457	Protein folding	5.61	0.010
GO:0006986	Response to unfolded protein	9.39	0.014
GO:0042493	Response to drug	3.18	0.029
BLOOD			
GO:0002376	Immune system process	6.51	2.29×10^{-25}
GO:0045087	Innate immune response	6.01	6.40×10^{-23}
GO:0006954	Inflammatory response	5.83	3.38×10^{-18}
GO:0052697	Xenobiotic glucuronidation	39.59	5.18×10^{-8}
GO:0032496	Response to lipopolysaccharide	4.97	1.61×10^{-6}
GO:0030593	Neutrophil chemotaxis	8.39	1.40×10^{-5}
GO:0006955	Immune response	3.93	1.72×10^{-5}
GO:0006935	Chemotaxis	6.04	1.70×10^{-5}
GO:0042742	Defense response to bacterium	4.66	1.54×10^{-5}
GO:0032760	Positive regulation of tumor necrosis factor production	9.06	1.47×10^{-5}
GO:0009813	Flavonoid biosynthetic process	16.97	4.82×10^{-5}
GO:0052696	Flavonoid glucuronidation	16.97	4.82×10^{-5}
GO:0071223	Cellular response to lipoteichoic acid	29.69	1.19×10^{-4}
GO:0009615	Response to virus	6.36	4.56×10^{-4}
GO:0050729	Positive regulation of inflammatory response	7.07	0.0017
GO:0032755	Positive regulation of interleukin-6 production	7.71	0.0028
GO:0002755	MyD88-dependent toll-like receptor signaling pathway	16.70	0.0028
GO:0019221	Cytokine-mediated signaling pathway	4.27	0.0033
GO:0055072	Iron ion homeostasis	8.48	0.0045
GO:0050830	Defense response to Gram-positive bacterium	5.27	0.0051
GO:0031663	Lipopolysaccharide-mediated signaling pathway	10.06	0.0062
GO:0042127	Regulation of cell proliferation	3.34	0.006
GO:0045766	Positive regulation of angiogenesis	4.42	0.009
GO:0050873	Brown fat cell differentiation	9.17	0.009
GO:0010628	Positive regulation of gene expression	2.57	0.009
GO:0050728	Negative regulation of inflammatory response	5.12	0.013
GO:0042535	Positive regulation of tumor necrosis factor biosynthetic process	17.13	0.013
GO:0002548	Monocyte chemotaxis	7.79	0.020
GO:0034341	Response to interferon-gamma	10.28	0.019
GO:0071222	Cellular response to lipopolysaccharide	3.20	0.021
GO:0008360	Regulation of cell shape	3.84	0.022
GO:0007165	Signal transduction	1.70	0.026
GO:0006898	Receptor-mediated endocytosis	5.94	0.026
GO:0051607	Defense response to virus	3.47	0.026
GO:0043123	Positive regulation of I-kappaB kinase/NF-kappaB signaling	3.59	0.035
GO:0032494	Response to peptidoglycan	22.27	0.036
GO:0050766	Positive regulation of phagocytosis	6.49	0.041
GO:0035456	Response to interferon-beta	19.79	0.050
GO:0045410	Positive regulation of interleukin-6 biosynthetic process	19.79	0.050

[a] *FE, Fold Enrichment.*
[b] *p-value following Benjamini-Hochberg correction for multiple testing.*

In response to fear conditioning, prior acute stress immobilization conducted the previous week, induces distinct gene expression differences involved in immune activation pathways in blood. Several studies have shown a strict causal association between immune response, inflammation, and PTSD (40). Compared to mice that underwent FC alone, mice exposed

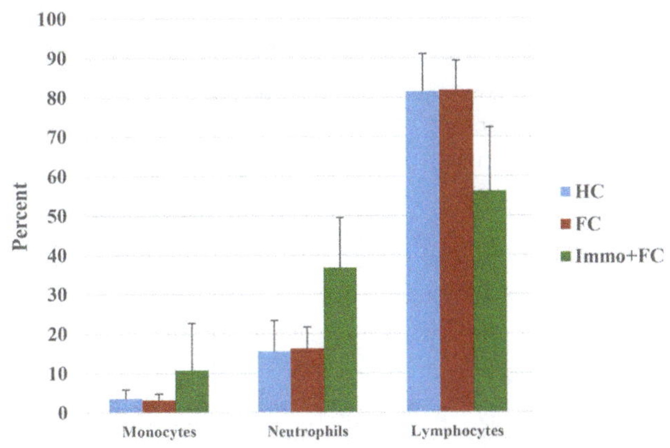

FIGURE 4 | Prior stress sensitization causes immune dysregulation. Percent of monocytes, neutrophils, and lymphocytes in the three different groups (HC, FC, and Immo+FC) are shown. Bars indicate standard errors.

to prior immobilization showed gene expression patterns consistent with immune dysregulation. This was supported by the observation that blood from Immo+FC mice had a higher proportion of neutrophils, an essential part of the innate immune system, and an indicator of inflammation. The neutrophil-lymphocyte ratio has recently been used as an indicator of chronic low-grade inflammation, and known to associate with clinical outcomes in neuropsychiatric disorders (41, 42). Our data suggested that immune response genes and pathways are responsive to prior immobilization stress both in the blood and amygdala.

In examining transcriptional differences in the amygdala of mice with and without prior stress exposure, we observed a number of genes that have previously been associated with PTSD. In particular, *DRD2*, and *HTR2a* are of interest as both the dopaminergic and serotonergic systems have been traditionally implicated in the pathophysiology of PTSD (28, 43, 44). Indeed, dopamine dysregulation has been implicated in various PTSD symptoms (e.g., attention, vigilance, arousal, sleep), and *DRD2* has been associated with PTSD diagnosis (26, 29). Similarly, as serotonin and norepinephrine reuptake inhibitors (SSRI and SNRI) remain the first line pharmacotherapy for PTSD, and numerous candidate gene studies have identified a link between variants in serotonin related genes, including *HTR2a* (27, 28), our observation of differential expression of *HTR2a* is consistent with the previous literature and support for this neurotransmitter system in the consequences of threat and trauma exposure. We also identified genes (*Igf2, Clock, Grm2, Trhr1*) that have been previously associated with stress-related phenotypes. Interestingly, *Igf2* methylation has been found to associate with PTSD (45), fear extinction (30), and more classically in chronic stress response (46). Among other differentially expressed genes in Immo+FC vs. FC, *Clock*, a gene involved in the circadian rhythms, is particularly interesting as mice with mutations of this gene have altered anxiety behaviors (31), and as sleep disturbances are commonly reported by PTSD patients (47). Similarly, *Grm2* (metatropic glutamate 2 receptor) has been associated with anxiety-like behaviors in several rodent models, and activation of these receptors in the amygdala has been found to be necessary for fear related behaviors. Highly selective mGluR2/3 agonists depress excitatory neurotransmission in the amygdala (48), suggesting that such agonists may be potentially therapeutic for PTSD patients by reducing amygdala hyperactivity (32, 49). Finally, we observed regulation of the Thyrotropin Releasing Hormone Receptor1 (*Trhr1*) in Immo+FC animals; a novel finding that is of interest given its role in the hypothalamic-pituitary-thyroid axis and the observation that clinical dysfunction of the thyroid hormone system can manifest with anxiety behaviors (50). These data support the utility of this approach in examining blood and brain-based alterations in threat exposure occurring with and without a prior stress history.

As one of our main objectives was to identify common biological responses to fear and stress in both brain and blood, we evaluated shared genes in amygdala and blood. Although there was a limited overlap in individual genes that responded to each condition (**Table 4**), we found six genes in which changes of expression were specifically associated with immobilization. Among these genes, *Pde7* encodes phosphodiesterase-7, known for its regulation of T-cell function and association with regulation of immune response, and its inhibitors may help patients with immunological and neuro-inflammatory disorders (51). In rodents, inhibition of Pde7 regulates anxiety behaviors, mediated by increasing levels of hypothalamic thyrotropin-releasing hormone (52). Notably, a dual Pde7 and GSK-3β inhibitor significantly improves episodic and spatial memory and enhances fear memory, as well as facilitating paired-pulse inhibition and latent inhibition, both behaviors that have been found to be impaired in psychosis, suggesting that inhibition of Pde7 and GSK-3β enhances cognition (53). Lipopolysaccharide Binding Protein (*Lbp*) and Lipocalin 2 (*Lnc2*) are involved in an acute phase of immunological response and metabolic inflammation (54). Sterol O-Acyltransferase 1 (*Soat1*) plays an important role in cholesterol homeostasis regulation and metabolism, and it has been extensively studied as a target for hypercholesterolemia and Alzheimer's disease (55). The observation of immune response and inflammation-related genes is of particular interest given the recent emerging appreciation of the role of immune-response and inflammatory pathways in psychiatric disorders, including depression, autism, and trauma-related disorders (56, 57). Recent work examining the consequences of early-life inflammation via lipopolysaccharide administration has revealed impairments in fear memory extinction during adulthood (58), in line with our observation that a prior history of stress results alterations in inflammation, might suggest that prolonged inflammatory responses contribute to impaired fear extinction. Further, it is of interest that inhibition of pro-inflammatory cytokines has been suggested to facilitate fear memory extinction (59). Taken together, these findings suggest that a closer examination of the induction of inflammation and cytokine pathways in stress and trauma

TABLE 4 | Overlap in amygdala and blood in Immo+FC vs. FC.

Gene	Amygdala			Blood		
	Fold change	***p*-value**	***q*-value**	**Fold change**	***p*-value**	***q*-value**
Dmxl2	0.39	5E-05	0.003	0.99	5E-05	0.002
Erdr1	−0.59	5E-05	0.003	−1.07	5E-05	0.002
Lcn2	3.36	5E-05	0.003	0.95	5E-05	0.002
Pde7b	0.33	4E-04	0.015	1.15	5E-05	0.002
Trps1	0.40	2E-04	0.007	0.81	5E-05	0.002
Sdf2l1	0.39	7E-04	0.024	0.64	2E-04	0.007
Soat1	0.34	5E-04	0.019	0.55	5E-04	0.015
Thbd	0.69	5E-05	0.003	0.69	7E-04	0.019
Fgd4	0.78	5E-05	0.003	0.84	8E-04	0.021
Lbp	0.83	5E-05	0.003	0.94	2E-03	0.047
Gh	−4.49	5E-04	0.019	−1.84	3E-03	0.058
Cers6	0.44	5E-05	0.003	0.55	4E-03	0.072
Rbm3	−0.30	1E-03	0.032	−0.46	4E-03	0.075
Stxbp6	−0.27	8E-04	0.025	0.74	7E-03	0.107
Lyst	0.53	5E-05	0.003	0.42	7E-03	0.110
Jhdm1d	0.35	5E-05	0.003	0.40	1E-02	0.154
Lnpep	3.10	5E-05	0.003	0.41	1E-02	0.178
Endou	1.01	5E-05	0.003	−0.76	2E-02	0.212
Cdk5rap2	0.72	5E-05	0.003	−0.44	2E-02	0.242
Polr2a	−0.26	7E-04	0.023	−0.36	3E-02	0.270
F5	0.60	3E-04	0.012	−0.38	3E-02	0.282
Prkdc	0.29	1E-03	0.031	−0.37	3E-02	0.310
Hpcal1	−0.31	5E-05	0.003	0.33	3E-02	0.311
Nr4a1	0.31	1E-04	0.005	−0.33	3E-02	0.312
Dnajb14	1.55	5E-05	0.003	0.54	4E-02	0.342
Pcnx	0.26	5E-04	0.017	0.33	5E-02	0.368
Pisd_ps3	−0.40	5E-05	0.003	−0.31	5E-02	0.373

Gene associated in both blood and amygdala. Gene Name: Dmxl2, Dmx-like 2; Erdr1, erythroid differentiation regulator 1; Fgd4, FYVE, RhoGEF, and PH domain containing 4; Lcn2, lipocalin 2; Lbp, lipopolysaccharide binding protein; Pde7b, phosphodiesterase 7B; Soat1, sterol O-acyltransferase 1; Sdf2l1, stromal cell-derived factor 2-like 1; Thbd, thrombomodulin; Trps1, trichorhinophalangeal syndrome I.

responses may yield new strategies for alleviating the deleterious consequences of stress and trauma.

While our data reveal transcriptional alterations in the amygdala and peripheral blood that accompany fear conditioning with and without prior stress history, it is important to note that other recent studies employing alternative models of rodent stress have examined gene expression in blood and brain (38, 60, 61). Our use of immobilization restraint stress is predicated on our prior experience with this paradigm resulting in altered fear memory processes, anxiety behaviors and HPA axis function (4, 15); as our primary goal was to examine the consequences of stress history on subsequent molecular alterations that accompany fear conditioning, we utilized this model to conduct this genetic discovery study. Importantly, while recent studies employing different stress procedures, 21-day variable stress, chronic restraint stress, repeated shock administration, and social defeat stress have been used to examine transcriptional processes in the amygdala, this single-session immobilization stress procedure is relatively acute in comparison (38, 61, 62). Coupled with our previous demonstration of altered fear and anxiety processes using this paradigm, the altered transcriptional processes observed in this current study suggest that even relatively brief exposures to stress prior to a threating situation, such as auditory fear conditioning, can be useful in revealing the lasting imprint of stress history on molecular events associated with traumatic memory formation. While it would be unwise to intensively interpret our data with relevance to those which have utilized different paradigms, it is important to highlight that many of these studies have also revealed alterations of genes that are associated with immune response, dopamine function, and glucocorticoid related signaling (38, 60, 61), which suggest that shared pathways altered by stress are emerging across a variety of behavioral models.

We acknowledge that this study has some limitations. First, although blood cell counts varied in the different groups, we were not able to account for such variation in the analysis but were able to capture the information related to that variation. Alternatively, as white blood cell counts change following immobilization, covarying for cell composition may obscure biological differences that accompany gene expression changes.

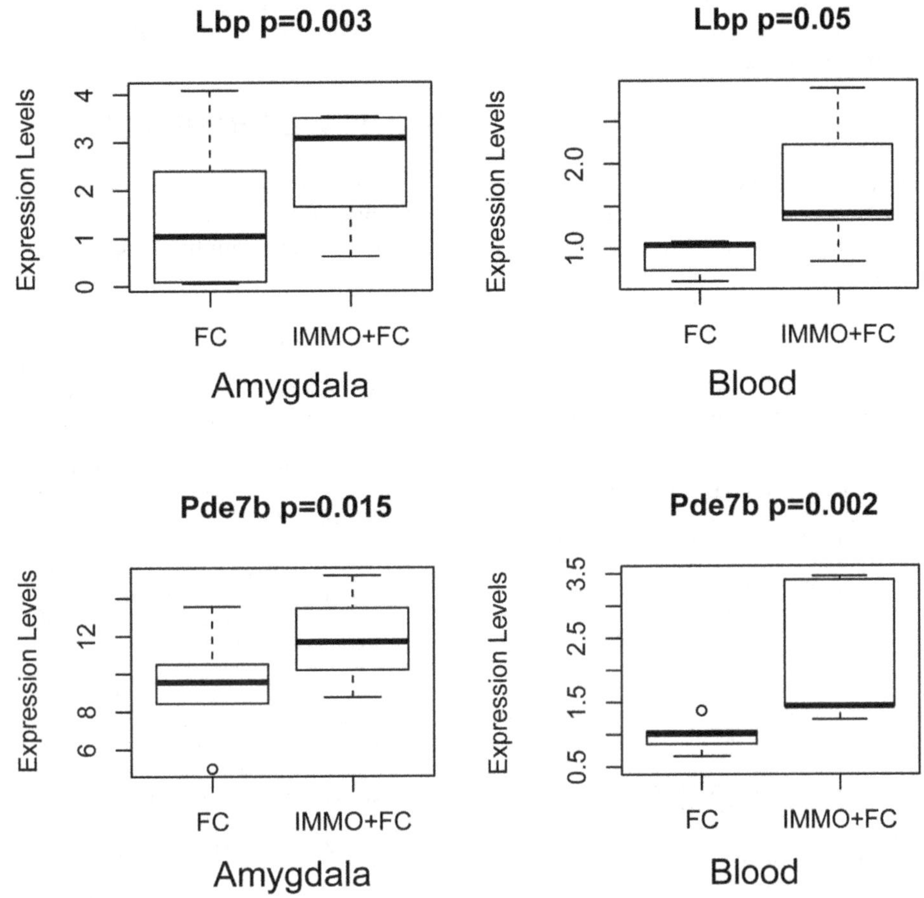

FIGURE 5 | Common Signals in Amygdala and Blood prior stress sensitization in representative genes. Box and Whiskers plots depict gene expression (y-axis) in FC and Immo+FC animals. Representative genes that associate with prior immobilization in both amygdala and blood are shown. On the y axis, gene expression values from the different animal group. The box represents their quartiles; whiskers the variability outside the upper, and lower quartiles; the horizontal line represents the median; outliers are indicated by single dots.

Second, we focused our analyses on the amygdala, because of its role in fear and threat response behaviors. As such, we utilized auditory fear conditioning as it is well established to rely on amygdala function. As a result, we cannot extrapolate these data to other brain regions that contribute to stress and traumatic memory (e.g., hippocampus, insula, cingulate, and prefrontal cortex). Additionally, this study was conducted exclusively in male rodents, which showed a higher response to shock-induced contextual fear conditioning than females in terms of behavioral phenotypes (freezing and rearing activity) (63). However, given the higher prevalence and heritability of PTSD in females in human population (64, 65), and the emerging role of circulating estrogen levels in relation to fear and anxiety behaviors, additional studies should specifically examine transcriptional changes in females with full regard to the estrus phase. Next, in order to get sufficient RNA for a comprehensive survey of the transcriptome, we pooled two animals per sample for each group. Though this does not limit our ability to identify overall similarities and differences in different tissues of the same animals in response to threat exposure or to interpret pathway analysis, caution should be taken in interpreting the results of individual genes. Finally, we are aware that different strains of mice may generate different patterns of expression in response to FC; a cumulative analysis in different strains of mice could eventually increase the power to detect additional genes relevant to PTSD-related phenotypes (66).

In conclusion, this study provides a translational framework for mouse and human studies aimed at examining the molecular correlates that inform studies of psychiatric disorders. We were able to identify, in the amygdala, several genes that specifically respond to the stress immobilization paradigm, some of which have been traditionally associated with PTSD, and anxiety disorders. Future studies will be needed to evaluate if these genes associate with PTSD or stress-related traits in human clinical studies.

AUTHOR CONTRIBUTIONS

AL performed statistical analyses and contributed to writing the manuscript. SM performed the mouse experiments and contributed to study design, and manuscript writing. SS and RA helped with the mouse experiments and manuscript editing. KR helped to design the experiment, interpret the data, and write the manuscript. AS helped to design the experiment, analyze and interpret the data, and write the manuscript.

FUNDING

This research was supported by NARSAD Young Investigator Grants (#19233 and #22434) from the Brain Behavior Foundation. Additional support for RA provided by Ramón y Cajal program RYC2014-15784, RETOS-MINECO SAF2016-76565-R, and FEDER funds.

ACKNOWLEDGMENTS

We would like to thank the Yerkes Genomics Core at Emory University, and in particular Dr. Gregory Tharp and Dr. Nirav Patel for their help with RNA sequencing.

REFERENCES

1. Daviss WB. The child trauma screening questionnaire predicts ptsd onset 6 months after traumatic accident better than the children's impact of events scale. *Evid Based Ment Health* (2007) 10:44. doi: 10.1136/ebmh.10.2.44
2. Powers A, Fani N, Cross D, Ressler KJ, Bradley B. Childhood trauma, PTSD, and psychosis: findings from a highly traumatized, minority sample. *Child Abuse Negl.* (2016) 58:111–8. doi: 10.1016/j.chiabu.2016.06.015
3. Orr SP, Pitman RK, Lasko NB, Herz LR. Psychophysiological assessment of posttraumatic stress disorder imagery in World War II and Korean combat veterans. *J Abnorm Psychol.* (1993) 102:152–9. doi: 10.1037/0021-843X.102.1.152
4. Andero R, Heldt SA, Ye K, Liu X, Armario A, Ressler KJ. Effect of 7,8-dihydroxyflavone, a small-molecule TrkB agonist, on emotional learning. *Am J Psychiatry* (2011) 168:163–72. doi: 10.1176/appi.ajp.2010.10030326
5. Fanselow MS, LeDoux JE. Why we think plasticity underlying Pavlovian fear conditioning occurs in the basolateral amygdala. *Neuron* (1999) 23:229–32. doi: 10.1016/S0896-6273(00)80775-8
6. Keifer OP Jr, Hurt RC, Ressler KJ, Marvar PJ. The physiology of fear: reconceptualizing the role of the central amygdala in fear learning. *Physiology* (2015) 30:389–401. doi: 10.1152/physiol.00058.2014
7. Rauch SL, Whalen PJ, Shin LM, McInerney SC, Macklin ML, Lasko NB, et al. Exaggerated amygdala response to masked facial stimuli in posttraumatic stress disorder: a functional MRI study. *Biol Psychiatry* (2000) 47:769–76. doi: 10.1016/S0006-3223(00)00828-3
8. Neumeister P, Feldker K, Heitmann CY, Buff C, Brinkmann L, Bruchmann M, et al. Specific amygdala response to masked fearful faces in post-traumatic stress relative to other anxiety disorders. *Psychol Med.* (2017) 48:1209–17. doi: 10.1017/S0033291717002513
9. Logue MW, Smith AK, Baldwin C, Wolf EJ, Guffanti G, Ratanatharathorn A, et al. An analysis of gene expression in PTSD implicates genes involved in the glucocorticoid receptor pathway and neural responses to stress. *Psychoneuroendocrinology* (2015) 57:1–13. doi: 10.1016/j.psyneuen.2015.03.016
10. Lamprecht R, Dracheva S, Assoun S, LeDoux JE. Fear conditioning induces distinct patterns of gene expression in lateral amygdala. *Genes Brain Behav.* (2009) 8:735–43. doi: 10.1111/j.1601-183X.2009.00515.x
11. Hayes JP, LaBar KS, McCarthy G, Selgrade E, Nasser J, Dolcos F, et al. Reduced hippocampal and amygdala activity predicts memory distortions for trauma reminders in combat-related PTSD. *J Psychiatr Res.* (2011) 45:660–9. doi: 10.1016/j.jpsychires.2010.10.007
12. Stevens JS, Jovanovic T, Fani N, Ely TD, Glover EM, Bradley B, et al. Disrupted amygdala-prefrontal functional connectivity in civilian women with posttraumatic stress disorder. *J Psychiatr Res.* (2013) 47:1469–78. doi: 10.1016/j.jpsychires.2013.05.031
13. Stevens JS, Almli LM, Fani N, Gutman DA, Bradley B, Norrholm SD, et al. PACAP receptor gene polymorphism impacts fear responses in the amygdala and hippocampus. *Proc Natl Acad Sci USA.* (2014) 111:3158–63. doi: 10.1073/pnas.1318954111
14. Kessler RC, Aguilar-Gaxiola S, Alonso J, Benjet C, Bromet EJ, Cardoso G, et al. Trauma and PTSD in the WHO world mental health surveys. *Eur J Psychotraumatol.* (2017) 8:1353383. doi: 10.1080/20008198.2017.1353383
15. Andero R, Daviu N, Escorihuela RM, Nadal R, Armario A. 7,8-dihydroxyflavone, a TrkB receptor agonist, blocks long-term spatial memory impairment caused by immobilization stress in rats. *Hippocampus* (2012) 22:399–408. doi: 10.1002/hipo.20906
16. Andero R, Brothers SP, Jovanovic T, Chen YT, Salah-Uddin H, Cameron M, et al. Amygdala-dependent fear is regulated by Oprl1 in mice and humans with PTSD. *Sci Transl Med.* (2013) 5:188ra173. doi: 10.1126/scitranslmed.3005656
17. Wingo AP, Velasco ER, Florido A, Lori A, Choi DC, Jovanovic T, et al. Expression of the PPM1F gene is regulated by stress and associated with anxiety and depression. *Biol Psychiatry* (2018) 83:284–95. doi: 10.1016/j.biopsych.2017.08.013
18. Stein MB, Yehuda R, Koverola C, Hanna C. Enhanced dexamethasone suppression of plasma cortisol in adult women traumatized by childhood sexual abuse. *Biol Psychiatry* (1997) 42:680–6. doi: 10.1016/S0006-3223(96)00489-1
19. Phassouliotis C, Garner BA, Phillips LJ, Bendall S, Yun Y, Markulev C, et al. Enhanced cortisol suppression following administration of low-dose dexamethasone in first-episode psychosis patients. *Aust N Z J Psychiatry* (2013) 47:363–70. doi: 10.1177/0004867412465125
20. Jovanovic T, Norrholm SD, Blanding NQ, Davis M, Duncan E, Bradley B, et al. Impaired fear inhibition is a biomarker of PTSD but not depression. *Depress Anxiety* (2010) 27:244–51. doi: 10.1002/da.20663
21. Sawamura T, Klengel T, Armario A, Jovanovic T, Norrholm SD, Ressler KJ, et al. Dexamethasone treatment leads to enhanced fear extinction and dynamic Fkbp5 regulation in amygdala. *Neuropsychopharmacology* (2016) 41:832–46. doi: 10.1038/npp.2015.210
22. Paxinos G, Franklin KBJ. *The Mouse Brain in Stereotaxic Coordinates.* 2nd Edn. San Diego, CA: Academic Press (2001).
23. Dobin A, Davis CA, Schlesinger F, Drenkow J, Zaleski C, Jha S, et al. STAR: ultrafast universal RNA-seq aligner. *Bioinformatics* (2013) 29:15–21. doi: 10.1093/bioinformatics/bts635
24. Trapnell C, Roberts A, Goff L, Pertea G, Kim D, Kelley DR, et al. Differential gene and transcript expression analysis of RNA-seq experiments with TopHat and Cufflinks. *Nat Protoc.* (2012) 7:562–78. doi: 10.1038/nprot.2012.016
25. Huang da W, Sherman BT, Lempicki RA. Systematic and integrative analysis of large gene lists using DAVID bioinformatics resources. *Nat Protoc.* (2009) 4:44–57. doi: 10.1038/nprot.2008.211
26. Segman RH, Cooper-Kazaz R, Macciardi F, Goltser T, Halfon Y, Dobroborski T, et al. Association between the dopamine transporter gene and posttraumatic stress disorder. *Mol Psychiatry* (2002) 7:903–7. doi: 10.1038/sj.mp.4001085
27. Lee HJ, Lee MS, Kang RH, Kim H, Kim SD, Kee BS, et al. Influence of the serotonin transporter promoter gene polymorphism on susceptibility to posttraumatic stress disorder. *Depress Anxiety* (2005) 21:135–9. doi: 10.1002/da.20064
28. Mellman TA, Alim T, Brown DD, Gorodetsky E, Buzas B, Lawson WB, et al. Serotonin polymorphisms and posttraumatic stress disorder in a trauma exposed African American population. *Depress Anxiety* (2009) 26:993–7. doi: 10.1002/da.20627

29. Li L, Bao Y, He S, Wang G, Guan Y, Ma D, et al. The association between genetic variants in the dopaminergic system and posttraumatic stress disorder: a meta-analysis. *Medicine* (2016) 95:e3074. doi: 10.1097/MD.0000000000003074
30. Agis-Balboa RC, Arcos-Diaz D, Wittnam J, Govindarajan N, Blom K, Burkhardt S, et al. A hippocampal insulin-growth factor 2 pathway regulates the extinction of fear memories. *EMBO J.* (2011) 30:4071–83. doi: 10.1038/emboj.2011.293
31. Lamont EW, Legault-Coutu D, Cermakian N, Boivin DB. The role of circadian clock genes in mental disorders. *Dialogues Clin Neurosci.* (2007) 9:333–42.
32. Baker DG, Nievergelt CM, Risbrough VB. Post-traumatic stress disorder: emerging concepts of pharmacotherapy. *Expert Opin Emerg Drugs* (2009) 14:251–72. doi: 10.1517/14728210902972494
33. Ogle CM, Rubin DC, Siegler IC. The impact of the developmental timing of trauma exposure on PTSD symptoms and psychosocial functioning among older adults. *Dev Psychol.* (2013) 49:2191–200. doi: 10.1037/a0031985
34. Blair HT, Schafe GE, Bauer EP, Rodrigues SM, LeDoux JE. Synaptic plasticity in the lateral amygdala: a cellular hypothesis of fear conditioning. *Learn Mem.* (2001) 8:229–42. doi: 10.1101/lm.30901
35. Mahan AL, Ressler KJ. Fear conditioning, synaptic plasticity and the amygdala: implications for posttraumatic stress disorder. *Trends Neurosci.* (2012) 35:24–35. doi: 10.1016/j.tins.2011.06.007
36. Ou LC, Yeh SH, Gean PW. Late expression of brain-derived neurotrophic factor in the amygdala is required for persistence of fear memory. *Neurobiol Learn Mem.* (2010) 93:372–82. doi: 10.1016/j.nlm.2009.12.003
37. Ressler KJ, Paschall G, Zhou XL, Davis M. Regulation of synaptic plasticity genes during consolidation of fear conditioning. *J Neurosci.* (2002) 22:7892–902. doi: 10.1523/JNEUROSCI.22-18-07892.2002
38. Daskalakis NP, Cohen H, Cai G, Buxbaum JD, Yehuda R. Expression profiling associates blood and brain glucocorticoid receptor signaling with trauma-related individual differences in both sexes. *Proc Natl Acad Sci USA.* (2014) 111:13529–34. doi: 10.1073/pnas.1401660111
39. Katz IK, Lamprecht R. Fear conditioning leads to alteration in specific genes expression in cortical and thalamic neurons that project to the lateral amygdala. *J Neurochem.* (2015) 132:313–26. doi: 10.1111/jnc.12983
40. Baker DG, Nievergelt CM, O'Connor DT. Biomarkers of PTSD: neuropeptides and immune signaling. *Neuropharmacology* (2012) 62:663–73. doi: 10.1016/j.neuropharm.2011.02.027
41. Rembach A, Watt AD, Wilson WJ, Rainey-Smith S, Ellis KA, Rowe CC, et al. An increased neutrophil-lymphocyte ratio in Alzheimer's disease is a function of age and is weakly correlated with neocortical amyloid accumulation. *J Neuroimmunol.* (2014) 273:65–71. doi: 10.1016/j.jneuroim.2014.05.005
42. Ivkovic M, Pantovic-Stefanovic M, Dunjic-Kostic B, Jurisic V, Lackovic M, Totic-Poznanovic S, et al. Neutrophil-to-lymphocyte ratio predicting suicide risk in euthymic patients with bipolar disorder: moderatory effect of family history. *Compr Psychiatry* (2016) 66:87–95. doi: 10.1016/j.comppsych.2016.01.005
43. Southwick SM, Paige S, Morgan CA III, Bremner JD, Krystal JH, Charney DS. Neurotransmitter alterations in PTSD: catecholamines and serotonin. *Semin Clin Neuropsychiatry* (1999) 4:242–8.
44. Lawford BR, Young R, Noble EP, Kann B, Ritchie T. The D2 dopamine receptor (DRD2) gene is associated with co-morbid depression, anxiety and social dysfunction in untreated veterans with post-traumatic stress disorder. *Eur Psychiatry* (2006) 21:180–5. doi: 10.1016/j.eurpsy.2005.01.006
45. Rusiecki JA, Byrne C, Galdzicki Z, Srikantan V, Chen L, Poulin M, et al. PTSD and DNA methylation in select immune function gene promoter regions: a repeated measures case-control study of U.S. military service members. *Front Psychiatry* (2013). 4:56. doi: 10.3389/fpsyt.2013.00056
46. Jung S, Lee Y, Kim G, Son H, Lee DH, Roh GS, et al. Decreased expression of extracellular matrix proteins and trophic factors in the amygdala complex of depressed mice after chronic immobilization stress. *BMC Neurosci.* (2012) 13:58. doi: 10.1186/1471-2202-13-58
47. Cox RC, Tuck BM, Olatunji BO. Sleep disturbance in posttraumatic stress disorder: epiphenomenon or causal factor? *Curr Psychiatry Rep.* (2017) 19:22. doi: 10.1007/s11920-017-0773-y
48. Muly EC, Mania I, Guo JD, Rainnie DG. Group II metabotropic glutamate receptors in anxiety circuitry: correspondence of physiological response and subcellular distribution. *J Comp Neurol.* (2007) 505:682–700. doi: 10.1002/cne.21525
49. Helton DR, Tizzano JP, Monn JA, Schoepp DD, Kallman MJ. Anxiolytic and side-effect profile of LY354740: a potent, highly selective, orally active agonist for group II metabotropic glutamate receptors. *J Pharmacol Exp Ther.* (1998) 284:651–60.
50. Montero-Pedrazuela A, Fernandez-Lamo I, Alieva M, Pereda-Perez I, Venero C, Guadano-Ferraz A. Adult-onset hypothyroidism enhances fear memory and upregulates mineralocorticoid and glucocorticoid receptors in the amygdala. *PLoS ONE* (2011) 6:e26582. doi: 10.1371/journal.pone.0026582
51. Safavi M, Baeeri M, Abdollahi M. New methods for the discovery and synthesis of PDE7 inhibitors as new drugs for neurological and inflammatory disorders. *Expert Opin Drug Discov.* (2013) 8:733–51. doi: 10.1517/17460441.2013.787986
52. Valdes-Moreno MI, Alcantara-Alonso V, Estrada-Camarena E, Mengod G, Amaya MI, Matamoros-Trejo G, et al. Phosphodiesterase-7 inhibition affects accumbal and hypothalamic thyrotropin-releasing hormone expression, feeding, and anxiety behavior of rats. *Behav Brain Res.* (2017) 319:165–73. doi: 10.1016/j.bbr.2016.11.027
53. Lipina TV, Palomo V, Gil C, Martinez A, Roder JC. Dual inhibitor of PDE7 and GSK-3-VP1.15 acts as antipsychotic and cognitive enhancer in C57BL/6J mice. *Neuropharmacology* (2013) 64:205–14. doi: 10.1016/j.neuropharm.2012.06.032
54. Gomes JM, Costa JA, Alfenas RC. Metabolic endotoxemia and diabetes mellitus: a systematic review. *Metabolism* (2017) 68:133–44. doi: 10.1016/j.metabol.2016.12.009
55. Shibuya Y, Chang CC, Chang TY. ACAT1/SOAT1 as a therapeutic target for Alzheimer's disease. *Future Med Chem.* (2015) 7:2451–67. doi: 10.4155/fmc.15.161
56. Miller MW, Lin AP, Wolf EJ, Miller DR. Oxidative stress, inflammation, and neuroprogression in chronic PTSD. *Harv Rev Psychiatry* (2017) 26:57–69. doi: 10.1097/HRP.0000000000000167
57. Queissner R, Pilz R, Dalkner N, Birner A, Bengesser SA, Platzer M, et al. The relationship between inflammatory state and quantity of affective episodes in bipolar disorder. *Psychoneuroendocrinology* (2018) 90:61–7. doi: 10.1016/j.psyneuen.2018.01.024
58. Doenni VM, Song CM, Hill MN, Pittman QJ. Early-life inflammation with LPS delays fear extinction in adult rodents. *Brain Behav Immun.* (2017) 63:176–85. doi: 10.1016/j.bbi.2016.11.022
59. Young MB, Howell LL, Hopkins L, Moshfegh C, Yu Z, Clubb L, et al. A peripheral immune response to remembering trauma contributes to the maintenance of fear memory in mice. *Psychoneuroendocrinology* (2018) 94:143–51. doi: 10.1016/j.psyneuen.2018.05.012
60. Cohen H, Zohar J. An animal model of posttraumatic stress disorder: the use of cut-off behavioral criteria. *Ann NY Acad Sci.* (2004) 1032:167–78. doi: 10.1196/annals.1314.014
61. Sillivan SE, Joseph NF, Jamieson S, King ML, Chevere-Torres I, Fuentes I, et al. Susceptibility and resilience to posttraumatic stress disorder-like behaviors in inbred mice. *Biol Psychiatry* (2017) 82:924–33. doi: 10.1016/j.biopsych.2017.06.030
62. Ponomarev I, Rau V, Eger EI, Harris RA, Fanselow MS. Amygdala transcriptome and cellular mechanisms underlying stress-enhanced fear learning in a rat model of posttraumatic stress disorder. *Neuropsychopharmacology* (2010) 35:1402–11. doi: 10.1038/npp.2010.10
63. Daviu N, Andero R, Armario A, Nadal R. Sex differences in the behavioural and hypothalamic-pituitary-adrenal response to contextual fear conditioning in rats. *Horm Behav.* (2014) 66:713–23. doi: 10.1016/j.yhbeh.2014.09.015
64. Kessler RC, Sonnega A, Bromet E, Hughes M, Nelson CB. Posttraumatic stress disorder in the national comorbidity survey. *Arch Gen Psychiatry* (1995) 52:1048–60. doi: 10.1001/archpsyc.1995.03950240066012

65. Duncan LE, Ratanatharathorn A, Aiello AE, Almli LM, Amstadter AB, Ashley-Koch AE, et al. Largest GWAS of PTSD (N=20 070) yields genetic overlap with schizophrenia and sex differences in heritability. *Mol Psychiatry* (2018) 23:666–73. doi: 10.1038/mp.2017.77

66. Keum S, Park J, Kim A, Park J, Kim KK, Jeong J, et al. Variability in empathic fear response among 11 inbred strains of mice. *Genes Brain Behav.* (2016) 15:231–42. doi: 10.1111/gbb.12278

2

Variations in Mitochondrial Respiration Differ in IL-1ß/IL-10 Ratio Based Subgroups in Autism Spectrum Disorders

Harumi Jyonouchi[1,2], Lee Geng[1], Shannon Rose[3,4], Sirish C. Bennuri[3,4] and Richard E. Frye[5,6]*

[1] Department of Pediatrics, Saint Peter's University Hospital, New Brunswick, NJ, United States, [2] Robert Wood Johnson Medical School-Rutgers, New Brunswick, NJ, United States, [3] Arkansas Children's Research Institute, Little Rock, AR, United States, [4] Department of Pediatrics, University of Arkansas of Medical Sciences, Little Rock, AR, United States, [5] Department of Child Health, University of Arizona College of Medicine-Phoenix, Phoenix, AZ, United States, [6] Barrow Neurological Institute at Phoenix Children's Hospital, Phoenix, AZ, United States

***Correspondence:**
Harumi Jyonouchi
hjyonouchi@saintpetersuh.com

Autism spectrum disorder (ASD)[7] is associated with multiple physiological abnormalities, including immune dysregulation, and mitochondrial dysfunction. However, an association between these two commonly reported abnormalities in ASD has not been studied in depth. This study assessed the association between previously identified alterations in cytokine profiles by ASD peripheral blood monocytes (PBMo) and mitochondrial dysfunction. In 112 ASD and 38 non-ASD subjects, cytokine production was assessed by culturing purified PBMo overnight with stimuli of innate immunity. Parameters of mitochondrial respiration including proton-leak respiration (PLR), ATP-linked respiration (ALR), maximal respiratory capacity (MRC), and reserve capacity (RC) were measured in peripheral blood mononuclear cells (PBMCs). The ASD samples were analyzed by subgrouping them into high, normal, and low IL-1ß/IL-10 ratio groups, which was previously shown to be associated with changes in behaviors and PBMo miRNA expression. MRC, RC, and RC/PLR, a marker of electron transport chain (ETC) efficiency, were higher in ASD PBMCs than controls. The expected positive associations between PLR and ALR were found in control non-ASD PBMCs, but not in ASD PBMCs. Higher MRC, RC, RC/PLR in ASD PBMCs were secondary to higher levels of these parameters in the high and normal IL-1ß/IL-10 ratio ASD subgroups than controls. Associations between mitochondrial parameters and monocyte cytokine profiles differed markedly across the IL-1ß/IL-10 ratio based ASD subgroups, rendering such associations less evident when ASD samples as a whole were compared to non-ASD controls. Our results indicate for the first time, an association between PBMC mitochondrial function and PBMo cytokine profiles in ASD subjects. This relationship differs across the IL-1ß/IL-10 ratio based ASD subgroups. Changes in mitochondrial function are likely due to adaptive changes or mitochondrial dysfunction, resulting from chronic oxidative stress. These results may indicate alteration in molecular pathways affecting both the immune system and mitochondrial function in some ASD subjects.

Keywords: autism spectrum disorders, IL-1ß/IL-10 ratio, mitochondrial respiration, monocytes, peripheral blood mononuclear cells (PBMCs)

INTRODUCTION

Autism spectrum disorder (ASD) is defined by behavioral symptomatology which results in a heterogeneous phenotype. ASD is also known to be associated with various co-morbid medical conditions, most notably gastrointestinal (GI) symptoms, and sleep disorders (1, 2).

We have previously identified a subset of ASD subjects who exhibit innate immune abnormalities (3). Our recent study revealed that the IL-1ß/IL-10 ratios produced by PBMo may serve as a marker of immune activation or immune mediated inflammation in individuals with ASD. Deviated IL-1ß/IL-10 ratios were seen in up to 40% of ASD subjects in our previous study (4). IL-1ß is a representative inflammatory cytokine, and IL-10 is a representative counter-regulatory cytokine. Thus, IL-1ß/IL-10 ratios are thought to reflect the balance of inflammatory vs. counter-regulatory responses by monocytes.

One knowledge gap in understanding the pathology of ASD is how the various medical comorbidities are related to each other and to abnormalities in brain function. Research has pointed to abnormalities in cellular systems that are common to cells in many organ systems. For example, studies have associated ASD with abnormalities in mitochondrial (5) and redox metabolism (6) that are systems important to varying extents to almost every cell in the body. Other possible connections between different organ systems include abnormalities in cellular regulatory pathways, such as those controlled by microRNA (miRNA). This is a prime area of research as we are learning that abnormalities in miRNA expressions are associated with a wide range of psychiatric diseases, including ASD (7). On the other hand, little is known regarding what changes in miRNA expression are linked to both innate immune and mitochondrial abnormalities in ASD and other neuropsychiatric disorders.

Our previous studies showed that changes in expression of miRNA in ASD PBMo differed in ASD subgroups when they were subdivided on the basis of the IL-1ß/IL-10 ratio produced by PBMo (high, low, and normal as defined in the method section) (4, 8). Namely, many miRNA were up-regulated in the high ratio ASD subgroup, while in the low ratio ASD subgroup, multiple miRNAs were down-regulated, as compared to non-ASD controls (4). Determining targeted genes by these miRNAs indicated that the changes in miRNA expression are expected to affect the key signaling pathways, including RAS, MAPK, and PI3K-AKT pathways: these signaling pathways regulate immune cell differentiation and activation, partly through altering metabolism. Interestingly, this analysis also revealed that changes in miRNA would affect the expression of molecules important for formation of synaptic junctions (4). These results may indicate that there exist alterations in the signaling pathways affecting both the nervous and the immune systems in the high and low IL-1ß/IL-10 ratio ASD subgroups. The above described signaling pathways are also known to affect mitochondrial functions. For example, activation of MAPK and PI3K-AKT pathways enhances glycolysis, but reduces mitochondrial fitness, rendering cells more vulnerable to oxidative stress (9). Therefore, there may be a possibility that mitochondrial function is altered in the high/low IL-1ß/IL-10 ratio ASD subgroups. miRNAs secreted from innate immune cells including monocytes serve as mediators of innate immune responses (10). In fact, platelets and PBMo are major secretary source of miRNAs in the serum. Secreted miRNAs are taken up by other cells and regulate their cellular functions (10). Therefore, changes in IL-1ß/IL-10 ratios by ASD PBMo can be reflected in mitochondrial dysfunction in multiple cell lineages in ASD.

Independent of studies linked to immune abnormalities in ASD, there is also mounting evidence of mitochondrial dysfunction and chronic oxidative stresses in multiple cell types in ASD (11–14). However, primary mitochondrial diseases with known gene mutations are rarely found in ASD subjects (5, 15). Nevertheless, mitochondrial dysfunctions have been reported in 30–80% of individuals with ASD (16), and evidence of oxidative stress may be diagnostic for ASD (17). Putative alterations in signaling pathways as described above, if present, could make some ASD subjects vulnerable to both immune mediated inflammation and mitochondrial dysfunction. However, little is known regarding associations between monocyte cytokine profiles and mitochondrial dysfunction in ASD and other neuropsychiatric diseases.

On the basis of findings described above, we postulated that changes in monocyte cytokine profiles, especially IL-1ß/IL-10 ratios in ASD PBMo, are associated with alterations in mitochondrial respiration. This study examines our hypothesis by evaluating associations between IL-1ß/IL-10 ratios produced by PBMo and variations in mitochondrial respiration in PBMCs, a mixture of multiple lineage cells, in ASD subjects. Associations between mitochondrial parameters and other monocyte cytokines were also determined, since IL-1ß and IL-10 production were often closely associated with production of inflammatory and counter-regulatory cytokine produced by monocytes. Typically developing (TD), age-matched non-ASD subjects served as controls.

Abbreviations: Ab, antibody; ABC, aberrant behavior checklist; AC, allergic conjunctivitis; ADI-R, autism diagnostic inventory, revisited; ADOS, autism diagnostic observational scale; Ag, antigen; Akt, protein kinase B activated through PI3K-Akt pathway; ALR, ATP-linked respiration; ANOVA, analysis of variance; AR, allergic rhinitis; ASD, autism spectrum disorder; CSHQ, Children's sleep habit questionnaire; ELISA, enzyme linked immune-sorbent assay; ETC, electron transport chain; FA, food allergy; IL, interleukin; MIA, maternal immune activation; miRNA, microRNA; MRC, maximum respiration capacity; NFA, non-IgE mediated food allergy; OCR, oxygen consumption rate; PBMCs, peripheral blood mononuclear cells; PBMo, peripheral blood monocytes; PI3K, phosphoinositide 3-kinase; PTEN, phosphatase and tension homolog; PLR, proton-linked respiration; PST, prick skin testing; RC, reserve capacity; SAD, specific antibody deficiency; SD, standard deviation; TGF, transforming growth factor; TLR, toll like receptor; TNF, tumor necrosis factor; Treg cells, regulatory T cells; VABS, Vineland adaptive behavioral scale.

MATERIALS AND METHODS

Study Subjects

The study followed the protocol approved by the Institutional Review Board at our institution, Saint Peter's University Hospital, New Brunswick, NJ, United States. In this study, both ASD and non-ASD, TD control subjects were enrolled, and the signed consent forms were obtained prior to entering the study. Consent was obtained from parents if participant was a minor (<18 years old) or parents had custody. For ASD subjects, we also assessed whether they had history of FA, asthma, allergic rhinitis (AR), and specific antibody deficiency (SAD), or seizure disorders. Any ASD or non-ASD subject diagnosed with chromosomal abnormalities or other genetic diseases, or well-characterized chronic medical conditions involving major organs was excluded from the study. Subjects with common minor medical conditions such as AR, mild to moderate asthma, eczema were not excluded from the study.

ASD Subjects

ASD subjects ($N = 112$) were recruited in the Pediatric Allergy/Immunology clinic. The ASD diagnosis was based on the Autism Diagnostic Observation Scale (ADOS) and/or Autism Diagnostic Interview-Revisited (ADI-R), and other standard measures at various autism diagnostic centers, including ours. ASD subjects were also evaluated for their behavioral symptoms and sleep habits with the Aberrant Behavior Checklist (ABC) (18) and the Children's Sleep Habits Questionnaires (CSHQ) (19), respectively. Information regarding cognitive activity and adaptive skills were obtained from previous school records, which documented cognitive ability (by standard measures such as Woodcock-Johnson III test), and adaptive skills (by standard measures such as Vineland Adaptive Behavior Scale (VABS) (20). These were data documented within 1 year of enrollment to the study.

Non-ASD Controls

TD, non-ASD control subjects ($N = 38$) were recruited from the pediatric Allergy/Immunology and General Pediatrics Clinics. These subjects were not reported to have any medical conditions included in the exclusion criteria and self-reported not to have seizure disorders or known immunodeficiency.

Demographic information of the study subjects is summarized in **Table 1**. There were no differences between females and males by two tailed Mann-Whitney test with regard to mitochondrial respiration parameters and monocyte cytokine profiles examined in this study.

Diagnosis of FA

IgE mediated FA was diagnosed with reactions to offending food, by affecting skin, GI, and/or respiratory tract immediately (within 2 h) after intake of offending food, supported by prick skin testing (PST) reactivity, and/or presence of food allergen-specific IgE in the serum. NFA was diagnosed if GI symptoms resolved, following implementation of a restricted diet (i.e., avoidance of offending food), and symptoms recurred upon re-introduction of offending food, following the Food Allergy Diagnostic Guidelines (21). NFA patients are per definition, non-reactive to PST, and negative for food allergen-specific, serum IgE (21).

TABLE 1 | Demographics of ASD children.

	ASD[a] subjects ($N = 112$)	Non-ASD controls ($N = 38$)
AGE (YEARS)		
Median (range)	12.3 (2.5–30.3)	13.4 (3.9–29.7)
Mean ± SD	12.6 ± 5.9	13.8 ± 7.2
Gender (M:F and %)	97:15 (86.6%: 13.4%)	26:12 (68.4%: 31.4%)
Ethnicity	AA 6, Asian 21, Mixed 2, C 83	Asian 3, Mixed 3, C 32
Cognitive activity <1%	83/112 (74.1%)	0
Disturbed sleep	34/112 (30.4%)	N/A
GI symptoms	75/112 (67.0%)	Unknown[c]
Seizure disorders	14/112 (12.5%)	0
Specific antibody deficiency	18/112 (16.1%)	0
Asthma[b]	12/112 (10.7%)	Unknown
Allergic rhinitis[b]	23/112 (20.5%)	Unknown

[a]*AA, African American; ASD, autism spectrum disorder; C, Caucasian; N/A, not applicable; SD, standard deviation.*

[b]*Frequencies of asthma and allergic rhinitis are equivalent for those reported in general population.*

[c]*No self-reported GI complaint by non-ASD controls*

Diagnosis of Asthma and Allergic Rhinitis

AR and allergic conjunctivitis (AC) were diagnosed with positive PST reactivity, and/or presence of allergen-specific IgE in the serum, accompanied by clinical features consistent with AR and AC (22, 23). Asthma diagnosis was based on the guidelines from the Expert Panel Report 3 (24). Asthma, without PST reactivity to allergens and/or allergen-specific IgE antibodies was categorized as non-atopic asthma (23).

Specific Antibody Deficiency (SAD)

SAD was diagnosed by the absence of protective levels of antibody (Ab) titers (>1.3 μg/mL) to more than 11 of 14 serotypes of *Streptococcus pneumonia,* following a booster dose of Pneumovax® (25) or PCV13, a standard diagnostic measure for SAD.

Sample Collection

Blood samples were obtained by venipuncture after obtainment of informed consent. Efforts were made to obtain the samples at the time of medically required blood work to minimize the numbers of venipuncture. For the non-ASD control subjects, only 1 sample was obtained. For select ASD subjects, samples were obtained at 2–3 time points to assess variability of parameters that we tested. Venipuncture was conducted by the physician and if requested, the site of venipuncture was numbed by applying a topical lidocaine/prilocaine cream (Emla cream®).

Cell Cultures

PBMCs were isolated by Ficoll-Hypaque density gradient centrifugation. PBMo were purified by negatively selecting PBMo depleting T, B, natural killer, and dendritic cells from PBMCs, using magnetic beads labeled with anti-CD3, CD7, CD16, CD19, CD56, CD123, and glycophorin A (monocyte separation kit II—human, MILTENYI BIOTEC, Cambridge, MA, United States).

PBMo cytokine production was assessed by incubating purified PBMo (2.5 × 10^5 cells/ml) overnight with a TLR4 agonist (LPS; 0.1 μg/ml, GIBCO-BRL, Gaithersburg, MD, USA), a TLR2/6 agonist (zymosan; 50 μg/ml, Sigma-Aldrich, St. Luis, Mo), and a TLR7/8 agonist (CL097, water-soluble derivative of imidazoquinoline, 20 μM, InvivoGen, San Diego, CA, Unites States) in RPMI 1640 with additives as previously described (26). Overnight incubation (16–20 h) was adequate to induce the optimal responses in this setting. The culture supernatant was used for cytokine assays. LPS is a representative endotoxin, reflecting a common pathway of innate immune responses by gram negative [G (−)] bacteria. Zymosan is a representative innate immune stimulus from G (+) bacteria and fungi. CL097 mimics stimuli from ssRNA viruses, common respiratory pathogens causing respiratory infection, such as influenza. These stimuli have been widely used for testing innate immune responses.

Levels of pro-inflammatory [tumor necrosis factor-α (TNF-α), IL-1β, IL-6, IL-12p40, and IL-23] and counter-regulatory [IL-10, transforming growth factor-ß (TGF-ß) and soluble TNF receptor II (sTNFRII)] cytokines were measured by enzyme-linked immuno-sorbent assay (ELISA);10–100 μl/well supernatant were used for ELISA, depending on culture conditions. The ELISA, OptEIA™ Reagent Sets for IFN-γ, IL-1ß, IL-5, IL-6, IL-10, IL-12p40, and TNF-α (BD Biosciences, San Jose, CA, USA), and for sTNFRII, IL-17 (IL-17A), and TGF-ß were obtained from BD Biosciences and R & D (Minneapolis, MN, United States), respectively. IL-23 ELISA kit was purchased from eBiosciences, San Diego, CA, United States. Intra- and inter-variations of cytokine levels were <5%.

Categorizing ASD Samples Based on IL-1ß/IL-10 Ratios

Previously, we observed both high and low IL-1ß/IL-10 ratios in subsets of ASD PBMo as compared to non-ASD controls (8). We found changes in IL-1ß/IL-10 ratios were associated with behavioral changes as well as changes in miRNA expression (4, 8). In this study, we also observed the presence of high and low IL-1ß/IL-10 ratios in some ASD PBMo, as compared to control PBMo (**Supplemental Figure 1**). To assess whether there was an association between IL-1ß/IL-10 ratios produced by PBMo and mitochondrial respiration exhibited by PBMCs, we subdivided ASD samples into subgroups based on the IL-1ß/IL-10 ratios produced by ASD PBMo as described below, following the criteria used in our previous study (4, 8).

High IL-1ß/IL-10 Ratio

IL-1ß/IL-10 ratios > +2 standard deviation (SD) than control cells under at least 1 culture condition and/or > +1 SD under more than 2 culture conditions.

Normal IL-1β/IL-10 Ratio

IL-1ß/IL-10 ratios between −1 SD < IL-1ß/IL-10 ratios < +1 SD under all the culture conditions, or +1 SD < IL-1ß/IL-10 ratios < +2 SD under only one culture condition.

Low IL-1β/IL-10 Ratios

IL-1ß/IL-10 ratios < −1 SD under at least 1 culture condition.

As for ASD subjects whose samples were taken at 2–3 time points, most subjects were categorized in the same group with analysis of samples taken at 2–3 time points. One ASD subject who was assessed at 3 time points revealed high ratios at 2 time points and normal ratio at 1 time point when his GI symptoms became under control. This patient was categorized as the high ratio group. Another subject revealed low ratios at 2 time points and a normal ratio at one time point, thus this subject was categorized as the low ratio group. Most non-ASD controls fall into the normal IL-1β/IL-10 group, except for 2 subjects who fall into the high ratio group and 1 subject who falls into the low ratio group, consistent with our previous study (4). Since our current hypothesis was developed based on this subgrouping definition, we used the same definition in this study.

Assays of Mitochondrial Function

PBMCs (2 × 10^6 cells) were suspended in bio-freezing medium (90% heat-inactivated fetal calf serum and 10% DMSO) and kept in −20°C for about 1 h and then transferred to −80°C degree freezer and kept until shipment. Then samples were sent to Dr. R. Frye's laboratory on dry ice where Seahorse Extracellular Flux (XF) 96 Analyzer (Seahorse Bioscience, Inc., North Billerica, MA, United States) was used for measurement of oxygen consumption ratio (OCR), which is an indicator of mitochondrial respiration, in real time in live PBMCs (14, 27). Several measures of mitochondrial respiration, including basal respiration, ALR, PLR, MRC, and RC, were derived by the sequential addition of pharmacological agents to the respiring cells. For each parameter, three repeated rates of oxygen consumption are made over an 18 min period. First, baseline cellular oxygen consumption is measured, from which basal respiration is derived by subtracting non-mitochondrial respiration. Next oligomycin, an inhibitor of complex V, is added, and the resulting OCR is used to derive ALR (by subtracting the oligomycin rate from baseline cellular OCR) and PLR subtracting non-mitochondrial respiration from the oligomycin rate). Next carbonyl cyanide-p-trifluoromethoxyphenyl-hydrazon (FCCP), a protonophore, is added to collapse the inner membrane gradient, driving the ETC to function to its maximal rate, and MRC is derived by subtracting non-mitochondrial respiration from the FCCP OCR. Lastly, antimycin A, a complex III inhibitor, and rotenone, a complex I inhibitor, are added to shut down ETC function, revealing the non-mitochondrial respiration. RC is calculated by subtracting basal respiration from maximal respiratory capacity.

Both ALR and MRC are measures of the ability of the electron transport chain (ETC) to produce ATP, the molecule that carries energy to other areas of the cell to support vital functions. However, the ETC is also a major source of the production of reactive oxygen species (ROS), which can damage the mitochondrial and the cell if produced in excess. The ETC can "leak" some of its energy to reduce ROS production. This "leak" is measured by PLR and makes the ETC less efficient at producing energy. In general, PLR should increase as more ATP is produced since the production of ATP does create ROS. The ratio of the measures of ATP production, specifically ALR and MRC, to PLR can provide a measure of efficiency of the ETC. Theoretically this ratio would be very high with very efficient mitochondrial function and very low in dysfunctional mitochondria where a great amount of ROS is produced to make energy.

Statistical Analysis

For comparison of two sets of numerical data, two tailed Mann-Whitney test was used. For comparison of several sets of numerical data, a one-way analysis of variance (ANOVA) was used if the data were distributed normally. If the data were not normally distributed, Kruskal-Wallis test was used. For differences in frequency between two groups, Fisher exact test was used. For differences in frequency among multiple groups, Chi-square test and Likelihood ratio were used. Co-variance of repeated measures and a linear association between two variables were assessed by regression analysis (mixed models—repeated measures) and Spearman test, respectively. NCSS12 (Kaysville, UT, United States) was used for analysis. A p-value of < 0.05 was considered nominally significant. Statistical measures used in this study are summarized in **Supplemental Figure 2**.

RESULTS

Mitochondrial Respiration in ASD PBMCs

When mitochondrial respiration parameters were compared between all the ASD and non-ASD control samples, MRC and RC were higher in ASD cells than non-ASD controls (**Figure 1**). There were no differences in PLR and ALR between ASD and non-ASD control PBMCs (**Figure 1**).

Non-ASD control PBMCs demonstrated the expected positive correlation between PLR and ALR (**Figure 2A**). MRC and PLR tended to show similar positive correlation, but not statistically significant (**Figure 2C**). However, these expected positive associations were not observed in ASD PBMCs (**Figures 2B,D**). For ALR, this was secondary to ASD PBMCs demonstrating low PLR despite high ALR, and those with high PLR demonstrating low ALR (**Figure 2B**). These cells are likely to have a tightly coupled ETC with very active mitochondrial respiration, or under mitochondrial dysfunction, respectively. Given these findings, we assessed differences in ALR/PLR, MRC/PLR, and RC/PLR ratios, as markers of ETC efficiency, between ASD and non-ASD PBMCs. As shown in **Table 2**, we observed nominally significant differences in RC/PLR ratios between ASD and non-ASD samples. This is secondary to presence of ASD subjects with high RC/PLR ratios, but some ASD subjects also showed low RC/PLR ratios.

Associations Between Mitochondrial Respiration and Monocyte Cytokine Profiles in ASD

As summarized in **Table 3**, we found several positive or negative associations in the ASD samples mainly between IL-1ß and IL-6 levels under LPS stimulated cultures, and mitochondrial respiratory parameters. Specifically, negative associations were observed between PLR and IL-1ß/IL-10 ratio and IL-1ß levels under LPS stimulated cultures in ASD samples. On the other hand, no significant associations between these parameters were

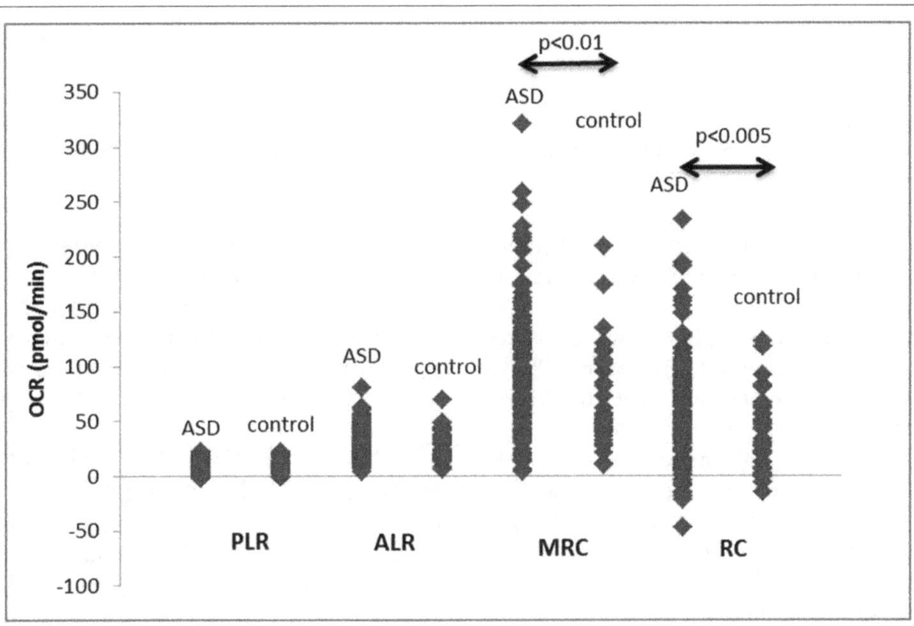

FIGURE 1 | PLR, ALR, MRC, and RC values in PBMCs from ASD subjects as well as control non-ASD subjects. F-ratios are 0.2971 (PLR), 0.2484 (ALR), 8.6833 ($p <$ 0.005), and 13.487 ($p < 0.001$) by Welch's test. P-values shown in the figure by two-tailed Mann-Whitney test.

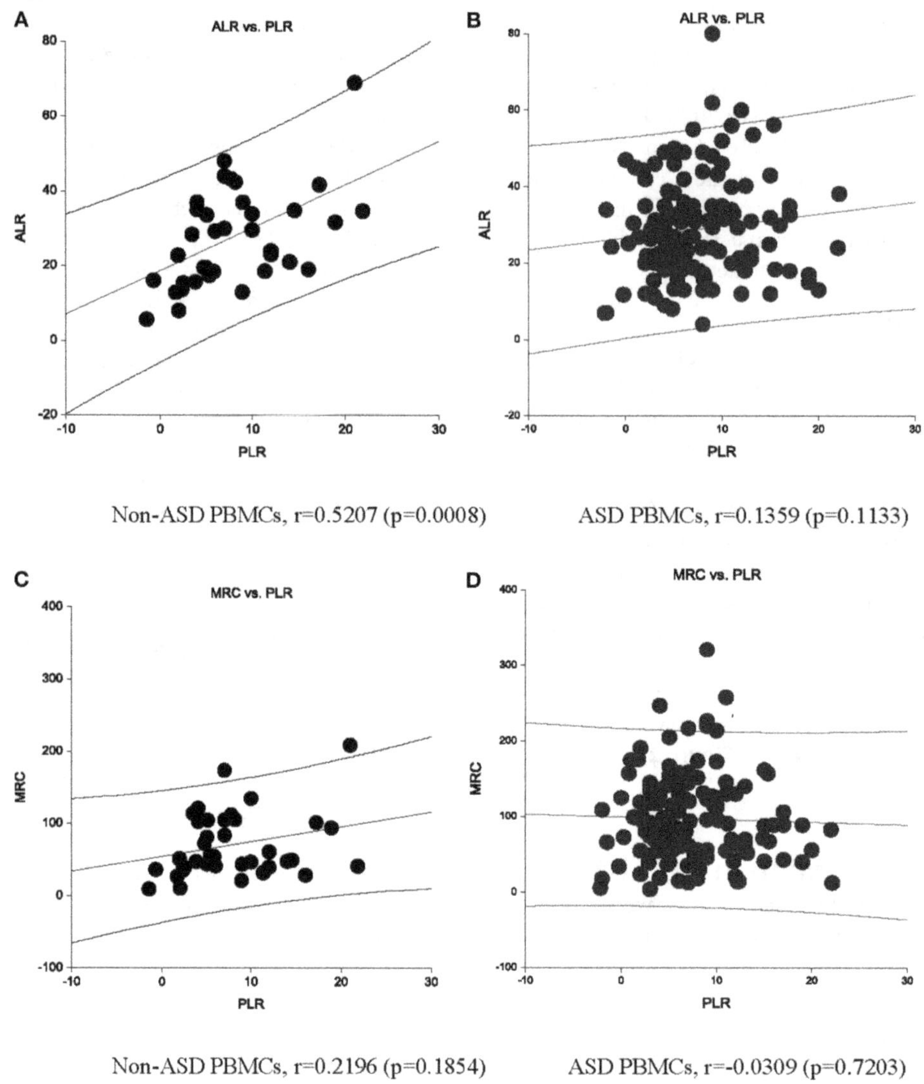

FIGURE 2 | An association between ALR and PLR OCR (pmol/min) are shown in non-ASD **(A)** and ASD **(B)** PBMCs. An association between MRC and PLR OCR (pmol/min) are also shown in non-ASD **(C)** and ASD **(D)** PBMCs. Correlation Co-efficient and *p*-values shown were by Spearman test.

observed in non-ASD controls, except for associations between MRC and TNF-α (under the zymosan-stimulated cultures) or CCL2 (without stimuli) (**Table 3**).

In 13 ASD subjects, mitochondrial respiration was measured at 2–3 time-points along with cytokine profiles by PBMo. Repeated measures regression demonstrated that IL-1ß/IL-10 ratios under CL097 stimulated cultures were positively associated with ALR ($p = 0.026$), MRC ($p = 0.014$), and RC ($p = 0.0294$). In these samples, mitochondrial respiration appeared to change in some ASD subjects, while these values remained stable in others (**Figure 3**). However, these numbers are too small to confirm this trend and further studies are required.

We also assessed the associations between monocyte cytokine profiles and ALR/PLR, MRC/PLR, and RC/PLR ratios, as markers of ETC efficiency. We observed positive associations mainly between these ETC efficiency markers and IL-1ß and IL-6 levels under LPS stimulated culture conditions (**Table 3**). The results of association analysis between RC/PLR and monocyte cytokine profiles are almost identical to those between MRC/PLR and cytokine profiles (data now shown). We did not observe significant associations between monocyte cytokine levels and ETC efficiency parameters in non-ASD controls.

Clinical Features of IL-1ß/IL-10 Ratio Based ASD Subgroups

Clinical features of ASD subjects in the ASD subgroups are summarized in **Table 4**. We found frequency of history of NFA differed across the ASD subgroups; frequency of history of NFA was higher in the low ratio ASD subgroup than normal ratio group ($p < 0.05$ by Fisher's exact test). Disturbed sleep was reported at a higher frequency in the lower ratio ASD subgroup than in normal ratio ASD subgroup ($p < 0.05$ by

TABLE 2 | Mitochondrial respiration ratios in the ASD cell subgroups based on IL-1ß/IL-10 ratios by PBMo.

	Total ASD samples ($N = 136$)	Non-ASD controls ($N = 38$)	Statistics (mann-whitney test)
ALR/PLR ratio[a,b]	5.4 ± 11.1	4.9 ± 3.1	$p = 0.8949$
MRC/PLR ratio	19.6 ± 37.7	8.8 ± 14.0	$p = 0.0558$
RC/PLR ratio[b]	13.2 ± 27.1	4.4 ± 8.6	$p = 0.01239$

[a]*F-ratios are 1.314 (ALR/PLR), 6.693 (MRC/PLR), and 9.009 (RC/PLR) by Welch's test.*
[b]*ALR, ATP-linked respiration; MRC, Maximum respiration capacity; PLR, proton-leak respiration; RC, reserve capacity.*

TABLE 3 | Mitochondrial respiration ratios in the ASD cell subgroups based on IL-1ß/IL-10 ratios by PBMo.

	Correlation coefficient ASD samples ($N = 136$)	Correlation coefficient non-ASD controls ($N = 38$)
PLR[c]		
Ratio (medium)	0.1855 ($p < 0.05$)[a,b]	*0.1133*
Ratio (LPS)	−0.3266 ($p < 0.0001$)	*0.1882*
IL-1ß (LPS)	−0.2742 ($p < 0.005$)	*0.1242*
TGF-ß (zymosan)	0.2067 ($p < 0.02$)	*−0.1636*
ALR		
IL-10 (LPS)	0.181 ($p < 0.05$)	0.188
MRC[d]		
IL-1ß (LPS)	0.2431 ($p < 0.005$)	0.0119
IL-10 (LPS)	0.251 ($p < 0.005$)	0.0219
IL-6 (medium)	0.1916 ($p < 0.05$)	−0.1224
IL-6 (LPS)	0.2999 ($p < 0.0005$)	0.1286
TNF-α (zymosan)	−0.2278 ($p < 0.01$)	−0.3681 ($p < 0.05$)
CCL2 (medium)	−0.1284	−0.4162 ($p < 0.01$)
ALR/PLR		
IL-1ß (LPS)	0.1938 ($p < 0.05$)	−0.1191
IL-6 (LPS)	0.1954 ($p < 0.05$)	0.3046
MRC/PL		
Ratio (LPS)	0.2034 ($p < 0.02$)	−0.1061
IL-1ß (LPS)	0.2462 ($p < 0.005$)	−0.1417
IL-6 (LPS)	0.2263 ($p < 0.01$)	0.1668

[a]*Values of Correlation coefficients revealed significant results in ASD and control samples are shown.*
[b]*Correlation coefficient by Spearman test; Statistically significant values are shown with p-values.*
[c]*ALR, ATP-linked respiration; LPS, lipopolysaccharide; MRC, Maximum respiration capacity; PLR, proton-leak respiration; RC, reserve capacity.*
[d]*Correlations between RC or RC/PLR and monocyte cytokine levels are almost identical as observed in MRC and MRC/PLR vs. monocyte cytokine levels and not included in this table.*

Fisher's exact test). No difference was found in frequency in seizures, SAD, asthma, or AR among the IL-1ß/IL-10 ratio based ASD subgroups.

Mitochondrial Respiration in IL-1ß/IL-10 Ratio ASD Subgroups

In this study, we found a distribution of ASD PBMo samples into the high, normal, or low IL-1ß/IL-10 ratio subgroups similar to our previous reports (**Table 5**) (4). Most non-ASD control samples (35/38 sample, 92%) were categorized as normal ratio subgroup. Consistent with our previous results (4), we observed differences in production of monocyte cytokines (IL-6, TNF-α, and CCL2) across the IL-1ß/IL-10 ratio based ASD subgroups (**Supplemental Table 1**).

Given these results, we then assessed mitochondrial parameters in the IL-1ß/IL-10 based ASD subgroups as summarized in **Table 5**. MRC and RC differed among the ASD subgroups. Specifically, the high and normal IL-1ß/IL-10 ratio ASD subgroups revealed a higher MRC and RC than non-ASD controls. MRC and RC in the low ratio ASD subgroup did not differ from those in non-ASD controls. Parameters of ETC efficiency (ALR/PLR, MRC/PLR, and RC/PLR ratios) were also assessed in these ASD subgroups. Only RC/PLR ratios revealed changes in association with the IL-1ß/IL-10 ratio based ASD subgrouping (**Table 6**). Specifically, the high and normal ratio ASD subgroups revealed higher RC/PLR ratios than non-ASD controls.

Associations Between Mitochondrial Respiration Parameters and Monocyte Cytokine Profiles in the IL-1ß/IL-10 Based ASD Subgroups

As shown in **Table 4**, ASD samples as a whole, revealed associations only between PLR and IL-1ß/IL-10 ratios. In contrast, in the IL-1ß/IL-10 based ASD subgroups, ALR and MRC revealed significant associations with the IL-1ß/IL-10 ratios, but not PLR (**Table 7**). Moreover, associations differed across the IL-1ß/IL-10 based ASD subgroups. Since MRC and RC revealed almost identical results, in this analysis, the results of associations between RC and IL-1ß/IL-10 ratios are not shown in the **Table 7**.

Multiple cytokines (IL-1ß, IL-10, IL-6, TNF-α, and TGF-ß) under various culture conditions revealed positive or negative associations with mitochondrial parameters in the IL-1ß/IL-10 ratio based ASD subgroups (**Table 8**). Moreover, associations differed markedly across the IL-1ß/IL-10 ratio based ASD subgroups (**Table 8**). Again, MRC and RC revealed almost identical associations (data not shown). Specifically, nominally significant associations between PLR and cytokine levels were observed only in the high ratio ASD group (**Table 8**) and *p*-values are not under 0.005. In contrast, ALR and MRC revealed significant associations with several cytokines across the ASD subgroups (**Table 8**). The high ratio ASD subgroup mainly revealed negative associations between ALR and spontaneously produced IL-1ß and IL-6. In contrast, the normal and low ratio ASD subgroups revealed positive associations between ALR and IL-1ß or IL-6 levels. MRC in the normal ratio ASD subgroup also showed similar results. The low ratio ASD subgroup revealed negative associations between ALR or MRC and levels of TNF-α under multiple culture conditions. It should be noted that associations between ALR or MRC and monocyte cytokine profiles revealed

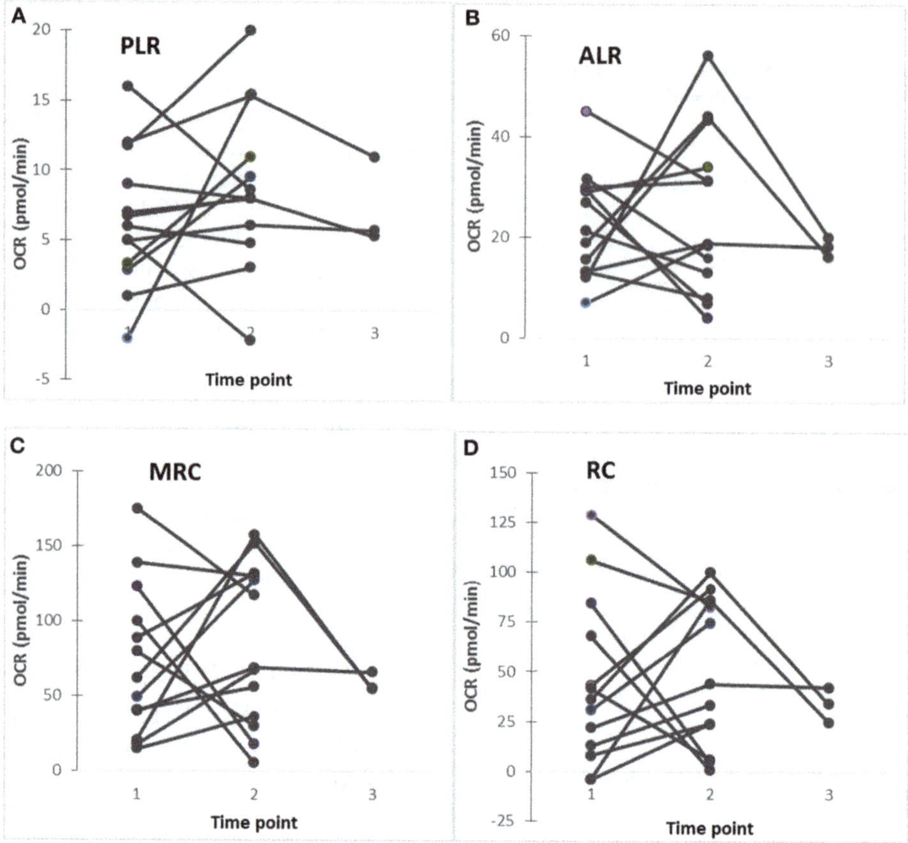

FIGURE 3 | (A–D) Changes in mitochondrial respiration (PLR, ALR, MRC, and RC) in ASD subjects studied at 2–3 time points, showing that in some ASD subjects revealed stable these parameters, while others show fluctuating these parameters. Five ASD subjects (4 males and 1 female) showed stable clinical conditions without fluctuating behavioral symptoms, while 8 ASD subjects (7 males and 1 female) revealed fluctuating behavioral symptoms (anxiety, irritability, OCD, and self-injurious behaviors) along with fluctuating GI (diarrhea alternating with constipation) symptoms.

higher *p*-values ($p < 0.005$ or lower) in the normal ratio ASD subgroup.

Next, we analyzed associations between monocyte cytokine profiles and ALR/PLR, MR/PLR, and RC/PLR ratios, as markers of ETC efficiency, among the IL-1ß/IL-10 ratio based ASD subgroups. The associations between monocyte cytokine profiles and ETC efficiency markers differed across the IL-1ß/IL-10 ratio based ASD subgroups (**Table 9**). The high ratio ASD subgroup revealed positive associations between ETC efficiency parameters and IL-10 levels under LPS stimulated cultures. In the ASD normal ratio subgroup, ETC efficiency parameters were positively associated with IL-1ß levels and IL-1ß/IL-10 ratios under LPS stimulated cultures. In the low ratio ASD subgroup, positive associations were observed between ETC efficiency parameters and IL-1ß levels under zymosan-stimulated cultures. The most striking positive associations were observed between IL-1ß/IL-10 ratios (under LPS stimulated cultures) and MRC/PLR as well as RC/PLR ratios ($p < 0.0005$) in the normal ratio ASD subgroup. While the low ratio ASD subgroup revealed a negative association between MRC/PLR or RC/PLR and IL-1ß/IL-10 ratios (under CL097 stimulated cultures).

DISCUSSION

The results of our results indicate associations exist between mitochondrial respiration by PBMCs and monocyte cytokine profiles in ASD subjects. Our findings may be the result of the presence of ASD subjects in whom adaptive changes triggered by environmental stimuli are dysregulated in both innate immunity and in mitochondrial function. In such subjects, maladapted changes may cause detrimental effects on the nervous system, leading to a puzzling array of clinical features in ASD subjects.

Mounting evidence indicates that there is abnormal or altered mitochondrial function in individuals with ASD (5, 28). There is also mounting evidence of mitochondrial dysfunction and chronic oxidative stresses in ASD (11–14). Interestingly, individuals with ASD seem to have unique types of mitochondrial dysfunction. For example, while it is estimated that 5% of individuals with ASD appear to have primary mitochondrial disease, the majority (~75%) do not have known genetic mutations to explain their mitochondrial disease (5, 15). What is more interesting is that 30% of more individuals with ASD have biomarkers of mitochondrial dysfunction, even though they may not have primary mitochondrial disease (16). In addition, up to

TABLE 4 | Demographics and clinical characteristics of the ASD study subjects, when ASD subjects subdivided into the high, normal, and low IL-1ß/IL-10 ratios groups.

	ASD subjects subgrouped based on IL-1ß/IL-10 ratios		
	High ratio (*N* = 51)	**Normal ratio (*N* = 47)**	**Low ratio (*N* = 14)**
AGE			
Median (range)	11.8 year (2.5–30.0)	13.4 year (3.8–30.0)	11.1 year (5.8–19.8)
Mean ± SD	12.3 ± 6.3 year	13.1 ± 5.9 year	11.8 ± 4.9 year
Gender (M:F and %)	43:8 (84.3%: 15.7%)	41:6 (87.2%: 12.8%)	13:1 (92.9%: 7.1%)
Ethnicity	AA[a] 5, Asian 10, C 36	AA 2, Asian 9, Mixed 2, C 34	AA 1, Asian 2, C 11
Cognitive activity (<1st %)	37/51 (72.5%)	32/47 (70.2%)	11/14 (78.6%)
Disturbed sleep	16/51 (31.4%)	11/47 (23.4%)	8/14 (57.1%)[c]
GI symptoms[d]	33/51 (64.7%)	32/47 (68.1%)	11/14 (78.6%)
History of NFA	29/51 (56.9%)	21/47 (44.7%)	11/14 (78.6%)[b]
Seizure disorders	5/51 (9.8%)	6/47 (12.8%)	3/14 (21.4%)
SAD	7/51 (14.9%)	9/47 (19.1%)	3/14 (21.4%)
Allergic rhinitis	11/51 (21.6%)	10/47 (21.3%)	2/14 (14.3%)
Asthma	8/51 (11.9%)	4/47 (8.5%)	0

[a]*AA, African American; ASD, autism spectrum disorder; C, Caucasian; GI, gastrointestinal; NFA, non-IgE mediated food allergy; SAD, specific antibody deficiency; SD, standard deviation.*
[b]*Significantly different in frequencies by Chi-Square test and Likelihood Ratio ($p < 0.05$). Frequency of history of NFA is higher in the low ratio ASD subgroup than in the normal ratio ASD subgroup ($p < 0.05$ by Fisher's exact test)*
[c]*Frequency of disturbed sleep was higher in the low ratio ASD subgroup than in the normal ratio ASD subgroup ($p < 0.05$ by Fisher's exact test).*
[d]*GI symptoms present at the time of sample obtainment: Constipation is the most common complaint.*

TABLE 5 | IL-1ß/IL-10 ratios and Mitochondrial function in ASD cells and non-ASD control cells.

	IL-1ß/IL-10 ratio[a] based ASD cell subgroups			Non-ASD controls (*N* = 38)	Krushkal wallis test
	High (*N* = 56)[e]	**Normal (*N* = 59)**	**Low (*N* = 22)**		
IL-1ß/IL-10 RATIOS CULTURED WITH *P*-VALUE					
medium	1.54 ± 2.03[d]	0.79 ± 1.12	0.32 ± 0.30	0.88 ± 0.92	<0.00001
LPS[c]	2.03 ± 1.43	1.19 ± 0.51	0.77 ± 0.56	1.81 ± 2.02	<0.00001
Zymosan	5.86 ± 3.94	2.53 ± 0.87	1.42 ± 0.74	3.25 ± 1.98	<0.00001
CL097	9.40 ± 16.84	2.89 ± 2.84	2.72 ± 2.19	3.95 ± 2.77	0.00061
MITOCHONDRIAL RESPIRATION[b] *P*-VALUE					
PLR	6.2 ± 5.2	8.3 ± 5.2	7.5 ± 3.8	7.9 ± 5.8	0.06771
ALR	27.2 ± 10.8	31.2 ± 14.0	27.3 ± 15.7	27.7 ± 13.2	0.5153
MRC[f]	93.3 ± 57.2	104.7 ± 59.0	84.6 ± 59.3	70.8 ± 44.4	0.0269
RC	59.9 ± 49.5	64.6 ± 48.5	49.7 ± 47.9	35.1 ± 33.6	0.00788

[a]*IL-1ß/IL-10 ratios are those obtained from purified ASD monocytes cultured with medium only, LPS (0.1 µg/ml), zymosan (50 µg/ml), or C097 (20 µM) as detailed in the materials and methods section. IL-1ß/IL-10 ratios were calculated as IL-1ß levels/IL-10 levels in each culture condition. The high ratio group revealed higher ratios than normal and low ratio groups under all the culture conditions than the normal and low ratio groups ($p < 0.005$ by two tailed Mann-Whitney test). The normal ratio group also revealed higher ratios than the low ratio group under the culture condition tested ($p < 0.005$, by two tailed Mann-Whitney test), except for the cultures under CL097.*
[b]*Mitochondrial respiration parameters were measured in PBMCs.*
[c]*Abbreviations used; ALR, ATP-linked respiration; LPS, lipopolysaccharide; MRC, Maximum respiration capacity; PLR, proton-leak respiration; RC, reserve capacity.*
[d]*All the data are expressed as a mean value ± SD.*
[e]*In 10 ASD subjects, samples were obtained at 2 time points, and in 3 ASD subjects. samples were obtained at 3 time points.*
[f]*MRC and RC were higher than non-ASD controls in the high ($p < 0.05$ for MRC, $p < 0.02$ for RC), and normal ($p < 0.005$ for both MRC and RC) ratio ASD subgroups by two tailed Mann Whitney test.*

80% of immune cells (lymphocytes and granulocytes) may show abnormalities in the respiratory chain when examined (29, 30). Furthermore, converging evidence from several human tissues (lymphoblastic cell lines, buccal endothelium muscle, fibroblasts, and postmortem brain) demonstrate that the mitochondria may have atypical over-activity of the respiratory chain which may result in a vulnerability to oxidative insults (16). References of mitochondrial dysfunction in ASD subjects are summarized in **Supplemental Table 2**. One important unanswered question is the reason for these alterations in mitochondrial function, especially given the fact that no clear genetic cause seems to explain these changes.

Apart from changes in mitochondrial functions, immune abnormalities are also frequently reported in ASD children

TABLE 6 | Mitochondrial respiration ratios in the ASD cell subgroups based on IL-1ß/IL-10 ratios by PBMo.

IL-1ß/IL-10 ratio			Non-ASD controls ($N = 38$)	Statistics (krushkal-wallis test)
High ($N = 56$)	Normal ($N = 59$)	Low ($N = 22$)		
ALR/PLR RATIO[a]				
4.3 ± 11.1[c]	6.8 ± 12.6	4.7 ± 4.8	*4.9 ± 3.1*	*p = 0.9186*
MRC/PLR RATIO				
17.3 ± 38.5	23.3 ± 42.0	15.6 ± 20.0	8.8 ± 14.0	*p* = 0.1583
RC/PLR RATIO[b]				
12.0 ± 27.7	15.6 ± 30.0	9.8 ± 15.3	4.4 ± 8.6	*p* = 0.0430

[a]*F-ratios are 0.7654 (p = 0.9153), 1.4245 (p = 0.1040), 3.559 (p = 0.0229) for ALR/PLR, MRC/PLR, and RC/PLR ratios, respectively, by Welch's test among the IL-1ß/IL-10 ratio ASD subgroups.*

[b]*RC/PLR ratios differ among the ASD subgroups and non-ASD controls. Specifically, the RC/PLR ratios are higher in the ASD high (p < 0.05) and normal (p < 0.01) ratio groups than non-ASD controls (by two-tailed Mann-Whitney test).*

[c] *The results were expressed as a mean ±SD.*

TABLE 7 | Associations between parameters of mitochondrial respiration (PLR, ALR, and MRC) and IL-1ß/IL-10 ratios by PBMo under various culture conditions.

IL-1ß/IL-10 ratio correlation with PLR, ALR, and MRC[a]	IL-1ß/IL-10 ratio[d] based ASD subgroups			Non-ASD control cells ($N = 38$)
	High ratio ($N = 56$)	Normal ratio ($N = 59$)	Low ratio ($N = 22$)	
PLR[c]	No association	No association	No association	No association
ALR				
Ratio (medium)	−0.4379 ($p < 0.001$)[b]	−0.0752	0.0594	0.1133
Ratio (LPS)	−0.3638 ($p < 0.01$)	0.3294 ($p < 0.02$)	0.117	0.1882
MRC[e]				
Ratio (medium)	−0.3275 ($p < 0.02$)	0.0676	0.0407	0.0783
Ratio (LPS)	−0.1612	0.4935 ($p < 0.0001$)	0.2333 ($p < 0.005$)	−0.1055
Ratio (CL097)	−0.0323	−0.1066	−0.5885 ($p < 0.005$)	−0.264

[a]*Values of Correlation coefficients revealed significant results in at least one of ASD subgroups or non-ASD controls are shown. Stimulants used for cultures of PBMo are shown in the parentheses.*

[b]*Correlation coefficient by Spearman test. Statistically significant values are shown with p-values.*

[c]*Abbreviations used: please see* ***Table 3***

[d]*Definition of high, normal, and low ratio groups are detailed in the method section.*

[e]*Correlations between RC and IL-1ß/IL-10 ratios are almost identical as observed in associations between MRC and ratios. Thus, not shown in the table.*

(31–35). Although immune abnormalities reported in ASD subjects affect almost every arm of the immune system, multiple researchers have reported innate immune abnormalities independently. This may not be surprising, since one of the most studied animal models of autism is the maternal immune activation (MIA) in rodents; in this model, sterile inflammation triggered by stimuli of innate immunity during pregnancy results in aberrant behaviors and impaired cognitive activity in offspring (36–39).

The findings in MIA models indicate that during critical period of pregnancy (2nd trimester), maternally derived inflammatory mediators affect developing fetal brain, resulting in ASD like behaviors and impaired cognitive activity in offspring (38, 40). Interestingly, several studies have linked the MIA model with mitochondrial dysfunction and abnormalities in redox metabolism (41–43). Therefore, it may be possible that changes in innate immune responses are inter-related with mitochondrial dysfunction and together, they impose detrimental effects on neurodevelopment in ASD children. Our previous study has also shown that changes in cytokine profiles of monocytes, major innate immune cells in the periphery, are associated with changes in behavioral symptoms in some ASD subjects (8).

Activation of innate immunity is known to shape subsequent changes in adaptive immunity via cell-cell interactions, as well as soluble mediators. Antigens (Ags) are typically taken up by innate immune cells, processed, and presented to T cells. Ag-triggered T cell activation is tightly regulated to avoid excessive immune responses. Recent research highlights the importance of metabolic control of the immune system in fine tuning of the immune responses. That is, upon immune activation, effector T cells are required to proliferate rapidly, preferentially producing ATP through glycolysis, while regulatory T (Treg) cells with anti-inflammatory natures require the generation of mitochondrial ATP (9). Therefore, adaptive changes in mitochondrial function in effector immune cells in ASD subjects could result in immune imbalances, postulated to be present in our hypotheses. In this study, we also postulated that metabolic changes reflected in changes in mitochondrial function of immune cells are associated

TABLE 8 | Associations between parameters of mitochondrial respiration (PLR, ALR, and MRC) and cytokine levels produced by PBMo.

Cytokine showed correlation with PLR, ALR, and MRC[a]	IL-1ß/IL-10 ratio[d] based ASD subgroups			Non-ASD control cells ($N = 38$)
	High ratio ($N = 56$)	Normal ratio ($N = 59$)	Low ratio ($N = 22$)	
PLR[c]				
IL-1ß (medium)[a]	−0.2875 ($p < 0.05$)[b]	0.1494	−0.0744	0.1741
IL-1ß (LPS)	−0.37 ($p < 0.01$)	−0.0795	−0.2572	0.1242
CCL2 (LPS)	0.324 ($p < 0.02$)	−0.2164	0.2668	0.1087
ALR				
IL-1ß (medium)	−0.422 ($p < 0.001$)	0.3825 ($p < 0.005$)	−0.0311	0.0988
IL-1ß (LPS)	−0.2535	0.4154 ($p < 0.005$)	0.1006	0.0551
IL-1ß (zymosan)	−0.155	0.1213	0.5139 ($p < 0.02$)	0.1864
IL-10 (LPS)	0.1696	0.3293 ($p < 0.02$)	0.0435	0.188
IL-6 (medium)	−0.3306 ($p < 0.02$)	0.4148 ($p < 0.005$)	0.0548	0.0755
IL-6 (LPS)	0.0111	0.3735 ($p < 0.005$)	0.1295	0.1902
IL-6 (zymosan)	0.0308	0.1863	0.5139 ($p < 0.02$)	0.207
TNF-α (medium)	−0.1248	0.0394	−0.6064 ($p < 0.005$)	−0.0422
TNF-α (LPS	−0.0696	0.0228	−0.5601 ($p < 0.01$)	−0.1003
TNF-α (zymosan)	−0.1351	−0.2718 ($p < 0.05$)	−0.2154	−0.3078
TNF-α (CL097)	0.1403	0.1842	−0.4354 ($p < 0.05$)	0.2563
TGF-ß (CL097)	0.0274	−0.077	0.5093 ($p < 0.02$)	−0.2786
MRC[e]				
IL-1ß (medium)	−0.2258	0.2971 ($p < 0.05$)	0.0184	−0.0078
IL-1ß (LPS)	−0.0302	0.524 ($p < 0.0001$)	0.1423	0.0119
IL-1ß (zymosan)	−0.1154	0.1638	0.5479 ($p < 0.01$)	0.1842
IL-10 (LPS)	0.2896 ($p < 0.05$)	0.4935 ($p < 0.0001$)	0.2101	0.0219
IL-6 (medium)	−0.0622	0.4286 ($p < 0.001$)	0.1209	−0.1224
IL-6 (LPS)	0.1178	0.4402 ($p < 0.005$)	0.3073	0.1286
TNF-α (medium)	−0.1054	0.0532	−0.5576 ($p < 0.01$)	−0.1702
TNF-α (LPS)	0.0072	0.1358	−0.4588 ($p < 0.05$)	−0.1959
TNF-α (zymosan)	−0.1528	−0.3308 ($p < 0.02$)	−0.1706	−0.3861 ($p < 0.05$)
TNF-α (CL097)	−0.1009	0.1082	−0.5800 ($p < 0.005$)	−0.3425
CCL2 (medium)	−0.1445	0.1689	0.0164	−0.4162 ($p < 0.01$)

[a]*Values of Correlation coefficients revealed significant results in at least one of ASD subgroups or non-ASD controls are shown. Stimulants used for cultures of PBMo are shown in the parentheses.*
[b]*Correlation coefficient by Spearman test; Statistically significant values are shown with p-values.*
[c]*Abbreviations used: please see **Table 3***
[d]*Definition of high, normal, and low ratio groups are detailed in the method section.*
[e]*Correlations between RC and monocyte cytokine levels are almost identical as observed in MRC and monocyte cytokine levels. Thus, not shown in the table.*

with changes in cytokine profiles by innate immune cells, such as monocytes.

In previous studies, we found that changes in IL-1ß/IL-10 ratios produced by PBMo from ASD subjects are closely associated with changes in miRNA expression in ASD PBMo (4). Namely, significant up-regulation of multiple miRNAs were observed in the high IL-1ß/IL-10 ratio ASD subgroup, while normal and low ratio ASD subgroups revealed down-regulation of multiple miRNAs, as compared to non-ASD control PBMo (4). Such changes were less evident when miRNA expression by ASD PBMo as a whole was compared to non-ASD controls. We also analyzed targeted genes by these miRNAs that revealed differences in expression in the IL-1ß/IL-10 based ASD subgroup. The results revealed that such changes in miRNA expression would modulate immune cell functions and mitochondrial fitness through several pathways, including mTOR-PI-3K pathways in the high or low ratio ASD subgroups (4). Interestingly, gene mutations in these pathways have also revealed an association between immune and mitochondrial dysfunction. Specifically, in a PTEN hamartoma tumor syndrome, deficiency of PTEN causes alteration in the mTOR-PI3K pathway, resulting in dysregulated T cell activation and impaired mitochondrial fitness (44). Moreover, patients with PTEN mutation exhibit a broad spectrum of neuropsychiatric syndromes, including ASD (45). Indeed, a new ASD mouse model was created by inducing germline mislocalization of PTEN (46). Taken together, it may be postulated that abnormalities found in ASD PBMo are closely associated with mitochondrial dysfunction reported in some ASD subjects.

TABLE 9 | Assessment of correlations between PBMo cytokine production and markers of ETC efficiency (ALR/PLR, MRC/PLR, and RC/PLR).

Cytokine showed correlation with ALR/PLR, MRC/PLR, and RC/PLR[a]	IL-1ß/IL-10 ratio[d] based ASD subgroups			Non-ASD controls ($N = 38$)
	High ratio ($N = 56$)	Normal ratio ($N = 59$)	Low ratio ($N = 22$)	
ALR/PLR[c]				
Ratio (LPS)	-0.1907[b]	−0.359 ($p < 0.01$)	0.4033	−0.0631
Ratio (zymosan)	−0.3285 ($p < 0.02$)	−0.0309	0.0932	0.2167
IL-1ß (LPS)	−0.0384	0.3122 ($p < 0.02$)	0.3303	−0.1191
IL-1ß (zymosan)	0.0289	0.0965	0.4783 ($p < 0.05$)	0.0379
IL-10 (LPS)	0.3468 ($p < 0.01$)	0.0506	0.2298	0.1267
MRC/PLR				
Ratio (LPS)	−0.1415	0.473 ($p < 0.0005$)	0.2569	−0.1251
Ratio (CL097)	−0.0679	−0.0954	−0.5089 ($p < 0.02$)	−0.0501
IL-1ß (LPS)	0.0019	0.392 ($p < 0.005$)	0.2976	−0.1587
IL-1ß (zymosan)	0.0267	0.1176	0.5088 ($p < 0.02$)	0.0333
IL-10 (LPS)	0.356 ($p < 0.01$)	−0.024	0.2863	0.0123
RC/PLR				
Ratio (LPS)	−0.1201	0.5029 ($p < 0.0005$)	0.1836	−0.1067
Ratio (CL097)	−0.0677	0.1154	−0.5345 ($p < 0.01$)	−0.0992
IL-1ß (LPS)	0.025	0.4204 ($p < 0.005$)	0.2677	−0.1417
IL-1ß (zymosan)	0.0355	0.1225	0.4607 ($p < 0.05$)	−0.0355
IL-10 (LPS)	0.3504 ($p < 0.01$)	0.0377	0.3321	−0.0278

[a] *The relationship between levels of cytokine produced by PBMo and ALR/PLR, MRC/PLR, or RC/PLR. Results are shown in cytokines that showed positive or negative associations with ETC efficiency parameters in at least one of ASD subgroups or non-ASD controls. Stimulants used for PBMo cultures are shown in the parentheses. The details of PBMo culture conditions are shown in the method section.*

[b] *Correlation coefficient by Spearman Test. When the results are significant, the values are shown with p-values.*

[c] *Abbreviations used: please see **Table 3**.*

[d] *Definition of high, normal, and low ratio groups are detailed in the method section.*

As briefly discussed in the introduction section, miRNAs are known to serve as mediators of innate immune cells, affecting functions of other immune and even non-immune cells not located in close proximity (10). This is because miRNAs secreted by secretary cells like monocytes are stable as a form of exosomal miRNA and circulate in the body fluid. They affect functions of other lineage cells when taken up. In our other study, we have already identified serum levels of miRNAs that are significantly altered across the IL-1ß/IL-10 based ASD subgroups (preliminary results and manuscript submitted for publication). Therefore, we postulated, if miRNAs serve as mediators of innate immune responses to other lineage cells, we will be able to detect associations between monocyte cytokine production profile and mitochondrial functions of PBMCs, a mixture of immune cells including lymphocytes, monocytes, dendritic cells, and natural killer cells.

First, we determined whether there is any evidence of adaptive changes in mitochondrial function in ASD PBMCs. Consistent with the previous report in transformed B lymphoblastoid cell lines derived from ASD subjects (14), we observed higher levels of MRC and RC in ASD PBMCs (**Figure 1**). We also observed altered association between PLR and ALR in ASD PBMCs. The expected positive association between PLR and ALR was lost in ASD PBMCs, due to the presence of ASD cells with high ALR despite low PLR, and those with low ALR despite high PLR. High ALR with low PLR is considered to reflect efficient ATP production, most likely reflecting adapted changes in mitochondrial function in response to chronic oxidative stresses, but this may lead to increase in production of ROS. While low ALR with increase in PLR indicates mitochondrial failure, being unable to compensate on-going oxidative stresses. These results indicate that a fair number of ASD PBMCs reveals changes in mitochondrial function that may reflect dysregulation of normal control mechanism, perhaps as consequences of adaptive changes and/or failure of mitochondrial function. Since ASD subjects recruited to this study were those without any known gene mutations, these changes are more likely to reflect physiological and/or pathological alterations in the regulatory pathways.

We then determined whether observed changes in mitochondrial functions in ASD PBMCs parallel changes in cytokine profiles produced by PBMo. In select ASD subjects, we simultaneously assessed mitochondrial function in PBMCs and monocyte cytokine production by PBMo at 2–3 time points. Similar to our previous time-course study (4, 8), we found variable levels of PLR, ALR, MRC, and RC in some ASD subjects, while these levels remained stable in others (**Figure 3**). Our results may indicate a possibility of a positive association between mitochondrial respiration and IL-1ß/IL-10 ratios in some ASD subjects, although further studies are necessary with the use of samples taken at multiple time points in a larger number of study subjects.

We then analyzed associations between ASD samples and monocyte cytokine profiles between ASD samples as a whole and non-ASD controls. Our results revealed some associations between these two groups of parameters, but these associations were not strong, partly reflecting variable values of mitochondrial parameters as revealed in **Figures 1, 2**. Since we did not find close associations between mitochondrial parameters and monocyte cytokine profiles in non-ASD controls either, these two variables may not be associated, not supporting our initial hypothesis. On the other hand, as detailed in the 2nd paragraph of the Discussion section, apparent unique mitochondrial dysfunction observed in ASD subjects may be associated with chronic oxidative stress mediated by immune mediated inflammation in some ASD subjects. To further address such a possibility, we turned assessing changes in mitochondrial parameters in the IL-1ß/IL-10 based ASD subgroups, since our previous results indicated that IL-1ß/IL-10 ratios are closely associated with behavioral changes and miRNA expression in ASD PBMo in our previous studies (4, 8).

Our results have shown that ASD PBMCs revealed higher MRC and RC, only when ASD PBMo revealed high or normal IL-1ß/IL-10 ratios (**Table 5**). We also determined whether ALR/PLR, MRC/PLR, and RC/PLR ratios, as markers of ETC efficiency, are altered in the IL-1ß/IL-10 ratio based ASD subgroups. Our results revealed differences in RC/PLR between specific ASD subgroups and non-ASD controls: these ratios were higher only in the high and normal IL-1ß/IL-10 ratio ASD subgroups than controls (**Table 6**). High RC/PLR may indicate efficient mitochondrial function or low generation of mitochondrial oxidative stress. However, given lack of expected positive associations between ALR and PLR in ASD subjects, increase in RC/PLR is more likely secondary to an adaptive increase in mitochondrial activity. Taken together, changes in RC/PLR ratios in the IL-1ß/IL-10 ratio based ASD subgroups indicated a possibility, that changes in monocytes cytokine profiles may affect mitochondrial function of PBMCs in ASD. Alternatively, this finding may indicate changes in regulatory mechanisms of immune metabolism affecting both PBMCs and PBMo in ASD. When we assessed associations between mitochondrial parameters and IL-1ß/IL-10 ratios under different culture conditions, we also observed differences of associations between these two groups of parameters across the IL-1ß/IL-10 based ASD subgroups (**Table 7**).

Cytokines produced by monocytes exert multiple functions and their actions are closely inter-related and they are often categorized as "proinflammatory" vs. "counter-regulatory" cytokines. Although we have used IL-1ß/IL-10 ratios as a surrogate marker for balanced immune responses, mitochondrial functions can also be affected by other monocyte cytokines. We, therefore, further determined if mitochondrial respiration in PBMCs were associated with representative proinflammatory (IL-1ß, IL-6, and TNF-α) and counter-regulatory (IL-10, TGF-ß, and TNFRII) cytokine levels produced by PBMo.

When associations between parameters of mitochondrial respiration (PLR, ALR, MRC, and RC) and cytokine levels produced by PBMo were examined, we also observed marked differences across the IL-1ß/IL-10 based ASD subgroups (**Table 8**). Namely, only the high ratio ASD subgroup revealed positive associations between PLR and IL-1ß. The above described results may indicate a compensatory increase in protein leak to reduce ROS with increase in production of IL-1ß, an inflammatory cytokine, in the high ratio ASD subgroup.

On the other hand, the normal ratio ASD subgroup revealed positive associations between ALR and MRC with IL-1ß, IL-6, and IL-10 levels. This finding may indicate that adapted mitochondrial responses are on-going in response to changes in innate immune responses. In the low ratio ASD subgroup, levels of TNF-α under multiple culture conditions revealed negative associations with ALR and MRC. TNF-α is a major inducer of apoptosis and autophagy, affecting mitochondrial functions (47). Inappropriate mitochondrial responses to TNF-α is associated with dysregulated apoptosis or clearance of cell organelles, leading to pathological conditions such as tumorigenesis (47). PBMCs in the low ratio ASD subgroup may be in the state of mitochondrial dysfunction, not adapting to changes in monocyte cytokine production. Such associations are not revealed in control non-ASD subjects. Since we found a high frequency of history of NFA in ASD subjects whose monocyte revealed low IL-1ß/IL-10 ratios than the normal ratio ASD subgroup (**Table 4**), a major source of chronic oxidative stress may be gut inflammation in these ASD subjects.

We then assessed associations between ETC efficiency parameters (ALR/PLR, MRC/PLR, and RC/PLR ratios) and cytokine levels produced by PBMo. Our results revealed that associations between parameters of ETC efficiency and monocyte cytokine levels produced by PBMo again markedly differed across the IL-1ß/IL-10 ratio based ASD subgroups (**Table 9**). Namely, the IL-1ß/IL-10 high ratio group revealed a positive association between ETC efficiency parameters and IL-10 levels produced by PBMo under LPS stimulated cultures. Given the fact that IL-10 is a counter-regulatory cytokine, it may be speculated that in the high ratio ASD subgroup, suppressive mechanisms may be in place. In contrast, the normal and low ratio ASD subgroups revealed positive associations between ETC efficiency markers and IL-1ß levels. IL-1ß is an inflammatory cytokine and implicated in the stress responses to the brain. Thus, in these two ASD subgroups, up-regulatory drive for ETC efficiency may be in place.

Taken together, the above described results indicate that associations between monocyte cytokine profiles and mitochondrial parameters in PBMCs differed significantly across the IL-1ß/IL-10 based ASD subgroups, and these changes also differed from non-ASD controls. Our findings support our initial hypothesis that innate immune abnormalities and mitochondrial abnormalities, two abnormalities frequently reported in ASD subjects, are closely inter-related and may exert detrimental effects on the brain. However, our results did not clarify whether innate immune responses cause secondary mitochondrial dysfunction or dysregulations of common pathways key to functions of innate immunity and mitochondrial respiration. It remains to be seen how these changes are associated with ASD clinical features and health outcomes in future studies.

Although many questions need to be answered in further studies, our results indicate that concurrent use of immune-modulating agents and mitochondrial rescue medications may be required in ASD subjects who exhibit innate immune abnormalities and mitochondrial dysfunction, possibly due to alterations in the signaling pathways affecting the both systems. In each such ASD individual, fine adjustment in doses and administration schedule will be required.

AUTHOR CONTRIBUTIONS

HJ was responsible for the study design, recruitment of the study subjects, collection of clinical information, and blood samples, analysis of the overall data, and preparation of most of this manuscript. LG conducted cytokine production assays with the use of purified monocytes and also prepared samples for mitochondrial function for shipping to RF's laboratory. She also adopted biofreezing methodology of PBMCs. SR and SB conducted assays for mitochondrial respiration with the use of PBMCs and helped prepare a manuscript. RF supervised SR and SB and discussed with HJ extensively, regarding data analysis, and helped extensively for manuscript preparation.

ACKNOWLEDGMENTS

This study was supported by funding from Autism Research Institute, San Diego, CA, Jonty Foundation, St. Paul, MN, United States, and the Governor's Council for Medical Research and Treatment of Autism, DHHS, Trenton, NJ, United States. We are thankful for grant office staff for helping conducting this study as well as Marc and Lisa Huguenin for helping us submitting clinical data to NDAR.

REFERENCES

1. Buie T, Campbell DB, Fuchs GJ III, Furuta GT, Levy J, Vandewater J, et al. Evaluation, diagnosis, and treatment of gastrointestinal disorders in individuals with ASDs: a consensus report. *Pediatrics* (2010) 125 (Suppl. 1):S1–18. doi: 10.1542/peds.2009-1878C
2. Cohen S, Conduit R, Lockley SW, Rajaratnam SM, Cornish KM. The relationship between sleep and behavior in autism spectrum disorder (ASD): a review. *J Neurodev Disord.* (2014) 6:44. doi: 10.1186/1866-1955-6-44
3. Jyonouchi H, Geng L, Davidow AL. Cytokine profiles by peripheral blood monocytes are associated with changes in behavioral symptoms following immune insults in a subset of ASD subjects: an inflammatory subtype? *J Neuroinflammation* (2014) 11:187. doi: 10.1186/s12974-014-0187-2
4. Jyonouchi H, Geng L, Streck DL, Dermody JJ, Toruner GA. MicroRNA expression changes in association with changes in interleukin-1ss/interleukin10 ratios produced by monocytes in autism spectrum disorders: their association with neuropsychiatric symptoms and comorbid conditions (observational study). *J Neuroinflammation* (2017) 14:229. doi: 10.1186/s12974-017-1003-6
5. Rossignol DA, Frye RE. Mitochondrial dysfunction in autism spectrum disorders: a systematic review and meta-analysis. *Mol Psychiatry* (2012) 17:290–314. doi: 10.1038/mp.2010.136
6. Frye RE, James SJ. Metabolic pathology of autism in relation to redox metabolism. *Biomark Med.* (2014) 8:321–30. doi: 10.2217/bmm.13.158
7. Alural B, Genc S, Haggarty SJ. Diagnostic and therapeutic potential of microRNAs in neuropsychiatric disorders: past, present, and future. *Prog Neuropsychopharmacol Biol Psychiatry* (2017) 73:87–103. doi: 10.1016/j.pnpbp.2016.03.010
8. Jyonouchi H, Geng L, Buyske S. Interleukin-1β/Interleukin10 ratio produced by monocytes as a biomarker of neuroinflammation in autism. *J Clin Cell Immunol.* (2017) 8:1000503. doi: 10.4172/2155-9899.1000503
9. Perl A. Review: metabolic control of immune system activation in rheumatic diseases. *Arthritis Rheumatol.* (2017) 69:2259–70. doi: 10.1002/art.40223
10. Roy S. miRNA in macrophage development and function. *Antioxid Redox Signal.* (2016) 25:795–804. doi: 10.1089/ars.2016.6728
11. Frye RE, Nankova B, Bhattacharyya S, Rose S, Bennuri SC, MacFabe DF. Modulation of immunological pathways in autistic and neurotypical lymphoblastoid cell lines by the enteric microbiome metabolite propionic acid. *Front Immunol.* (2017) 8:1670. doi: 10.3389/fimmu.2017.01670
12. Rose S, Bennuri SC, Murray KF, Buie T, Winter H, Frye RE. Mitochondrial dysfunction in the gastrointestinal mucosa of children with autism: a blinded case-control study. *PLoS ONE* (2017) 12:e0186377. doi: 10.1371/journal.pone.0186377
13. Rose S, Bennuri SC, Wynne R, Melnyk S, James SJ, Frye RE. Mitochondrial and redox abnormalities in autism lymphoblastoid cells: a sibling control study. *FASEB J.* (2017) 31:904–9. doi: 10.1096/fj.201601004R
14. Rose S, Frye RE, Slattery J, Wynne R, Tippett M, Pavliv O, et al. Oxidative stress induces mitochondrial dysfunction in a subset of autism lymphoblastoid cell lines in a well-matched case control cohort. *PLoS ONE* (2014) 9:e85436. doi: 10.1371/journal.pone.0085436
15. Marin SE, Saneto RP. Neuropsychiatric features in primary mitochondrial disease. *Neurol Clin.* (2016) 34:247–94. doi: 10.1016/j.ncl.2015.08.011
16. Rose S, Niyazov DM, Rossignol DA, Goldenthal M, Kahler SG, Frye RE. Clinical and molecular characteristics of mitochondrial dysfunction in autism spectrum disorder. *Mol Diagn Ther.* (2018) 22:571–93. doi: 10.1007/s40291-018-0352-x
17. Howsmon DP, Vargason T, Rubin RA, Delhey L, Tippett M, Rose S, et al. Multivariate techniques enable a biochemical classification of children with autism spectrum disorder versus typically-developing peers: a comparison and validation study. *Bioeng Transl Med.* (2018) 3:156–65. doi: 10.1002/btm2.10095
18. Aman MG, Singh NN, Stewart AW, Field CJ. The aberrant behavior checklist: a behavior rating scale for the assessment of treatment effects. *Am J Ment Defic.* (1985) 89:485–91.
19. Owens JA, Spirito A, McGuinn M. The Children's Sleep Habits Questionnaire (CSHQ): psychometric properties of a survey instrument for school-aged children. *Sleep* (2000) 23:1043–51. doi: 10.1093/sleep/23.8.1d
20. Sparrow SB, Balla DA, Cicchetti DV. *Adaptive Behavior Scales Survey Form Manual.* Cirde Pines, MN: American Guidance Service (1985).
21. Boyce JA, Assa'ad A, Burks AW, Jones SM, Sampson HA, Wood RA, et al. Guidelines for the diagnosis and management of food allergy in the United States: report of the NIAID-sponsored expert panel. *J Allergy Clin Immunol.* (2010) 126 (Suppl. 6):S1–58. doi: 10.1016/j.jaci.2010.10.008
22. Butrus S, Portela R. Ocular allergy: diagnosis and treatment. *Ophthalmol Clin North Am.* (2005) 18:485–92. doi: 10.1016/j.ohc.2005.07.007
23. Nassef M, Shapiro G, Casale TB. Identifying and managing rhinitis and its subtypes: allergic and nonallergic components–a consensus report and materials from the Respiratory and Allergic Disease Foundation. *Curr Med Res Opin.* (2006) 22:2541–8. doi: 10.1185/030079906X158057
24. National Asthma Education and Prevention Program. Expert Panel Report 3 (EPR-3): guidelines for the diagnosis and management of asthma-summary report 2007. *J Allergy Clin Immunol.* (2007) 120 (Suppl. 5): S94–138. doi: 10.1016/j.jaci.2007.09.043
25. Orange JS, Ballow M, Stiehm ER, Ballas ZK, Chinen J, De La Morena M, et al. Use and interpretation of diagnostic vaccination in primary immunodeficiency: a working group report of the basic and clinical immunology interest section of the american academy of allergy, asthma & immunology. *J Allergy Clin Immunol.* (2012) 130(Suppl. 3): S1–24. doi: 10.1016/j.jaci.2012.07.002

26. Jyonouchi H, Geng L, Ruby A, Zimmerman-Bier B. Dysregulated innate immune responses in young children with autism spectrum disorders: their relationship to gastrointestinal symptoms and dietary intervention. *Neuropsychobiology* (2005) 51:77–85. doi: 10.1159/000084164
27. Burger BJ, Rose S, Bennuri SC, Gill PS, , Tippett ML, Delhey L, et al. Autistic siblings with novel mutations in two different genes: insight for genetic workups of autistic siblings and connection to mitochondrial dysfunction. *Front Pediatr.* (2017) 5:219. doi: 10.3389/fped.2017.00219
28. Rossignol DA, Frye RE. A review of research trends in physiological abnormalities in autism spectrum disorders: immune dysregulation, inflammation, oxidative stress, mitochondrial dysfunction and environmental toxicant exposures. *Mol Psychiatry* (2012) 17:389–401. doi: 10.1038/mp.2011.165
29. Giulivi C, Zhang YF, Omanska-Klusek A, Ross-Inta C, Wong S, Hertz-Picciotto I, et al. Mitochondrial dysfunction in autism. *JAMA* (2010) 304:2389–96. doi: 10.1001/jama.2010.1706
30. Napoli E, Wong S, Hertz-Picciotto I, Giulivi C. Deficits in bioenergetics and impaired immune response in granulocytes from children with autism. *Pediatrics* (2014) 133:e1405–10. doi: 10.1542/peds.2013-1545
31. Careaga M, Rogers S, Hansen RL, Amaral DG, Van de Water J, Ashwood P. Immune endophenotypes in children with autism spectrum disorder. *Biol Psychiatry* (2017) 81:434–41. doi: 10.1016/j.biopsych.2015.08.036
32. Edmiston E, Ashwood P, Van de. Water J. Autoimmunity, autoantibodies, and autism spectrum disorder. *Biol Psychiatry* (2017) 81:383–90. doi: 10.1016/j.biopsych.2016.08.031
33. Gladysz D, Krzywdzinska A, Hozyasz KK. Immune abnormalities in autism spectrum disorder-could they hold promise for causative treatment? *Mol Neurobiol.* (2018) 55:6387–435. doi: 10.1007/s12035-017-0822-x
34. Jyonouchi H. Immunological abnormalities in autism spectrum disorders. *Adv Neuroimmune Biol.* (2013) 4:141–59. doi: 10.3233/NIB-130061
35. Masi A, Glozier N, Dale R, Guastella AJ. The immune system, cytokines, and biomarkers in autism spectrum disorder. *Neurosci Bull.* (2017) 33:194–204. doi: 10.1007/s12264-017-0103-8
36. Careaga M, Murai T, Bauman MD. Maternal immune activation and autism spectrum disorder: from rodents to nonhuman and human primates. *Biol Psychiatry* (2017) 81:391–401. doi: 10.1016/j.biopsych.2016.10.020
37. Estes ML, McAllister AK. Maternal immune activation: Implications for neuropsychiatric disorders. *Science* (2016) 353:772–7. doi: 10.1126/science.aag3194
38. Pendyala G, Chou S, Jung Y, Coiro P, Spartz E, Padmashri R, et al. Maternal immune activation causes behavioral impairments and altered cerebellar cytokine and synaptic protein expression. *Neuropsychopharmacology* (2017) 42:1435–46. doi: 10.1038/npp.2017.7
39. Rose DR, Careaga M, Van de Water J, McAllister K, Bauman MD, Ashwood P. Long-term altered immune responses following fetal priming in a non-human primate model of maternal immune activation. *Brain Behav Immun.* (2017) 63:60–70. doi: 10.1016/j.bbi.2016.11.020
40. Straley ME, Van Oeffelen W, Theze S, Sullivan AM, O'Mahony SM, Cryan JF, et al. Distinct alterations in motor & reward seeking behavior are dependent on the gestational age of exposure to LPS-induced maternal immune activation. *Brain Behav Immun.* (2017) 63:21–34. doi: 10.1016/j.bbi.2016.06.002
41. Giulivi C, Napoli E, Schwartzer J, Careaga M, Ashwood P. Gestational exposure to a viral mimetic poly(I:C) results in long-lasting changes in mitochondrial function by leucocytes in the adult offspring. *Mediators Inflamm.* (2013) 2013:609602. doi: 10.1155/2013/609602
42. Naviaux JC, Wang L, Li K, Bright AT, Alaynick W, Williams KR, et al. Antipurinergic therapy corrects the autism-like features in the Fragile X (Fmr1 knockout) mouse model. *Mol Autism* (2015) 6:1. doi: 10.1186/2040-2392-6-1
43. Naviaux RK, Zolkipli Z, Wang L, Nakayama T, Naviaux JC, Le TP, et al. Antipurinergic therapy corrects the autism-like features in the poly(IC) mouse model. *PLoS ONE* (2013) 8:e57380. doi: 10.1371/journal.pone.0057380
44. Chen HH, Handel N, Ngeow J, Muller J, Huhn M, Yang H, et al. Immune dysregulation in patients with PTEN hamartoma tumor syndrome: analysis of FOXP3 regulatory T cells. *J Allergy Clin Immunol.* (2017) 139:607–20 e615. doi: 10.1016/j.jaci.2016.03.059
45. Balci TB, Davila J, Lewis D, Boafo A, Sell E, Richer J, et al. Broad spectrum of neuropsychiatric phenotypes associated with white matter disease in PTEN hamartoma tumor syndrome. *Am J Med Genet B Neuropsychiatr Genet.* (2018) 177:101–9. doi: 10.1002/ajmg.b.32610
46. Tilot AK, Bebek G, Niazi F, Altemus JB, Romigh T, Frazier TW, et al. Neural transcriptome of constitutional Pten dysfunction in mice and its relevance to human idiopathic autism spectrum disorder. *Mol Psychiatry* (2016) 21:118–25. doi: 10.1038/mp.2015.17
47. Tummers B, Green DR. Caspase-8: regulating life and death. *Immunol Rev.* (2017) 277:76–89. doi: 10.1111/imr.12541

3

The Therapeutic Potential of Mangosteen Pericarp as an Adjunctive Therapy for Bipolar Disorder and Schizophrenia

Melanie M. Ashton [1,2,3], Olivia M. Dean [1,2,4], Adam J. Walker [1], Chiara C. Bortolasci [5], Chee H. Ng [3], Malcolm Hopwood [6], Brian H. Harvey [7], Marisa Möller [7], John J. McGrath [8,9,10], Wolfgang Marx [1], Alyna Turner [1,4], Seetal Dodd [1,4,11], James G. Scott [8,12,13], Jon-Paul Khoo [1,12], Ken Walder [5], Jerome Sarris [3,14] and Michael Berk [1,2,4,11,15]*

[1] IMPACT Strategic Research Centre, School of Medicine, Barwon Health, Deakin University, Geelong, VIC, Australia, [2] Florey Institute for Neuroscience and Mental Health, University of Melbourne, Parkville, VIC, Australia, [3] Professorial Unit, The Melbourne Clinic, Department of Psychiatry, University of Melbourne, Richmond, VIC, Australia, [4] Department of Psychiatry, Royal Melbourne Hospital, University of Melbourne, Parkville, VIC, Australia, [5] Centre for Molecular and Medical Research, School of Medicine, Deakin University, Geelong, VIC, Australia, [6] Professorial Psychiatry Unit, Albert Road Clinic, University of Melbourne, Melbourne, VIC, Australia, [7] Centre of Excellence for Pharmaceutical Sciences, School of Pharmacy (Pharmacology), North West University, Potchefstroom, South Africa, [8] Queensland Centre for Mental Health Research, The Park Centre for Mental Health, Wacol, QLD, Australia, [9] Queensland Brain Institute, University of Queensland, St. Lucia, QLD, Australia, [10] National Centre for Register-Based Research, Aarhus University, Aarhus, Denmark, [11] Centre of Youth Mental Health, University of Melbourne, Parkville, VIC, Australia, [12] Faculty of Medicine, The University of Queensland, Herston, QLD, Australia, [13] Metro North Mental Health, Royal Brisbane and Women's Hospital, Brisbane, QLD, Australia, [14] NICM Health Research Institute, Western Sydney University, Westmead, NSW, Australia, [15] Orygen Youth Health Research Centre, Parkville, VIC, Australia

***Correspondence:**
Melanie M. Ashton
m.ashton@deakin.edu.au*

New treatments are urgently needed for serious mental illnesses including bipolar disorder and schizophrenia. This review proposes that *Garcinia mangostana Linn.* (mangosteen) pericarp is a possible adjunctive therapeutic agent for these disorders. Research to date demonstrates that neurobiological properties of the mangosteen pericarp are well aligned with the current understanding of the pathophysiology of bipolar disorder and schizophrenia. Mangosteen pericarp has antioxidant, putative neuroprotective, anti-inflammatory, and putative mitochondrial enhancing properties, with animal studies demonstrating favorable pharmacotherapeutic benefits with respect to these disorders. This review summarizes evidence of its properties and supports the case for future studies to assess the utility of mangosteen pericarp as an adjunctive treatment option for mood and psychotic disorders.

Keywords: mangosteen pericarp, bipolar disorder, schizophrenia, psychiatry, oxidative stress, inflammation, mitochondria

INTRODUCTION

Serious mental illness, generally defined as disorders with psychotic or high severity symptoms (such as bipolar disorder and schizophrenia), contribute significantly toward disease burden worldwide (1). Importantly, those living with serious mental illnesses often experience suboptimal responses to conventional treatments (2, 3), and treatment options are limited (2, 4). The developmental pipeline for conventional psychiatric medications, historically driven by large pharmaceutical companies, is dwindling (5, 6); as such, the investigation of novel therapeutics is both warranted, and needed. One promising avenue of research is in the potential use of nutraceutical agents, as adjunctive therapies, that target biological pathways known to be dysregulated in neuropsychiatric disorders (7).

This narrative review explores the neurobiological properties and therapeutic potential of an extract derived from the pericarp of *Garcinia mangostana Linn.* (mangosteen) for serious mental illness. Due to its bioactive components and the parallels with the current understanding of the pathophysiology of both schizophrenia and bipolar disorder, the mangosteen pericarp may be or may contain a useful adjunctive therapeutic agent for these disorders. The salient neurobiological targets that overlap in serious mental illness include; oxidative stress, neuroinflammation, neurogenesis and apoptosis, and mitochondrial dysfunction. The potential therapeutic value of mangosteen pericarp will be explored within the context of these factors.

BIPOLAR DISORDER AND SCHIZOPHRENIA: SHARED PHYSIOLOGY

Major neuropsychiatric disorders appear to share much of their basic neurobiology, suggesting that nutraceutical and other agents may have broad utility. Schizophrenia and bipolar disorder exhibit shared genetic and neurocognitive factors and clinical symptoms (8, 9). Similarly, schizophrenia and bipolar disorder have overlapping biological aberrations demonstrated by the use of some drugs to treat both conditions (e.g., atypical antipsychotics) (10).

Monoamine Disturbances

Monoamines play a critical role in the pathophysiology of bipolar disorder and schizophrenia (11, 12). Glutamatergic dysregulation has also been implicated in the pathophysiology of bipolar disorder (13–15) and schizophrenia (16). Excess mesolimbic dopaminergic activity is implicated in the pathophysiology of psychosis (17). Serotonergic dysregulation has also been implicated in bipolar disorder and schizophrenia including alterations in 5-HT_{2A}, 5-HT_{1A}, and 5-HT_{1B} receptors in the prefrontal cortex and hippocampus (18). Some common psychotropic medications target these pathways but are not effective for everyone. Therefore, new therapies should aim to address critical biological targets which are not addressed by this common monoamine theory (19), but instead mediate changes through the biological processes outlined from here in.

Oxidative Stress

Altered oxidative biology in serious mental illness is indicated by a reduction in antioxidant levels, including glutathione and glutathione transferase (20, 21) and increased reactive oxygen species (ROS) and reactive nitrogen species (RNS) (20). There may also be a rise in oxidative stress markers such as malondialdehyde (MDA) and thiobarbituric acidic reactive substances (TBARS). Redox markers (20), including nitric oxide, superoxide dismutase, catalase, and glutathione peroxidase are altered in serious mental illness (20, 22, 23). It has been suggested that the variability in redox markers may to some extent be due to differences between early and late stages of the disorder (19).

The high levels of oxidative stress may, in part, originate in mitochondria and are associated with mitochondrial dysfunction (19). Aberrations in neurotransmitters such as glutamate are also associated with altered redox state and this ties into changes in monoamines seen in serious mental illness (13). Targeting redox imbalance has been shown to be a useful therapeutic pathway, exemplified by agents such as N-acetyl cysteine that have conferred some benefits in schizophrenia and bipolar disorder (20, 24–27).

Inflammation and Neurogenesis

In both schizophrenia and bipolar disorder, there is evidence of raised inflammatory cytokines both in the central nervous system and peripheral circulation (21, 28–32). The effects of neuroinflammation include lowering mitochondrial energy generation, increased free radicals and lipid peroxidation and increased neuroexcitation which may lead to neurodegeneration and apoptosis through raising intracellular calcium and glutamate levels (21, 33, 34). Inflammation can also lead to higher levels of NO being produced by inducible nitric oxide synthase (iNOS) (35). A recent meta-analysis found that acute illness in schizophrenia was associated with elevated levels of the peripheral proinflammatory cytokines interleukin (IL) 6 and tumor necrosis factor alpha (TNF-α), and elevated levels of cytokine receptor antagonist (IL-1Ra) and soluble cytokine receptor (36). In chronically ill patients, peripheral IL-6, IL-1β, and soluble cytokine receptor levels were persistently elevated (36).

Serious mental illnesses are also associated with higher rates of programmed cell death or apoptosis than healthy controls (37, 38), with irregularities in apoptotic and metabolic markers observed in schizophrenia (39). For example, evidence indicates activated apoptotic programmed cell death pathways in the anterior cingulate cortex and hippocampus of patients with schizophrenia (40). Alterations in neurotrophins, which protect against neuronal apoptosis, have been reported in bipolar disorder. For example, brain derived neurotrophic factor, B-cell lymphoma 2 (bcl-2), and vascular endothelial growth factor (VEGF) are decreased during acute phases of bipolar disorder (both mania and depression) (21).

Mitogen-activated protein kinases (MAPK) regulate cell survival and apoptosis via gene expression, cell proliferation,

Abbreviations: 3-NP, 3-nitropropionic acid; Bcl-2, B-cell lymphoma 2; COX-2, Cyclooxygenase-2; CRP, C-reactive protein; DPPH, 11-diphenyl-2-picrylhydrazyl; ENA, Epithelial Cell-Derived Neutrophil-Activating Protein; ERK, Extracellular Signal-regulated Kinase; GPx, Glutathione peroxidase; GSH, Glutathione peroxidase; H_2O_2, Hydrogen peroxide; IBA-1, Ionized calcium binding adaptor molecule 1; IL, Interleukin; iNOS, Inducible nitric oxide synthase; JNK, c-Jun N-terminal; LPS, Lipopolysaccharide; MAPK, Mitogen-activated protein kinases; MDA, Malondialdehyde; MIA, Maternal immune-activation; MTT, 3-(2,5-dimethylthiazol-1-yl)2,5-; NF-kB, Nuclear factor kappa B; NO, Nitric oxide; NOS, Nitric oxide synthase; NOX, NADPH-oxidase; PGE_2, Prostaglandin E_2; ROS, Reactive oxygen species; SOD, Superoxide dismutase; TBARS, Thiobarbituric acidic reactive substances; TNF-α, Tumor necrosis factor; VEGF, Vascular endothelial growth factor.

cell survival, and death, and thus, are important for neuronal plasticity (37). Other MAPKs, including p38 and c-Jun N-terminal (JNK), are also possible mediators of mitochondrial-induced apoptosis (41). Neuroleptic medications used in bipolar disorder and schizophrenia (e.g., olanzapine and haloperidol) can activate the MAPK pathway (42).

Heightened neuroinflammation, and indeed microglial activation are associated with inhibition of neurogenesis (43, 44). Some evidence suggests that altered neurogenesis, particularly in the hippocampus, occurs in schizophrenia. For example, a significant reduction in Ki67+ cells (a marker for cell proliferation) was observed in post-mortem hippocampal tissue of patients with schizophrenia (45, 46). Altered postnatal neurogenesis in the striatum was also proposed as an explanation for the dopaminergic deficits commonly reported in schizophrenia (43), in addition to gross hypodopaminergia in the frontal cortex, and hyperdopaminergia in the striatum (16).

Adjunctive treatments targeting inflammation (and consequently neuroprotection), for example celecoxib (COX-2 inhibitor) and minocycline (tetracyclic antibiotic), have shown some efficacy in treating schizophrenia and bipolar disorder [see Müller (47); Sommer et al. (48) for discussion]. Other adjuncts with anti-inflammatory effects, including aspirin, *N*-acetylcycteine, and estrogen modulating treatments were also shown to have potential efficacy (48–51).

Mitochondrial Dysfunction

Mitochondria are essential contributors to cellular energy metabolism, synaptic transmission and neuronal growth and are involved in oxidative stress and apoptotic pathways. Overproduction of ROS can cause mitochondrial dysfunction by damaging mitochondrial DNA and mitochondrial respiratory chain (leading to a reduction in energy production). Lipid peroxidation can also occur due to ROS and increase the mitochondrial membrane permeability leading to a disruption in Ca^{2+} homeostasis (52). Elevation in intracellular Ca^{2+} levels can cause neuronal degeneration and cell death and can lead to the production of superoxide ion radicals, forming a vicious cycle (52, 53). Differences in the size, shape, and distribution of mitochondria has been reported in post-mortem prefrontal cortex of participants with bipolar disorder compared to healthy controls (54). There is a shift toward glycolysis within the mitochondria which is associated with an impairment of oxidative phosphorylation with lactate accumulation and decreased energy production (55).

Accumulating evidence suggests that differences in mitochondrial abundance, function, and morphology are associated with the onset and pathophysiology of schizophrenia (56, 57). Post-mortem studies of schizophrenia patients have reported region-specific differences in mitochondrial abundance, localization, size, and function across a number of cell types and brain regions [see Roberts (58) for review]. There is also some evidence to suggest a link between schizophrenia symptoms and mitochondrial pathology in the periphery, for example altered microstructure as well as a decreased density of mitochondria in blood lymphocytes, corresponding to dysregulated energy metabolism (59, 60). Medications targeting mitochondria, such as L-acetyl-carnitine (61) and methylene blue (62, 63), have demonstrated therapeutic utility as antidepressants, antipsychotics, and mood stabilizers.

In bringing together the aforementioned relevant information regarding the known pathophysiology of serious mental illness and the known bioactivity of mangosteen pericarp, this review sets the scene for exploring the potential use of mangosteen pericarp for the treatment of serious mental illness. The wide variety of pathophysiological targets discussed, likely combined, may highlight one of the most important and still unsolved problems in the development of psychotropic medications. New developments targeting these pathways in combination, may help to improve treatment response and fill the gap left by conventional treatments.

GARCINIA MANGOSTANA LINN. (MANGOSTEEN) PERICARP

Garcinia mangostana Linn, more commonly known as mangosteen, is a tropical fruit affectionately referred to as the "Queen of the Fruits" (64, 65). The flesh of the fruit is contained within a husk (pericarp). Mangosteen pericarp has historically been used for its antimicrobial effects in South East Asia to treat skin infections, wounds and dysentery (64). The mangosteen pericarp contains at least 50 different bioactive compounds including polyphenol-subclasses, xanthones and catechins (64). Several of these compounds are reported in this review, including α-mangostin, γ-mangostin, gartanin, 8-deoxygartanin, garciniafuran, garcinone C, and garcinone D (66), 7-O-demethyl mangostanin (67), mangostenone F (68, 69), and mangostenone G (69). Compared to the edible aril part of the fruit, the pericarp contains 10 times more phenolic compounds and 20 times more antioxidant activity (70). It is noteworthy that xanthones are tricyclic compounds and their biological activities might be associated with this chemical structure (64). The most prominent xanthones in the mangosteen pericarp are α-mangostin and γ-mangostin (64). There have been many reports of the potential benefits of xanthones of the mangosteen pericarp, including properties that are antioxidant, anti-inflammatory and anti-apoptotic (64, 71). The properties of mangosteen pericarp have been summarized in **Table 1**.

To further illustrate the biomarkers and mechanistic pathways mangosteen pericarp may have an effect on, **Figure 1** provides a summary of the molecular pathways implicated in oxidative stress, inflammation and mitochondrial function and which may be targeted by mangosteen pericarp.

The Neuroreceptor Profile of Mangosteen Pericarp Extract

Studies have demonstrated that α- and γ-mangostin have anti-histaminergic properties and can selectively block serotonin type 2A ($5\text{-}HT_{2A}$) receptors in rabbit aorta, a pathway that is a feature of some atypical antipsychotics (96, 97). Furthermore,

TABLE 1 | Summary of neurobiological activity of *Garcinia mangostana Linn*. (mangosteen).

Paper	Mangosteen compound	Pathway/marker	Method	Interpretation
Marquez-Valadez et al. (72)	α-mangostin	↓TBARs ↓ mitochondrial dysfunction	Rats received pro-oxidant agents: ferrous sulfate, quinolinic acid and 3-NP ($n = 60$)	Antioxidant properties, reduced mitochondrial dysfunction
Marquez-Valadez et al. (73)	α-mangostin CH2Cl2–MeOH (dichloromethane) solution extraction	↓GSH ↓GPx ~ Glutathione S-transferase	*In vitro* Rats administered ferrous sulfate, or 3-NP, in addition to α-mangostin and compared to control of only α-mangostin	Selective modulation of GSH system, antioxidant properties
Moongkarndi et al. (65)	α-mangostin Comparing ethyl acetate vs. water extract	↓DPPH (↑ROS scavenging; water extract only) ↓ cancer cell production	*In vitro* Breast cancer (SKBR3) cells	Antioxidant properties
Lee et al. (74)	α-mangostin	↓Bcl-2 ↑Bax ↓MAPk and ERK pathways, ↑apoptosis	*In vitro*—tongue carcinoma cells	
Yang et al. (67)	7-O-Demethyl mangostanin	↑apoptosis	*In vitro* Cancer cells	
Shin-Yu et al. (75)	α-mangostin	↓TBARs ↑ GSH, GPx, glutathione reductase, SOD, and catalase	*In vitro*. High fat diet with mangosteen vs. High fat diet without mangosteen and compared to regular diet control.	Antioxidant properties
Oberholzer et al. (76)	Mangosteen pericarp extract	↓ hippocampal lipid peroxidation	*In vivo*: Flinders sensitive line rats, compared with imipramine (tricyclic antidepressant)	Antioxidant properties
Harvey et al. (77); Lotter et al. (78)	Raw mangosteen pericarp (50 mg/kg)	↓IL-6 and TNF-α ↓ cortico-striatal lipid peroxidation	*In vivo* inflammatory rat model of schizophrenia *cf.* haloperidol	Antioxidant and Anti-inflammatory properties
Wang et al. (66)	α-Mangostin, 8-Deoxygartanin, Gartanin, Garciniafuran, Garcinone C, Garcinone D, and γ-Mangostin	↓β-amyloid build up ↓ DPPH ↑ROS scavenging (↓ oxidative stress) ↑neuroprotective properties	*In vitro*	Antioxidant and Neuroprotective properties
Catorce et al. (79)	α-Mangostin	↓IL-6 and COX-2 ~IL-β and TNF-α,	*In vivo* 18 mice with LPS induced neuroinflammation.	Anti-inflammatory properties
Gutierrez-Orozco et al. (80)	α-mangostin	↓IL-8 and TNF-α ↑ TNF-α in monocyte-derived macrophages cells	*In vitro*. LPS-induced inflammation in human cells.	Anti-inflammatory properties
Tewtrakul et al. (81)	Mangosteen pericarp (ethanoic extract) α-mangostin γ-mangostin	↓NO, PGE_2, TNF-α, IL-4 ↓iNOS (α- and γ-mangostin) ↓ COX-2 (α-mangostin only)	*In vitro*. LPS-induced inflammation in murine RAW264.7 macrophage cells.	Anti-inflammatory properties
Chen et al. (82)	α- and γ-mangostin (ethyl acetate extract)	↓NO, PGE_2 ↓ iNOS ~ COX-2	*In vitro*. LPS-induced inflammation in murine RAW264.7 macrophage cells.	Anti-inflammatory properties
Cho et al. (68)	Mangostenone F	↓ NO, TNF-α, IL6 and IL-1β, ↓ iNOS ↓ NF-κB (via p65 and IκB-α) ↓ MAPK (vis AP-1)	*In vitro*. LPS-induced inflammation in murine RAW264.7 macrophage cells.	Anti-inflammatory properties
Bumrungpert et al. (83)	α- and γ-mangostin	↓IL-6, IL1β, interferon-γ and TNF-α ↓ MAPK, NF-κB	*In vitro*	Anti-inflammatory properties
Hu et al. (84)	α-mangostin (1, 10, and 100 nM).	↓ IBA-1 and iNOS production ↓ H_2O_2 (reduced ROS) ↑ Dopamine uptake	*In vitro*—wild-type Sprague-Dawley rat cells treated with α-synuclein induced inflammation.	Anti-inflammatory properties
Weecharangsan et al. (85)	Mangosteen pericarp extracted by: Water vs. 50% ethanol vs. 95% ethanol vs. ethyl acetate	↓ DPPH free radical scavenging. ↓NG108-15 (water and 50% ethanol superior) ↓ H_2O_2 Cell death	*In vitro* NG108-15 cells treated with H_2O_2	Neuroprotective and antioxidant properties

(Continued)

TABLE 1 | Continued

Paper	Mangosteen compound	Pathway/marker	Method	Interpretation
Janhom et al. (86)	α-mangostin	↓ apoptosis and ROS ↓Bax, Bax/Bcl-2, p53, and caspase 3 ↑ Bcl-2	*In vitro* human SH-SY5Y neuroblastoma cells in an MPP^{+} Parkinson's Disease like state	Neuroprotective and anti-apoptotic properties
Phyu and Tangpong (87)	Xanthones from aqueous extract of mangosteen pericarp	↓acetylcholinesterase ↓MDA	$N = 42$ lead-poisoned mice	Antioxidant and neuroprotective properties
Sattayasai et al. (88)	Mangosteen pericarp extract	↓ROS	*In vivo* and *In vitro* memory impaired mice	Antioxidant and neuroprotective properties
Wihastuti et al. (89)	Mangosteen pericarp extracted by ethanol solution	↓ VEGFR-1, NF-κB	*In vivo* 20 male rats-–5 groups: Normal diet High cholesterol diet High cholesterol and mangosteen pericarp 200 mg/kg High cholesterol and mangosteen pericarp 400 mg/kg High cholesterol and mangosteen pericarp 800 mg/kg	Neurogenesis, anti-oxidative and anti-inflammatory properties
Huang et al. (90)	Mangosteen pericarp extract	~ JNK, ERK ↓ROS, COX-2 and IL-6 ↑GSH, brain derived neurotropic factor, and serotonin	*In vivo* and *In vitro*: 3xTg-AD mouse model of Alzheimer's Disease. Hippocampal cells and serum.	Antioxidant and neuroprotective properties
Jariyapongskul et al. (91)	α-mangostin	↓ VEGF, TNF-α, MDA, and fasting glucose	*In vivo*: 56 type 2 diabetic rats, retinal blood.	Neurogenesis, anti-inflammatory, antioxidant, and anti-hyperglycemic properties
Aisha et al. (92)	combination of α- and γ-mangostin (81 and 16%, respectively)	↑caspases-3/7 ↑MAPK, ERK and p52	*In vitro*: human colon cancer cells	Activate mitochondrial pathway of apoptosis
Tang et al. (93)	Commercially available Mangosteen juice (Mangosteen Plus™ with Essential Minerals®), main xanthone: β-mangostin	↓IL-1α ↓CRP ~ IL-β and IL-2	Randomized, double-blind, placebo-controlled trial ($n = 60$)	Anti-inflammatory properties
Xie et al. (94)	Mangosteen-based drink (Verve®)	↓Peroxyl radical scavenging capacity (antioxidant activity) ↓CRP ~ IL- 1α, IL- 1β, and IL- 2	Randomized, double-blind, placebo-controlled trial ($n = 60$)	Antioxidant and anti-inflammatory properties
Udani et al. (95)	Mangosteen juice from whole fruit, combined with other fruit juices (XanGo Juice™)	↓CRP (18 oz/day group only), IL-12p70 ↓ Body mass index (for 6oz group only) ~ENA-78 and lipid peroxidation	Randomized, double blind placebo-controlled pilot of obese participants ($n = 40$)	Anti-inflammatory properties

3-NP, 3-nitropropionic acid; Bcl-2, B-cell lymphoma 2; COX-2, cyclooxygenase-2; CRP, C-reactive protein; DPPH, 1,1-diphenyl-2-picrylhydrazyl; ENA, epithelial Cell-Derived Neutrophil-Activating Protein; ERK, extracellular Signal-regulated Kinase; GPx, glutathione peroxidase; GSH, glutathione peroxidase; H_2O_2, hydrogen peroxide; IBA-1, ionized calcium binding adaptor molecule 1; IL, interleukin; iNOS, inducible nitric oxide synthase; JNK, c-Jun N-terminal; LPS, lipopolysaccharide; MAPK, Mitogen-activated protein kinases; MDA, malondialdehyde; NF-kB, nuclear factor kappa B; NO, nitric oxide; PGE_2, prostaglandin E_2; ROS, reactive oxygen species; SOD, superoxide dismutase; TBARS, thiobarbituric acidic reactive substances; TNF-α, tumor necrosis factor; VEGF, vascular endothelial growth factor.

α- and γ-mangostin have demonstrated some inhibitory effects on cyclic adenosine monophosphate (cAMP) phosphodiesterase (98, 99), a property shared with another putatively psychoactive plant, sceletium tortuosum (100). Indeed, cyclic adenosine monophosphate cAMP phosphodiesterase inhibitors, such as rolipram, have antidepressant and anti-inflammatory activity (101). Targeting these pathways is implicated in antidepressant and antipsychotic treatments (97).

Antioxidant Properties of Mangosteen Pericarp

Marquez-Valadez et al. (72) explored α-mangostin as a treatment to reduce oxidative damage in homogenized rat brain tissue (cerebellum removed) and synaptosomal P2 fractions, in a model of neurotoxicity. Following administration of various neurotoxins, *viz.* ferrous sulfate, quinolinic acid, and 3-nitropropionic acid (3-NP), administration of α-mangostin

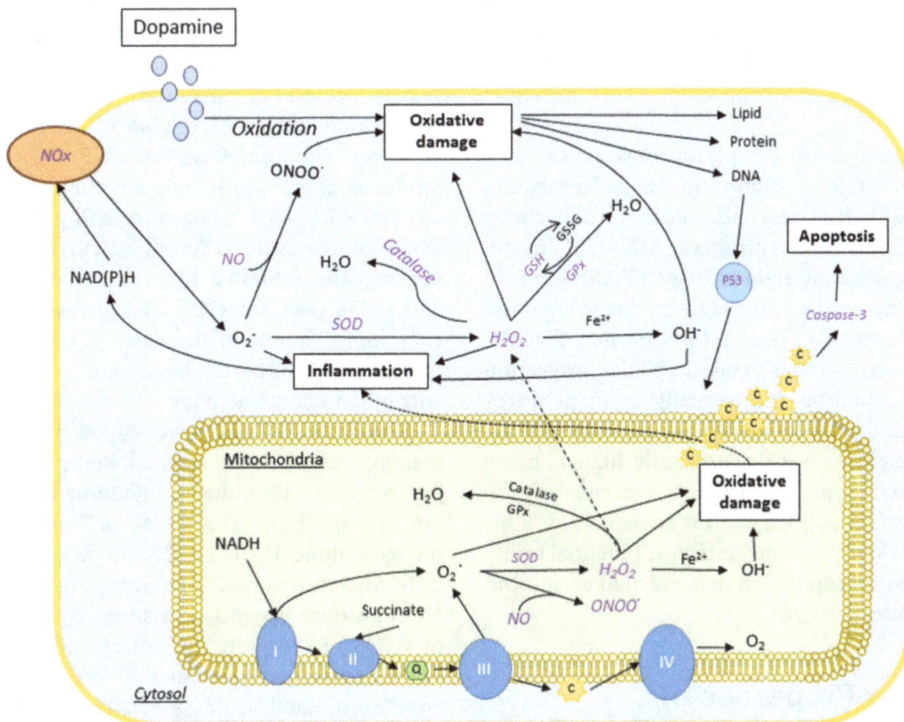

FIGURE 1 | Proposed neurobiology of bipolar disorder and schizophrenia and associated mechanisms of mangosteen pericarp (purple italics). These major psychiatric disorders have been shown to have aberrations in oxidative biology, mitochondrial function and neurogenesis/apoptosis. The purple italicized text indicates the points at which mangosteen pericarp has mechanistic actions that may benefit these disorders. Complexes I, II, II, and IV; CoQ, Coenzyme Q; C, cytochrome C; Fe^{2+}, ferrous ion; GPx, glutathione peroxidase; GSH, reduced glutathione; GSSG, oxidized glutathione; H_2O, water; H_2O_2, hydrogen peroxide; NADH, nicotinamide adenine dinucleotide (phosphate); NO, nitric oxide; Nox, NADH, Reduced Nicotinamide adenine; O2, Superoxide anion; OH, Hydroxyl radical; ONOO, peroxynitrite; SOD, Superoxide dismutase.

(25–500 uM) resulted in a reduction in toxin-induced oxidative stress as measured by TBARs formation, with all doses being effective. α-Mangostin also reduced quinolinic acid and 3-nitropropionic acid induced mitochondrial dysfunction as assessed by 3-(2,5-dimethylthiazol-1-yl)2,5-diphenyltetrazolium (MTT) reduction. It was concluded that α-mangostin was effective as a broad-spectrum antioxidant.

Marquez-Valadez et al. (73) then examined α-mangostin modulation of the GSH system and antioxidant properties in rat brain tissue prepared as above (72). Rats ($n = 4$–5 per group) received varying doses of α-mangostin (10, 25, and 50 μM) either alone or with ferrous sulfate or with 3-NP. Synaptosomal fractions were analyzed for glutathione (GSH), glutathione peroxidase GPx, and glutathione S-transferase (GST) levels. All doses of α-mangostin reduced GSH levels compared to controls when tested alone (no ferrous sulfate or 3-NP). In the ferrous sulfate studies, α-mangostin at doses of 25 and 50 μM returned GSH levels to control levels and were significantly higher than that of the ferrous sulfate group. Similar results were found with respect to GSH levels following 3-NP challenge for all doses of α-mangostin. GPx activity was increased only in the α-mangostin 25 and 50 μM doses compared to controls, but this effect was lost when administered alongside ferrous sulfate. There were no differences in glutathione S-transferase activity across any of the groups. Due to the varying effects of α-mangostin on redox activity, the authors concluded that α-mangostin was selectively modulating the GSH system to preferentially raise protective GSH levels, thereby highlighting a putative mechanism for α-mangostin's antioxidant properties.

Moongkarndi et al. (65) compared 25 μg/ml doses of purified α-mangostin with mangosteen pericarp extracts using two different solvents—ethyl acetate and water to explore the bioactive components in SKBR3 cells, a breast cancer cell line. The ethyl acetate-soluble extract, noted to contain low polar constituents, appeared to inhibit cancer cell proliferation. The purified α-mangostin and the water extract of mangosteen pericarp that contains high polar constituents both demonstrated antioxidant activity. In particular, the water-soluble extract demonstrated the most pronounced free-radical scavenging activity against 1,1-diphenyl-2-picrylhydrazyl (DPPH). It was concluded that purified α-mangostin showed superior activity in reducing cytotoxicity, apoptosis, and antioxidative activity in cancer cells, compared to the water extract. Previous cancer studies have shown mangosteen pericarp to be pro-apoptotic in certain laboratory conditions [e.g., Lee et al. (74) and Yang et al. (67)]. Differences in tissue type (e.g., cancer cells), dosing and other parameters complicate the interpretation of these studies within the context of neurobiology. Similarly, biological agents often have both beneficial and detrimental effects, dependent on these factors. For example, in an environment of oxidative stress, *N*-acetylcycteine has beneficial effects but can be toxic (due to oversupply of cysteine) under conditions of normal redox homeostasis (102).

Shin-Yu et al. (75) fed mangosteen pericarp extract (85% α-mangostin; 25 mg/day) to rats in addition to a high-fat diet and compared changes in oxidative stress and mitochondrial activity among rats fed a high fat diet and a group on AIN-93M control diet. Results showed significantly reduced liver TBARS levels in mangosteen fed rats compared with the high-fat diet group (and were similar levels to controls). The authors posited that the reduction in oxidative stress and increased cellular protection (measured by TBARS) could be due to mangosteen pericarp-induced increases in cellular oxidative defense mechanisms. All antioxidant enzymes explored were significantly higher in the mangosteen pericarp extract group than that described in the high-fat diet group (i.e., GSH, GPx, glutathione reductase, SOD, and catalase; CAT). This study also suggested the potential utility of mangosteen pericarp in a population that has high co-morbid obesity and metabolic disorders (30).

Anti-inflammatory Properties of Mangosteen Pericarp

Catorce et al. (79) explored the anti-inflammatory properties of α-mangostin in a murine model. They administered lipopolysaccharide (LPS) to mice ($n = 18$) to induce neuroinflammation. Results showed that oral gavage administration of α-mangostin significantly inhibited the LPS-induced increase in IL-6 in the brain. The levels of other inflammatory cytokines studied (IL-1β and TNF-α) were not affected by α-mangostin administration. This study further demonstrated α-mangostin-associated reduction in the levels of the inflammation-associated enzyme COX-2, in the brain.

The anti-inflammatory effects of α-mangostin have also been observed in human cells challenged with LPS (80), where α-mangostin was found to significantly reduce the release of pro-inflammatory cytokines IL-8 and TNF-α. Interestingly, these results were only true for THP-1 (monocyte-like leukemia), HepG2 (hepatocellular carcinoma), and Caco-2 HTB-37 (colorectal adenocarcinoma with enterocyte-like phenotype) cells, but not for other cell-lines such as monocyte-derived macrophages. These results suggest the effects of α-mangostin may differ depending on cell type. In contrast, α-mangostin stimulated the release of TNF-α in monocyte-derived macrophages cells.

In a study by Tewtrakul et al. (81), an ethanolic extraction of mangosteen pericarp and α- and γ-mangostin isolations were administered to murine RAW264.7 macrophage cells to explore the pathway of anti-inflammatory action of the compounds. LPS was first used to produce an increase in inflammatory molecules NO, prostaglandin E_2 (PGE_2), TNF-α, and IL-4, with mangosteen pericarp and its isolates administered in different concentrations (0, 0.3, 1, 3, 10, 30, and 100 μM). Release of NO was significantly inhibited by α-mangostin (3, 10, 30, and 100 μM), and by γ-mangostin and mangosteen pericarp (10, 30, and 100 μM). Release of PGE_2 was significantly inhibited by all compounds at all doses. Pro-inflammatory cytokine TNF-α release was inhibited by mangosteen pericarp (10 and 30 μM) and by α- and γ-mangostin (30 and 100 μM). All extracts significantly inhibited release of IL-4 (10, 30, and 100 μM). However, the inhibition of TNF-α and IL-4 were only of moderate effect. Lastly, inducible iNOS and COX-2 expression were inhibited by α-mangostin, with γ-mangostin only inhibiting iNOS. Similar studies found an ethyl acetate extract of α- and γ-mangostin inhibited LPS induced NO and PGE_2 production and iNOS (but not COX-2) expression in murine RAW264.7 cells (82). Therefore, the authors concluded that mangosteen pericarp and, in particular, α- and γ-mangostin have potential anti-inflammatory activity.

Cho et al. (68) also investigated the effects of the xanthone, mangostenone F, an isolated compound of the mangosteen pericarp, on LPS-induced inflammation in murine RAW264.7 macrophage cells. The RAW264.7 cells were pre-treated with mangostenone F (0, 10, 20, 30, 40, 60, 80, and 100 μM) for 24 h. Mangostenone F significantly inhibited the production of NO in a dose dependent manner by decreasing the expression of iNOS. To explore the effects of mangostenone F on the pro-inflammatory cytokines TNF-α, IL6, and IL-1β, the cells were pre-treated at doses of 20, 40, and 60 μM. There was a dose dependent reduction in all pro-inflammatory cytokines by mangostenone F. There was also a dose dependent reduction in NF-κB DNA binding activity, via p65 and IκB-α. Lastly, AP-1 reporter activity was inhibited by the mangostenone F, suggesting suppression of the MAPK signaling pathway. Therefore, it was suggested that the anti-inflammatory response was via suppression of MAPK and NF-κB activation. In agreement with afore-noted findings, an *in vitro* study in human cells examined whether α- and γ-mangostin could reduce obesity-associated inflammation (83). The study found that the reduction in inflammation was possibly due to the mangosteen pericarp extract preventing MAPK and NF-κB activation which in turn reduced levels of IL-6, IL-1β, interferon-γ and TNF-α (83).

A study investigating a cell culture model of Parkinson's disease included investigations of NO and iNOS response to α-mangostin (84). There was a significant dose-dependent reduction of iNOS by α-mangostin, showing the effects of α-mangostin to reduce immunologically-induced NO release. The authors also explored the NF-κB signaling pathway via IκB-α and p65 in the cytosol and found α-mangostin had a concentration dependent beneficial effect on these pathways. Therefore, this may be a pathway for α-mangostin reduction of pro-inflammatory cytokines and NO production. In addition, they noted that ROS was significantly reduced by α-mangostin in a dose dependent manner in microglial cells, demonstrated by reduction of H_2O_2. The authors posited that this may be due to α-mangostin targeting NADPH-oxidase (NOX). Reduced dopamine uptake induced by α-synuclein was also increased by α-mangostin, with α-mangostin significantly protecting dopamine neurons from apoptosis in a dose-dependent manner. It was concluded that α-mangostin has demonstrated capacity as a neuroprotective agent in neurodegenerative disorders via microglial activation pathways of neuroinflammation and serves as an anti-inflammatory and antioxidant agent.

Production of NO through iNOS and inflammatory process have been implicated in both psychosis and depression (23, 103). It is relevant to note that diverse antidepressants (104) and antipsychotics (105) target the NO system, while selectively targeting the NO system has been implicated in the antidepressant and antipsychotic actions of methylene blue (62, 63).

Neuroprotective and Anti-apoptotic Properties of Mangosteen Pericarp

Effective neuroprotective compounds will impede or stop the progression of an illness (44). Neuroprotective compounds can modulate antioxidant systems (85) and inflammatory systems (44). Weecharangsan et al. (85) investigated the neuroprotective properties of four mangosteen pericarp extractions: distilled water, 50% ethanol, 95% ethanol or ethyl acetate. Each treatment group was assessed for antioxidant activity through DPPH free radical scavenging and for neuroprotective activity in NG108-15 cells treated with hydrogen peroxide (H_2O_2). Both the water and 50% ethanol extracts dose-dependently exhibited superior free radical-scavenging activities and inhibited H_2O_2-induced cell death, compared to the other extracts.

Xanthones extracted from mangosteen pericarp (aqueous extraction) were explored for neuroprotective properties in lead-poisoned mice (87). Lead results in cognitive impairments by inhibiting antioxidant function and increasing free radical production. This is achieved by lead competitively inhibiting calcium binding sites on acetylcholinesterase, leading to oxidative damage. Xanthone treatment (administered orally, in drinking water) had a significant dose-dependent effect on increasing acetylcholinesterase activity in the blood and brain of lead-treated mice. Oxidative stress in the mangosteen pericarp treatment groups was significantly reduced as shown by MDA reduction. Thus, the authors concluded that the xanthone component of mangosteen pericarp has neuroprotective properties while reducing cognitive impairment by inhibiting oxidative stress. In addition to these results, depressive-like behavior in lead-intoxicated mice as demonstrated using the forced swim test was significantly reversed by the xanthone extract group compared to control groups (87).

In an *in vivo* study by Wihastuti et al. (89), the effect of mangosteen pericarp on neurogenesis was explored. Varying doses (200, 400, and 800 mg/kg) of mangosteen pericarp extracted by an ethanol solution were trialed via gavage in rats fed a high-cholesterol diet (and compared to a normal diet, negative control group and high-cholesterol diet, positive control group). The VEGF receptor 1 and NF-κB were measured. VEGF receptor 1 is expressed in inflammatory cells including macrophages and monocytes. The protein NF-κB responds to free radicals and is involved in the production of cytokines and influences synaptic plasticity and memory. Mangosteen pericarp extract significantly inhibited the formation of VEGF receptor 1, and reduced NF-κB, iNOS, H_2O_2, and H1F1-α expression. The highest dose (800 mg/kg) was most effective in terms of anti-oxidative and anti-inflammatory activities.

Huang et al. (90) investigated the effects of a mangosteen pericarp extract rich in xanthones and polyphenols in a 3xTg-AD mouse model of Alzheimer's Disease to explore neuroprotective and anti-apoptotic properties. Mice received the mangosteen pericarp extract in addition to a regular diet and were compared to a control group fed only the regular diet. Analyses were conducted both *in vitro* in hippocampal cells and *in vivo* with respect to serum markers. In hippocampal cells, no differences in JNK or ERK pathways were noted in the hippocampal cells, although an increase in GSH levels was observed. However, the results in serum showed a reduction in ROS, cyclooxygenase-2 (COX-2), and IL-6, as well as an increase in GSH and serotonin. Lastly, mice treated with the mangosteen pericarp dietary supplement presented with reduced cognitive impairment and spatial memory retrieval deficit compared to untreated controls. It was concluded the mangosteen pericarp extract demonstrated antioxidative, anti-inflammatory and neuroprotective properties.

To test for anti-inflammatory, antioxidant, and anti-hyperglycemic properties of the mangosteen pericarp, Jariyapongskul et al. (91) investigated the effects of α-mangostin on inflammatory cytokines, oxidative stress markers, and neurotrophins in the retina of streptozotocin-induced diabetic mice. In an *in vivo* study, within 8 weeks of intraperitoneally injecting rats with streptozotocin, α-mangostin was administered via gavage to type-2 diabetic rats ($n = 56$). The treatment with α-mangostin reduced ocular degeneration, a manifestation that can occur in early stages of type 2 diabetes. The authors found that α-mangostin treatment reduced levels of VEGF, TNF-α, and MDA. Whilst α-mangostin significantly reduced fasting glucose levels of the diabetic rats, there was no difference between non-diabetic rats and control rats, suggesting a role in glucose regulation. Whilst this study illustrates some promise as a treatment option in type 2 diabetes, further research is needed to determine if it may also be a preventative strategy for the disorder and for the development of vascular abnormalities. Due to the relationship between general medical conditions, including metabolic disorders such as diabetes and bipolar disorder and schizophrenia, this study highlights the potential symbiosis of treating the disorders together (41).

Mitochondrial Enhancing Properties of Mangosteen Pericarp

Many of the biological targets for mangosteen pericarp and its isolates involve the mitochondria. For example, when mitochondrial dysfunction was induced *in vitro* via 3-NP, increased oxidative stress was mitigated by α-mangostin (72, 73, 75). It was further suggested that α-mangostin may modulate apoptosis associated with mitochondrial pathways (86). This shows how complex and inter-related the mitochondrial, oxidative stress, and inflammation pathways are, and suggests the potential of treatments that can target these pathways.

To better inform the therapeutic potential of mangosteen pericarp in psychiatry, we investigated other fields where mangosteen pericarp has been shown to have relevant actions.

Cancer cells studies can demonstrate the relationship between apoptosis and the mitochondria, relevant to psychiatry. Aisha et al. (92) explored the anti-colon cancer effects of a combination of α- and γ-mangostin (81 and 16%, respectively) through *in vitro* and *in vivo* experiments. For the *in vitro* study, human colon cancer cells were treated with the xanthone extract of mangosteen pericarp and α-mangostin and compared to the chemotherapy medication, cisplatin as a positive control. The treatment with xanthones killed the cancer cells and did so at a lower concentration than cisplatin. Their findings suggested an action mediated by enhancing executioner caspases-3/7 and by activating the initiator caspase-9 leading to apoptosis of cancer cells. The authors postulated that mitochondria-mediated cytotoxicity was involved. Apoptosis was further analyzed through the upregulation of the MAPK/ERK and p53 pathways, showing potent, selective, and dose dependent cytotoxicity due to the enhancement and activation of mitochondrial pathways of apoptosis.

This review outlines pathways implicated in oxidative stress, inflammation and mitochondrial function. Importantly, these pathways are also directly or indirectly linked to monoamine release and/or function. As previously mentioned, α-mangostin has a tricyclic structure (64) which is relevant to existing medications (e.g., tricyclic antidepressants) which block serotonin re-uptake. However, we believe that because mangosteen has other important biological properties in addition to potentially modulating monoamines, mangosteen pericarp may be a novel and indeed highly efficacious adjunctive therapy.

THERAPEUTIC POTENTIAL OF MANGOSTEEN PERICARP

Mangosteen Pericarp as an Antidepressant

Recent preclinical evidence has demonstrated the antidepressant and memory enhancing actions of mangosteen pericarp, together with a suppression of hippocampal lipid peroxidation, in a rodent model of depression (76). In this study, an extract of mangosteen pericarp at an acute dose of 50 mg/kg administered by oral gavage was found to be an effective antidepressant in Flinder's Sensitive Line rats (a model of depression). The raw pericarp extract contained predominantly α- and γ-mangostin. A 14-day treatment regimen of mangosteen pericarp extract (50 mg/kg per day) displayed sustained antidepressant and pro-cognitive effects in the forced swim test and novel object recognition test, respectively, while demonstrating parity with the reference tricyclic antidepressant, imipramine (76). Behavioral and regional brain monoamine assessments suggested a more prominent serotonergic action for mangosteen pericarp extract as opposed to the noradrenergic action of imipramine, with both imipramine and mangosteen pericarp extract reversing hippocampal lipid peroxidation in rats. Indeed, the hippocampus is highly vulnerable to oxidative stress while being a key factor in memory. Moreover, both memory and hippocampal structure and function are compromised in patients with depression (106). This work confirms the antidepressant activity of raw mangosteen pericarp, while linking this therapeutic action to correction of disordered brain monoamines as well as the restoration of cellular damage brought on by oxidative stress (76). Interestingly, disordered redox status is known to mediate changes in brain monoamines (107) that in turn can drive changes in behavior (108).

Mangosteen Pericarp as an Antipsychotic

Concerning schizophrenia, preclinical findings in a maternal immune-activation (MIA) rat model of schizophrenia found that chronic oral dosing of haloperidol (2 mg/kg for 14 days) and raw mangosteen pericarp (50 mg/kg for 14 days) were equally effective in reversing MIA-induced deficits in sensorimotor gating and depressive-like behavior, with haloperidol plus mangosteen showing a more pronounced response (77, 78). MIA-induced elevations in IL-6 and TNF-α levels and cortico-striatal lipid peroxidation were reversed by haloperidol, mangosteen, and haloperidol plus mangosteen. The authors suggested that, at least in this model, depressive manifestations are more responsive to mangosteen than sensorimotor gating deficits, implicating promise in the management of mood-related deficits in schizophrenia (77, 78).

Mangosteen Pericarp as a Treatment for Neurodegenerative Disorders

The neuroprotective effects of α-mangostin were investigated in a cellular model of Parkinson's disease (86) by exposing human SH-SY5Y neuroblastoma cells to 1-methyl-4-phenylpyridinium (MPP^+). α-mangostin was then administered for 24 h (doses 2.5, 5, 10, 20, and 40 μM). Doses of 20 and 40 μM α-mangostin induced significant loss of cell viability and were excluded from further experiments. All other doses of α-mangostin significantly decreased ROS induced apoptosis in an MPP^+ model designed to trigger apoptosis. α-mangostin also significantly reduced MPP^+ induced Bax, Bax/Bcl-2, p53, and caspase-3 expression. Therefore, the study suggests the ability of α-mangostin to reduce apoptosis, potentially via mitochondrial pathways and reduction of oxidative stress. Of interest, Parkinson's disease has been viewed as a biological parallel to bipolar disorder because of the dopaminergic pathology and the cyclical nature of depression which occurs in the on-off phenomenon in Parkinson's disease (11). In fact, novel methylene blue analogs which inhibit nitric oxide synthase (NOS) and inhibit monoamine oxidase have been synthesized to address such a comorbid condition by virtue of their neuroprotective actions and restoration of mitochondrial function (62).

In the study utilizing a Parkinson's disease model, the effects of α-mangostin on neuroinflammation via the microglial activation pathway was investigated (84). In this study, wild-type Sprague-Dawley rat cells were treated with α-synuclein to induce inflammation and then treated for 24 h with α-mangostin at 1, 10, and 100 nM doses. Results showed a significant dose dependent reduction in pro-inflammatory cytokines IL-6, IL-1β, and TNF-α in the α-mangostin treated group. The 100 nM dose of α-mangostin reduced microglial activation by inhibiting production of a marker of ionized calcium binding adaptor molecule 1(IBA-1), a microglial specific protein.

Mangosteen pericarp has been investigated as a treatment for Alzheimer's disease (66). In one *in vitro* study, the seven most common xanthones were isolated (α-mangostin, 8-deoxygartanin, gartanin, garciniafuran, garcinone C, garcinone D, and γ-mangostin) and assessed for their ability to inhibit β-amyloid-related cell damage, as well as their metal chelating, antioxidant and neuroprotective properties in an Alzheimer's Disease model (66). Results demonstrated that mangosteen pericarp reduced β-amyloid build up and reduced glutamate-induced cell damage by scavenging ROS (assessed by DPPH). Of the isolated xanthones, α-mangostin, gartanin, garcinone C, and γ-mangostin showed the greatest antioxidant properties.

Similar protective effects of mangosteen pericarp extract were explored *in vitro* and *in vivo* in mice in a study by Sattayasai et al. (88). Mice were administered scopolamine to induce memory impairments in an attempt to model the cognitive symptoms of Alzheimer's disease through central cholinergic muscarinic receptor antagonism. Afflicted mice were administered either mangosteen pericarp extract at 100 mg/kg via oral gavage or water as a control. Results obtained using the Morris water maze test for spatial memory and passive avoidance (fear) tests showed mangosteen pericarp extract protected mice from the memory degrading effects of scopolamine, leading to improved memory retention. In the *in vitro* arm of the study, mangosteen pericarp was protective against H_2O_2 and polychlorinated biphenyl induced oxidative stress in SK-N-SH (human blastoma cells) cells pre-incubated with mangosteen pericarp extract as shown by reduced ROS. This study demonstrated not only the anti-oxidative and neuroprotective properties of mangosteen pericarp extract, but also its memory protecting capacity, and thus is congruent with the *in vivo* depression model data described in Flinder's Sensitive Line rats by Oberholzer et al. (76).

CLINICAL TRIALS OF MANGOSTEEN PERICARP

Mangosteen pericarp, as well as isolated compounds such as α-mangostin, have been demonstrated in both animal and *in vitro* studies to favorably modulate pathways relevant to mitochondrial function, inflammation, and oxidative stress. However, clinical trials are required to confirm whether these properties are clinically relevant. The following sections will provide an overview of the existing clinical trial data and its relevance to psychiatry, in particular bipolar disorder and schizophrenia. The behavioral effects of mangosteen pericarp are summarized in **Table 2**.

Use of Mangosteen Pericarp in General Health

Mangosteen pericarp has been investigated in general medicine. Given these data are predominantly in healthy individuals, caution needs to be taken regarding the specific applicability to psychiatric disorders. However, to provide a comprehensive overview of the potential mechanisms by which mangosteen pericarp may be beneficial for psychiatric disorders these data have been included in this review.

A randomized, placebo-controlled, double blind trial studied the effects of 30 days of treatment with a commercially available mangosteen juice (Mangosteen Plus™ with Essential Minerals®; mixed with vitamins A, B-6, C, D, E, selenium, folate, and thiamine; 59 ml) on immunity in 60 healthy human participants aged 40–60 years (93). Fructose liquid (59 ml) was used as a placebo control. The most prominent bioactive substances in the juice were β-mangostin and catechins. The mangosteen juice group had significantly higher levels of inflammatory cytokines IL-1α and IL-1b compared to placebo. To note, anti-inflammatory medications are adept at reducing heightened inflammation. If there is no inflammation in the system then adding anti-inflammatories may be detrimental, or even toxic (e.g., as with *N*-acetylcycteine (102). The mangosteen juice group also reported a reduction in inflammatory biomarker C-reactive protein (CRP) compared to baseline. There were no significant group differences with respect to IL-1β and IL-2. Interestingly, all participants in the mangosteen juice group self-reported an increase in subjective health status compared to the placebo group.

A randomized, double-blind, placebo controlled clinical trial explored antioxidant and anti-inflammatory biomarkers in healthy adults who were administered a mangosteen-based drink (94). Whilst mainly containing mangosteen, the drink also included vitamins, green tea, aloe vera, and a caffeinated energy blend. A total of 60 adult participants (30 men, 30 women) were administered 245 ml of either the mangosteen-based drink or placebo (fructose liquid) daily for 30 days together with pre- and post-administration blood analyses. After 30 days, results showed significantly more antioxidant activity, as measured by an increase in the peroxyl radical scavenging capacity, in the mangosteen-based drink group compared to the placebo arm. CRP levels significantly decreased in the mangosteen-based drink group and were not changed in the placebo group. There was no significant change in immunity markers IgA, IgG, IgM, C3, C4; and no significant change in inflammatory markers IL- 1α, IL-1β, and IL- 2 across groups and time points.

Udani et al. (95) conducted a randomized, double-blind, controlled pilot study of commercially available mangosteen juice (XanGo Juice™), a whole fruit juice blended with other fruit juices, in obese participants. A combination of fruit juices and sucrose was used as a control. A total of 40 participants who agreed to not change any current diet or exercise regimes and ceased any anti-inflammatory agents completed the study, all of whom were obese and had an elevated CRP score of $\geq$3. This was a 4-arm study: control, 3, 6, or 9 oz XanGo™ juice whereby participants drank the intervention or control juice twice a day for 8 weeks. The combination juice used as a control was added to each of the lower mangosteen doses so each total individual serving volume was 9 oz liquid. As a result, participant received total daily doses of XanGO™ juice at 6 oz, 12 oz or 18 oz, or control juice. Results showed a non-significant increase in CRP for the placebo group as well as a non-significant decrease in CRP for all doses of the mangosteen juice. There was a significant difference between changes in CRP across the 8 weeks in the control and the 18 oz/day group. Changes in body mass index and body fat were only significantly reduced

TABLE 2 | Summary of behavioral evidence for *Garcinia mangostana Linn*. (mangosteen).

Paper	Mangosteen compound	Outcome	Method
Oberholzer et al. (76)	Mangosteen pericarp extract	↓ Depressive-like behaviors, ↑ Recognition memory	*In vivo*: Flinders sensitive line rats, compared with imipramine (tricyclic antidepressant)
Harvey et al. (77); Lotter et al. (78)	Raw mangosteen pericarp (50 mg/kg)	↓ Depressive-like behaviors	*In vivo* inflammatory rat model of schizophrenia cf. haloperidol
Phyu et al. (87)	Xanthones from aqueous extract of mangosteen pericarp	↓ Depressive-like behaviors	*In vivo* lead-poisoned mice ($n = 42$)
Sattayasai et al. (88)	Mangosteen pericarp extract	↑ Memory	*In vivo* and *In vitro* memory impaired mice
Huang et al. (90)	Mangosteen pericarp extract	↓ Cognitive impairment and spatial memory recall	*In vivo* and *In vitro*: 3xTg-AD mouse model of Alzheimer's Disease. Hippocampal cells and serum.
Chang et al. (109)	Mangosteen-based juice blend (containing 305 mg of α-mangostin and 278 mg of hydroxycitric acid)	~ Physical fatigue, heart rate, ↓ Mental fatigue	Randomized, double-blind, placebo-controlled trial healthy adults ($n = 12$)
Watanabe et al. (110)	Mangosteen pericarp (40% α- and γ-mangostin)	↓ Insulin levels and insulin resistance ~ Glucose levels, weight loss, waist circumference, body composition, LDL, HDL, triglycerides	Randomized controlled pilot study ($n = 20$)
Kudiganti et al. (111)	Meratrim (Sphaeranthus indicus flower and mangosteen pericarp at 3:1 ratio)	↓ Total mood disturbance	Randomized, double-blind, placebo-controlled trial in healthy overweight subjects ($n = 60$)
Laupu (112)	1,000 mg/day Mangosteen pericarp	↓ Depressive-like behaviors, positive and negative symptoms of schizophrenia, ↑ Life satisfaction and general functioning	Randomized, double-blind, placebo-controlled trial in schizophrenia/schizoaffective population ($n = 80$)

in the 6 oz/day group compared to placebo. There were no significant differences between groups for lipid peroxidation and Epithelial Cell-Derived Neutrophil-Activating Protein (ENA)-78. There was a significant reduction of IL-12p70 levels across time in all active groups.

Due to the association between ROS and fatigue during exercise, Chang et al. (109) trialed mangosteen in 12 healthy adults. Participants were randomized to receive an acute dose of either a mangosteen juice blend or a diluted drink that replaced 50% mangosteen juice with water. There was no significant difference in time to exhaustion or other measures of physical performance (e.g., heart rate).

Mangosteen pericarp has been trialed in a combination treatment for weight loss in two human trials (111, 113) and mangosteen pericarp alone in one insulin resistance study (110) and all showed some promising results. In a population of obese female adults with insulin resistance (but not diabetes) mangosteen pericarp was trialed as a treatment for insulin resistance, reducing inflammatory markers and participant weight in a 26-week randomized controlled pilot study (110). All participants in the study ($n = 20$) received a lifestyle intervention delivered by a dietician focusing on physical activity and caloric restriction. Participants were randomized to receive either 400 mg/day mangosteen pericarp (40% α- and γ-mangostin) in addition to the intervention or no additional study medication. Participants in the mangosteen pericarp group showed significantly reduced insulin levels and demonstrated reduced insulin resistance. However, there were no significant differences in body fat percentage, waist circumference, or weight loss between participants in the mangosteen pericarp arm and control arm. There were no significant differences in glucose markers or in cholesterol markers and triglycerides levels when comparing the mangosteen pericarp and control groups. This study would have benefited from a placebo control to include blinding and reduce placebo response from the mangosteen administration. Given the lack of placebo, small sample size and female only sample, results from this study are cautiously interpreted as showing some efficacy in reducing insulin and insulin resistance and appears to be well tolerated.

These trials provide preliminary clinical evidence to suggest that mangosteen juice and mangosteen pericarp extract can alter inflammatory markers *in vivo*. However, due to most studies providing mangosteen in combination with other bioactive compounds, further trials are required to determine the effect of mangosteen pericarp or mangosteen juice as a standalone intervention for inflammation. Furthermore, the small sample sizes and predominately healthy populations included in these studies suggest that they may be underpowered.

It has been highlighted that the anti-inflammatory and antioxidant properties of varying extracts of mangosteen pericarp can also help to reduce co-morbid metabolic disorders common in those with bipolar disorder (114). Shandiz et al. (114) discussed this in their review on the metabolic effects of mangosteen pericarp extract *in vitro* and *in vivo*. Their review concluded that the reduction in metabolic disorders may occur by inhibiting inflammatory cytokines, reducing body weight and fat storage, and altering glucose metabolism.

Use of Mangosteen Pericarp in Mental Health

In the study by Chang et al. (109) where the effect of mangosteen juice was explored in a small placebo-controlled trial for exercise fatigue in healthy adults, self-reported mood, and fatigue were assessed as a secondary outcome using the Profile of Mood States. There were no significant differences between depression scores of the mangosteen juice vs. placebo groups at any time point. Whilst both groups had an increase in fatigue following the exercise, those who received mangosteen had significantly less mental fatigue (measured on the Profile of Mood States scale) compared to the control intervention. Both groups also reported improvements in vigor and fatigue compared to baseline (109).

Mental health was assessed as a secondary outcome in a randomized controlled trial of a combination herbal treatment containing mangosteen pericarp (Meratrim®) in a healthy overweight human sample (111). The primary outcomes of the study were reduction in weight, body mass index, waist, and hip size which were all significantly improved in the Meratrim ® group compared to placebo. Participants ($n = 60$) were randomized to receive 400 mg, twice a day Meratrim (combination of Sphaeranthus indicus flower and mangosteen pericarp extract in a 3:1 ratio) or placebo. Participants receiving Meratrim reported reduced mood disturbances as measured by the Short form of the Profile of Mood States when compared to placebo.

In a double-blind placebo-controlled randomized trial, adjunctive mangosteen pericarp (1,000 mg) was investigated in participants with schizophrenia receiving second generation antipsychotic treatment ($n = 80$) (112). The mangosteen pericarp group performed significantly better than the placebo group across all outcomes including the primary outcome, the Positive and Negative Syndrome Scale and secondary outcomes including Montgomery Åsberg Depression Rating Scale, positive, negative, and general subscales of the Positive and Negative Syndrome Scale, Clinical Global Impression Severity and Improvement, Self-rated Life Satisfaction Scale, and Global Assessment of Functioning. Therefore, the study concluded there was a significant reduction in symptoms of depression and symptomatology of schizophrenia and schizoaffective disorder. The study was limited due to its small sample size, and while symptoms of depression were a secondary outcome, participants on average had mild depression at baseline as measured by the Montgomery Åsberg Depression Rating Scale. To date, this is the only study which directly assesses the potential of mangosteen pericarp at treating a serious mental illness. Due to the small sample size combined with promising results, this study provides significant impetus for further research of mangosteen pericarp for the treatment of bipolar disorder, schizophrenia, and other psychiatric disorders.

Safety Profile of Mangosteen Pericarp

Whilst current clinical evidence is limited, several studies demonstrate that mangosteen pericarp appears to have a good safety profile and is well-tolerated. In animal models, mangosteen pericarp has been shown to reduce blood glucose levels, suggesting it could be used as a treatment for diabetes mellitus and that consumption of mangosteen pericarp may need to be supervised in patients undergoing insulin therapy (91, 115). In the insulin resistance study (110), gastrointestinal upset were the only reported adverse events and this occurred across both groups.

Suthammarak et al. (116) investigated the safety and antioxidant effects of mangosteen pericarp. Participants were orally administered polar (water-soluble) fractions of mangosteen pericarp in capsule form for 24 weeks. For the first three months, participants weighing under 55 kg received a 220 mg dose and those over 55 kg received 280 mg. After 3 months, all participants had their doses doubled. Participants were monitored at weeks 0, 1, 4, 12, 16, and 24. The study was limited by the lack of a placebo control group and a small sample size ($n = 11$) making it difficult to relate the emergence of adverse events to an association with the mangosteen pericarp. In addition, a small dose of mangosteen pericarp was used. Nevertheless, no major adverse events or medical issues were reported.

In a pilot study of 1,000 mg mangosteen pericarp for the adjunctive treatment of schizophrenia, there was no significant difference of reported adverse events between the placebo and the active groups (112). Only 2 adverse events were reported in this study (viz. headache and thoughts of self-harm). However, given the nature of the population, it is probable that adverse events could have been under-reported.

No adverse events were reported in a placebo-controlled randomized control trial of mangosteen juice in adults aged 40–60 years (93). Nor were there any adverse events in a similar study with a mangosteen-based drink (Verve®) (94). The mangosteen-based drink study also showed no significant difference compared to the placebo group for weight, body mass index, heart rate or blood pressure (94). Another mangosteen juice study again had no side effects reported and no clinically significant changes in electrocardiograms (95). In a study of 400 mg/day capsules of Meratrim for weight loss ($n = 60$), there was no significant difference in adverse events or liver, heart, kidney, or metabolic function, compared to the placebo group (113). This safety profile held true for another study of Meratrim at 800 mg/day (111). Interestingly, mangosteen pericarp has also been associated with increased renoprotection due to reduction in inflammation and oxidative and/or nitrosative stress (117). Hence, the current evidence suggests that mangosteen pericarp is well-tolerated with no known side effects. However, given the limited evidence base, particularly within clinical populations and those with polypharmacy, future trials are required to evaluate the long-term safety of this intervention across a range of doses and treatment durations. This is especially true when considering that the clinical application for mangosteen will be adjunctive to conventional treatments. With the recent study in animals suggesting increased serotonergic activity in mangosteen pericarp-treated depressed rats (76), and given the unknown interactions of mangosteen pericarp with conventional serotonergic agents, the possibility of drug-drug interactions should be considered.

Use of Mangosteen Pericarp as an Adjunctive Treatment for Serious Mental Disorders

In summary, this review has summarized a number of properties of the mangosteen pericarp that could target known aberrations in bipolar disorder and schizophrenia. In terms of biological processes, bipolar disorder, and schizophrenia share heightened oxidative stress including an increase in ROS, RNS, TBARS, and MDA which may be modulated by the glutamatergic system. Mangosteen pericarp in animal models reduces ROS, TBARS, MDA, and has demonstrated effects on the glutamatergic system. Inflammation is present in bipolar disorder and schizophrenia indexed by inflammatory cytokines IL-6, IL-1Ra, IL-1β TNF-α, and also by NO production via iNOS, superoxide dismutase catalase, and glutathione peroxidase. Our review collates results showing mangosteen pericarp can also have an effect on IL-6, IL-1β TNF- α, NO, catalase, and glutathione peroxidase, in addition to IL-2, IL-8, COX-2, and NF-κB. Alterations in apoptosis and neurogenesis are demonstrated by changes in Ki67+ cells as well as relevant markers including VEGF, bcl-2, MAPK, and JNK. Mangosteen pericarp has demonstrated effects on VEGF, bcl-2, and MAPK. However, there were no significant demonstrated effects of mangosteen pericarp on JNK. Lastly, the mitochondrial disturbances observed in bipolar disorder and schizophrenia may be targeted by mangosteen via the mitochondrial pathway to apoptosis. In addition to the biological pathways, mangosteen pericarp has demonstrated potential in reducing depression which is a key phase in bipolar disorder and in negative symptoms of schizophrenia. However, future research is required to observe the efficacy of mangosteen pericarp across the scope of the disorders and in human participants.

FUTURE DIRECTIONS

Mangosteen pericarp is a potential adjunctive treatment option in bipolar disorder and schizophrenia. Given only one randomized controlled trial has been completed in the field (112), future work could target the limitations of research such as the small sample sizes, lack of comparable outcomes, and non-standardization in the extraction process. Currently, a range of mangosteen pericarp extracts have been utilized which are either whole compound or isolated components (such as α- and γ-mangostin). Further research must be undertaken to discern the optimal dosing and extraction of the bioactive components, if separate, or if the bioactivity comes from a combination of the components working together in the compound. Mangosteen pericarp has been posited for use in neurodegenerative disorders such as Alzheimer's (66, 88, 90) and Parkinson's disease (84, 86). In animal models, mangosteen pericarp has been trialed for cognitive decline (87) and memory impairments (88). More recently, mangosteen pericarp displayed marked antidepressant and pro-cognitive effects in the Flinders Sensitive Line rat, a genetic animal model of depression (76). In addition, a reduction of hippocampal lipid peroxidation and correction of disordered regional brain monoamines and sensorimotor gating and depressive-like symptoms were reduced in an inflammatory rat model of schizophrenia (77, 78). Future directions could directly trial mangosteen pericarp as an adjunctive antidepressant in human trials for major depressive disorder and bipolar disorder. There are no animal studies utilizing the effects of mangosteen pericarp in a bipolar disorder model, however, due to the psychosis overlap with schizophrenia models, and the depressive phase of the illness, symbiotic benefits may be inferred. There is a need to demonstrate these findings from animal models in human studies. There are currently two studies directly trialing the effect of mangosteen pericarp on schizophrenia (118) (Trial registry ID: ACTRN12616000859482) and bipolar depression (119) (Trial registry ID: ACTRN12616000028404), both in adult populations.

CONCLUSION

The evidence of the bioactivity and neurobiology of mangosteen pericarp is rapidly emerging. Mangosteen pericarp has produced promising results in animals, and has been demonstrated to have antioxidant, anti-inflammatory, anti-apoptotic, neuroprotective, and mitochondrial enhancing properties. Taken together, the theoretical biological rationale of psychiatric disorders, bioactivity of mangosteen pericarp extract and the available preclinical data, support the therapeutic potential as an adjunctive psychiatric treatment. As the clinical evidence base for mangosteen pericarp as an adjunctive psychiatric treatment is scarce, future research requires human clinical trials to explore the risks and benefits of treatment and assess the potential for translation into clinical care.

AUTHOR CONTRIBUTIONS

Initial planning of the paper was conducted by MA, OD, and MB. MA conducted the literature search and wrote the first draft. MA, CB, and AW created the descriptive figure. OD, AW, CB, CN, MH, BH, MM, JM, WM, AT, SD, JGS, J-PK, KW, JS, and MB contributed to and edited drafts of the paper.

ACKNOWLEDGMENTS

The authors would like to acknowledge the NHMRC Project Grant Scheme (APP1121510) for supporting this review. MA would further like to acknowledge the support of Australian Rotary Health/Ian Parker Bipolar Research Fund PhD scholarship and the ASBDD/Lundbeck PhD neuroscience scholarship. OD is supported by a NHMRC R.D. Wright Biomedical Research Fellowship (APP1145634). AW is supported by a Trisno Family Fellowship. CB is supported by an Alfred Deakin Postdoctoral Research Fellowship. BH declares that the work referred to in this manuscript has been funded by Deakin University and the South African National

Research Foundation (grant number 77323). The NRF grant-holder acknowledges that opinions, findings and conclusions or recommendations expressed in any publication generated by NRF supported research are those of the authors, and that the NRF accepts no liability whatsoever in this regard. JM is supported by a NHMRC John Cade Fellowship (APP1056929) and Niels Bohr Professorship from the Danish National Research Foundation. JGS is supported by a National Health and Medical Research Council Practitioner Fellowship Grant APP1105807 and employed by The Queensland Center for Mental Health Research which receives core funding from the Queensland Health. JS is funded by an NHMRC Clinical Research Fellowship APP1125000. MB is supported by NHMRC Senior Principal Research Fellowship (APP1059660 and APP1156072).

REFERENCES

1. World Health Organisation (WHO). *Global Burden of Disease: 2004 Update*. Geneva: World Health Organisation (2004).
2. Fountoulakis KN. An update of evidence-based treatment of bipolar depression: where do we stand? *Curr Opin Psychiatry.* (2010) 23:19–24. doi: 10.1097/YCO.0b013e328333e132
3. Rossler W, Salize HJ, van Os J, Riecher-Rossler A. Size of burden of schizophrenia and psychotic disorders. *Eur Neuropsychopharmacol.* (2005) 15:399–409. doi: 10.1016/j.euroneuro.2005.04.009
4. Malhi GS, Bassett D, Boyce P, Bryant R, Fitzgerald PB, Fritz K, et al. Royal Australian and New Zealand College of Psychiatrists clinical practice guidelines for mood disorders. *Aust N Z J Psychiatry.* (2015) 49:1087–206. doi: 10.1177/0004867415617657
5. Hyman SE. Psychiatric drug development: diagnosing a crisis. *Cerebrum.* (2013) 2013:5.
6. Miller G. Is pharma running out of brainy ideas? *Science.* (2010) 329:502–4. doi: 10.1126/science.329.5991.502
7. Sarris J, Logan AC, Akbaraly TN, Amminger GP, Balanzá-Martínez V, Freeman MP, et al. Nutritional medicine as mainstream in psychiatry. *Lancet Psychiatry.* (2015) 2:271–4. doi: 10.1016/S2215-0366(14)00051-0
8. Yüksel C, McCarthy J, Shinn A, Pfaff DL, Baker JT, Heckers S, et al. Gray matter volume in schizophrenia and bipolar disorder with psychotic features. *Schizophr Res.* (2012) 138:177–82. doi: 10.1016/j.schres.2012.03.003
9. Maggioni E, Crespo-Facorro B, Nenadic I, Benedetti F, Gaser C, Sauer H, et al. Common and distinct structural features of schizophrenia and bipolar disorder: the European Network on Psychosis, Affective disorders and Cognitive Trajectory (ENPACT) study. *PLoS ONE.* (2017) 12:e0188000. doi: 10.1371/journal.pone.0188000
10. Anttila V, Bulik-Sullivan B, Finucane HK, Walters RK, Bras J, Duncan L, et al. Analysis of shared heritability in common disorders of the brain. *Science.* (2018) 360:6395. doi: 10.1126/science.aap8757
11. Berk M, Dodd S, Kauer-Sant'Anna M, Malhi GS, Bourin M, Kapczinski F, et al. Dopamine dysregulation syndrome: implications for a dopamine hypothesis of bipolar disorder. *Acta Psychiatr Scand.* (2007) s434:41–9. doi: 10.1111/j.1600-0447.2007.01058.x
12. Brugue E, Vieta E. Atypical antipsychotics in bipolar depression: neurobiological basis and clinical implications. *Prog Neuro Psychopharmacol Biol Psychiatry.* (2007) 31:275–82. doi: 10.1016/j.pnpbp.2006.06.014
13. Dager SR, Friedman SD, Parow A, Demopulos C, Stoll AL, Lyoo IK, et al. Brain metabolic alterations in medication-free patients with bipolar disorder. *Arch General Psychiatry.* (2004) 61:450–8. doi: 10.1001/archpsyc.61.5.450
14. Yoon SJ, Lyoo IK, Haws C, Kim TS, Cohen BM, Renshaw PF. Decreased glutamate/glutamine levels may mediate cytidine's efficacy in treating bipolar depression: a longitudinal proton magnetic resonance spectroscopy study. *Neuropsychopharmacology.* (2009) 34:1810–8. doi: 10.1038/npp.2009.2
15. Frye MA, Watzl J, Banakar S, O'Neill J, Mintz J, Davanzo P, et al. Increased anterior cingulate/medial prefrontal cortical glutamate and creatine in bipolar depression. *Neuropsychopharmacology.* (2007) 32:2490–9. doi: 10.1038/sj.npp.1301387
16. Howes O, McCutcheon R, Stone J. Glutamate and dopamine in schizophrenia: an update for the 21(st) century. *J Psychopharmacol.* (2015) 29:97–115. doi: 10.1177/0269881114563634
17. Howes OD, Kapur S. The dopamine hypothesis of schizophrenia: version III—the final common pathway. *Schizophr Bull.* (2009) 2009:35. doi: 10.1093/schbul/sbp006
18. López-Figueroa AL, Norton CS, López-Figueroa MO, Armellini-Dodel D, Burke S, Akil H, et al. Serotonin 5-HT1A, 5-HT1B, and 5-HT2A receptor mRNA expression in subjects with major depression, bipolar disorder, and schizophrenia. *Biol Psychiatry.* (2004) 55:225–33. doi: 10.1016/j.biopsych.2003.09.017
19. Data-Franco J, Singh A, Popovic D, Ashton M, Berk M, Vieta E, et al. Beyond the therapeutic shackles of the monoamines: new mechanisms in bipolar disorder biology. *Prog Neuropsychopharmacol Biol Psychiatry.* (2017) 72:73–86. doi: 10.1016/j.pnpbp.2016.09.004
20. Ng F, Berk M, Dean O, Bush AI. Oxidative stress in psychiatric disorders: evidence base and therapeutic implications. *Int J Neuropsychopharmacol.* (2008) 11:851–76. doi: 10.1017/S1461145707008401
21. Berk M, Kapczinski F, Andreazza AC, Dean OM, Giorlando F, Maes M, et al. Pathways underlying neuroprogression in bipolar disorder: focus on inflammation, oxidative stress and neurotrophic factors. *Neurosci Biobehav Rev.* (2011) 35:804–17. doi: 10.1016/j.neubiorev.2010.10.001
22. Andreazza AC, Kauer-Sant'anna M, Frey BN, Bond DJ, Kapczinski F, Young LT, et al. Oxidative stress markers in bipolar disorder: a meta-analysis. *J Affect Disord.* (2008) 111:135–44. doi: 10.1016/j.jad.2008.04.013
23. Brand SJ, Moller M, Harvey BH. A review of biomarkers in mood and psychotic disorders: a dissection of clinical vs. preclinical correlates. *Curr Neuropharmacol.* (2015) 13:324–68. doi: 10.2174/1570159X13666150307004545
24. Berk M, Copolov D, Dean O, Lu K, Jeavons S, Schapkaitz I, et al. N-acetyl cysteine as a glutathione precursor for schizophrenia—a double-blind, randomized, placebo-controlled trial. *Biol Psychiatry.* (2008) 2008:64. doi: 10.1016/j.biopsych.2008.03.004
25. Farokhnia M, Azarkolah A, Adinehfar F, Khodaie-Ardakani MR, Hosseini SM, Yekehtaz H, et al. N-acetylcysteine as an adjunct to risperidone for treatment of negative symptoms in patients with chronic schizophrenia: a randomized, double-blind, placebo-controlled study. *Clin Neuropharmacol.* (2013) 36:185–92. doi: 10.1097/wnf.0000000000000001
26. Breier A, Liffick E, Hummer TA, Vohs JL, Yang Z, Mehdiyoun NF, et al. Effects of 12-month, double-blind N-acetyl cysteine on symptoms, cognition and brain morphology in early phase schizophrenia spectrum disorders. *Schizophr Res.* (2018) 199:395–402. doi: 10.1016/j.schres.2018.03.012
27. Rossell SL, Francis PS, Galletly C, Harris A, Siskind D, Berk M, et al. N-acetylcysteine (NAC) in schizophrenia resistant to clozapine: a double blind randomised placebo controlled trial targeting negative symptoms. *BMC Psychiatry.* (2016) 16:320. doi: 10.1186/s12888-016-1030-3
28. Najjar S, Pearlman DM, Alper K, Najjar A, Devinsky O. Neuroinflammation and psychiatric illness. *J Neuroinflamm.* (2013) 10:43. doi: 10.1186/1742-2094-10-43
29. Réus GZ, Fries GR, Stertz L, Badawy M, Passos IC, Barichello T, et al. The role of inflammation and microglial activation in the pathophysiology of psychiatric disorders. *Neuroscience.* (2015) 300:141–54. doi: 10.1016/j.neuroscience.2015.05.018
30. SayuriYamagata A, Brietzke E, Rosenblat JD, Kakar R, McIntyre RS. Medical comorbidity in bipolar disorder: the link with metabolic-inflammatory systems. *J Affect Disord.* (2017) 211:99–106. doi: 10.1016/j.jad.2016.12.059
31. Munkholm K, Brauner JV, Kessing LV, Vinberg M. Cytokines in bipolar disorder vs. healthy control subjects: a systematic review and meta-analysis. *J Psychiatr Res.* (2013) 47:1119–33. doi: 10.1016/j.jpsychires.2013.05.018

32. Modabbernia A, Taslimi S, Brietzke E, Ashrafi M. Cytokine alterations in bipolar disorder: a meta-analysis of 30 studies. *Biol Psychiatry.* (2013) 74:15–25. doi: 10.1016/j.biopsych.2013.01.007
33. Berk M, Plein H, Belsham B. The specificity of platelet glutamate receptor supersensitivity in psychotic disorders. *Life Sci.* (2000) 66:2427–32. doi: 10.1016/S0024-3205(00)80002-8
34. Berk M, Plein H, Csizmadia T. Supersensitive platelet glutamate receptors as a possible peripheral marker in schizophrenia. *Int Clin Psychopharmacol.* (1999) 14:119–22. doi: 10.1097/00004850-199903000-00009
35. Colasanti M, Suzuki H. The dual personality of NO. *Trends Pharmacol Sci.* (2000) 21:249–52. doi: 10.1016/S0165-6147(00)01499-1
36. Goldsmith D, Rapaport M, Miller B. A meta-analysis of blood cytokine network alterations in psychiatric patients: comparisons between schizophrenia, bipolar disorder and depression. *Mol Psychiatry.* (2016) 21:1696. doi: 10.1038/mp.2016.3
37. McKernan DP, Dinan TG, Cryan JF. "Killing the Blues": a role for cellular suicide (apoptosis) in depression and the antidepressant response? *Prog Neurobiol.* (2009) 88:246–63. doi: 10.1016/j.pneurobio.2009.04.006
38. Sheng M, Ertürk A. Long-term depression: a cell biological view. *Philos Trans R Soc B Biol Sci.* (2014) 369:20130138. doi: 10.1098/rstb.2013.0138
39. Morris G, Walder K, Carvalho AF, Tye SJ, Lucas K, Berk M, et al. The role of hypernitrosylation in the pathogenesis and pathophysiology of neuroprogressive diseases. *Neurosci Biobehav Rev.* (2018) 84:453–69. doi: 10.1016/j.neubiorev.2017.07.017
40. Boyajyan A, Chavushyan A, Zakharyan R, Mkrtchyan G. Markers of apoptotic dysfunctions in schizophrenia. *Mol Biol.* (2013) 47:587–91. doi: 10.1134/S002689331304002X
41. Xie N, Wang C, Lin Y, Li H, Chen L, Zhang T, et al. The role of p38 MAPK in valproic acid induced microglia apoptosis. *Neurosci Lett.* (2010) 482:51–6. doi: 10.1016/j.neulet.2010.07.004
42. Jozwiak-Bebenista M, Jasinska-Stroschein M, Kowalczyk E. Involvement of vascular endothelial growth factor (VEGF) and mitogen-activated protein kinases (MAPK) in the mechanism of neuroleptic drugs. *Pharmacol Rep.* (2018) 70:1032–9. doi: 10.1016/j.pharep.2018.05.005
43. Inta D, Lang UE, Borgwardt S, Meyer-Lindenberg A, Gass P. Microglia activation and schizophrenia: lessons from the effects of minocycline on postnatal neurogenesis, neuronal survival and synaptic pruning. *Schizophr Bull.* (2017) 43:493–6. doi: 10.1093/schbul/sbw088
44. Dodd S, Maes M, Anderson G, Dean OM, Moylan S, Berk M. Putative neuroprotective agents in neuropsychiatric disorders. *Prog Neuro-Psychopharmacol Biol Psychiatry.* (2013) 2013:42. doi: 10.1016/j.pnpbp.2012.11.007
45. Allen KM, Fung SJ, Shannon Weickert C. Cell proliferation is reduced in the hippocampus in schizophrenia. *Austr N Zeal J Psychiatry.* (2016) 50:473–80. doi: 10.1177/0004867415589793
46. Reif A, Fritzen S, Finger M, Strobel A, Lauer M, Schmitt A, et al. Neural stem cell proliferation is decreased in schizophrenia, but not in depression. *Mol Psychiatry.* (2006) 11:514. doi: 10.1038/sj.mp.4001791
47. Müller N. Immunological aspects of the treatment of depression and schizophrenia. *Dialogues Clin Neurosci.* (2017) 19:55.
48. Sommer IE, van Westrhenen R, Begemann MJ, de Witte LD, Leucht S, Kahn RS. Efficacy of anti-inflammatory agents to improve symptoms in patients with schizophrenia: an update. *Schizophr Bull.* (2014) 40:181–91. doi: 10.1093/schbul/sbt139
49. Kulkarni J, Gavrilidis E, Wang W, Worsley R, Fitzgerald PB, Gurvich C, et al. Estradiol for treatment-resistant schizophrenia: a large-scale randomized-controlled trial in women of child-bearing age. *Mol Psychiatry.* (2015) 20:695–702. doi: 10.1038/mp.2014.33
50. Kulkarni J, Gavrilidis E, Gwini SM, Worsley R, Grigg J, Warren A, et al. Effect of adjunctive raloxifene therapy on severity of refractory schizophrenia in women: a randomized clinical trial. *JAMA Psychiatry.* (2016) 73:947–54. doi: 10.1001/jamapsychiatry.2016.1383
51. Laan W, Grobbee DE, Selten J-P, Heijnen CJ, Kahn RS, Burger H. Adjuvant aspirin therapy reduces symptoms of schizophrenia spectrum disorders: results from a randomized, double-blind, placebo-controlled trial [CME]. *J Clin Psychiatry.* (2010) 71:520. doi: 10.4088/JCP.09m05117yel
52. Guo C, Sun L, Chen X, Zhang D. Oxidative stress, mitochondrial damage and neurodegenerative diseases. *Neural Regenerat Res.* (2013) 8:2003–14. doi: 10.3969/j.issn.1673-5374.2013.21.009
53. Bhat AH, Dar KB, Anees S, Zargar MA, Masood A, Sofi MA, et al. Oxidative stress, mitochondrial dysfunction and neurodegenerative diseases; a mechanistic insight. *Biomed Pharmacother.* (2015) 74:101–10. doi: 10.1016/j.biopha.2015.07.025
54. Cataldo AM, McPhie DL, Lange NT, Punzell S, Elmiligy S, Ye NZ, et al. Abnormalities in mitochondrial structure in cells from patients with bipolar disorder. *Am J Pathol.* (2010) 177:575–85. doi: 10.2353/ajpath.2010.081068
55. Stork C, Renshaw PF. Mitochondrial dysfunction in bipolar disorder: evidence from magnetic resonance spectroscopy research. *Mol Psychiatry.* (2005) 10:900. doi: 10.1038/sj.mp.4001711
56. Konradi C, Ongur D. Role of mitochondria and energy metabolism in schizophrenia and psychotic disorders. *Schizophr Res.* (2017) 187:1–2. doi: 10.1016/j.schres.2017.07.007
57. Rajasekaran A, Venkatasubramanian G, Berk M, Debnath M. Mitochondrial dysfunction in schizophrenia: pathways, mechanisms and implications. *Neurosci Biobehav Rev.* (2015) 48:10–21. doi: 10.1016/j.neubiorev.2014.11.005
58. Roberts RC. Postmortem studies on mitochondria in schizophrenia. *Schizophr Res.* (2017) 187:17–25. doi: 10.1016/j.schres.2017.01.056
59. Inuwa IM, Peet M, Williams MA. QSAR modeling and transmission electron microscopy stereology of altered mitochondrial ultrastructure of white blood cells in patients diagnosed as schizophrenic and treated with antipsychotic drugs. *Biotech Histochem.* (2005) 80:133–7. doi: 10.1080/10520290500303349
60. Uranova N, Bonartsev P, Brusov O, Morozova M, Rachmanova V, Orlovskaya D. The ultrastructure of lymphocytes in schizophrenia. *World J Biol Psychiatry.* (2007) 8:30–7. doi: 10.1080/15622970600960207
61. Nasca C, Xenos D, Barone Y, Caruso A, Scaccianoce S, Matrisciano F, et al. L-acetylcarnitine causes rapid antidepressant effects through the epigenetic induction of mGlu2 receptors. *Proc Natl Acad Sci USA.* (2013) 110:4804–9. doi: 10.1073/pnas.1216100110
62. Delport A, Harvey BH, Petzer A, Petzer JP. Methylene blue and its analogues as antidepressant compounds. *Metabol Brain Dis.* (2017) 32:1357–82. doi: 10.1007/s11011-017-0081-6
63. Delport A, Harvey BH, Petzer A, Petzer JP. Methylene blue analogues with marginal monoamine oxidase inhibition retain antidepressant-like activity. *ACS Chem Neurosci.* (2018) 9:2917–28. doi: 10.1021/acschemneuro.8b00042
64. Pedraza-Chaverri J, Cárdenas-Rodríguez N, Orozco-Ibarra M, Pérez-Rojas JM. Medicinal properties of mangosteen (Garcinia mangostana). *Food Chem Toxicol.* (2008) 46:3227–39. doi: 10.1016/j.fct.2008.07.024
65. Moongkarndi P, Jaisupa N, Samer J, Kosem N, Konlata J, Rodpai E, et al. Comparison of the biological activity of two different isolates from mangosteen. *J Pharm Pharmacol.* (2014) 66:1171–9. doi: 10.1111/jphp.12239
66. Wang SN, Li Q, Jing MH, Alba E, Yang XH, Sabate R, et al. Natural xanthones from garcinia mangostana with multifunctional activities for the therapy of Alzheimer's disease. *Neurochem Res.* (2016) 41:1806–17. doi: 10.1007/s11064-016-1896-y
67. Yang R, Li P, Li N, Zhang Q, Bai X, Wang L, et al. Xanthones from the pericarp of garcinia mangostana. *Molecules.* (2017) 22:1–10. doi: 10.3390/molecules22050683
68. Cho BO, Ryu HW, So Y, Lee CW, Jin CH, Yook HS, et al. Anti-inflammatory effect of mangostenone F in lipopolysaccharide-stimulated RAW264.7 macrophages by suppressing NF-κB and MAPK activation. *Biomol Ther.* (2014) 22:288–94. doi: 10.4062/biomolther.2014.052
69. Ryu HW, Curtis-Long MJ, Jung S, Jin YM, Cho JK, Ryu YB, et al. Xanthones with neuraminidase inhibitory activity from the seedcases of Garcinia mangostana. *Bioorg Med Chem.* (2010) 18:6258–64. doi: 10.1016/j.bmc.2010.07.033
70. Karim AA, Azlan A. Fruit pod extracts as a source of nutraceuticals and pharmaceuticals. *Molecules.* (2012) 17:11931–46. doi: 10.3390/molecules171011931
71. Suttirak W, Manurakchinakorn S. *In vitro* antioxidant properties of mangosteen peel extract. *J Food Sci Technol.* (2014) 51:3546–58. doi: 10.1007/s13197-012-0887-5
72. Marquez-Valadez B, Lugo-Huitron R, Valdivia-Cerda V, Miranda-Ramirez LR, Perez-De La Cruz V, Gonzalez-Cuahutencos O, et al. The natural

xanthone alpha-mangostin reduces oxidative damage in rat brain tissue. *Nutr Neurosci.* (2009) 12:35–42. doi: 10.1179/147683009X388850

73. Marquez-Valadez B, Maldonado PD, Galvan-Arzate S, Mendez-Cuesta LA, Perez-De La Cruz V, Pedraza-Chaverri J, et al. Alpha-mangostin induces changes in glutathione levels associated with glutathione peroxidase activity in rat brain synaptosomes. *Nutr Neurosci.* (2012) 15:13–9. doi: 10.1179/147683012x13327575416400
74. Lee HN, Jang HY, Kim HJ, Shin SA, Choo GS, Park YS, et al. Antitumor and apoptosis-inducing effects of [alpha]-mangostin extracted from the pericarp of the mangosteen fruit (Garcinia mangostana L.) in YD-15 tongue mucoepidermoid carcinoma cells. *Int J Mol Med.* (2016) 4:939. doi: 10.3892/ijmm.2016.2517
75. Shin-Yu T, Pei-Chin C, Owaga EE, Tsai IJ, Pei-Yuan W, Jeng IT, et al. Alpha-mangostin from mangosteen (pericarp extract *Garcinia mangostana* Linn.) reduces high fat-diet induced hepatic steatosis in rats by regulating mitochondria function and apoptosis. *Nutr Metabol.* (2016) 13:1–10. doi: 10.1186/s12986-016-0148-0
76. Oberholzer I, Möller M, Holland B, Dean O, Berk M, Harvey B. Garcinia mangostana Linn diplay antidepressant-like and pro-coginitve effects in a genetic animal model of depresssion. *Metabol Brain Dis.* (2018) 33:467–80. doi: 10.1007/s11011-017-0144-8
77. Harvey B, Oberholzer I, Lotter J, Möller M, Holland B, Dean O, et al. Garcinia mangostana Linn displays antidepressant, antipsychotic and pro-cognitive effects in translational models of depression and schizophrenia: role of serotonin and immune-inflammatory cascades. In: *19th Congress of the International Serotonin Society*; 15-19 July 2018; University College Cork, Cork (2018).
78. Lotter J. *Studies on Garcinia mangostana Linn as a Therapeutic Intervention in an Immune-Inflammatory Model of Schizophrenia* [Master's thesis]. Potchefstroom: North-West University (2017).
79. Nava Catorce M, Acero G, Pedraza-Chaverri J, Fragoso G, Govezensky T, Gevorkian G. Alpha-mangostin attenuates brain inflammation induced by peripheral lipopolysaccharide administration in C57BL/6J mice. *J Neuroimmunol.* 297:20–7. doi: 10.1016/j.jneuroim.2016.05.008
80. Gutierrez-Orozco F, Chitchumroonchokchai C, Lesinski GB, Suksamrarn S, Failla ML. alpha-Mangostin: anti-inflammatory activity and metabolism by human cells. *J Agric Food Chem.* (2013) 61:3891–900. doi: 10.1021/jf4004434
81. Tewtrakul S, Wattanapiromsakul C, Mahabusarakam W. Effects of compounds from Garcinia mangostana on inflammatory mediators in RAW264.7 macrophage cells. *J Ethnopharmacol.* (2009) 121:379–82. doi: 10.1016/j.jep.2008.11.007
82. Chen L-G, Yang L-L, Wang C-C. Anti-inflammatory activity of mangostins from Garcinia mangostana. *Food Chem Toxicol.* (2008) 2:688. doi: 10.1016/j.fct.2007.09.096
83. Bumrungpert A, Kalpravidh RW, Chuang CC, Overman A, Martinez K, Kennedy A, et al. Xanthones from mangosteen inhibit inflammation in human macrophages and in human adipocytes exposed to macrophage-conditioned media. *J Nutr.* (2010) 140:842–7. doi: 10.3945/jn.109.120022
84. Hu Z, Wang W, Ling J, Jiang C. α-mangostin inhibits alpha-synuclein-induced microglial neuroinflammation and neurotoxicity. *Cell Mol Neurobiol.* (2016) 36:811–20. doi: 10.1007/s10571-015-0264-9
85. Weecharangsan W, Opanasopit P, Sukma M, Ngawhirunpat T, Sotanaphun U, Siripong P. Antioxidative and neuroprotective activities of extracts from the fruit hull of mangosteen (Garcinia mangostana Linn.). *Med Principles Pract.* (2006) 15:281–7. doi: 10.1159/000092991
86. Janhom P, Dharmasaroja P. Neuroprotective effects of alpha-mangostin on MPP(+)-induced apoptotic cell death in neuroblastoma SH-SY5Y cells. *J Toxicol.* (2015) 2015:919058. doi: 10.1155/2015/919058
87. Phyu MP, Tangpong J. Neuroprotective effects of xanthone derivative of Garcinia mangostana against lead-induced acetylcholinesterase dysfunction and cognitive impairment. *Food chemical Toxicol.* (2014) 70:151–6. doi: 10.1016/j.fct.2014.04.035
88. Sattayasai J, Chaonapan P, Arkaravichie T, Soi-Ampornkul R, Junnu S, Charoensilp P, et al. Protective effects of mangosteen extract on H2O2-induced cytotoxicity in SK-N-SH cells and scopolamine-induced memory impairment in mice. *PLoS ONE.* (2013) 8:e85053. doi: 10.1371/journal.pone.0085053
89. Wihastuti TA, Sargowo D, Tjokroprawiro A, Permatasari N, Widodo MA, Soeharto S. Vasa vasorum anti-angiogenesis through H(2)O(2), HIF-1alpha, NF-kappaB, and iNOS inhibition by mangosteen pericarp ethanolic extract (*Garcinia mangostana Linn*) in hypercholesterol-diet-given Rattus norvegicus Wistar strain. *Vasc Health Risk Manag.* (2014) 10:523–31. doi: 10.2147/vhrm.s61736
90. Huang HJ, Chen WL, Hsieh RH, Hsieh-Li HM. Multifunctional effects of mangosteen pericarp on cognition in C57BL/6J and triple transgenic alzheimer's mice. *Evid Based Complement Alternat Med.* (2014) 2014:813672. doi: 10.1155/2014/813672
91. Jariyapongskul A, Areebambud C, Suksamrarn S, Mekseepralard C. Alpha-mangostin attenuation of hyperglycemia-induced ocular hypoperfusion and blood retinal barrier leakage in the early stage of type 2 diabetes rats. *BioMed Res Int.* (2015) 2015:785826. doi: 10.1155/2015/785826
92. Aisha AF, Abu-Salah KM, Ismail Z, Majid AM. *In vitro* and *in vivo* anti-colon cancer effects of Garcinia mangostana xanthones extract. *BMC Complement Alternat Med.* (2012) 12:104. doi: 10.1186/1472-6882-12-104
93. Tang YP, Li PG, Kondo M, Ji HP, Kou Y, Ou B. Effect of a mangosteen dietary supplement on human immune function: a randomized, double-blind, placebo-controlled trial. *J Med Food.* (2009) 12:755–63. doi: 10.1089/jmf.2008.0204
94. Xie Z, Sintara M, Chang T, Ou B. Daily consumption of a mangosteen-based drink improves *in vivo* antioxidant and anti-inflammatory biomarkers in healthy adults: a randomized, double-blind, placebo-controlled clinical trial. *Food Sci Nutr.* (2015) 3:342–8. doi: 10.1002/fsn3.225
95. Udani JK, Singh BB, Barrett ML, Singh VJ. Evaluation of Mangosteen juice blend on biomarkers of inflammation in obese subjects: a pilot, dose finding study. *Nutr J.* (2009) 8:48. doi: 10.1186/1475-2891-8-48
96. Chairungsrilerd N, Furukawa K, Ohta T, Nozoe S, Ohizumi Y. Histaminergic and serotonergic receptor blocking substances from the medicinal plant Garcinia mangostana. *Plant Med.* (1996) 62:471–2. doi: 10.1055/s-2006-957943
97. Celada P, Puig MV, Amargós-Bosch M, Adell A, Artigas F. The therapeutic role of 5-HT(1A) and 5-HT(2A) receptors in depression. *J Psychiatry Neurosci.* (2004) 29:252–65.
98. Garrity AR, Morton GA, Morton JC. *Nutraceutical Mangosteen Composition.* Google Patents (2013).
99. Chin YW, Kinghorn AD. Structural characterization, biological effects, and synthetic studies on xanthones from mangosteen (*Garcinia mangostana*), a popular botanical dietary supplement. *Mini Rev Organic Chem.* (2008) 5:355–64. doi: 10.2174/157019308786242223
100. Krstenansky JL. Mesembrine alkaloids: review of their occurrence, chemistry, and pharmacology. *J Ethnopharmacol.* (2017) 195:10–9. doi: 10.1016/j.jep.2016.12.004
101. Zhu J, Mix E, Winblad B. The antidepressant and antiinflammatory effects of rolipram in the central nervous system. *CNS Drug Rev.* (2001) 7:387–98. doi: 10.1111/j.1527-3458.2001.tb00206.x
102. Harvey BH, Joubert C, du Preez JL, Berk M. Effect of chronic N-acetyl cysteine administration on oxidative status in the presence and absence of induced oxidative stress in rat striatum. *Neurochem Res.* (2008) 33:508–17. doi: 10.1007/s11064-007-9466-y
103. Harvey BH. Affective disorders and nitric oxide: a role in pathways to relapse and refractoriness? *Hum Psychopharmacol.* (1996) 11:309–19. doi: 10.1002/(SICI)1099-1077(199607)11:4<309::AID-HUP775>3.0.CO;2-B
104. Wegener G, Volke V, Harvey BH, Rosenberg R. Local, but not systemic, administration of serotonergic antidepressants decreases hippocampal nitric oxide synthase activity. *Brain Res.* (2003) 959:128–34. doi: 10.1016/S0006-8993(02)03738-1
105. Nel A, Harvey BH. Haloperidol-induced dyskinesia is associated with striatal NO synthase suppression: reversal with olanzapine. *Behav Pharmacol.* (2003) 14:251–5. doi: 10.1097/01.fbp.0000073700.15098.b3
106. Cao B, Bauer IE, Sharma AN, Mwangi B, Frazier T, Lavagnino L, et al. Reduced hippocampus volume and memory performance in bipolar disorder patients carrying the BDNF val66met met allele. *J Affect Disord.* (2016) 198:198–205. doi: 10.1016/j.jad.2016.03.044

107. Möller M, Du Preez JL, Viljoen FP, Berk M, Harvey BH. N-Acetyl cysteine reverses social isolation rearing induced changes in cortico-striatal monoamines in rats. *Metabol Brain Dis.* (2013) 28:687–96. doi: 10.1007/s11011-013-9433-z
108. Möller M, Du Preez JL, Viljoen FP, Berk M, Emsley R, Harvey BH. Social isolation rearing induces mitochondrial, immunological, neurochemical and behavioural deficits in rats, and is reversed by clozapine or N-acetyl cysteine. *Brain Behav Immun.* (2013) 30:156–67. doi: 10.1016/j.bbi.2012.12.011
109. Chang C-W, Huang T-Z, Chang W-H, Tseng Y-C, Wu Y-T, Hsu M-C. Acute Garcinia mangostana (mangosteen) supplementation does not alleviate physical fatigue during exercise: a randomized, double-blind, placebo-controlled, crossover trial. *J Int Soc Sports Nutr.* (2016) 13:1–8. doi: 10.1186/s12970-016-0132-0
110. Watanabe M, Gangitano E, Francomano D, Addessi E, Toscano R, Costantini D, et al. Mangosteen extract shows a potent insulin sensitizing effect in obese female patients: a prospective randomized controlled pilot study. *Nutrients.* (2018) 10:586. doi: 10.3390/nu10050586
111. Kudiganti V, Kodur RR, Kodur SR, Halemane M, Deep DK. Efficacy and tolerability of Meratrim for weight management: a randomized, double-blind, placebo-controlled study in healthy overweight human subjects. *Lipids Health Dis.* (2016) 15:136. doi: 10.1186/s12944-016-0306-4
112. Laupu WK. *The Efficacy of Garcinia mangostana L. (mangosteen) Pericarp as an Adjunctive to Second Generation Antipsychotics for the Treatment of Schizophrenia: A Double Blind, Randomised, Placebo-Controlled Trial* [Doctoral Dissertation]: James Cook University (2014).
113. Stern JS, Peerson J, Mishra AT, Sadasiva Rao MV, Rajeswari KP. Efficacy and tolerability of a novel herbal formulation for weight management. *Obesity.* (2013) 21:921–7. doi: 10.1002/oby.20211
114. Tousian Shandiz H, Razavi BM, Hosseinzadeh H. Review of Garcinia mangostana and its xanthones in metabolic syndrome and related complications. *Phytother Res.* (2017) 31:1173–82. doi: 10.1002/ptr.5862
115. Taher M, Tg Zakaria TM, Susanti D, Zakaria ZA. Hypoglycaemic activity of ethanolic extract of Garcinia mangostana Linn. in normoglycaemic and streptozotocin-induced diabetic rats. *BMC Complement Alternat Med.* (2016) 16:135. doi: 10.1186/s12906-016-1118-9
116. Suthammarak W, Numpraphrut P, Charoensakdi R, Neungton N, Tunrungruangtavee V, Jaisupa N, et al. Antioxidant-enhancing property of the polar fraction of mangosteen pericarp extract and evaluation of its safety in humans. *Oxid Med Cell Longevity.* (2016) 2016:1293036. doi: 10.1155/2016/1293036
117. Perez-Rojas JM, Cruz C, Garcia-Lopez P, Sanchez-Gonzalez DJ, Martinez-Martinez CM, Ceballos G, et al. Renoprotection by alpha-Mangostin is related to the attenuation in renal oxidative/nitrosative stress induced by cisplatin nephrotoxicity. *Free Radic Res.* (2009) 43:1122–32. doi: 10.1080/10715760903214447
118. Turner A, McGrath JJ, Dean OM, Dodd S, Baker A, Cotton SM, et al. Protocol and rationale: a 24-week double-blind, randomised, placebo controlled trial of the efficacy of adjunctive *Garcinia mangostana* Linn.(mangosteen) pericarp for schizophrenia. *Clin Psychopharmacol Neurosci.* (2018). [Epub ahead of print].
119. Ashton MM, Berk M, Ng CH, Hopwood M, Dodd S, Turner A, et al. Efficacy of adjunctive Garcinia mangostana Linn (mangosteen) pericarp for bipolar depression: study protocol for a proof-of-concept trial. *Braz J Psychiatry.* (2018) 2018:114. doi: 10.1590/1516-4446-2018-0114

4

Microglial Phagocytosis of Neurons: Diminishing Neuronal Loss in Traumatic, Infectious, Inflammatory, and Autoimmune CNS Disorders

*Samuel F. Yanuck**

Program on Integrative Medicine, Department of Physical Medicine and Rehabilitation, University of North Carolina School of Medicine, Chapel Hill, NC, United States

Correspondence:
Samuel F. Yanuck
syanuck@yanuckcenter.com

Errors in neuron-microglial interaction are known to lead to microglial phagocytosis of live neurons and excessive neuronal loss, potentially yielding poorer clinical outcomes. Factors that affect neuron-microglial interaction have the potential to influence the error rate. Clinical comorbidities that unfavorably impact neuron-microglial interaction may promote a higher rate of neuronal loss, to the detriment of patient outcome. This paper proposes that many common, clinically modifiable comorbidities have a common thread, in that they all influence neuron-microglial interactions. Comorbidities like traumatic brain injury, infection, stress, neuroinflammation, loss of neuronal metabolic integrity, poor growth factor status, and other factors, all have the potential to alter communication between neurons and microglia. When this occurs, microglial phagocytosis of live neurons can increase. In addition, microglia can shift into a morphological form in which they express major histocompatibility complex II (MHC-II), allowing them to function as antigen presenting cells that present neuronal debris as antigen to invading T cells. This can increase risk for the development of CNS autoimmunity, or can exacerbate existing CNS autoimmunity. The detrimental influence of these comorbidities has the potential to contribute to the mosaic of factors that determine patient outcome in some CNS pathologies that have neuropsychiatric involvement, including TBI and CNS disorders with autoimmune components, where excessive neuronal loss can yield poorer clinical outcomes. Recognition of the impact of these comorbidities may contribute to an understanding of the common clinical observation that many seemingly disparate factors contribute to the overall picture of case management and clinical outcome in these complex disorders. In a clinical setting, knowing how these comorbidities can influence neuron-microglial interaction can help focus surveillance and care on a broader group of potential therapeutic targets. Accordingly, an interest in the mechanisms underlying the influence of these factors on neuron-microglial interactions is appropriate. Neuron-microglial interaction is reviewed, and the various mechanisms by which these potential comorbidities influence neuro-microglial interaction are described.

Keywords: depression, microglia, neuron, autoimmunity, inflammation, traumatic brain injury, cytokine, excitotoxicity

INTRODUCTION

Impaired neuronal function (1–4), from neuroinflammation or other causes, is a known driver of depression and related neuropsychiatric problems (5–11) that often accompany complex CNS disorders, including TBI (12, 13) and CNS disorders with autoimmune components (14), such as multiple sclerosis (MS) (15, 16), Parkinson's disease (PD) (17–19), and Pediatric Acute-onset Neuropsychiatric Syndrome (PANS)/Pediatric Autoimmune Neuropsychiatric Disorders Associated with Streptococcal Infections (PANDAS) (20). A recent twin study by Huang, et al, suggests that the causal connection between depression and neuroinflammation may be bidirectional. (21)

Neuronal impairment can occur with insults to brain function from trauma, as with TBI (reviewed in 22), or can be metabolic or immunological, as with neuroinflammation (5–11), loss of neuronal cellular metabolic integrity [reviewed in Ref. (23)], infection [reviewed in Ref. (24)], or autoimmune response to neuronal targets.

Neuronal impairment can also occur due to dysfunction of neuronal autophagy, the mechanism by which neurons repair themselves *via* autodigestive recycling of damaged organelles and other cellular constituents (25). The association between impaired neuronal autophagy and Alzheimer's disease (AD) has been reviewed by Uddin, et al. (26). The association between impaired autophagy and PD has been reviewed by Sheehan and Yue (27), and with neurodegeneration by Menzies (28). Plaza-Zabala et al, have proposed that the dysregulation of autophagy in microglia affects their capacity for phagocytosis and affects whether they adopt an inflammatory morphology, with implications for aging and neurodegenerative diseases (29). Yoshii and Mizushima have reviewed the practical impediments to measuring autophagy in humans (30).

Both traumatic and non-traumatic insults to brain can trigger mechanisms of ongoing neuronal destruction that are inherently immunological, as microglial cells phagocytize live but marginally functioning neurons (31). Details of the signaling mechanisms that instigate this process have been described by Fricker et al. (32) and by Neher et al. (33), cited in Galloway et al. (34).

Neuron – microglial signaling can be influenced by neuroinflammation, metabolic impairment, and microglial activation. In cases involving autoimmune processes, the clinical outcome also depends on appropriate ongoing immune modulation. In cases involving an infectious etiology, maintenance of a non-infected status may be crucial to favorable patient outcome. These processes are themselves influenced by a group of known comorbidities, whose biological influences have been described.

It is this author's contention that, in a clinical setting, knowing how comorbidities that affect neuron-microglial signaling can influence patient biology may create the potential for clinical advantage in patients with neuropsychiatric disorders, through clinical attention to seemingly disparate factors like exercise, reducing inflammation, neurotransmitter (NT) support, stress reduction, and inhibition of autoimmune attack of self-tissue. While these clinical interventions involve many complex factors, they share an influence on the fundamentally convergent core mechanisms governing neuron-microglial interaction, some by supporting intact neuronal metabolism in support of adequate neuronal firing rate (frequency of action potentials) and NT release (exercise, NT support, glycemic control, oxygenation, etc.), some by reducing neuroinflammation (stress reduction, elimination of infection, etc.), some by other mechanisms. Understanding the details of neuron-microglial interactions may be of use in identifying specific factors involved in a given patient's case and matching clinical interventions to specific targets that appear to be involved in dysregulating neuron-microglial interaction. This may help sharpen efforts to help patients with difficult neuroimmunological disorders, for whom prognosis is often suboptimal.

NEURON-MICROGLIAL INTERACTIONS IN THE HEALTHY BRAIN

Many studies acknowledge the role of neuroinflammation as a causal factor in the biology of depression (5–11). Neuroinflammation has profound effects on neuron - microglial interactions. To better understand the clinical implications of neuron - microglial interactions and their application in neuropsychiatric disorders, we discuss here the biology of neuron - microglial interactions and the factors affecting these interactions that can be influenced in the clinical setting.

The origin and development of microglia have been reviewed in detail by Ginhoux et al. (35). Microglial cells are specialized macrophages (36). They are the predominant immune cells in the healthy brain (37). They arise from CD45+ bone marrow precursors that colonize the fetal brain, where they migrate from the periphery during fetal development. Parenchymal microglia are uncommitted myeloid progenitors of immature dendritic cells and macrophages (38). Once established in the CNS parenchyma, microglia are sustained by proliferation of resident progenitors, independent of blood cells (39). It has been estimated that 13% of the CNS white matter consists of microglial cells (40). The functional plasticity of microglial cells that allows them to carry out a broad repertoire of activities has been reviewed by Gomez-Nicola and Perry (41). Microglia perform continuous surveillance on neurons (34, 35, 42, 43). The pruning of synapses by microglia is an essential part of normal brain development (44).

Normal pruning of synapses during brain development involves the elimination of excess or inappropriate neuronal connections, in support of a properly organized brain (44). In adulthood, synaptic pruning is part of the neural plasticity involved in learning (45). Galván describes the synaptic pruning that occurs in brain development and that of adults as occurring on a continuum (45). These are normal processes, in contrast with the excessive microglial phagocytosis of live neurons that is a primary effect of the altered neuron-microglial signaling with which this paper chiefly concerns itself (31).

Errors yielding excessive or deficient synaptic pruning during childhood brain development have been associated with neurodevelopmental disorders, including autism, epilepsy, and schizophrenia (46). Stress and its potential to induce neuroinflammation has been discussed by O'Connor, et al, as playing a potentially damaging role in brain development, increasing susceptibility to behavioral disorders in the pediatric population (47). Kariuki et al. have shown that infection early in life is associated with impairment of multiple aspects of childhood development (48). A meta-analysis by Khandaker et al. has shown an association between childhood CNS viral infection and later development of schizophrenia, which they describe as involving either direct pathogen influences or influences of the inflammatory process associated with the infection (49). Miller et al. have shown an association between dyslexia, a developmental disorder, and later development of some variants of progressive aphasia, a form of dementia (50). Neurons are also continuously lost in the healthy adult brain. Among several functions provided by microglial surveillance is the elimination by phagocytosis of the apoptotic bodies of these dead and dying neurons. Sowell et al. state that "A decline in gray matter volume is prominent between adulthood and old age, whereas white matter volume increases between 19 and 40 years, after which it steadily declines" [Ref. (51), citing Refs. (52–54)]. The normal process of neuronal loss thus presents a requirement for phagocytosis and clearance of apoptotic neurons by microglia, so that the neurons do not progress into secondary necrosis, a state that is highly inflammatory (55). Just as stone is removed during the creation of a sculpture, the daily loss of neurons during brain development is a normal function, leading to the emergence of the healthy adult brain. This pattern of neuronal loss continues in the adult. If the rate of neuronal loss is modest, the adult brain can maintain healthy function.

However, at any age, microglial morphology can change, disrupting the healthy homeostatic balance between neurons and microglia, and leading to excessive neuroinflammation, triggering or promoting the progression of neuronal loss and brain-based autoimmune processes such as MS, PD, dementia, PANS/PANDAS, and chronic traumatic encephalopathy (CTE) (56–60).

The Error Rate

There are billions of neurons in the brain, and a comparable number of microglial cells (61, 62). Microglia perform continuous surveillance on neurons (34, 35, 42, 43). Using *in vivo* two-photon imaging of the neocortex, Nimmerjahn et al. (43), observed that "microglial cells are highly active in their presumed resting state, continually surveying their microenvironment with extremely motile processes and protrusions." Kierdorf, describing both Nimmerjahn (43) and another two photon imaging study by Davalos et al. (63), states that, "two-photon microscopy imaging revealed a strict territorial organization of microglia *in vivo*... the processes of each microglial cell are highly dynamic, and retract and extend to sample the surrounding CNS. The sampling is highly random and has a high turnover rate, such that each microglia can sample the CNS parenchyma once in a few hours."

The presence of billions of neurons, a comparable number of microglia, and the observation that microglia are "continually surveying" neurons, with microglia surveying the CNS parenchyma once in a few hours, suggests a number of surveillance events per day that is also in the billions.

In each of these surveillance events, a microglial cell senses a neuron *via* multiple signals. The microglial cell will either phagocytize or be inhibited from phagocytizing the neuron, based on the balance of these activating and inhibiting signals (32–34, 63–65). As Brown and Neher have described, microglial cells can incorrectly phagocytize "stressed but viable neurons," an event they have termed "phagoptosis," citing evidence that suggests phagoptosis can contribute to neuronal loss during brain development, inflammation, ischemia and neurodegeneration. The number of times that microglial cells commit these errors in phagocytic execution is a function of all of the inputs that determine the extent of phagoptosis. The higher the error rate, the more live neurons are inappropriately phagocytized, yielding a greater expression of dysfunction [reviewed by Brown and Neher (31)]. In some patients, this may be expressed as neuronal loss leading to dementia, CTE, or other inflammatory disorders. In other patients, the chief feature may be an expression of autoimmune process, discussed below. In either case, the expression of dysfunction centers on the change in neuron-microglial interaction, the change in microglial morphology, and the interactions of these two processes.

BIOLOGY OF NEURON-MICROGLIAL INTERACTIONS

Neuron-microglial interaction is bidirectional and involves two key mechanisms. The first is the set of factors driven by neuronal membrane bound factors like phosphatidyl-serine (PS) and substances released by neurons, like cytokines, neurotransmitters, and other immunological factors. These factors determine the extent of microglial phagocytosis of neurons and determine other features of microglial morphology.

The second key mechanism regulated *via* neuron-microglial interaction is the expression of major histocompatibility complex II (MHC-II) on the surface of microglia. This step enables microglia to function as antigen-presenting cells (APCs) and potentially activate T cell immunity. In the normal brain, microglia induce apoptosis (programmed cell death) in T cells that enter the brain, *via* ligation of CD95, aka FAS (FS-7-associated surface antigen) (66).

Macrophages are capable of substantial plasticity and can change their physiology in response to environmental cues, yielding populations of cells with distinct functions, which can promote or suppress inflammation (36). Of particular interest is the transformation of a microglial cell from a phagocytic macrophage morphology to an APC morphology. Antigen presentation capability in the brain is provided by microglial cells, not by the dendritic cells that serve this function in the periphery (40). This capability is necessary for proper immune surveillance against pathogenic organisms in the brain. However, if the microglial cell presents fragments of neuronal debris as antigen to T cells that have invaded the brain, autoimmune process in the brain can be initiated or promoted.

Microglia in the Healthy Brain

In the healthy brain, microglial cells phagocytize apoptotic neurons and prune synapses of live neurons in a way that promotes neuronal function and brain health (31). As is the case with macrophage phagocytosis of apoptotic cells in the periphery, phagocytosis of apoptotic neurons by microglia yields production and secretion of anti-inflammatory cytokines that are released into the local brain parenchyma (66). During neuronal repair, phagocytic microglia clean up debris from injured neurites and secrete neurotrophic substances, such as brain derived neurotrophic factor (BDNF), to enhance repair (67). Ayata et al. have recently found evidence that the polycomb repressive complex 2 (PRC2) epigenetically restricts the expression of genes that support microglial clearance of neurons in the striatum and cortex (68). Brown and Neher point out that the healthy brain is relatively free of invading T cells, which are kept out of the brain by the intact blood brain barrier (BBB). Brain inflammation, which occurs behind the BBB, therefore differs from inflammation in the periphery by the relative absence of leukocytes (including neutrophils, monocytes, B cells, and T cells) and antibodies (37).

In addition to the maintenance of a healthy non-inflammatory brain parenchymal environment, glial cells, along with neurons, express cellular death signals including CD95Fas/CD95L (aka FasL), tumor necrosis factor-related apoptosis-inducing ligand (TRAIL) and TNF receptor (TNFR). These cellular death signals trigger apoptosis of T cells and other infiltrating cells (66). In the healthy brain, microglia and astrocytes also express FasL, which also induces apoptosis in T cells that migrate from the periphery into the brain (69). Induction of T cell apoptosis is an important housekeeping mechanism by which microglial cells eliminate invading T cells that could otherwise participate in the autoimmune activation processes.

Microglia in the Dysfunctioning Brain

The first activity of microglia that adversely affects neurons occurs when microglia are acting as phagocytic cells, engaging in inappropriate phagocytosis of neurons. Brown and Neher have shown that microglia can execute neuronal death by phagocytizing stressed-but-viable neurons, which they have termed "phagoptosis" (31). It is noteworthy that mast cell-microglial interactions can play an important role in microglial activity. This has been reviewed by Skaper et al. (70).

The second activity of microglia that adversely affects neurons occurs when microglia act as APCs, presenting neuronal debris as antigen to invading T cells. In inflammatory and neurodegenerative diseases, including MS, infections, trauma, stroke, neoplasia, and Alzheimer's disease, glial cells such as microglia gain antigen-presenting capacity through the expression of MHC molecules (71).

Experimental autoimmune encephalomyelitis (EAE) is the mouse model used to study MS. In an EAE model, Ponomarev et al. found that microglial activation occurred before the onset of disease symptoms and infiltration of peripheral myeloid cells into the CNS, suggesting that resident glial cells were involved in the initiation of disease. They found further that activated microglial cells underwent proliferation and up-regulated the expression of CD45, MHC-II, CD40, CD86, and the dendritic cell marker CD11c. At the peak of EAE disease, activated microglial cells comprised 37% of the total macrophage and dendritic cell populations and co-localized with infiltrating leukocytes in inflammatory lesions (72).

MHC-II, CD40, and CD86 are all required for antigen presentation and co-activation in the signaling between microglial cells and T cells. Expression of these markers and of the dendritic cell marker CD11c, clearly demonstrates the shift in microglial morphology to a dendritic-cell-like APC morphology, in which presentation of neuronal debris as antigen can trigger or promote brain-based autoimmunity. Co-localization of invading T cells with microglia is a hallmark of microglial APC behavior (40). An antigen presentation capacity is necessary to the clearance of pathogens from the brain, and experimental inhibition of these functions yields catastrophic effects in animal models (73). Nonetheless, imbalance in this mechanism can yield up-regulation of neuro-autoimmunity (see **Table 1**).

Mechanisms of Neuron-Microglial Regulation

The key feature of healthy neuron microglial homeostasis is that microglial cells correctly identify and phagocytize only the neurons going through normal, apoptotic cell death. Viable neurons are left alone or repaired if necessary. Apoptosis of dying neurons is non-inflammatory (74).

In the healthy brain, regulation of this process is accomplished by signals produced by neurons that affect microglial cell behavior. However, changes in either neurological or immunological factors can disrupt this homeostasis.

Neural Self-Control

Neurons control the behavior of microglial cells through a repertoire of signals, some membrane bound and some released into the surrounding environment. At the center of this moving multi-variable equation is phosphatidylserine (PS). PS in the normal cell sits on the inner wall of the cell membrane. When the cell undergoes apoptosis, PS is flipped to the outer cell membrane, where it is visible to other cells (32–34, 63, 65). This change signals macrophages that the cell is undergoing apoptosis, and is a candidate for phagocytosis by the macrophage. Throughout the body, macrophages perform surveillance on cells in the surrounding environment by palpating them. This is true of microglial surveillance of neurons as well. When neurons flip PS to their outer membrane, where it is then encountered *via* microglial cell palpation, the microglial cell is triggered to phagocytize the neuron. PS is normally confined to the inner cell membrane in intact neurons because the neurons continuously move it from the outer to the inner membrane using a group of phosphatidylserine translocases, which have been identified as the type 4 P-type ATPases (31).

In addition to PS and factors related to its recognition, other signal molecules affect neuron-microglial interaction. Biber et al. describe neuronal "Off" signals that keep microglia in their

TABLE 1 | Microglial functions in the inflamed and non-inflamed brain.

Normal non-inflamed brain	Inflamed brain
Housekeeping microglial functions	Potentially problematic microglial functions
• Repair damaged neurons • Phagocytize apoptotic neurons • Inhibit inflammation • Induce apoptosis in invading T cells	• Phagocytize live but impaired neurons • Express MHC II • Present fragments of neuronal debris to invading T cells • Promote autoimmune process in brain

resting state and reduce pro-inflammatory activity, and "On" signals that are inducible, including purines, chemokines, and glutamate. Thus, Biber et al. describe neurons as key immune modulators in the brain (64).

Microglial uptake of pathogen associated molecular patterns (PAMPs) from pathogens in the brain or damage associated molecular patterns (DAMPs) from neuronal debris contributes to NFκB activation. Simultaneous activation of phagocyte NADPH oxidase (PHOX) and inducible nitric oxide synthase (iNOS) in microglia resulted in the disappearance of nitric oxide (NO), appearance of peroxynitrite and apoptosis. However, the chronic state of activation may progress to "resolution phase" where microglia are amoeboid, highly phagocytic, and produce anti-inflammatory cytokines (including IL-10 and TGFβ) in order to resolve the inflammation and clear up the debris (36).

In a healthy brain, the interplay of neurons and microglia is balanced. Healthy, viable neurons produce adequate "OFF" signals to repel microglial phagocytic interest. These include TGFβ, which inhibits effector T cell activation, neurotransmitters, which constitute a signal that a neuron is active, BDNF and other trophic factors, as well as factors that inhibit microglial inflammation and neurotoxicity. Neurons undergoing apoptosis in the normal brain produce "ON" signals, attracting microglial cells and promoting phagocytosis of the apoptotic neurons. These include glutamate that drives tumor necrosis factor alpha (TNFα) release and neuroexcitotoxicity, microglial chemoattractants like CCL21 and CXCL10, ATP that promotes chemoattraction and interleukin-1β (IL-1β) release, and others. When microglia phagocytize apoptotic neurons, they secrete TGFβ, which promotes a tolerogenic, anti-inflammatory tissue environment (74).

Normally, the non-phlogistic (non-inflammatory) microglial phagocytosis of apoptotic neurons involves engulfment and digestion of the neuron without release of additional neuronal debris into the tissue environment. The microglial cell produces anti-inflammatory cytokines that shift the surrounding tissue toward resolution of inflammation. If instead the neuron undergoes primary necrosis through direct or indirect trauma, or exposure to a pathogen or toxin, its death releases cell fragments and cytosolic contents into the tissue environment. The extracellular appearance of ATP and other intracellular contents triggers a pro-inflammatory response in surrounding microglia. In addition, incompletely digested/disassembled neuronal debris can be taken up by microglia and presented as antigen to invading T cells, promoting brain-based autoimmunity.

FACTORS AFFECTING THE BIOCHEMISTRY OF "ON" AND "OFF" SIGNALING IN NEURONS AND MICROGLIA

Each of the factors described in this section affect the biochemistry of "On" and "Off" signaling through impacts on the underlying biology of neurons and microglial cells, shifting the function of neurons or microglia in a way that alters the overall sum of influences.

Changes Affecting Outer Membrane PS Expression

Brown and Neher (31) describe several factors that can drive PS exposure, promoting apoptosis of neurons by microglia. These include ATP depletion, inhibition of phosphatidylserine translocases by oxidative stress, and increased calcium levels. All three of these conditions are commonly found in the clinical setting, including in patients with neuropsychiatric issues arising from head trauma, chronic neuroinflammation, or autoimmune disorders affecting brain. These biological processes represent potentially modifiable treatment targets.

Brown and Neher go on to assert that reversible phosphatidylserine exposure can occur in stressed-but-viable neurons as a result of non-toxic levels of glutamate, oxidative stress, or growth-factor withdrawal (31).

Brown and Neher state that phagocytosis of neurons with exposed phosphatidylserine can be mediated *via* several microglial receptors and opsonins, some of which are strongly upregulated by inflammation (31). This suggests again that modulation of brain inflammation represents a potentially modifiable treatment target. Brown and Neher state that, "...during inflammation, microglia and astrocytes release increased amounts of milk fat globule EGF factor 8 (MFG-E8; also known as lactadherin or SED1), which tightly binds to exposed phosphatidylserine through its C1 and C2 domains and to microglial vitronectin receptors (VNRs)—αvβ3 or αvβ5 integrins—through an RGD motif. The resulting activation of VNRs induces phagocytosis by activating a CRKII–DOCK180–RAC1 signaling pathway that causes remodeling of the microglial actin cytoskeleton." They further state that, "On neurons, calreticulin exposure promotes their phagocytosis by binding to microglial low-density lipoprotein receptor-related protein (LRP), probably in association with other signals. In addition, the complement components C1q and C3, which are produced by microglia and astrocytes, may induce phagocytosis by binding to altered neuronal surfaces" (31).

Lunnon et al. have shown that systemic inflammation upregulates Fc receptors, including activating FcγRIII and FcγRIV, but not the inhibitory FcγRII. They conclude that, "systemic inflammation during chronic neurodegeneration increases the expression levels of activating FcγR on microglia and thereby lowers the signaling threshold for Ab-mediated cell activation" (75).

Huizinga et al. have shown that, in MS, fragments of axonal debris are taken up by microglial cells and degraded, a process that appears to support neuronal debris clearance, but that the authors describe as potentially playing a role in augmenting autoimmunity to neuronal antigens (76).

Changes in Neuronal Metabolic Integrity Affecting Multiple Factors

Mitochondrial ATP production stands at the center of cellular function in all cells, including neurons. The success of the neuron in carrying out ATP production determines the success of all other cellular functions. If the neuron cannot produce ATP, it cannot continue to pump PS from its outer membrane to its inner membrane; nor can it produce adequate neurotransmitters, growth factors, or other "OFF" signals. If this occurs, the likelihood of apoptosis of live but metabolically compromised neurons is increased. This may increase the rate of phagocytosis errors, favoring more frequent microglial phagocytosis of live neurons whose ATP production is compromised (31).

Inflammation, oxidative stress, and persistently excessive production of epinephrine associated with stress have all been shown to be associated with mitochondrial dysfunction (77–79).

At the simplest level, neurons require stimulation, oxygen, and glucose. Impairment of any of these functions will diminish metabolic integrity.

Adequate glucose is required for the normal function of all cells, including neurons. Glycemic dysregulation in diabetes, hypoglycemia, insulin resistance and other such conditions can impair systemic and consequently CNS glucose levels. Many diabetic patients also have microcirculatory problems, compounding blood glucose issues with poor circulatory delivery of oxygen and glucose.

Likewise, CNS oxygen levels can be impaired by respiratory disorders like asthma and COPD, by cerebrovascular disorders, or by systemic microcirculatory disorders that also affect brain.

Fumagalli et al. reviewed changes that occur with hypoperfusion in the brain, such as can occur with stroke or TIA, leading to hypoxia, which causes excitotoxicity, oxidative stress, BBB dysfunction, microvascular injury, hemostatic activation, post-ischemic inflammation and neuronal death. Fumagalli et al. go on to say that these events contribute to changing the ischemic environment over time and, consequently, the behavior of microglia and macrophages (80).

Changes Driving Brain Inflammation

Brain inflammation differs from inflammation in the periphery because of the relative absence of leukocytes and antibodies. There is a limited traffic across the BBB and this traffic can be increased by inflammation, which can recruit leukocytes into the brain (36).

As discussed, brain inflammation induces unfavorable changes to microglial morphology, yielding a state in which microglia phagocytize viable neurons, express MHC-II, and present fragments of neuronal debris to T cells instead of inducing the T cells to undergo apoptosis. This is in contrast to the normal brain, in which microglia induce apoptosis of invading T cells *via* FAS/FASL interactions (66). The result of the inflammation-induced shift in microglial morphology and behavior can be excessive neuronal loss and upregulation of brain autoimmunity (66) (see **Figure 1**).

Inflammation also causes impaired neuronal metabolic integrity. It is noteworthy that TNFα and IL-1β, two important "ON" signals, are both primary pro-inflammatory cytokines that are upregulated in the context of brain inflammation. The theme of neuroinflammation driving deleterious effects in brain suggests the importance of identifying and addressing causes of brain inflammation in the clinical setting.

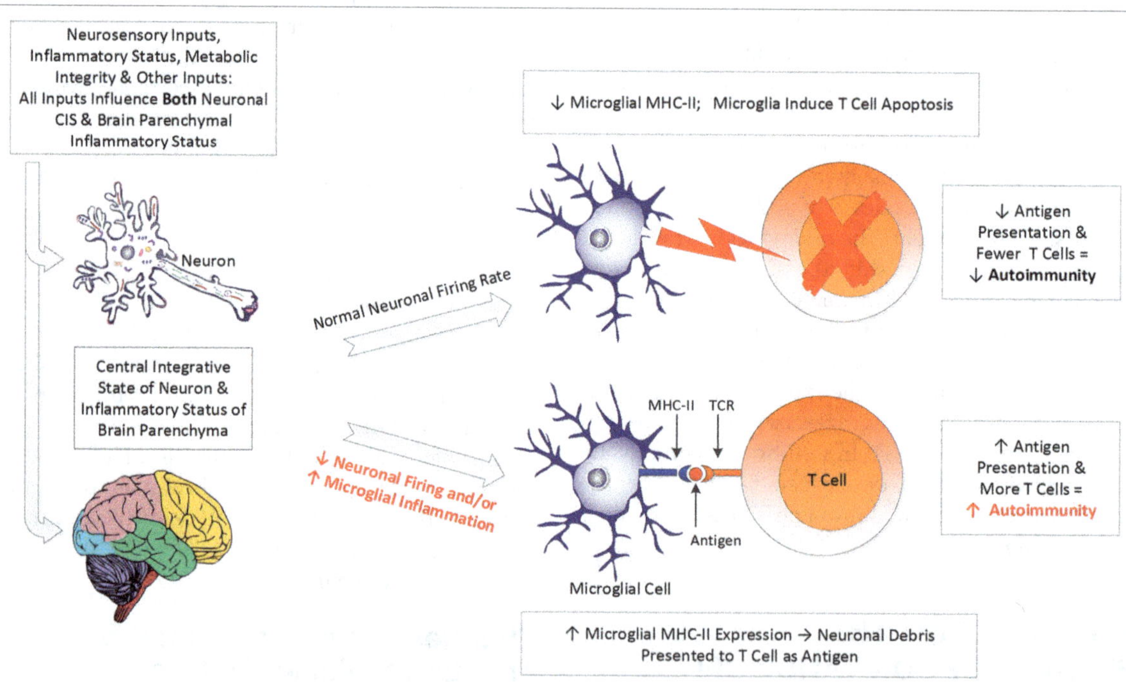

FIGURE 1 | Impact of neuronal CIS and inflammation on microglial function. A host of inputs determine both the central integrative state (CIS) of neurons and the extent of neuroinflammation (see text). These two factors determine whether the neuronal firing rate (frequency of action potentials) will be rapid enough to generate the electrical activity necessary to inhibit microglial expression of major histocompatibility complex II (MHC-II) on their cell membranes. If neuronal electrical activity is adequate, microglial expression of MHC-II will be inhibited, and microglia will be prevented from presenting antigen to T cells. Instead, microglia will be kept in their resting/ramified state, in which they induce apoptosis in T cells that enter the brain, *via* FAS/FASL interactions. This diminishes the risk of expression of autoimmune process in the brain. If neuronal signaling is inadequate, or if neuroinflammation is increased, it becomes more likely that microglia will express MHC-II and will perform antigen presentation of neuronal debris to the T cell receptors (TCR) of invading T cells. This increases the risk of developing autoimmune process with neuronal tissue as the target of the autoimmune process.

One of the primary drivers of brain inflammation is body inflammation (81). Increases in pro-inflammatory cytokines in the periphery yield upregulation of brain inflammation and potentiate neuronal death (71, 82–84). Systemic IL-1β can cause CNS inflammation once it enters the brain, thus linking systemic inflammation and immune activation with brain inflammation (56).

Perry et al. state that microglial phenotype is modified by systemic infection or inflammation. They go on to say that the fact that diseases with a chronic systemic inflammatory component are risk factors for AD implies that crosstalk occurs between systemic inflammation and microglia in the CNS (85). AD risk has been shown to be increased in patients with metabolic syndrome and adiposity (86), decreased diversity of the intestinal microbiome (87), periodontal disease (88), infection (89), and vascular risk factors like type 2 diabetes, smoking, hypertension and heart disease (90), and stroke (91).

With regard to arthritides, Fusco et al. have reviewed contributions to neuroinflammation from osteoarthritis and rheumatoid arthritis (RA), suggesting contributions from both *via* upregulation of IL-1β and mast cell mediated microglial activation (92). In patients with RA, neuroinflammation, and AD, Schrepf et al. using multimodal MRI, have demonstrated patterns of CNS connectivity that predicted fatigue, pain and cognitive dysfunction during phases of RA flare (93). Chou et al. in a case control trial of 8.5 million patient records from the US, Puerto Rico, and the USVI, found that AD was more prevalent among RA patients (0.79%) than among those without RA (0.11%), that relative AD risk was increased by the presence of comorbidities like diabetes and peripheral vascular disease, and that relative AD risk was lowered by etanercept, but not by the other anti-TNF agents studied or other immunosuppressive medications (94). Cao et al. analyzing a Taiwanese patient database, found an inverse association between prior RA and AD (95). Contrastingly, Policicchio et al. in a meta-analysis and Mendelian randomization study, found that an apparent inverse correlation between RA and AD identified in previous studies is not causal (96). Cai et al. analyzing a large GWAS dataset of patients of European descent, also found no association between RA and AD (97).

van Langenberg et al. in a human trial, found that patients with Crohn's disease had cognitive impairment attributable to systemic inflammation (98). McCaulley and Grush have reviewed evidence for the clinical utility of TNFα inhibitors in AD, noting that etanercept has shown a clinical benefit. They point out that etanercept has not shown benefit in inflammatory bowel disease (99).

Ajami et al. describe two distinct pools of monocytic cells in MS and EAE: infiltrating monocytes and resident microglial cells. They observed a strong correlation between monocyte infiltration from the periphery into the brain and progression to the paralytic stage of EAE. They go on to state that increases in circulating inflammatory monocytes have been shown to correlate with relapses in EAE mice (100).

Lipopolysaccharide (LPS), aka endotoxin, is a PAMP found in the outer membrane of gram-negative bacteria that is a known B cell mitogen. Increasing the peripheral LPS level can induce the activation of central pro-inflammatory mechanisms, even when the amount of LPS used for stimulation is minimal or when the peripheral inflammatory cytokine levels are suppressed artificially. Both central and peripheral inflammation can exacerbate local brain inflammation and neuronal death (101).

Rivest (73) citing others (102–105) observed "a single systemic injection of LPS (1 mg/kg intraperitoneally) results in the robust induction of expression in microglial cells of genes that encode pro-inflammatory cytokines and chemokines, as well as proteins of the complement system" (73). This suggests that a bodily infection with gram negative bacteria can drive brain inflammation (73).

Other authors have also discussed the impact of factors involved in systemic inflammation on CNS inflammation. LaFlamme et al. (106) showed that, in a mouse model of sterile inflammation but not in endotoxemia, IL-1β is necessary for the activation of NF-kappaB and prostaglandins in the endothelial cells of the BBB.

Varatharaj and Galea (107) have reviewed mechanisms by which both sterile and infectious systemic inflammation can affect the BBB, with inflammatory consequences in the CNS, reflected in sickness behavior and other factors. They describe a heightened sensitivity of the diseased BBB to systemic inflammation, and a greater progression of AD and MS in patients with systemic inflammation. Kuhlmann et al. have described mechanisms by which c-reactive protein (CRP) promotes degradation of BBB integrity (108), though mention of CRP is notably absent in Varatharaj and Galea (107). Sproston and Ashworth, describe CRP as associated with both inflammation and infection (109).

Banks et al. have discussed the transport of IL-1β, a microglial "ON" signaling molecule, across the BBB in sickness behavior (110). Lin et al. (111) showed in a human trial that increased serum oxidative stress was associated with declined perceptual functioning in patients with PD. A meta-analysis by Peng et al. (112) found that post-operative cognitive dysfunction was correlated with the concentrations of peripheral inflammatory markers, particularly interleukin-6 and S-100β.

Denes et al. (113) in a mouse middle cerebral artery occlusion (MCAo) model of stroke, found that both LPS and anaphylaxis (induced by ovalbumin exposure in sensitized mice) induced inflammatory changes in the blood and in the brain prior to induction of stroke. After MCAo, both LPS and anaphylaxis increased microglial interleukin-1a (IL-1a) expression and blood-brain barrier breakdown, with profound impairment of survival in the first 24 h after stroke in the presence of systemic inflammatory challenges. They concluded that these finding "suggest that systemic inflammatory conditions induce cerebrovascular inflammation," and that "increased brain inflammation, BBB injury and brain edema formation can be major contributors to impaired outcome in mice after experimental stroke with systemic inflammatory stimuli, independently of infarct size."

Taken together, the work of these authors suggests a connection between factors contributing to systemic inflammation and the promotion of neuroinflammation. In the clinical setting, targeting biological factors outside the CNS that have been shown to upregulate neuroinflammation may present an opportunity to influence outcomes in cases involving neuroinflammation. Particularly in cases where other approaches have not yielded improvement, further study of a clinical inventory of factors that have the potential to impact systemic inflammation may be warranted.

Infection (73, 114, 115), stress and depression (6, 116–118), altered microbiota (120) and other forms of digestive dysregulation (119–122), dysglycemia, insulin resistance, and obesity (123–126), tissue hypoxia [80, 127 (review), 128, 129], poor diet (130–134), lack of exercise (135–139), environmental or other toxic exposure (140–144), and autoimmune processes (145, 146) are all potential drivers of body inflammation. As such, these factors may be worthy of attention in patients with neuropsychiatric disorders associated with neuroinflammation, patients with head trauma, neuroinflammation, or any condition known to be worsened by neuroinflammation and changes in microglial activation, including PD, AD or other dementias, ALS, MS, and PANS/PANDAS.

Bredesen et al. report significant reversal of cognitive decline, including some patients who returned to work, in a series of patients diagnosed with AD, assessed *via* quantitative MRI and neuropsychological testing. The approach, described as personalized rather than monotherapeutic, focused on identifying and modifying factors like neuroinflammation, infection, oxidative stress, dysglycemia, hypoxia and poor diet (147). The effect of the MS medication glatiramer acetate is partly attributed to its ability to modify microglial morphology and the resulting impacts on neuron-microglial interactions (148). Feinstein et al. have reviewed treatment approaches focused on restoration of noradrenaline to influence both neurons and microglia (149). Other human studies (150–153) and reviews (154–156) have described improvements in neurological function using clinical approaches that target oxidative stress, BDNF, and neuroinflammation. Regarding biomarkers, Hirad et al. have demonstrated that reduced midbrain white matter integrity, demonstrated on MRI, correlates with post-concussion deficit severity and with serum tau levels, a marker of blood-brain barrier disruption (157). Strawbridge, et al, have reviewed biomarkers of depression (158). Though some biomarkers related to neuron-microglial signaling, such as serum TGF beta, IL-6 or TNFα levels, or the extent of midbrain white matter loss observed on MRI, are obtainable in a clinical setting, most of the markers involved in direct measurement of the mechanisms described in research on neuron-microglial signaling interactions are not available to the clinician.

It is noteworthy that there are also mechanisms by which disorders whose primary locus of dysfunction is in the CNS can impact systemic inflammation, such that the arrow of causation does not always point from the periphery to the CNS. For example, efferent neuronal signaling from the dorsal motor nucleus (DMN) of the vagus nerve is known to inhibit sympathetic outflow (159) and to inhibit the production of inflammatory cytokines in the spleen (TNFα), liver (IL-6), and small intestine (TNFα) (160–162). Support for vagus nerve motor activity has been shown to inhibit kidney damage in an ischemia-reperfusion model (163). Any CNS disorder that involves diminished DMN signaling thus has the potential to influence the patient toward increased systemic inflammation.

MICROGLIAL PRIMING

The pattern of inflammatory activation of microglia has been referred to as microglial priming. The hallmark of primed microglia is a shift from the resting or ramified state to one in which they swell and fill with pro-inflammatory cytokines (55, 67, 164, 165). Priming can be induced by aging, trauma, infection, or other stimuli. Microglia can remain in the primed state for long periods of time, without returning to the ramified state, but without releasing their bolus of cytokines. In a clinical setting, the concern is that any new trauma or insult introduced into a brain containing primed microglia will result in a flooding release of pro-inflammatory cytokines that can be damaging to the brain (55, 67, 164, 165). The first injury shifts microglia into the primed state. When the second TBI or non-traumatic brain insult occurs, the microglia release a flood of pro-inflammatory cytokines, yielding more deleterious effects. This is the basis for the common observation that a second or subsequent traumatic brain injury often yields more serious consequences and carries the potential for a poorer prognosis.

Since systemic inflammation can drive brain inflammation, factors capable of driving body inflammation predispose the microglia to a shift into the primed state. If body inflammation and thus brain inflammation is already present at the time of a new brain insult, whether that new insult is a TBI, or a biochemical insult associated with autoimmune process, metabolic insult, infection, or other factors, the prognosis is likely to be worse.

This suggests that, for individuals already affected by neuropsychiatric disorders, neuro-autoimmunity, or an existing head trauma, there may be utility in taking steps to prevent systemic and neuroinflammation, oxidative stress, loss of metabolic integrity, and related factors, with the twin goals of diminishing existing neuronal impairment and protecting against the eventuality of additional insults.

It is especially noteworthy that a new brain insult can result from causes other than trauma. As referenced above, upregulation of inflammation can occur from a new infection in the body, an upsurge of stress due to a change in life circumstance, overtraining syndrome, glycemic dysregulation, immunological reactions to environmental factors like chemicals, pollens, pollutants or other antigenic burdens, or a host of other instigating factors. Any of these factors, if they induce neuroinflammation and affect microglial function sufficiently, can instigate a flooding release of inflammatory mediators into the brain parenchyma, resulting in a worsening of symptoms. Introduction of any of these comorbidities can change the ongoing equation in the brain in a way that can tip the balance of neuron-microglial interaction toward a higher error rate or, in more severe cases, constitute a biological second hit. This "two hit" or "multiple hit" theory has been described in TBI (67, 166, 167) and in non-traumatic forms of brain insult, including aging (164, 167), neurodegenerative diseases (167–170), and perinatal white matter injury (171).

Thus, clinical measures taken to reduce systemic inflammation accomplish the triple agenda of reducing current impairment, reducing the potential effect of a second hit from actual trauma (like head banging in autism or sport-related impact), and reducing the risk of a second hit effect occurring from a non-traumatic pro-inflammatory insult.

ELECTRICAL CELL-SIGNALING EFFECTS

The Role of Neuronal Electrical Activity in Maintenance of Neuron-Microglial Homeostasis

Microglial antigen presentation capability depends on microglial MHC-II expression. As Neumann points out; the electrical activity of healthy neurons suppresses MHC-II expression in surrounding glial cells. Hence, the antigen presentation process that leads to autoimmunity is counter-regulated in intact CNS areas by the electrical activity of neurons (101). Similarly, Grieb et al. observed that when high frequency electrical stimulation was applied to the subthalamic nucleus of freely moving animals, gene enrichment analysis showed the strongest regulation occurred in MHC-encoding genes (172).

The repertoire of neuronal control mechanisms regulating microglial function thus includes both biochemical factors (neurotransmitters and other "Off" signals produced as a consequence of normal neurotransmission) and neuronal-firing-rate-dependent electrical inhibition of microglial MHC-II expression.

This implies that there are two distinct immune consequences to reductions in neuronal firing rate. These are: diminished production of NT's and other "OFF" signals, and a reduction in electrical activity that allows greater microglial MHC-II expression. The microglia in this situation are not adequately inhibited from phagocytizing live neurons (31, 64), nor are they adequately inhibited from functioning as APCs (101, 172).

The capacity of neurons to maintain robust firing rate depends in large part on two factors. The first, metabolic integrity of the neuron (the neuron as a cell) is discussed above. The second is the central integrative state (CIS) of the neuron, which depends on the sum of its excitatory and inhibitory presynaptic stimuli. CIS is the sum of all activity within the neuron, partly resulting from external forces and synaptic signaling. CIS can be summarized as the combination of two factors: how close the neuron is to the firing threshold and how much metabolic integrity the neuron has, with which to maintain firing before fatigue.

Loss of neuronal firing rate will at some point yield a loss of the neuron's ability to generate enough electrical activity to adequately inhibit microglial MHC-II expression in microglial cells affected by that neuron's contribution to the electrical environment within the local brain parenchyma. This can occur as a consequence of impaired neuronal metabolic integrity, such that the neuron cannot generate enough ATP to sustain its firing rate. Or this can occur through direct neuronal injury, as with a TBI, or with diminished presynaptic stimulation from whatever area of the brain normally fires into the neuronal pool in question.

Afferent stimulation from the body to the brain plays a significant role in the maintenance of the CIS of CNS neurons. Thus, factors like lack of exercise, destruction of joint mechanoreceptors in arthritic conditions, poor muscular tone, diminished rib movement with respiratory disorders and other such changes can alter the neurosensory environment, altering the CIS of neurons. This process of reduced CIS in initially uninjured brain areas due to processes conceptually similar to dysafferentation or deafferentation coming from truly damaged areas has historically been called focal or non-focal diaschisis based on distance and connectivity (173, 174). Carrera and Tononi define diaschisis as a change in structural and functional connectivity between brain areas distant to a lesion (173).

Discrete areas of the brain more affected by these or other factors will have relatively greater reductions in the firing rates of their neurons, yielding a reduction in electrically mediated inhibition of microglial MHC-II expression on the surface of microglia doing surveillance on those neurons. Accordingly, areas of the brain more affected by factors that lower neuronal firing rates will be more vulnerable to the expression of autoimmune processes. As Neumann states, "in a variety of inflammatory and neurodegenerative diseases, including MS, infections, trauma, stroke, neoplasia, and AD, glial cells such as microglia gain antigen-presenting capacity through the expression of MHC molecules. Further, proinflammatory cytokines, such as TNF, IL-1β, and IFNγ, as well as chemokines, are synthesized by resident brain cells and T lymphocytes invading the affected brain tissue... The pro-inflammatory cytokines stimulate microglial MHC expression in the lesioned CNS areas only" (71).

MORE INFLAMMATION YIELDS FURTHER CONSEQUENCES

The damage to neurons that results from autoimmune attack yields the release of pro-inflammatory DAMPS. This yields two effects that can be considered as occurring in a second wave of effects:

First, the increased levels of neuroinflammation will include increased levels of TNFα and IL-1β. These cytokines are neuronal "ON" signals, influencing neuron-microglial signaling in favor of the likelihood of additional microglial phagocytosis of live neurons (64).

Second, increased inflammation further impairs neuronal metabolic integrity, further diminishing the capacity of neuronal mitochondria to make ATP, further diminishing the capacity of neurons to sustain their firing rates. Loss of neuronal firing rates allows further microglial MHC-II expression. While this may appear to simply be a restating of the mechanism by which new brain autoimmunity can develop (40, 56–60, 71, 72), the presence of additional neuronal tissue debris, which can be taken up by microglia and presented as antigen, risks the development of distinct antibody reactions to new neuronal tissue epitopes, an effect known as epitope spreading (175, 176). Munz et al. define epitope spreading as, "... a mechanism by which an immune response that is initiated by various stimuli, including microbial infection, trauma, transplanted tissue or autoimmunity, 'spreads' to include responses directed against a different portion of the same protein (intramolecular spreading) or a different protein (intermolecular spreading)" (177).

Thus, the loss of neuronal firing rates, itself a consequence of the inflammatory damage that occurs with brain insults, predisposes the affected brain areas to the development of new microglial antigen presentation events and opportunities for either new autoimmune process when the initial brain insult does not already involve autoimmunity (177), or epitope spreading

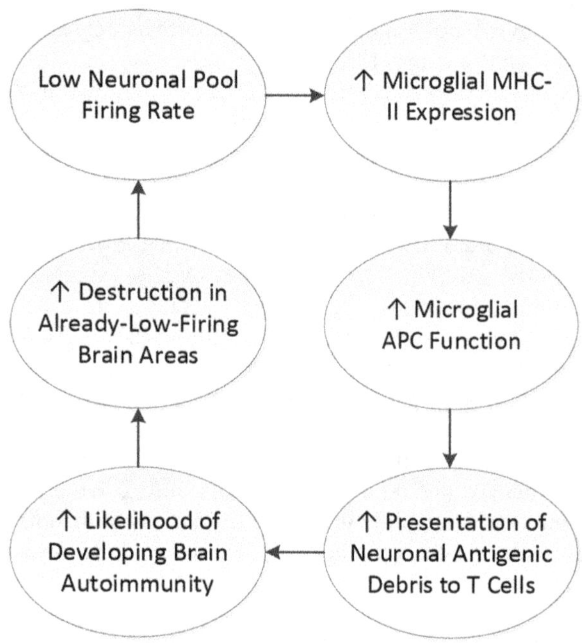

FIGURE 2 | Feedback loop of low neuronal firing rate. When neuronal firing rate is diminished, microglial major histocompatibility complex II (MHC-II) expression is increased. MHC-II is the cell surface mechanism by which microglial cells present fragments of neuronal debris as antigen to T cells. Presentation of neuronal debris as antigen increases the likelihood of expression of brain autoimmunity, which creates destruction of neurons and increases neuroinflammation of those neurons that are not destroyed. Neuroinflammation diminishes neuronal firing rate, yielding a loop.

and worsening of autoimmune-mediated damage in existing autoimmune brain disorders (177) (see **Figure 2**).

Still More Consequences

When an autoimmune brain disorder, PD or MS, for example, is already present, there are two important clinical implications:

First, the introduction of a new event or process that increases neuroinflammation can trigger a worsening of the pre-existing autoimmune disorder, through both accelerated neuronal loss and epitope spreading. This suggests that, in cases involving brain based autoimmune diseases, it's useful for clinicians to be particularly persistent in their attention to drivers of inflammation, including infection, stress, mood issues, digestive dysregulation, dysglycemia, hypoxia, dietary factors, immune responses to foods, haptens and environmental triggers, and other such factors. Clinical steps to mitigate these factors, and their pro-inflammatory effects, may be worthy of consideration.

Second, the introduction of either abrupt or evolving diaschisis, resulting in loss of neuronal firing rates, might increase the risk of further microglial antigen presentation, development of epitope spreading, worsening of existing disease, and expansion of involvement in areas most affected by the diaschisis (see **Figure 3**).

Clinicians must be alert to changes that might trigger an evolving diaschisis. These might include changes in the patient's capacity for voluntary movement, whether driven by pain, mechanical restriction, or changes in energy level; changes in respiratory patterns, or changes in the character of a tremor. Clinical steps to mitigate these factors, and to restore appropriate neuronal firing rates and CIS to affected central nervous system areas, are worthy of consideration. The proper clinical approach would depend upon the individual case. The aim in all cases would be to identify the change in afferent barrage to the area of diaschisis and to restore normal afferent stimulation to that area, with the goal of restoration of the normal central integrative state. Examples would include appropriate post-stroke rehabilitation, post-concussion rehabilitation, or restoration of afferent barrage of a CNS target from a hip, shoulder, or other sensory source after an injury or other dysfunctional change has taken place.

FURTHER NEUROIMMUNE TRIGGERS

Pathogens or Damaged Neuronal Debris Evoke Excitotoxicity and Neuronal Cell Death

Pathogens in tissue create pathogen-associated molecular patterns (PAMPs) (178). Damaged tissue creates damage associated molecular patterns (DAMPs) (179). As specialized macrophages, microglial cell membranes contain pattern recognition receptors (PRRs) that sense PAMPS and DAMPS, triggering phagocyte NADPH oxidase (PHOX), which turns molecular oxygen into reactive oxygen species (ROS). This conversion depletes the tissue of molecular oxygen, yielding hypoxia, driving hypoxia inducible factor 1α (HIF-1α). Under normal circumstances, HIF-1α induction by hypoxia promotes useful effects like the growth of blood vessels in hypoxic tissue (180, 181), as well as the activation of neutrophils that have migrated into tissue (182). However, HIF-1α also up regulates NFκB (182, 183), causing gene expression of IL-1β and TNFα (184). Since they are neuronal "ON" signals, increased IL-1β and TNFα promotes the activation of microglial phagocytosis of neurons (64). IL-1β and TNFα activation also promotes further NFκB upregulation, with this loop activation originally described by Barnes and Karin as the "amplifying loop" of the inflammatory process (184). NFκB induces iNOS expression, yielding abundant nitric oxide (NO) production (43). Though NO can be cytoprotective (43), the combination of NO and hypoxia impair cellular respiration (43), yielding excitotoxicity and resulting neuronal death (185). The formation of ROS like singlet oxygen (O_2^-) and hydrogen peroxide (H_2O_2) drives microglial activation (43). O_2^- and H_2O_2 in combination with NO yields peroxynitrite ($ONOO^-$), driving neuronal apoptotic cell death (43). Activated microglia release neurotoxic factors like glutamate, TNFα, and FASL, increasing neurotoxicity and increasing the likelihood of neuronal cell death (43). Nocella et al. have suggested that, in athletes, antioxidant depletion from single nucleotide polymorphisms or other factors may have an impact on the long-term risk for developing neurodegenerative disease (186) (see **Figure 4**).

Block et al. state that microglial activation can occur through recognition of inflammatory signals such as LPS from

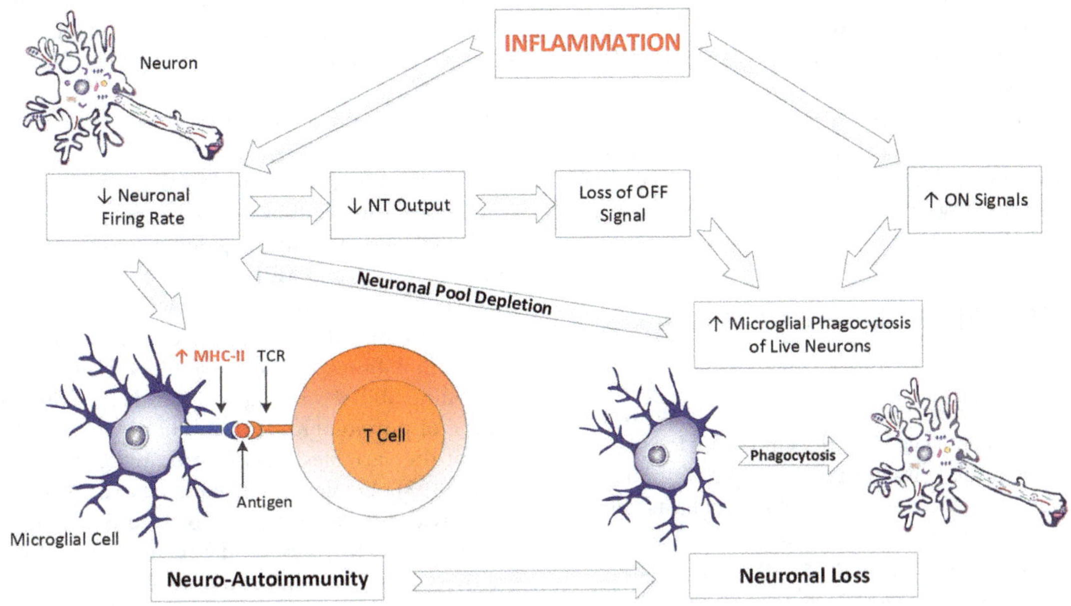

FIGURE 3 | Inflammation drives both neuro-autoimmunity and excessive neuronal loss. Inflammation impairs neuronal firing rate, allowing microglial MHC-II expression, yielding presentation of neuronal antigenic debris to T cells, driving neuro-autoimmunity. Decreased neuronal firing rate also decreases neuronal NT output. Since NT's are a significant OFF signal, diminished NT production constitutes the loss of an OFF signal. IL-1β and TNFα, two inflammatory cytokines, are part of the ON signal milieu. Loss of NT output and increased IL-1β and TNFα yield a tissue environment more favorable to microglial phagocytosis of live neurons. Depletion of neurons from a neuronal pool yields diminished electrical activity in that pool and greater vulnerability to MHC-II expression by microglial cells performing surveillance on those neurons. Hence, inflammation and subsequent loss of neurons increases the likelihood of developing subsequent neuro-autoimmunity. This promotes further neuronal loss. NT, neurotransmitter; MHC-II, major histocompatibility complex II; TCR, T cell receptor.

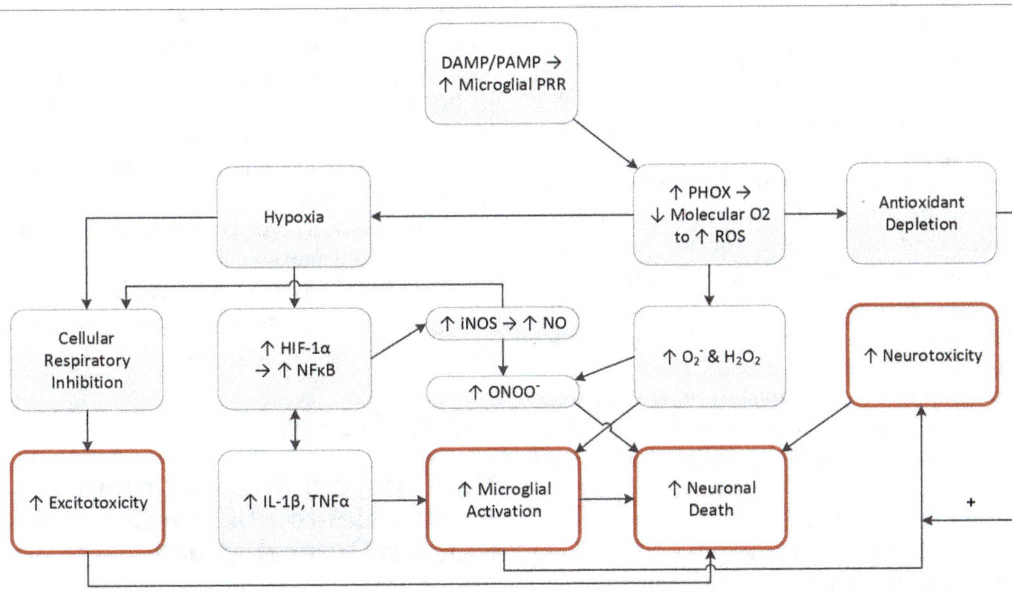

FIGURE 4 | PAMPs and DAMPs drive neuronal destruction. DAMPs and/or PAMPs trigger PRR's on microglia. Microglia generate PHOX, driving down O_2 levels, as the O_2 is consumed to make ROS. This yields three consequences: hypoxia, increased ROS (O_2– and H_2O_2), and antioxidant depletion as a result of the increased ROS. Hypoxia raises the level of hypoxia inducible factor 1 alpha (HIF-1α), a substance that induces the formation of blood vessels in areas of inadequate oxygen. HIF-1α upregulates inflammatory NFκB, which induces gene expression of IL-1β and TNFα. Thus, hypoxia drives microglial activation, promoting neuronal death. NFκB upregulation also promotes activation of NO *via* iNOS induction. NO drives up ONOO–, which combines with the ROS to activate microglia, again promoting neuronal death. NO also combines with hypoxia to induce excitotoxicity, promoting neuronal death. Microglial activation also increases neurotoxicity, *via* production of glutamate and other substances, an effect that may be amplified by antioxidant depletion. Red circles connote key downstream effects. DAMP, damage associated molecular pattern; PAMP, pathogen associated molecular pattern; PRR, pattern recognition receptor; PHOX, phagocyte NADPH oxidase; O_2, oxygen; ROS, reactive oxygen species; O_2–, singlet oxygen; H_2O_2, hydrogen peroxide; HIF-1α, hypoxia inducible factor 1 alpha; iNOS, inducible nitric oxide synthase; NO, nitric oxide; ONOO–, peroxynitrite; NFκB, nuclear factor kappa B; IL-1β, interleukin 1 beta; TNFα, tumor necrosis factor alpha.

gram-negative bacteria, causing the microglia to produce neurotoxic pro-inflammatory mediators. Microglia can also be activated by debris from neuronal damage (DAMPs), yielding reactive microgliosis, which is then toxic to neighboring neurons, which they describe as resulting in a perpetuating cycle of neuron death. Block et al. describe microgliosis as a "potential underlying mechanism of progressive neuron damage across numerous neurodegenerative diseases, regardless of the instigating stimuli" (56).

OTHER VIEWS AND QUESTIONS GOING FORWARD

The history of research on microglial cells has not been without controversy. Disagreement regarding the embryologic origin of microglial cells, now settled, has been reviewed by Ginhoux and Prinz (187). The evolving view of the role of microglia as villains or protectors, has been reviewed by Fernandez et al. (188). What has emerged is a view of microglial cells that is more complex, with the potential for both supportive and deleterious functions, depending upon a complex array of factors.

That neurons and microglial cells interact, that key components of these interactions are understood, and that these interactions are relevant biologically, appear to be supported by a substantial body of evidence. However, the clinical relevance of these neuroimmunological processes and the extent of their universality in patient populations are important questions that broaden our understanding and improve our perspectives for future study.

With regard to the effect size and clinical relevance of neuron-microglial interactions, the following papers discuss other relevant processes that precede neuron-microglial signaling and may play important roles: Culmsee et al. discuss the role of immunometabolic factors that influence mitochondria, with the potential to substantially alter function in both neurons and microglial cells (189). Chang et al. present evidence of an association between corticotrophin releasing hormone (CRH) polymorphisms and major depressive disorder (MDD) (190). Kelly and O'Neil have described the influence of glycolysis and tricarboxylic acid cycle function in influencing macrophage polarization to M1 and M2 morphologies, respectively (191). Corcoran and O'Neil have shown that HIF1α, induced by hypoxia, is a primary driver of microglial activation and also of Th17 cell activation, a primary mechanism by which tissue destruction is upregulated in autoimmunity (192).

These examples suggest that, even if changes in neuron-microglial signaling are a neuroimmunological bottleneck, larger therapeutic impacts on the clinical picture in a given patient might be accomplished by addressing other upstream issues, such as those described above that could be immunometabolic, neuroendocrine, or related to hypoxia/oxygenation *via* problems that are circulatory, respiratory, or hematologic. Addressing clinical factors mentioned previously, such as infection, stress, depression, GI dysfunction, poor diet, lack of exercise, and autoimmunity, to the extent present in a given case, may also yield greater impact on the clinical picture. The presence of each of these factors, and their relevance in each case, is a matter of individual clinical discernment. The work of Bredesen suggests that such clinical discernment can be embedded into a structured process that provides for reliably useful clinical outcomes (147).

With regard to the question of whether neuron-microglial dysfunction is a universally applicable feature of cases with CNS involvement, focusing on depression as a well-defined example of a neuroimmunological process involving neuron-microglial interactions, the following papers are useful to consider. Raison and Miller review evidence for two competing views. In one view, inflammation only contributes to depression in a subset of patients. In the other, the inducing influence of inflammation on depression is more widespread, but with vulnerability varying in accordance with the status of a pattern of physiological variables unique to each patient, with each of the variables known to be involved in the etiology of MDD (193). Dooley et al. have described a greater role for inflammation, a key influence on neuron-microglial signaling, in some core features of depression, including exaggerated reactivity to negative information, altered reward reactivity, and somatic symptoms, but has less clear evidence for an involvement in cognitive control (194).

These papers suggest that there is variability from one patient to another in the extent to which neuroimmunological factors influence depression and that there may be variability in the extent to which some features of depression are affected in a given patient. This suggests that the focus on neuron-microglial interaction described in this paper may not apply with equal utility in all cases, or to all features of a given case. Consistent with this view, Kopschina Feltes et al. have suggested that a clinical approach that addresses neuroimmunological factors might have greatest utility in MDD patients with elevated inflammatory cytokines, particularly IL-6, TNF-α and IL-1β, who have been resistant to treatment aimed at monoamine repletion (195, 196).

More research is needed to clarify the above questions and others, with regard to depression, TBI, neurodegenerative conditions, and neuro-autoimmunity, to ensure that in both research and clinical settings, sufficient attention and efforts are focused on areas that could provide significant returns.

CONCLUSION

Neuropsychiatric Disorders Involve Neuroinflammatory and Related Comorbidities

The presence of depression and related neuropsychiatric phenomena in a patient may reflect the presence of an underlying neuroinflammatory state and/or other comorbidities that can affect neuron - microglial interactions, with consequences for neuronal loss and neuro-autoimmunity. The clinician faced with the neuropsychiatric patient may be well served to assess the extent of systemic and neuroinflammation and the other comorbidities discussed and look for potential biological causes that could be instigating or worsening the patient's neuropsychiatric disorder. It is especially important when a patient presents with neuropsychiatric disorders that the neuropsychiatric nature of the disorder not decrease the clinicians' inclination to focus on underlying biology but rather increase the clinician's interest in identifying biological causes of neuroinflammation and related biological factors discussed here.

Time-Course Issues Matter for Patients With Brain Insults

Once a brain insult develops, the key question is whether it will resolve quickly or progress to a brain in a chronically inflamed state, resulting in greater neuronal loss, greater risk of developing autoimmune responses against brain tissue targets, and expanded loss of function for the patient. The time sequence can yield a cascade of further disease elaboration, including ongoing neuronal loss, epitope spreading, and increasing vulnerability of affected neuronal pools, all yielding further functional loss downstream.

Ongoing case management may need to include a focus on reducing comorbidities that are known to diminish neuronal metabolic integrity, promote neuroinflammation, trigger or perpetuate autoimmune process, increase oxidative burden, or drive other related processes. When expected levels of clinical improvement do not occur, it may be necessary to review the case in light of the known mechanisms by which neuron-microglial interaction can become dysregulated.

AUTHOR CONTRIBUTIONS

Conception and authorship of all sections, tables and figures, references, and final edited versioning and approval: SY.

ACKNOWLEDGMENTS

The author wishes to acknowledge the contribution of Michael Pierce to the discussion of diaschisis.

REFERENCES

1. Clarkson BDS, Kahoud RJ, McCarthy CB, Howe CL. Inflammatory cytokine-induced changes in neural network activity measured by waveform analysis of high-content calcium imaging in murine cortical neurons. *Sci Rep* (2017) 7(1):9037. doi: 10.1038/s41598-017-09182-5
2. Wu XB, Liang B, Gao YJ. The increase of intrinsic excitability of layer V pyramidal cells in the prelimbic medial prefrontal cortex of adult mice after peripheral inflammation. *Neurosci Lett* (2016) 611:40–5. doi: 10.1016/j.neulet.2015.11.030
3. Chung G, Kim SJ, Kim SK. Metabotropic glutamate receptor 5 in the medial prefrontal cortex as a molecular determinant of pain and ensuing depression. *Front Mol Neurosci* (2018) 11:376. doi: 10.3389/fnmol.2018.00376
4. Leonard BE. Impact of inflammation on neurotransmitter changes in major depression: an insight into the action of antidepressants. Prog. *Neuropsychopharmacol Biol Psychiatry* (2014) 48:261–7. doi: 10.1016/j.pnpbp.2013.10.018
5. Licht CM, de Geus EJ, Zitman FG, Hoogendijk WJ, van Dyck R, Penninx BW. Association between major depressive disorder and heart rate variability in the Netherlands Study of Depression and Anxiety (NESDA). *Arch Gen Psychiatry* (2008) 65(12):1358–67. doi: 10.1001/archpsyc.65.12.1358
6. Miller AH, Maletic V, Raison CL. Inflammation and its discontents: the role of cytokines in the pathophysiology of major depression. *Biol Psychiatry* (2009) 65(9):732–41. doi: 10.1016/j.biopsych.2008.11.029
7. Raison CL, Lowry CA, Rook GA. Inflammation, sanitation, and consternation loss of contact with coevolved, tolerogenic microorganisms and the pathophysiology and treatment of major depression. *Arch Gen Psychiatry* (2010) 67(12):1211–24. doi: 10.1001/archgenpsychiatry.2010.161
8. Young JJ, Bruno D, Pomara N. A review of the relationship between proinflammatory cytokines and major depressive disorder. *J Affect Disord* (2014) 169:15–20. doi: 10.1016/j.jad.2014.07.032
9. Dahl J, Ormstad H, Aass HC, Malt UF, Bendz LT, Sandvik L, et al. The plasma levels of various cytokines are increased during ongoing depression and are reduced to normal levels after recovery. *Psychoneuroendocrinology* (2014) 45:77–86. doi: 10.1016/j.psyneuen.2014.03.019
10. Eswarappa M, Neylan TC, Whooley MA, Metzler TJ, Cohen BE. Inflammation as a predictor of disease course in posttraumatic stress disorder and depression: a prospective analysis from the Mind Your Heart Study. *Brain Behav Immun* (2019) 75:220–7. doi: 10.1016/j.bbi.2018.10.012
11. Leonard BE. Inflammation and depression: a causal or coincidental link to the pathophysiology? *Acta Neuropsychiatr* (2018) 30(1):1–16. doi: 10.1017/neu.2016.69
12. Lavoie S, Sechrist S, Quach N, Ehsanian R, Duong T, Gotlib IH, et al. Depression in men and women one year following traumatic brain injury (TBI): a TBI model systems study. *Front Psychol* (2017) 8:634. doi: 10.3389/fpsyg.2017.00634
13. Bodnar CN, Morganti JM, Bachstetter AD. Depression following a traumatic brain injury: uncovering cytokine dysregulation as a pathogenic mechanism. *Neural Regen Res* (2018) 13(10):1693–704. doi: 10.4103/1673-5374.238604
14. Liu Y, Tang X. Depressive syndromes in autoimmune disorders of the nervous system: prevalence, etiology, and influence. *Front Psychiatry* (2018) 9:451. doi: 10.3389/fpsyt.2018.00451
15. Bhattacharjee S, Goldstone L, Ip Q, Warholak T. Depression treatment among adults with multiple sclerosis and depression in ambulatory care settings in the United States. *Mult Scler Int* (2017) 2017:3175358. doi: 10.1155/2017/3175358
16. Greeke EE, Chua AS, Healy BC, Rintell DJ, Chitnis T, Glanz BI. Depression and fatigue in patients with multiple sclerosis. *J Neurol Sci* (2017) 380:236–41. doi: 10.1016/j.jns.2017.07.047
17. Hely MA, Morris JG, Reid WG, Trafficante R. Sydney multicenter study of Parkinson's disease: non-L-dopa-responsive problems dominate at 15 years. *Mov Disord* (2005) 20(2):190–9. doi: 10.1002/mds.20324
18. van der Hoek TC, Bus BA, Matui P, van der Marck MA, Esselink RA, Tendolkar I. Prevalence of depression in Parkinson's disease: effects of disease stage, motor subtype and gender. *J Neurol Sci* (2011) 310(1–2):220–4. doi: 10.1016/j.jns.2011.07.007
19. Bhattacharjee S, Vadiei N, Goldstone L, Alrabiah Z, Sherman SJ. Patterns and predictors of depression treatment among older adults with Parkinson's disease and depression in ambulatory care settings in the United States. *Parkinsons Dis* (2018) 2018:3402983. doi: 10.1155/2018/3402983
20. Thienemann M, Murphy T, Leckman J, Shaw R, Williams K, Kapphahn C, et al. Clinical management of pediatric acute-onset neuropsychiatric syndrome: part I-psychiatric and behavioral interventions. *J Child Adolesc Psychopharmacol* (2017) 27(7):566–73. doi: 10.1089/cap.2016.0145
21. Huang M, Su S, Goldberg J, Miller AH, Levantsevych OM, Shallenberger L, et al. Longitudinal association of inflammation with depressive symptoms: a 7-year cross-lagged twin difference study. *Brain Behav Immun* (2019) 75:200–7. doi: 10.1016/j.bbi.2018.10.007
22. Sharma B, Lawrence DW. Top-cited articles in traumatic brain injury. *Front Hum Neurosci* (2014) 8:879. doi: 10.3389/fnhum.2014.00879
23. Amaral AI. Effects of hypoglycaemia on neuronal metabolism in the adult brain: role of alternative substrates to glucose. *J Inherit Metab Dis* (2013) 36(4):621–34. doi: 10.1007/s10545-012-9553-3
24. Tyler KL. Emerging viral infections of the central nervous system: part 1. *Arch Neurol.* (2009) 66(8):939–48. doi: 10.1001/archneurol.2009.153

25. Nixon RA. The role of autophagy in neurodegenerative disease. *Nat Med* (2013) 19(8):983–97. doi: 10.1038/nm.3232
26. Uddin MS, Stachowiak A, Mamun AA, Tzvetkov NT, Takeda S, Atanasov AG, et al. Autophagy and Alzheimer's disease: from molecular mechanisms to therapeutic implications. *Front Aging Neurosci* (2018) 10:04. doi: 10.3389/fnagi.2018.00004
27. Sheehan P, Yue Z. Deregulation of autophagy and vesicle trafficking in Parkinson's disease. *Neurosci Lett* (2019) 697:59–65. doi: 10.1016/j.neulet.2018.04.013
28. Menzies FM, Fleming A, Caricasole A, Bento CF, Andrews SP, Ashkenazi A, et al. Autophagy and neurodegeneration: pathogenic mechanisms and therapeutic opportunities. *Neuron* (2017) 93(5):1015–34. doi: 10.1016/j.neuron.2017.01.022
29. Plaza-Zabala A, Sierra-Torre V, Sierra A. Autophagy and microglia: novel partners in neurodegeneration and aging. *Int J Mol Sci* (2017) 18(3):E598. doi: 10.3390/ijms18030598
30. Yoshii SR, Mizushima N. Monitoring and measuring autophagy. *Int J Mol Sci* (2017) 18(9):E1865. doi: 10.3390/ijms18091865
31. Brown GC, Neher JJ. Microglial phagocytosis of live neurons. *Nat Rev Neurosci* (2014) 15(4):209–16. doi: 10.1038/nrn3710
32. Fricker M, Neher JJ, Zhao JW, Théry C, Tolkovsky AM, Brown GC. MFG-E8 mediates primary phagocytosis of viable neurons during neuroinflammation. *J Neurosci* (2012) 32(8):2657–66. doi: 10.1523/JNEUROSCI.4837-11.2012
33. Neher JJ, Emmrich JV, Fricker M, Mander PK, Théry C, Brown GC. Phagocytosis executes delayed neuronal death after focal brain ischemia. *Proc Natl Acad Sci USA* (2013) 110(43):E4098–107. doi: 10.1073/pnas.1308679110
34. Galloway DA, Phillips AEM, Owen DRJ, Moore CS. Phagocytosis in the brain: homeostasis and disease. *Front Immunol* (2019) 10:790. doi: 10.3389/fimmu.2019.01575
35. Ginhoux F, Lim S, Hoeffel G, Low D, Huber T. Origin and differentiation of microglia. *Front Cell Neurosci* (2013) 7:45. doi: 10.3389/fncel.2013.00045
36. Mosser DM, Edwards JP. Exploring the full spectrum of macrophage activation. *Nat Rev Immunol* (2008) 30:958–69. doi: 10.1038/nri2448
37. Brown GC, Neher JJ. Inflammatory neurodegeneration and mechanisms of microglial killing of neurons. *Mol Neurobiol* (2010) 41:242–7. doi: 10.1007/s12035-010-8105-9
38. Santambrogio L, Belyanskaya SL, Fischer FR, Cipriani B, Brosnan CF, Ricciardi-Castagnoli P. Developmental plasticity of CNS microglia. *Proc Natl Acad Sci USA* (2001) 98(11):6295–300. doi: 10.1073/pnas.111152498
39. Ransohoff RM, Brown MA. Innate immunity in the central nervous system. *J Clin Invest* (2012) 122(4):1164–71. doi: 10.1172/JCI58644
40. Ulvestad E, Williams K, Bjerkvig R, Tiekotter K, Antel J, Matre R. Human microglial cells have phenotypic and functional characteristics in common with both macrophages and dendritic antigen-presenting cells. *J Leukoc Biol* (1994) 56(6):732–40. doi: 10.1002/jlb.56.6.732
41. Gomez-Nicola D, Perry VH. Microglial dynamics and role in the healthy and diseased brain: a paradigm of functional plasticity. *Neuroscientist* (2015) 21(2):169–84. doi: 10.1177/1073858414530512
42. Kierdorf K, Prinz M. Microglia in steady state. *J Clin Invest* (2017) 127(9):3201–9. doi: 10.1172/JCI90602
43. Nimmerjahn A, Kirchhoff F, Helmchen F. Resting microglial cells are highly dynamic surveillants of brain parenchyma *in vivo*. *Science* (2005) 308(5726):1314–8. doi: 10.1126/science.1110647
44. Stogsdill JA, Eroglu C. The interplay between neurons and glia in synapse development and plasticity. *Curr Opin Neurobiol* (2017) 42:1–8. doi: 10.1016/j.conb.2016.09.016
45. Galván A. Neural plasticity of development and learning. *Hum Brain Mapp* (2010) 31(6):879–90. doi: 10.1002/hbm.21029
46. Neniskyte U, Gross CT. Errant gardeners: glial-cell-dependent synaptic pruning and neurodevelopmental disorders. *Nat Rev Neurosci* (2017) 18(11):658–70. doi: 10.1038/nrn.2017.110
47. O'Connor TG, Moynihan JA, Caserta MT. Annual research review: the neuroinflammation hypothesis for stress and psychopathology in children—developmental psychoneuroimmunology. *J Child Psychol Psychiatry* (2014) 55(6):615–31. doi: 10.1111/jcpp.12187
48. Kariuki M, Raudino A, Green MJ, Laurens KR, Dean K, Brinkman SA, et al. Hospital admission for infection during early childhood influences developmental vulnerabilities at age 5 years. *J Paediatr Child Health* (2016) 52(9):882–8. doi: 10.1111/jpc.13239
49. Khandaker GM, Zimbron J, Dalman C, Lewis G, Jones PB. Childhood infection and adult schizophrenia: a meta-analysis of population-based studies. *Schizophr Res* (2012) 139(1–3):161–8. doi: 10.1016/j.schres.2012.05.023
50. Miller ZA, Mandelli ML, Rankin KP, Henry ML, Babiak MC, Frazier DT, et al. Handedness and language learning disability differentially distribute in progressive aphasia variants. *Brain* (2013) 136(Pt 11):3461–73. doi: 10.1093/brain/awt242
51. Sowell ER, Peterson BS, Thompson PM, Welcome SE, Henkenius AL, Toga AW. Mapping cortical change across the human life span. *Nat Neurosci* (2003) 6(3):309–15. doi: 10.1038/nn1008
52. Bartzokis G, Beckson M, Lu PH, Nuechterlein KH, Edwards N, Mintz J. Age-related changes in frontal and temporal lobe volumes in men: a magnetic resonance imaging study. *Arch Gen Psychiatry* (2001) 58:461–5. doi: 10.1001/archpsyc.58.5.461
53. Good CD, Johnsrude IS, Ashburner J, Henson RN, Friston KJ. Frackowiak RS. A voxel-based morphometric study of ageing in 465 normal adult human brains. *Neuroimage* (2001) 14:21–36. doi: 10.1006/nimg.2001.0786
54. Jernigan TL, Archibald SL, Fennema-Notestine C, Gamst AC, Stout JC, Bonner J, et al. Effects of age on tissues and regions of the cerebrum and cerebellum. *Neurobiol Aging* (2001) 22:581–94. doi: 10.1016/S0197-4580(01)00217-2
55. Block ML, Zecca L, Hong JS. Microglia-mediated neurotoxicity: uncovering the molecular mechanisms. *Nat Rev Neurosci* (2007) 8(1):57–69. doi: 10.1038/nrn2038
56. Appel SH, Beers DR, Henkel JS. T cell-microglial dialogue in Parkinson's disease and amyotrophic lateral sclerosis: are we listening? *Trends Immunol* (2010) 31(1):7–17. doi: 10.1016/j.it.2009.09.003
57. Neher JJ, Neniskyte U, Zhao JW, Bal-Price A, Tolkovsky AM, Brown GC. Inhibition of microglial phagocytosis is sufficient to prevent inflammatory neuronal death. *J Immunol* (2011) 186(8):4973–83. doi: 10.4049/jimmunol.1003600
58. Neniskyte U, Neher JJ, Brown GC. Neuronal death induced by nanomolar amyloid ß is mediated by primary phagocytosis of neurons by microglia. *J Biol Chem* (2011) 286(46):39904–13. doi: 10.1074/jbc.M111.267583
59. Ling H, Hardy J, Zetterberg H. Neurological consequences of traumatic brain injuries in sports. *Mol Cell Neurosci* (2015) 66(Pt B):114–22. doi: 10.1016/j.mcn.2015.03.012
60. Kumar A, Williams MT, Chugani HT. Evaluation of basal ganglia and thalamic inflammation in children with pediatric autoimmune neuropsychiatric disorders associated with Streptococcal infection and Tourette syndrome: a positron emission tomographic (PET) study using 11C-[R]-PK11195. *J Child Neurol* (2014) 30(6):749–56. doi: 10.1177/0883073814543303
61. Szepesi Z, Manouchehrian O, Bachiller S, Deierborg T. Bidirectional microglia-neuron communication in health and disease. *Front Cell Neurosci* (2018) 12:323. doi: 10.3389/fncel.2018.00323
62. Eyo UB, Wu LJ. Bidirectional microglia-neuron communication in the healthy brain. *Neural Plast* (2013) 2013:456857. doi: 10.1155/2013/456857
63. Davalos D, Grutzendler J, Yang G, Kim JV, Zuo Y, Jung S, et al. ATP mediates rapid microglial response to local brain injury *in vivo*. *Nat Neurosci* (2005) 8(6):752–8. doi: 10.1038/nn1472
64. Biber K, Neumann H, Inoue K, Boddeke HW. Neuronal 'On' and 'Off' signals control microglia. *Trends Neurosci* (2007) 30(11):596–602. doi: 10.1016/j.tins.2007.08.007
65. Ravichandran K. Find-me and eat-me signals in apoptotic cell clearance: progress and conundrums. *J Exp Med* (2010) 207(9):1807–17. doi: 10.1084/jem.20101157
66. Griffiths MR, Gasque P, Neal JW. The multiple roles of the innate immune system in the regulation of apoptosis and inflammation in the brain. *J Neuropathol Exp Neurol* (2009) 68(3):217–26. doi: 10.1097/NEN.0b013e3181996688
67. Blaylock RL, Maroon J. Immunoexcitotoxicity as a central mechanism in chronic traumatic encephalopathy—a unifying hypothesis. *Surg Neurol Int* (2011) 2:107. doi: 10.4103/2152-7806.83391
68. Ayata P, Badimon A, Strasburger HJ, Duff MK, Montgomery SE, Loh YE, et al. Epigenetic regulation of brain region-specific microglia clearance activity. *Nat Neurosci* (2018) 21(8):1049–60. doi: 10.1038/s41593-018-0192-3
69. Wraith DC, Nicholson LB. The adaptive immune system in diseases of the central nervous system. *J Clin Invest* (2012) 122(4):1172–9. doi: 10.1172/JCI58648

70. Skaper SD, Facci L, Zusso M, Giusti P. An inflammation-centric view of neurological disease: beyond the neuron. *Front Cell Neurosci* (2018) 12:72. doi: 10.3389/fncel.2018.00072
71. Neumann H. Control of glial immune function by neurons. *Glia* (2001) 236:191–9. doi: 10.1002/glia.1108
72. Ponomarev ED, Shriver LP, Maresz K, Dittel BN. Microglial cell activation and proliferation precedes the onset of CNS autoimmunity. *J Neurosci Res* (2005) 81(3):374–89. doi: 10.1002/jnr.20488
73. Rivest S. Regulation of innate immune responses in the brain. *Nat Rev Immunol* (2009) 9(6):429–39. doi: 10.1038/nri2565
74. Neumann H, Kotter MR, Franklin RJ. Debris clearance by microglia: an essential link between degeneration and regeneration. *Brain* (2008) 132(Pt 2):288–95. doi: 10.1093/brain/awn109
75. Lunnon K, Teeling JL, Tutt AL, Cragg MS, Glennie MJ, Perry VH. Systemic inflammation modulates Fc receptor expression on microglia during chronic neurodegeneration. *J Immunol* (2011) 186(12):7215–24. doi: 10.4049/jimmunol.0903833
76. Huizinga R, van der Star BJ, Kipp M, Jong R, Gerritsen W, Clarner T, et al. Phagocytosis of neuronal debris by microglia is associated with neuronal damage in multiple sclerosis. *Glia* (2012) 60(3):422–31. doi: 10.1002/glia.22276
77. Urrutia PJ, Mena NP, Nunez MT. The interplay between iron accumulation, mitochondrial dysfunction, and inflammation during the execution step of neurodegenerative disorders. *Front Pharmacol* (2014) 5:38. doi: 10.3389/fphar.2014.00038
78. Ruskovska T, Bernlohr DA. Oxidative stress and protein carbonylation in adipose tissue—implications for insulin resistance and diabetes mellitus. *J Proteomics* (2013) 92:10.1016. doi: 10.1016/j.jprot.2013.04.002
79. Hunter RL, Dragicevic N, Seifert K, Choi DY, Liu M, Kim HC, et al. Inflammation induces mitochondrial dysfunction and dopaminergic neurodegeneration in the nigrostriatal system. *J Neurochem* (2005) 100(5):1375–86. doi: 10.1111/j.1471-4159.2006.04327.x
80. Fumagalli S, Perego C, Pischiutta F, Zanier ER, De Simoni MG. The ischemic environment drives microglia and macrophage function. *Front Neurol* (2015) 6:81. doi: 10.3389/fneur.2015.00081
81. Perry VH. The influence of systemic inflammation on inflammation in the brain: implications for chronic neurodegenerative disease. *Brain Behav Immun* (2004) 18(5):407–13. doi: 10.1016/j.bbi.2004.01.004
82. Cunningham C, Campion S, Lunnon K, Murray CL, Woods JF, Deacon RM, et al. Systemic Inflammation induces acute behavioral and cognitive changes and accelerates neurodegenerative disease. *Biol Psychiatry* (2009) 65(4):304–12. doi: 10.1016/j.biopsych.2008.07.024
83. Perry VH, Cunningham C, Holmes C. Systemic infections and inflammation affect chronic neurodegeneration. *Nat Rev Immunol* (2007) 7(2):161–7. doi: 10.1038/nri2015
84. Perry VH. Contribution of systemic inflammation to chronic neurodegeneration. *Acta Neuropathol* (2010) 120(3):277–86. doi: 10.1007/s00401-010-0722-x
85. Perry VH, Nicoll JA, Holmes C. Microglia in neurodegenerative disease. *Nat Rev Neurol* (2010) 6(4):193–201. doi: 10.1038/nrneurol.2010.17
86. Butterfield DA, Halliwell B. Oxidative stress, dysfunctional glucose metabolism and Alzheimer disease. *Nat Rev Neurosci* (2019) 20(3):148–60. doi: 10.1038/s41583-019-0132-6
87. Vogt NM, Kerby RL, Dill-McFarland KA, Harding SJ, Merluzzi AP, Johnson SC, et al. Gut microbiome alterations in Alzheimer's disease. *Sci Rep* (2017) 7(1):13537. doi: 10.1038/s41598-017-13601-y
88. Harding A, Gonder U, Robinson SJ, Crean S, Singhrao SK. Exploring the association between Alzheimer's disease, oral health, microbial endocrinology and nutrition. *Front Aging Neurosci* (2017) 9:398. doi: 10.3389/fnagi.2017.00398
89. Giridharan VV, Masud F, Petronilho F, Dal-Pizzol F, Barichello T. Infection-induced systemic inflammation is a potential driver of Alzheimer's disease progression. *Front Aging Neurosci* (2019) 11:122. doi: 10.3389/fnagi.2019.00122
90. Luchsinger JA, Reitz C, Honig LS, Tang MX, Shea S, Mayeux R. Aggregation of vascular risk factors and risk of incident Alzheimer disease. *Neurology* (2005) 65(4):545–51. doi: 10.1212/01.wnl.0000172914.08967.dc
91. Honig LS, Tang MX, Albert S, Costa R, Luchsinger J, Stern Y, et al. Stroke and the risk of Alzheimer disease. *Arch Neurol* (2003) 60(12):1707–12. doi: 10.1001/archneur.60.12.1707
92. Fusco M, Skaper SD, Coaccioli S, Varrassi G, Paladini A. Degenerative joint diseases and neuroinflammation. *Pain Pract* (2017) 17(4):522–32. doi: 10.1111/papr.12551
93. Schrepf A, Kaplan CM, Ichesco E, Larkin T, Harte SE, Harris RE, et al. A multimodal MRI study of the central response to inflammation in rheumatoid arthritis. *Nat Commun* (2018) 9(1):2243. doi: 10.1038/s41467-018-04648-0
94. Chou RC, Kane M, Ghimire S, Gautam S, Gui J. Treatment for rheumatoid arthritis and risk of Alzheimer's disease: a nested case-control analysis. *CNS Drugs* (2016) 30(11):1111–20. doi: 10.1007/s40263-016-0374-z
95. Kao LT, Kang JH, Lin HC, Huang CC, Lee HC, Chung SD. Rheumatoid arthritis was negatively associated with Alzheimer's disease: a population-based case-control study. *PLoS One* (2016) 11(12):e0168106. doi: 10.1371/journal.pone.0168106
96. Policicchio S, Ahmad AN, Powell JF, Proitsi P. Rheumatoid arthritis and risk for Alzheimer's disease: a systematic review and meta-analysis and a Mendelian Randomization study. *Sci Rep* (2017) 7(1):12861. doi: 10.1038/s41598-017-13168-8
97. Cai Q, Xin Z, Zuo L, Li F, Liu B. Alzheimer's disease and rheumatoid arthritis: a Mendelian randomization study. *Front Neurosci* (2018) 12:627. doi: 10.3389/fnins.2018.00627
98. van Langenberg DR, Yelland GW, Robinson SR, Gibson PR. Cognitive impairment in Crohn's disease is associated with systemic inflammation, symptom burden and sleep disturbance. United European. *Gastroenterol J* (2017) 5(4):579–87. doi: 10.1177/2050640616663397
99. McCaulley ME, Grush KA. Alzheimer's disease: exploring the role of inflammation and implications for treatment. *Int J Alzheimers Dis* (2015) 2015:515248. doi: 10.1155/2015/515248
100. Ajami B, Bennett JL, Krieger C, McNagny KM, Rossi FM. Infiltrating monocytes trigger EAE progression, but do not contribute to the resident microglia pool. *Nat Neurosci* (2011) 14(9):1142–9. doi: 10.1038/nn.2887
101. Cunningham C, Wilcockson DC, Campion S, Lunnon K, Perry VH. Central and systemic endotoxin challenges exacerbate the local inflammatory response and increase neuronal death during chronic neurodegeneration. *J Neurosci* (2005) 25(40):9275–84. doi: 10.1523/JNEUROSCI.2614-05.2005
102. Chakravarty S, Herkenham M. Toll-like receptor 4 on nonhematopoietic cells sustains CNS inflammation during endotoxemia, independent of systemic cytokines. *J Neurosci* (2005) 25:1788–96. doi: 10.1523/JNEUROSCI.4268-04.2005
103. Lacroix S, Feinstein D, Rivest S. The bacterial endotoxin lipopolysaccharide has the ability to target the brain in upregulating its membrane CD14 receptor within specific cellular populations. *Brain Pathol* (1998) 8:625–40. doi: 10.1111/j.1750-3639.1998.tb00189.x
104. Quan N, Whiteside M, Herkenham M. Time course and localization patterns of interleukin-1ß mRNA expression in the brain and pituitary after peripheral administration of lipopolysaccharide. *Neuroscience* (1997) 83:281–93. doi: 10.1016/S0306-4522(97)00350-3
105. Quan N, Whiteside M, Kim L, Herkenham M. Induction of inhibitory factor κBα mRNA in the central nervous system after peripheral lipopolysaccharide administration: an in situ hybridization histochemistry study in the rat. *Proc Natl Acad Sci USA* (1997) 94:10985–90. doi: 10.1073/pnas.94.20.10985
106. Laflamme N, Lacroix S, Rivest S. An essential role of interleukin-1beta in mediating NF-kappaB activity and COX-2 transcription in cells of the blood-brain barrier in response to a systemic and localized inflammation but not during endotoxemia. *J Neurosci* (1999) 19(24):10923–30. doi: 10.1523/JNEUROSCI.19-24-10923.1999
107. Varatharaj A, Galea I. The blood-brain barrier in systemic inflammation. *Brain Behav Immun* (2017) 60:1–12. doi: 10.1016/j.bbi.2016.03.010
108. Kuhlmann CR, Librizzi L, Closhen D, Pflanzner T, Lessmann V, Pietrzik CU, et al. Mechanisms of C-reactive protein-induced blood-brain barrier disruption. *Stroke* (2009) 40(4):1458–66. doi: 10.1161/STROKEAHA.108.535930
109. Sproston NR, Ashworth JJ. Role of C-reactive protein at sites of inflammation and infection. *Front Immunol* (2018) 9:754. doi: 10.3389/fimmu.2018.00754

110. Banks WA, Farr SA, Morley JE. Entry of blood-borne cytokines into the central nervous system: effects on cognitive processes. *Neuroimmunomodulation* (2002-2003) 10(6):319–27. doi: 10.1159/000071472
111. Lin WC, Chou KH, Lee PL, Huang YC, Tsai NW, Chen HL, et al. Brain mediators of systemic oxidative stress on perceptual impairments in Parkinson's disease. *J Transl Med* (2015) 13:386. doi: 10.1186/s12967-015-0749-9
112. Peng L, Xu L, Ouyang W. Role of peripheral inflammatory markers in postoperative cognitive dysfunction (POCD): a meta-analysis. *PLoS One* (2013) 8(11):e79624. doi: 10.1371/journal.pone.0079624
113. Dénes A, Ferenczi S, Kovács KJ. Systemic inflammatory challenges compromise survival after experimental stroke *via* augmenting brain inflammation, blood- brain barrier damage and brain oedema independently of infarct size. *J Neuroinflammation* (2011) 8:164. doi: 10.1186/1742-2094-8-164
114. Combrinck MI, Perry VH, Cunningham C. Peripheral infection evokes exaggerated sickness behaviour in pre-clinical murine prion disease. *Neuroscience* (2002) 112(1):7–11. doi: 10.1016/S0306-4522(02)00030-1
115. Cardoso FL, Kittel A, Veszelka S, Palmela I, Tóth A, Brites D, et al. Exposure to lipopolysaccharide and/or unconjugated bilirubin impair the integrity and function of brain microvascular endothelial cells. *PLoS One* (2012) 7(5):e35919. doi: 10.1371/journal.pone.0035919
116. Marsland AL, Walsh C, Lockwood K, John-Henderson NA. The effects of acute psychological stress on circulating and stimulated inflammatory markers: a systematic review and meta-analysis. *Brain Behav Immun* (2017) 64:208–19. doi: 10.1016/j.bbi.2017.01.011
117. Cohen S, Janicki-Deverts D, Doyle WJ, Miller GE, Frank E, Rabin BS, et al. Chronic stress, glucocorticoid receptor resistance, inflammation, and disease risk. *Proc Natl Acad Sci USA* (2012) 109(16):5995–9. doi: 10.1073/pnas.1118355109
118. Cole SW. Social regulation of leukocyte homeostasis: the role of glucocorticoid sensitivity. *Brain Behav Immun* (2008) 22(7):1049–55. doi: 10.1016/j.bbi.2008.02.006
119. Erny D, Hrabe de Angelis AL, Jaitin D, Wieghofer P, Staszewski O, David E, et al. Host microbiota constantly control maturation and function of microglia in the CNS. *Nat Neurosci* (2015) 18(7):965–77. doi: 10.1038/nn.4030
120. Thevaranjan N, Puchta A, Schulz C, Naidoo A, Szamosi JC, Verschoor CP, et al. Age-associated microbial dysbiosis promotes intestinal permeability, systemic inflammation, and macrophage dysfunction. *Cell Host Microbe* (2017) 21(4):455–466.e4. doi: 10.1016/j.chom.2017.03.002
121. Andersen K, Kesper MS, Marschner JA, Konrad L, Ryu M, Kumar Vr S, et al. Intestinal dysbiosis, barrier dysfunction, and bacterial translocation account for CKD-related systemic inflammation. *J Am Soc Nephrol* (2017) 28(1):76–83. doi: 10.1681/ASN.2015111285
122. de Jong PR, González-Navajas JM, Jansen NJ. The digestive tract as the origin of systemic inflammation. *Crit Care* (2016) 20(1):279. doi: 10.1186/s13054-016-1458-3
123. Cai D, Liu T. Inflammatory cause of metabolic syndrome *via* brain stress and NF-κB. *Aging.* (2012) 4(2):98–115. doi: 10.18632/aging.100431
124. Müller S, Martin S, Koenig W, Hanifi-Moghaddam P, Rathmann W, Haastert B, et al. Impaired glucose tolerance is associated with increased serum concentrations of interleukin 6 and co-regulated acute-phase proteins but not TNF-alpha or its receptors. *Diabetologia* (2002) 45(6):805–12. doi: 10.1007/s00125-002-0829-2
125. Temelkova-Kurktschiev T, Siegert G, Bergmann S, Henkel E, Koehler C, Jaross W, et al. Subclinical inflammation is strongly related to insulin resistance but not to impaired insulin secretion in a high risk population for diabetes. *Metabolism* (2002) 51(6):743–9. doi: 10.1053/meta.2002.32804
126. Yudkin JS, Stehouwer CD, Emeis JJ. Coppack SW. C-reactive protein in healthy subjects: associations with obesity, insulin resistance, and endothelial dysfunction: a potential role for cytokines originating from adipose tissue? *Arterioscler Thromb Vasc Biol* (1999) 19(4):972–8. doi: 10.1161/01.ATV.19.4.972
127. Eltzschig HK, Carmeliet P. Hypoxia and inflammation. *N Engl J Med* (2011) 364(7):656–65. doi: 10.1056/NEJMra0910283
128. Fujisaka S, Usui I, Ikutani M, Aminuddin A, Takikawa A, Tsuneyama K, et al. Adipose tissue hypoxia induces inflammatory M1 polarity of macrophages in an HIF-1α-dependent and HIF-1α-independent manner in obese mice. *Diabetologia* (2013) 56(6):1403–12. doi: 10.1007/s00125-013-2885-1
129. Walmsley SR, Print C, Farahi N, Peyssonnaux C, Johnson RS, Cramer T, et al. Hypoxia-induced neutrophil survival is mediated by HIF-1alpha-dependent NF-kappaB activity. *J Exp Med* (2005) 201(1):105–15. doi: 10.1084/jem.20040624
130. Giugliano D, Ceriello A, Esposito K. The effects of diet on inflammation: emphasis on the metabolic syndrome. *J Am Coll Cardiol* (2006) 48(4):677–85. doi: 10.1016/j.jacc.2006.03.052
131. vel Szic KS, Ndlovu MN, Haegeman G, Berghe WV. Nature or nurture: let food be your epigenetic medicine in chronic inflammatory disorders. *Biochem Pharmacol* (2010) 80(12):1816–32. doi: 10.1016/j.bcp.2010.07.029
132. Fisher G, Hyatt TC, Hunter GR, Oster RA, Desmond RA, Gower BA. Effect of diet with and without exercise training on markers of inflammation and fat distribution in overweight women. *Obesity (Silver Spring)* (2011) 19(6):1131–6. doi: 10.1038/oby.2010.310
133. Nicklas BJ, Ambrosius W, Messier SP, Miller GD, Penninx BW, Loeser RF, et al. Diet-induced weight loss, exercise, and chronic inflammation in older, obese adults: a randomized controlled clinical trial. *Am J Clin Nutr.* (2004) 79(4):544–51. doi: 10.1093/ajcn/79.4.544
134. Heilbronn LK, Noakes M, Clifton PM. Energy restriction and weight loss on very-low-fat diets reduce C-reactive protein concentrations in obese, healthy women. *Arterioscler Thromb Vasc Biol* (2001) 21(6):968–70. doi: 10.1161/01.ATV.21.6.968
135. Horsburgh S, Robson-Ansley P, Adams R, Smith C. Exercise and inflammation-related epigenetic modifications: focus on DNA methylation. *Exerc Immunol Rev* (2015) 21:26–41.
136. Vieira VJ, Valentine RJ, Wilund KR, Antao N, Baynard T, Woods JA. Effects of exercise and low-fat diet on adipose tissue inflammation and metabolic complications in obese mice. *Am J Physiol Endocrinol Metab* (2009) 296(5):E1164–71. doi: 10.1152/ajpendo.00054.2009
137. Ford ES. Does exercise reduce inflammation? Physical activity and C-reactive protein among U.S. adults. *Epidemiology* (2002) 13(5):561–8. doi: 10.1097/00001648-200209000-00012
138. You T, Berman DM, Ryan AS, Nicklas BJ. Effects of hypocaloric diet and exercise training on inflammation and adipocyte lipolysis in obese postmenopausal women. *J Clin Endocrinol Metab* (2004) 89(4):1739–46. doi: 10.1210/jc.2003-031310
139. Zoppini G, Targher G, Zamboni C, Venturi C, Cacciatori V, Moghetti P, et al. Effects of moderate-intensity exercise training on plasma biomarkers of inflammation and endothelial dysfunction in older patients with type 2 diabetes. *Nutr Metab Cardiovasc Dis* (2006) 16(8):543–9. doi: 10.1016/j.numecd.2005.09.004
140. Møller P, Danielsen PH, Karottki DG, Jantzen K, Roursgaard M, Klingberg H, et al. Oxidative stress and inflammation generated DNA damage by exposure to air pollution particles. *Mutat Res Rev Mutat Res* (2014) 762:133–66. doi: 10.1016/j.mrrev.2014.09.001
141. Yang SN, Hsieh CC, Kuo HF, Lee MS, Huang MY, Kuo CH, et al. The effects of environmental toxins on allergic inflammation. *Allergy Asthma Immunol Res* (2014) 6(6):478–84. doi: 10.4168/aair.2014.6.6.478
142. Klein CL, Köhler H, Kirkpatrick CJ. Increased adhesion and activation of polymorphonuclear neutrophil granulocytes to endothelial cells under heavy metal exposure *in vitro*. *Pathobiology* (1994) 62(2):90–8. doi: 10.1159/000163883
143. Dong W, Simeonova PP, Gallucci R, Matheson J, Flood L, Wang S, et al. Toxic metals stimulate inflammatory cytokines in hepatocytes through oxidative stress mechanisms. *Toxicol Appl Pharmacol* (1998) 151(2):359–66. doi: 10.1006/taap.1998.8481
144. Majkova Z, Smart E, Toborek M, Hennig B. Up-regulation of endothelial monocyte chemoattractant protein-1 by coplanar PCB77 is caveolin-1-dependent. *Toxicol Appl Pharmacol* (2009) 237(1):1–7. doi: 10.1016/j.taap.2009.02.016
145. Kebir H, Kreymborg K, Ifergan I, Dodelet-Devillers A, Cayrol R, Bernard M, et al. Human TH17 lymphocytes promote blood-brain barrier disruption and central nervous system inflammation. *Nat Med* (2007) 13(10):1173–5. doi: 10.1038/nm1651
146. Langrish CL, Chen Y, Blumenschein WM, Mattson J, Basham B, Sedgwick JD, et al. IL-23 drives a pathogenic T cell population that induces autoimmune inflammation. *J Exp Med* (2005) 201(2):233–40. doi: 10.1084/jem.20041257
147. Bredesen DE, Amos EC, Canick J, Ackerley M, Raji C, Fiala M, et al. Reversal of cognitive decline in Alzheimer's disease. *Aging (Albany NY).* (2016) 8(6):1250–8. doi: 10.18632/aging.100981

148. Aharoni R. Immunomodulation neuroprotection and remyelination—the fundamental therapeutic effects of glatiramer acetate: a critical review. *J Autoimmun* (2014) 54:81–92. doi: 10.1016/j.jaut.2014.05.005
149. Feinstein DL, Kalinin S, Braun D. Causes, consequences, and cures for neuroinflammation mediated *via* the locus coeruleus: noradrenergic signaling system. *J Neurochem* (2016) 139 Suppl 2:154–78. doi: 10.1111/jnc.13447
150. Jayedi A, Rashidy-Pour A, Shab-Bidar S. Vitamin D status and risk of dementia and Alzheimer's disease: a meta-analysis of dose-response. *Nutr Neurosci* (2018) 15:1–10. doi: 10.1080/1028415X.2018.1436639
151. Mrówczynski W. Health benefits of endurance training: implications of the brain-derived neurotrophic factor—a systematic review. *Neural Plast* (2019) 2019:5413067. doi: 10.1155/2019/5413067
152. Miyauchi T, Tokura T, Kimura H, Ito M, Umemura E, Sato Boku A, et al. Effect of antidepressant treatment on plasma levels of neuroinflammation-associated molecules in patients with somatic symptom disorder with predominant pain around the orofacial region. *Hum Psychopharmacol* (2019) 34(4):e2698. doi: 10.1002/hup.2698
153. Aftanas LI, Gevorgyan MM, Zhanaeva SY, Dzemidovich SS, Kulikova KI, Al'perina EL, et al. Therapeutic effects of repetitive transcranial magnetic stimulation (rTMS) on neuroinflammation and neuroplasticity in patients with Parkinson's disease: a placebo-controlled study. *Bull Exp Biol Med* (2018) 165(2):195–9. doi: 10.1007/s10517-018-4128-4
154. Deardorff WJ, Grossberg GT. Targeting neuroinflammation in Alzheimer's disease: evidence for NSAIDs and novel therapeutics. *Expert Rev Neurother* (2017) 17(1):17–32. doi: 10.1080/14737175.2016.1200972
155. De Virgilio A, Greco A, Fabbrini G, Inghilleri M, Rizzo MI, Gallo A, et al. Parkinson's disease: autoimmunity and neuroinflammation. *Autoimmun Rev* (2016) 15(10):1005–11. doi: 10.1016/j.autrev.2016.07.022
156. Rommer PS, Milo R, Han MH, Satyanarayan S, Sellner J, Hauer L, et al. Immunological aspects of approved MS therapeutics. *Front Immunol* (2019) 10:1564. doi: 10.3389/fimmu.2019.01564
157. Hirad AA, Bazarian JJ, Merchant-Borna K, Garcea FE, Heilbronner S, Paul D, et al. A common neural signature of brain injury in concussion and subconcussion. *Sci Adv* (2019) 5:eaau3460. doi: 10.1126/sciadv.aau3460
158. Strawbridge R, Young AH, Cleare AJ. Biomarkers for depression: recent insights, current challenges and future prospects. *Neuropsychiatr Dis Treat* (2017) 13:1245–62. doi: 10.2147/NDT.S114542
159. Clancy JA, Mary DA, Witte KK, Greenwood JP, Deuchars SA, Deuchars J. Non-invasive vagus nerve stimulation in healthy humans reduces sympathetic nerve activity. *Brain Stimul.* (2014) 7(6):871–7. doi: 10.1016/j.brs.2014.07.031
160. Andersson U, Tracey KJ. Neural reflexes in inflammation and immunity. *J Exp Med* (2012) 209(6):1057–68. doi: 10.1084/jem.20120571
161. Kimura K, Tanida M, Nagata N, Inaba Y, Watanabe H, Nagashimada M, et al. Central insulin action activates Kupffer cells by suppressing hepatic vagal activation *via* the nicotinic alpha 7 acetylcholine receptor. *Cell Rep* (2016) 14(10):2362–74. doi: 10.1016/j.celrep.2016.02.032
162. Di Giovangiulio M, Verheijden S, Di Giovangiulio M, Verheijden S, Bosmans G, Stakenborg N, et al. The neuromodulation of the intestinal immune system and its relevance in inflammatory bowel disease. *Front Immunol* (2015) 6:590. doi: 10.3389/fimmu.2015.00590
163. Inoue T, Abe C, Sung SS, Moscalu S, Jankowski J, Huang L, et al. Vagus nerve stimulation mediates protection from kidney ischemia-reperfusion injury through α7nAChR+ splenocytes. *J Clin Invest* (2016) 126(5):1939–52. doi: 10.1172/JCI83658
164. Dilger RN, Johnson RW. Aging, microglial cell priming, and the discordant central inflammatory response to signals from the peripheral immune system. *J Leukoc Biol* (2008) 84(4):932–9. doi: 10.1189/jlb.0208108
165. Mangano EN, Hayley S. Inflammatory priming of the substantia nigra influences the impact of later paraquat exposure: neuroimmune sensitization of neurodegeneration. *Neurobiol Aging* (2009) 30(9):1361–78. doi: 10.1016/j.neurobiolaging.2007.11.020
166. Hunter LE, Branch CA, Lipton ML. The neurobiological effects of repetitive head impacts in collision sports. *Neurobiol Dis* (2019) 123:122–6. doi: 10.1016/j.nbd.2018.06.016
167. Norden DM, Muccigrosso MM, Godbout JP. Microglial priming and enhanced reactivity to secondary insult in aging, and traumatic CNS injury, and neurodegenerative disease. *Neuropharmacology* (2015) 96(Pt A):29–41. doi: 10.1016/j.neuropharm.2014.10.028
168. Carvey PM, Punati A, Newman MB. Progressive dopamine neuron loss in Parkinson's disease: the multiple hit hypothesis. *Cell Transplant* (2006) 15(3):239–50. doi: 10.3727/000000006783981990
169. Patrick KL, Bell SL, Weindel CG, Watson RO. Exploring the "multiple-hit hypothesis" of neurodegenerative disease: bacterial infection comes up to bat. *Front Cell Infect Microbiol* (2019) 9:138. doi: 10.3389/fcimb.2019.00138
170. Fiebich BL, Akter S, Akundi RS. The two-hit hypothesis for neuroinflammation: role of exogenous ATP in modulating inflammation in the brain. *Front Cell Neurosci* (2014) 8:260. doi: 10.3389/fncel.2014.00260
171. Barnett ML, Tusor N, Ball G, Chew A, Falconer S, Aljabar P, et al. Exploring the multiple-hit hypothesis of preterm white matter damage using diffusion MRI. *Neuroimage Clin* (2017) 17:596–606. doi: 10.1016/j.nicl.2017.11.017
172. Grieb B, Engler G, Sharott A, von Nicolai C, Streichert T, Papageorgiou I, et al. High-frequency stimulation of the subthalamic nucleus counteracts cortical expression of major histocompatibility complex genes in a rat model of Parkinson's disease. *PLoS One* (2014) 9(3):e91663. doi: 10.1371/journal.pone.0091663
173. Carrera E, Tononi G. Diaschisis: past, present, future. *Brain* (2014) 137(9):2408–22. doi: 10.1093/brain/awu101
174. Silasi G, Murphy TH. Stroke and the connectome: how connectivity guides therapeutic intervention. *Neuron* (2014) 83(6):1354–68. doi: 10.1016/j.neuron.2014.08.052
175. Lehmann PV, Forsthuber T, Miller A, Sercarz EE. Spreading of T-cell autoimmunity to cryptic determinants of an autoantigen. *Nature* (1992) 358(6382):155–7. doi: 10.1038/358155a0
176. McRae BL, Vanderlugt CL, Dal Canto MC, Miller SD. Functional evidence for epitope spreading in the relapsing pathology of experimental autoimmune encephalomyelitis. *J Exp Med* (1995) 182(1):75–85. doi: 10.1084/jem.182.1.75
177. Münz C, Lünemann JD, Getts MT, Miller SD. Antiviral immune responses: triggers of or triggered by autoimmunity? *Nat Rev Immunol* (2009) 9(4):246–58. doi: 10.1038/nri2527
178. Akira S, Uematsu S, Takeuchi O. Pathogen recognition and innate immunity. *Cell* (2006) 124(4):783–801. doi: 10.1016/j.cell.2006.02.015
179. Schaefer L. Complexity of danger: the diverse nature of damage-associated molecular patterns. *J Biol Chem* (2014) 289(51):35237–45. doi: 10.1074/jbc.R114.619304
180. Semenza GL. Hypoxia-inducible factor 1 (HIF-1) pathway. *Sci STKE* (2007) 2007(407):cm8. doi: 10.1126/stke.4072007cm8
181. Semenza GL. Hypoxia-inducible factor 1 and cardiovascular disease. *Annu Rev Physiol* (2014) 76:39–56. doi: 10.1146/annurev-physiol-021113-170322
182. Nizet V, Johnson RS. Interdependence of hypoxic and innate immune responses. *Nat Rev Immunol* (2009) 9(9):609–17. doi: 10.1038/nri2607
183. D'Ignazio L, Bandarra D, Rocha S. NF-κB and HIF crosstalk in immune responses. *FEBS J* (2016) 283(3):413–24. doi: 10.1111/febs.13578
184. Barnes PJ, Karin M. Nuclear factor-kappaB: a pivotal transcription factor in chronic inflammatory diseases. *N Engl J Med* (1997) 336(15):1066–71. doi: 10.1056/NEJM199704103361506
185. Mander P, Brown GC. Activation of microglial NADPH oxidase is synergistic with glial iNOS expression in inducing neuronal death: a dual-key mechanism of inflammatory neurodegeneration. *J Neuroinflammation* (2005) 2:20. doi: 10.1186/1742-2094-2-20
186. Nocella C, Cammisotto V, Pigozzi F, Borrione P, Fossati C, D'Amico A, et al. Impairment between oxidant and antioxidant systems: short- and long-term implications for athletes' health. *Nutrients* (2019) 11(6):E1353. doi: 10.3390/nu11061353
187. Ginhoux F, Prinz M. Origin of microglia: current concepts and past controversies. *Cold Spring Harb Perspect Biol* (2015) 7(8):a020537. doi: 10.1101/cshperspect.a020537
188. Fernandes A, Miller-Fleming L, Pais TF. Microglia and inflammation: conspiracy, controversy or control? *Cell Mol Life Sci* (2014) 71(20):3969–85. doi: 10.1007/s00018-014-1670-8
189. Culmsee C, Michels S, Scheu S, Arolt V, Dannlowski U, Alferink J. Mitochondria, microglia, and the immune system—how are they linked in affective disorders? *Front Psychiatry* (2019) 99:739. doi: 10.3389/fpsyt.2018.00739

190. Chang HS, Won E, Lee HY, Ham BJ, Lee MS. Association analysis for corticotropin releasing hormone polymorphisms with the risk of major depressive disorder and the response to antidepressants. *Behav Brain Res* (2015) 292:116–24. doi: 10.1016/j.bbr.2015.06.005

191. Kelly B, O'Neill LA. Metabolic reprogramming in macrophages and dendritic cells in innate immunity. *Cell Res* (2015) 25(7):771–84. doi: 10.1038/cr.2015.68

192. Corcoran SE, O'Neill LA. HIF1α and metabolic reprogramming in inflammation. *J Clin Invest* (2016) 126(10):3699–707. doi: 10.1172/JCI84431

193. Raison CL, Miller AH. Is depression an inflammatory disorder? *Curr Psychiatry Rep* (2011) 13(6):467–75. doi: 10.1007/s11920-011-0232-0

194. Dooley LN, Kuhlman KR, Robles TF, Eisenberger NI, Craske MG, Bower JE. The role of inflammation in core features of depression: insights from paradigms using exogenously-induced inflammation. *Neurosci Biobehav Rev* (2018) 94:219–37. doi: 10.1016/j.neubiorev.2018.09.006

195. Kopschina Feltes P, Doorduin J, Klein HC, Juárez-Orozco LE, Dierckx RA, Moriguchi-Jeckel CM, et al. Anti-inflammatory treatment for major depressive disorder: implications for patients with an elevated immune profile and non-responders to standard antidepressant therapy. *J Psychopharmacol* (2017) 31(9):1149–65. doi: 10.1177/0269881117711708

196. Heninger GR, Delgado PL, Charney DS. The revised monoamine theory of depression: a modulatory role for monoamines, based on new findings from monoamine depletion experiments in humans. *Pharmacopsychiatry* (1996) 29(1):2–11 doi: 10.1055/s-2007-979535.

5

A Subset of Patients with Autism Spectrum Disorders Show a Distinctive Metabolic Profile by Dried Blood Spot Analyses

Rita Barone [1,2*†], *Salvatore Alaimo* [3†], *Marianna Messina* [2], *Alfredo Pulvirenti* [3], *Jean Bastin* [4,5], *MIMIC-Autism Group, Alfredo Ferro* [3], *Richard E. Frye* [6,7] *and Renata Rizzo* [1]

[1] Child Neurology and Psychiatry, Department of Clinical and Experimental Medicine, University of Catania, Catania, Italy, [2] Referral Centre for Inherited Metabolic Disorders, Department of Clinical and Experimental Medicine, University of Catania, Catania, Italy, [3] Bioinformatics Unit, Department of Clinical and Experimental Medicine, University of Catania, Catania, Italy, [4] Sorbonne Paris Cité, Faculté des Sciences Fondamentales et Biomédicales, Université Paris Descartes, Paris, France, [5] INSERM, UMR-S 1124, Toxicologie, Pharmacologie et Signalisation Cellulaire, Paris, France, [6] University of Arizona College of Medicine, Phoenix, AZ, United States, [7] Phoenix Children's Hospital, Phoenix, AZ, United States

***Correspondence:**
Rita Barone
rbarone@unict.it

†These authors have contributed equally to this work

Autism spectrum disorder (ASD) is currently diagnosed according to behavioral criteria. Biomarkers that identify children with ASD could lead to more accurate and early diagnosis. ASD is a complex disorder with multifactorial and heterogeneous etiology supporting recognition of biomarkers that identify patient subsets. We investigated an easily testable blood metabolic profile associated with ASD diagnosis using high throughput analyses of samples extracted from dried blood spots (DBS). A targeted panel of 45 ASD analytes including acyl-carnitines and amino acids extracted from DBS was examined in 83 children with ASD (60 males; age 6.06 ± 3.58, range: 2–10 years) and 79 matched, neurotypical (NT) control children (57 males; age 6.8 ± 4.11 years, range 2.5–11 years). Based on their chronological ages, participants were divided in two groups: younger or older than 5 years. Two-sided *T*-tests were used to identify significant differences in measured metabolite levels between groups. Näive Bayes algorithm trained on the identified metabolites was used to profile children with ASD vs. NT controls. Of the 45 analyzed metabolites, nine (20%) were significantly increased in ASD patients including the amino acid citrulline and acyl-carnitines C2, C4DC/C5OH, C10, C12, C14:2, C16, C16:1, C18:1 (P: < 0.001). Näive Bayes algorithm using acyl-carnitine metabolites which were identified as significantly abnormal showed the highest performances for classifying ASD in children younger than 5 years (n: 42; mean age 3.26 ± 0.89) with 72.3% sensitivity (95% CI: 71.3;73.9), 72.1% specificity (95% CI: 71.2;72.9) and a diagnostic odds ratio 11.25 (95% CI: 9.47;17.7). Re-test analyses as a measure of validity showed an accuracy of 73% in children with ASD aged ≤5 years. This easily testable, non-invasive profile in DBS may support recognition of metabolic ASD individuals aged ≤5 years and represents a potential complementary tool to improve diagnosis at earlier stages of ASD development.

Keywords: autism spectrum disorders, dried blood spots, ESI-MS/MS, mitochondrial fatty acid β-oxidation, machine learning

INTRODUCTION

Autism spectrum disorder (ASD) is a neurodevelopmental disorder that affects approximately 16.8 per 1,000 (one in 59) children aged 8 years in the US and with a male/female ratio of 4:1 (1). In Italy, a recent study reported an overall prevalence rate of one in 100 children at age 7–8 years (2). ASD is characterized by significant defects of social communication and interaction and by restricted and repetitive patterns of interests and activities with onset in early childhood (3). The etiology remains poorly understood. Increasing evidence has converged on possible interactions among pleiotropic genetic background conferring vulnerabilities to environmental inputs leading to multiple systemic co-morbidities including metabolic disarrangement (4). Classic inborn errors of metabolism (IEM) affect a subgroup of ASD patients accounting for 1–3% of patients (5). Acquired symptoms featuring autism or childhood disintegrative disorder may occur in the neuronopathic lysosomal storage disorders (6, 7). Among IEM, primary mitochondrial diseases affect nearly 5% of patients with ASD, however the occurrence of abnormal biomarkers indicating mitochondrial dysfunction is higher in patients with ASD than in the general population (8). On a clinical ground, children with ASD may exhibit features of a mitochondrial disease such as hypotonia and delayed motor development as well as gastrointestinal disturbances and regression following fever or other environmental triggers (9).

Clinical diagnosis of ASD relies on behavioral tests. Early recognition and specialized intervention improve the outcome and are most effective if initiated early in life (10). Thus, the development of multiple laboratory markers that can assist in the early and accurate diagnosis of ASD is envisaged. Urinary metabolomic studies (11–16) and a few studies performed on blood samples (17–19) collectively showed modification of amino acid, purine and fatty acid metabolic pathways, increased oxidative stress, gut dysbiosis and altered gut permeability in individuals with ASD. Multiplatform analytical methodology and multivariate analysis may provide the best models discriminating between ASD and typically developing (TD) children. Through this approach, a rigorous analysis for the discovery of ASD biomarkers combined several mass spectrometry (MS)-based analyses of blood. This combined analysis resulted in 40 features could differential ASD and TD samples with an accuracy of 70% (17). More recently, a study in 38 children with ASD reported increased advanced glycation endproducts, Nε-carboxymethyllysine and Nω-carboxymethylarginine, and increased oxidation damage marker, dityrosine, in plasma proteins, capable to classify the disease status (19).

Since the 1980s, electrospray ionization (ESI) and tandem MS/MS technology endorsed high throughput analyses of samples extracted from dried blood spots (DBS) for newborn screening of IEM as health care standard (20). Thus, we hypothesized that ESI-MS/MS analyses of different metabolites in DBS might represent a high throughput method for metabolic profiling of individuals with ASD by a single injection, in a rapid, low-cost, and suitable procedure. To test this hypothesis, we used a standardized ESI-MS/MS analyses in DBS to systematically examine the levels of a large panel of highly selective biochemical analytes in patients with ASD and healthy TD, matched-control subjects. The targeted metabolites include acyl-carnitines and amino acids representing a set of ASD candidate metabolic markers. We propose a novel approach applying machine learning methods to assess differences in the metabolic profile between ASD and age-matched healthy TD controls. This represents a promising novelty in the field given that previous analyses of multiple analytes in ASD often resort to a one-at-a-time approach that does not consider the data as a whole. Using univariate and multivariate data modeling, we outlined a metabolic risk profile capable to classify a subset of ASD patients from TD children. The study supports identification of metabolic ASD subtype whose distinguishing features suggest a reduced flux through the mitochondrial fatty acid β-oxidation (FAO) pathway.

METHODS

A total of 162 Caucasian subjects with age ranging from 30 months to 11 years were included in a case-control study during an 18-month period (January 1, 2016–June 30, 2017) at the Child Neurology and Psychiatry Unit of the University Children Hospital Catania, Italy. Participants comprised 83 children with the ASD diagnosis (60 males, 23 females; age 6.06 ± 3.6; range: 2–10 years) and 79 healthy TD controls, with a similar age and gender distribution as the patients (57 males, 22 females; age 6.8 ± 4.1; range 2.5–11 years) (**Table 1**). The Institutional Review Board at University Hospital of Catania approved the study that was performed in accordance with the ethical standards laid down in the 1964 Declaration of Helsinki and its later amendments (Helsinki Declaration 1975, revision 2013). Written informed consent was obtained from all ASD participants' parent or legal guardian in order to enter clinical and laboratory data from the clinical files into the present study. Diagnosis of ASD was obtained according to strict criteria using standardized diagnostic tests including the Autism Diagnostic Interview-Revised (ADI-R) (21) and Autism Diagnostic Observation Schedule (ADOS) (22). The Calibrated Severity Score (CSS) from 4 to 10 was used as a measure of autism severity (23). Developmental quotient (DQ) and/or Intellectual quotient (IQ) were measured in all participants by a comprehensive, standardized neuropsychological assessment battery administered according to age. Among ASD individuals, exclusion criteria were the presence of

---

Abbreviations: ASD, autism spectrum disorders; IEM, inborn errors of metabolism; ESI-MS/MS, electrospray ionization-tandem mass spectrometry. DBS, dried blood spots; TD, typically developing; FAO, fatty acid β-oxidation; ADI-R, Autism Diagnostic Interview-Revised; ADOS, Autism Diagnostic Observation Schedule; CSS, Calibrated Severity Score; DD, developmental delay; ID, intellectual disability; PPV, Positive Predictive Value; NPV, Negative Predictive Value; DOR, Diagnostic Odds Ratio.; RF, Random Forest, SVM, Support Vector Machine; LM, Linear Regression; PART, Recursive Partition Tree; SCAD, short chain acyl-CoA dehydrogenase; MCAD, medium chain acyl-CoA dehydrogenase, VLCAD, very long chain acyl-CoA dehydrogenase; LCHAD, long chain 3-hydroxyacyl-CoA dehydrogenase; PA, propionic academia; PPA, propionic acid; NSC, neural stem cells; CPT, carnitine palmitoyl transferase.

TABLE 1 | Demographic and clinical characteristics of ASD patients and TD controls divided by age.

	ASD				TD			
Participant characteristics	**Total sample (n = 83)**	**Age ≤ 5 (n = 42)**	**Age > 5 (n = 41)**	***P*-value***	**Total sample (n = 79)**	**Age ≤ 5 (n = 35)**	**Age > 5 (n = 44)**	***P*-value***
Age (years)	6.06 ± 3.58	3.26 ± 0.89	8.9 ± 2.98	n.a.	6.8 ± 4.11	3.06 ± 1.5	9.7 ± 2.86	n.a.
Boys (%)	60 (72.3)	29 (69.04)	31 (75.6)	0.653	57 (72.1%)	24 (68.5%)	33(75%)	0.692
DQ/IQ	63.2 ± 20.8	56.8 ± 17.1	69.6 ± 22.4	0.022	93.9 ± 14.2	89.6 ± 11.2	95.3 ± 10.5	0.752
DD/ID (%)	54 (65.1)	32 (76.2)	22 (53.6)	0.035	n.a	n.a.	n.a.	n.a.
Regression (%)	29 (35)	19 (45.2)	10 (24.4)	0.065	n.a	n.a.	n.a.	n.a.
Autism severity (ADOS CSS)°	6.7 ± 1.8	6.6 ± 1.8	6.8 ± 1.8	0.845	n.a.	n.a	n.a.	n.a.

**Fisher's Exact Test was performed for discrete variables gender, DD/ID and regression. T-test was performed for continuous variables DQ/IQ and ADOS-CSS. ° The Social Communication Questionnaire was used to screen and exclude autism in TD children. DQ, developmental quotient; IQ, intelligence quotient; DD, developmental disability; ID, intellectual disability; ADOS, Autism Diagnostic Observation Schedule. CSS, Calibrated Severity Score. n.a., not applicable.*

an associated monogenic disease (i.e., Fragile-X syndrome, Tuberous Sclerosis), positive chromosomal microarray analysis, positive history for mitochondrial disease or known medical conditions including autoimmune disease and inflammatory bowel diseases (IBD)/celiac disease.

TD children were recruited among subjects that underwent morning fasting blood analyses screening for sideropenic anemia that was definitely ruled out in all included TD participants. Full informed consent was signed from parents to participate in the study. TD participants' exclusion criteria included positive history for inherited metabolic diseases, intellectual disability or other developmental, neurological, or behavioral problems and inflammatory bowel diseases/celiac disease. The Social Communication Questionnaire (24) was used to screen and exclude autism in TD children. Since artifacts in plasma acylcarnitine levels are possible due to diet enriched with fatty acids (MCT-oil, ketogenic diet) (25), we ensured that no participants underwent fatty acids enriched diet, such as ketogenic diet or MCT-oil, at least 6 months before sample collection.

Metabolic Work-Up in ASD Subjects

ASD patients underwent blood and urine collection in the morning between 8.00 and 8.30 a.m. after nocturnal fasting. Routine blood analyses including glucose, transaminases, cholesterol, triglycerides, creatine kinase, electrolytes and thyroid hormones were normal. Morning fasting lactate and ammonia blood levels were increased in 12.5 and 22.2% of patients, respectively in line with previous reported rates of increased markers of mitochondrial dysfunction in ASD (8). Twenty-five out of 40 studied subjects (62.5%) had significantly decreased blood Vitamin D3 levels with normal Ca/P ratio. Urinary organic acids by using Gas Chromatography/MS detected increased excretion of ketone bodies in five patients. One patient showed increased urinary 3-hydroxy-isovaleric acid with normal plasma biotinidase activity. In two sibs with ASD, the acylcarnitine profile showed increase of C8, C10, C10:1 carnitine levels suggesting medium-chain acyl-CoA dehydrogenase deficiency (MCAD). Molecular analyses was not significant for any mutations associated to MCAD in these patients.

Biospecimen Collection, Processing and MS/MS Analysis

To avoid systematic differences related to the time of sample collection, blood spots on filter paper card (Whatman card Specimen 903) were collected from each participant in the ASD and TD groups in the morning between 8.00 and 8.30 a.m. after nocturnal fasting. Samples from the NT children were prospectively collected in the same period, along with ASD children samples. Once dried, blood spots were stored at 4°C in a unique refrigerator with controlled humidity rate and processed within 2 weeks after sampling.

A 3.2 mm diameter blood dot of each individual was used for the analyses. Underivatized specimens were analyzed using electrospray ionization (ESI)-Tandem MS/MS system. Forty-five metabolites including amino acids, free carnitine and acyl-carnitines (saturated, unsaturated, hydroxylated, and dicarboxylated) were simultaneously measured in DBS. The analyte concentration was quantified by comparison with known concentration of corresponding stable-isotope internal standards. Results of targeted 45 metabolites in ASD participants were considered in comparison with age-matched reference ranges obtained from studied TD healthy subjects.

Statistical Analyses

Blood levels of forty-five targeted analytes (μmol/L) obtained from 162 subjects, 83 ASD patients and 79 TD healthy controls, were evaluated. Metabolites, with statistically significant different blood levels between ASD and healthy TD control children were identified by using the R package limma (26). Since data supports equal population variances together with normal distributions, a T-test was applied. The p-value produced by the two-sided T-test, employed by limma, was corrected using the Benjamini & Hochberg method in order to estimate the False Discovery Rate (27). All differences were considered to be statistically significant at a 5% probability level. Possible associations between the identified metabolites and clinical features of ASD patients were verified by Spearman correlations analyses.

Classification Modeling

Model development was performed with the aim to detect metabolic features useful to profile ASD patients vs. healthy NT controls. For this purpose we trained an algorithm on the discriminant metabolites identified as described. The methodology was evaluated in terms of Sensitivity = TP/(TP + FN), Specificity = TN/(TN + FP), where TP is the number of true positives, i.e., the number of patients correctly classified; TN is the number of true negatives, i.e., number of controls correctly classified; FP is the number of false positives, i.e., number of controls classified as patients; and FN is the number of false negatives, i.e., number of patients classified as controls. Diagnostic odds ratios and 95% confidence intervals were evaluated.

The workflow of the study is depicted in **Figure 1**. Our dataset, comprising 83 ASD patients and 79 healthy controls, was randomly partitioned into a training set of 124 samples (67 ASD patients and 57 healthy controls) for identification of the classification modeling, and 38-sample holdout set (16 ASD patients and 22 healthy controls). Due to the small cohort size, keeping a large part of the samples in the training set is needed to proper identify the classification model (28). For this reason, we kept two third of the samples in the training set and the remainder was used as a holdout validation set. Samples were properly randomized using diagnosis, age and gender to establish a similar proportion of factors on both training and holdout sets. Such holdout strategy was repeated 1,000 times to estimate average performances together with a 95% CI of the classification model. In addition, a validation test was performed in an independent set of 29 ASD participants randomly recruited for re-test analyses. Neurotypical controls were not included in this analysis because further blood sampling was not achieved in the TD group. Finally, classification performance was evaluated by permutation testing in order to establish a distribution of chance estimates. For this purpose, we trained the classifier with the 124-sample training set with randomized group labels (ASD vs. TD) many times ($\approx$ 1,000). This allowed establishing a chance distribution that could be used for comparison.

RESULTS

Participant Characteristics

Based on their chronological ages, participants were divided in two groups: younger (ASD n.42; TD n.35) or older than 5 years (ASD n.41; TD n.44). Demographic data and clinical features of all participants in the two age groups, such as presence of developmental delay (DD), intellectual disability (ID) (IQ < 70) and symptoms of regressive autism are presented in **Table 1**. The rate and extent of DD/ID were higher in children with ASD younger than 5 years (*P*: 0.035 and *P*: 0.0228, respectively). No significant differences were found in the rate of patients with regressive autism and in the degree of autism severity (CSS) between the two age groups (*P*: 0.065 and *P*: 0.845, respectively). ASD patients did not fulfill diagnostic criteria for probable or definite mitochondrial disorder according to Morava mitochondrial disease criteria system (29). Less than 5% of studied ASD children had hypotonia and/or epileptic seizures. None presented with ataxia, peripheral neuropathy, sensorineural deafness, cardiomyopathy or endocrinological problems which are common features of mitochondrial diseases.

Metabolic Profile of Target Analytes by ESI-MS/MS of Blood Spots in Patients With ASD and Healthy Control Subjects

Over 45 analyzed metabolites in DBS, nine (20%) were significantly increased in ASD patients with respect to healthy, age-matched subjects (**Table 2**). The increased metabolites in ASD patients included eight acyl-carnitines such as short-chain (2-5 carbon length) C2 and C4DC\C5OH, medium-chain (6–12 carbon length) C10 and C12, and long-chain acyl-carnitines (13-18 carbon length) C14:2, C16, C16:1, C18:1. Among eleven studied amino acids, citrulline levels were increased in ASD patients (**Table 2**). Volcano plot showing the distribution of log-fold-changes vs. statistical significance (*p*-value) of the metabolites and individual swarm plots for the subject data, split by diagnosis, for the nine changed metabolites are reported in supplementary materials (**Figures S1–S4**). We estimated an effect size of 0.6 as the absolute difference between the mean of the most discriminant metabolites (short chain C2 and C4DC/C5OH acylcarnitines and long chain C10, C12, C14:2, C16, C16:1, C18:1 acylcarnitines, citrulline) within each class divided by the pooled variance observed between the two classes. This yielded a power of 0.93 at significance level of 0.05 suggesting a high practical significance. The power was also estimated within the two age groups at 0.79 for patient younger than 5 y. o. and 0.78 for older patients.

Spearman correlations showed that in the ASD sample metabolite levels did not correlate with age, developmental or intellectual quotient and autism severity score (CSS) (**Table 3**).

Training and Testing Set Model Performance

Next, we trained a classifier based on the Naïve Bayes algorithm making use of the training set and adopting as predictor variables only the nine metabolites differing significantly between ASD and TD subjects (*P*: < 0.001) (**Table 2**). The results were verified on the holdout set with the purpose of checking the robustness of the procedure.

To assess the model and the predictive power of the selected metabolites, we compared the Naïve Bayes algorithm, with other classification techniques such as C-tree, Random Forest (RF), Support Vector Machine (SVM), Linear Regression (LM), and Recursive Partition Tree (PART) (online methods). Our final choice fell on the Naïve Bayes algorithm due to its robustness and stability. The training procedure led to the selection of acyl-carnitines C2 and C4DC\C5OH, C10, C12, C14:2, C16, C16:1, C18:1 as the most promising classification variables. Naïve Bayes algorithm, using a 8 feature set, reaches an overall classification

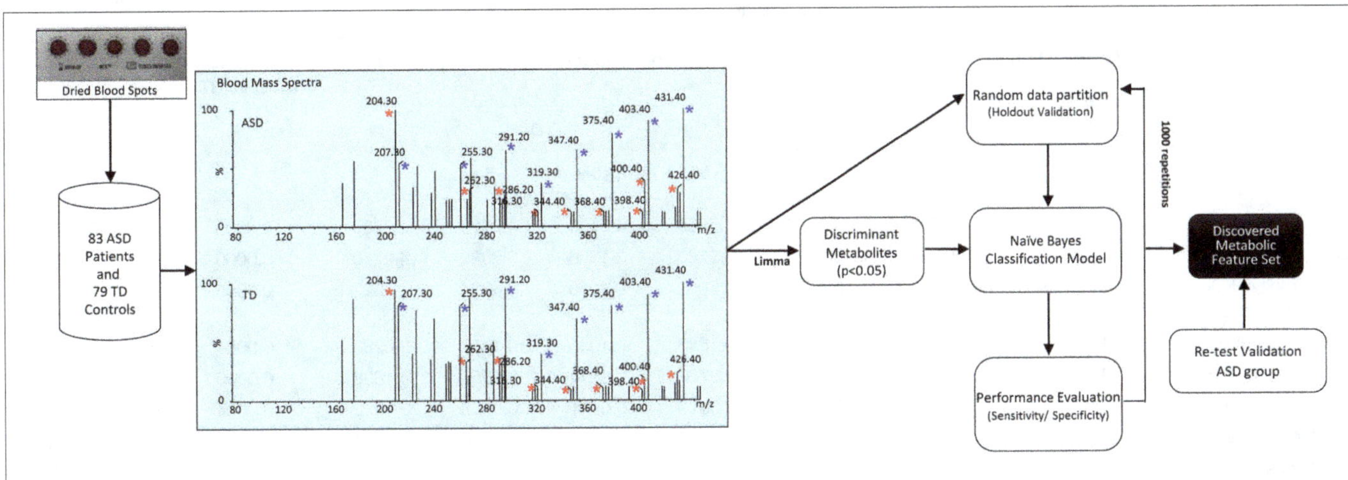

FIGURE 1 | Workflow of the study. Blood acylcarnitines (m/z) C2 (204.3); C4DC\C5OH (262.2); C10 (316.2); C12 (344.3); C14:2 (368.3); C16 (400.3); C16:1 (398.3); C18:1 (286.2) (red asterisks) measured in DBS are increased in patients with ASD. Näive Bayes algorithm trained on the identified metabolites was used to profile children with ASD vs. healthy controls. Blue asterisks indicate correspondent stable-isotope internal standards.

performance with 73.3% sensitivity (95% CI 72.6–73.9), 63.4% specificity (95% CI 62.8–64), 6.78 DOR (95% CI, 6.39–7.16).

Predictive Performances of the Metabolic Profile for Participants Divided by Age

Taking into account that ASD are neurodevelopmental disorders we considered closely possible interactions of measured metabolites with participant ages. For this purpose, we divided the sample into two groups according to age (≤5 years and >5 years) and we applied the classifier to discriminate among ASD and TD control subjects in each age group. **Table 4** presents the predictive performances of the metabolic profile (measures and 95% CI), using Naïve Bayes and other compared classifiers, for all participants; participants aged ≤5 years and >5 years.

We found an increased competitiveness of the framework for classifying ASD in toddlers (n: 42 subjects mean age 3.26 ± 0.89) 72.3% sensitivity (95% CI: 71.3;73.9), 72.1% specificity (95% CI: 71.2;72.9), and diagnostic odds ratio (DOR) 11.25 (95% CI: 9.47;17.74). Furthermore, by applying our classification framework to subjects older than 5 years of age, we found a reduction in performance compared to younger subjects: Sensitivity 67.5% (95% CI: 66.6; 68.4) Specificity 56.9% (56.1;57.7), DOR 4.29% (95% CI: 4.09;4.56).

Validation Test

Results were confirmed on independent validation test. For validation analyses, a set of 29 ASD participants was randomly recruited for re-test analyses. For this purpose, blood spot collection for metabolite analyses was repeated at the same conditions a second time after a mean time interval of 6.86 ± 3.8 months. Data from re-test were used as validation set. The initial values from total 132 subjects were used as training set. The results show an overall accuracy of 69% (20 patients correctly classified as ASD, and 9 misclassified as healthy). Splitting the re-test set by age we found a greater accuracy in younger subjects (≤5 years of age) ($n = 11$ samples, 73% accuracy) compared to individuals older than 5 years ($n = 18$ samples, 67% accuracy). It should be noted that the re-test validation set only includes participants with an ASD diagnosis. Therefore, the validation can only test for true positive and false negative ASD classifications.

Permutation Testing

Classifier performance was evaluated using permutation testing. Permutation testing can be used to evaluate the probability of getting specificity and sensitivity values higher than the ones obtained during the cross-validation procedure by chance. In order to establish a distribution of chance estimates, we trained the classifier with the 124-sample training set each time randomly assigning patient and control labels to each sample many times (≈ 1,000) and repeated the cross-validation procedure. The results show that the quality of the classification in such a case is even lower than expected values in the case of a random classifier model with 43.9% accuracy (95% CI: 43.3;44.5) (**Table S1**). We definitely demonstrated that the accuracy of the classifier (73%) is significantly better than expected by chance alone as the classification algorithms are actually able to extract molecular patterns that distinguish patients, with respect to a chance distribution.

DISCUSSION

ASD is a polygenic multifactorial disorder with variable underlying mechanisms including energy metabolism disarrangement among others (30). Recognition of specific classes of ASD patients by biological markers has been considering effective for better understanding molecular mechanisms and to guide tailored therapeutic strategies in patient subset (31). In the current study we pursued to set up an easily testable blood metabolic profile in DBS to support early recognition of metabolic subtype patients at risk for ASD diagnosis. We found in an ASD population without clinical relevant features secondary to primary mitochondrial disease,

TABLE 2 | Statistical significant metabolites in ASD participants with respect to TD participants.

Metabolite	Abbreviation	Log-FC	Average concentration				t	*p*-Value (ASD vs. TD)	Adjusted *p*-Value
			ASD		TD				
			≤5 y	>5 y	≤5 y	>5 y			
Citrulline	CIT	0.3601	4.7594	4.5606	4.3556	4.2129	3.7337	0.0003	0.0020
Acetylcarnitine	C2	0.3318	3.5333	3.5503	3.1886	3.2330	4.2770	0.0000	0.0007
Methylmalonyl/3-OH-isovalerylcarnitine*	C4DC\C5OH	0.0762	0.4734	0.5062	0.4058	0.4224	4.4927	0.0000	0.0006
Decanoylcarnitine	C10	0.0395	0.1468	0.1643	0.1035	0.1352	2.6288	0.0004	0.0470
Dodecanoylcarnitine	C12	0.0246	0.0714	0.0762	0.0414	0.0556	4.1838	0.0000	0.0007
Tetradecadienoylcarnitine	C14:2	0.0109	0.0398	0.0377	0.0211	0.0322	3.5912	0.0004	0.0025
Hexadecanoylcarnitine	C16	0.1409	1.0594	1.0934	0.9499	0.9180	3.7904	0.0002	0.0019
Hexadecenoylcarnitine	C16:1	0.0145	0.0758	0.0805	0.0634	0.0637	3.6726	0.0003	0.0021
Octadecenoylcarnitine	C18:1	0.1302	1.0725	1.1304	0.9295	0.9945	3.8526	0.0002	0.0019

*Logarithm of the fold-change (Log-FC) between the classes, average concentration in each age subgroup, t-test statistic with its p-value and Benjamini & Hochberg adjusted p-value. *Isomers or isobars metabolites. ASD, Autism Spectrum Disorders; TD, Typical Development; y, year.*

TABLE 3 | Spearman correlations computed for the metabolites listed in **Table 2** in relation to the quantitative clinical variables Age, DQ/IQ, and CSS.

Metabolite	Age		DQ/IQ		CSS	
		p-Value		*p*-Value		*p*-Value
C5OH\C4DC*	0.0771	0.4939	0.1176	0.2959	−0.1122	0.3188
C2	−0.1497	0.1821	−0.0634	0.5741	−0.0083	0.9414
C12	0.1103	0.3271	−0.0415	0.7129	−0.1488	0.1850
C18:1	0.0093	0.9341	−0.0986	0.3814	0.0155	0.8906
C16	−0.0130	0.9084	−0.0380	0.7362	−0.1340	0.2328
CIT	−0.1751	0.1180	−0.0685	0.5434	−0.1230	0.2741
C16:1	0.1286	0.2526	−0.0818	0.4677	−0.0795	0.4803
C14:2	−0.0410	0.7163	0.0060	0.9578	−0.0842	0.4551
C10	0.0843	0.4545	−0.0649	0.5647	−0.0607	0.5906

*For each metabolite we report the computed correlation together with a p-value, which indicates whether the observed correlation is statistically significant, under the null hypothesis that values are uncorrelated. *Isomers or isobars metabolites. DQ, developmental quotient; IQ, intelligence quotient; CSS, Calibrated Severity Score.*

a significant increase of blood short-chain, long-chain acyl-carnitines and, to a lesser extent, medium-chain acyl-carnitines. Our findings in a Sicilian ASD population (Mediterranean area) confirm the same, unique pattern of acyl-carnitine profile, which has been first systematically detected in ASD individuals from US, (32) defining a broadest coverage of ethnic and regional groups.

It is worth noting that distinct metabolite differences could be related to co-morbid undiagnosed medical conditions such as gastrointestinal disturbances that are frequently observed in ASD. In the present study we found significantly increased citrulline levels in children with ASD. Citrulline is an intermediate metabolic amino acid produced primarily by enterocytes. Blood citrulline level is considered a biomarker of gastrointestinal mucosal surface and enterocyte integrity. Previous studies showed that citrulline levels are inversely correlated with severity of intestinal malabsorption disease (i.e., coeliac disease) and inflammatory bowel disease (IBD) such as Crohn's disease (33). Patients with classic citrullinemia (type I) (argininosuccinate synthetase 1 gene mutation) present with elevated citrulline levels along with hyperammonemia and variable neurological symptoms in the neonatal period or later on. Interestingly, it was demonstrated that cumulative exposure to ammonia and citrulline are the most reliable indicators of poorer cognitive functioning in patients with classic citrullinemia (34).

Moreover, the existence of distinct metabolite differences could relate to concurrent vitamin D deficiency that was observed in a large proportion of patients with ASD (62%) in this study. Vitamin D has a pivotal role in neurodevelopment through several mechanisms including gene regulation and anti-inflammation/immunological modulation. Lower Vitamin D levels were consistently reported in subsets of patients with ASD compared to healthy controls (35). Carnitine is mainly provided in the diet, but is synthesized at extremely low rates from trimethyl-lysine residues generated during protein

TABLE 4 | Classifiers performances for all participants **(A)**; participants aged ≤ 5 years **(B)** and >5 years **(C)**.

Classifier	Sensitivity	Specificity	DOR
(A) All participants			
Naïve Bayes	0.7332 [0.7267; 0.7397]	0.6345 [0.6287; 0.6404]	6.7823 [6.3956; 7.1690]
C-tree	0.6715 [0.6590; 0.6841]	0.4942 [0.4824; 0.5060]	2.7437 [2.6171; 2.8703]
RF	0.7296 [0.7229; 0.7364]	0.5670 [0.5608; 0.5731]	4.8079 [4.5668; 5.0490]
SVM	0.7319 [0.7250; 0.7388]	0.5939 [0.5875; 0.6003]	5.5428 [5.2650; 5.8207]
LM	0.6324 [0.6250; 0.6397]	0.6585 [0.6523; 0.6646]	4.4804 [4.2328; 4.7280]
PART	0.6281 [0.6196; 0.6365]	0.5657 [0.5576; 0.5738]	2.9980 [2.8474; 3.1486]
(B) ≤age 5 years			
Naïve Bayes	0.7237 [0.7137; 0.7337]	0.7209 [0.7125; 0.7293]	10.1235 [9.4725; 10.7746]
C-tree	0.7590 [0.7441; 0.7739]	0.3574 [0.3399; 0.3749]	2.8163 [2.6411; 2.9914]
RF	0.8270 [0.8187; 0.8353]	0.5464 [0.5358; 0.5569]	7.1375 [6.5862; 7.6888]
SVM	0.8017 [0.7925; 0.8109]	0.6202 [0.6105; 0.6300]	8.1844 [7.6207; 8.7481]
LM	0.6567 [0.6450; 0.6684]	0.6871 [0.6771; 0.6972]	7.1923 [6.6648; 7.7198]
PART	0.7031 [0.6914; 0.7149]	0.4532 [0.4407; 0.4658]	2.9037 [2.6924; 3.1150]
(C) >age 5 years			
Naïve Bayes	0.6757 [0.6665; 0.6849]	0.5692 [0.5610; 0.5775]	4.2905 [4.0193; 4.5616]
C-tree	0.5071 [0.4867; 0.5275]	0.5468 [0.5290; 0.5645]	1.6693 [1.5826; 1.7559]
RF	0.5881 [0.5780; 0.5982]	0.5248 [0.5157; 0.5339]	2.3622 [2.2069; 2.5175]
SVM	0.5878 [0.5780; 0.5976]	0.6295 [0.6208; 0.6382]	3.9369 [3.6500; 4.2238]
LM	0.6039 [0.5939; 0.6139]	0.6022 [0.5933; 0.6112]	3.7105 [3.4456; 3.9755]
PART	0.5264 [0.5143; 0.5386]	0.5367 [0.5260; 0.5474]	2.0030 [1.8714; 2.1347]

Compared classification algorithms: Naïve Bayes, C-tree, Random Forest (RF), Support Vector Machine (SVM), Linear Regression Model (LM), and Recursive Partition Tree (PART). For each classifier sensitivity, specificity, of the model and diagnostic odds ratio (DOR) are shown. All the measures are reported together with the bounds of the 95% CI.

catabolism and is excreted in the urine. In patients with nutritional rickets (vitamin D deficiency), an increased urinary excretion of carnitine may occur that is reversed by vitamin D supplementation (36). It may be argued that carnitine metabolism may be involved in patients with nutritional rickets. Possible links between vitamin D deficiency and carnitine deficiency should be further investigated also in view of the higher prevalence of both these conditions in patients with ASD.

As ASD is developmental in nature, we considered possible interactions of measured metabolites with participant ages. Profiles of carnitine and acyl-carnitines change significantly during the first year of life, but kept at the same level between 2 and 15 years (37). We split the sample in two age categories (< 5 y.o. and ≥ 5 y.o.) to understand possible predictive metabolic signatures capable of distinguishing ASD and TD individuals at early stages of ASD development. This threshold is consistent with reliable ASD diagnosis and effectiveness of early intervention. Indeed, the definite diagnosis of ASD is generally made between 3 and 5 years (38). Moreover, increasing evidences support the effectiveness of early interventions (behavioral, developmental and educational approaches) in pre-schoolers (aged 24–71 months) with ASD (39).

The results show higher classification performance (sensitivity 72.3%, specificity 72.1%) at younger ages and potential application to improve diagnosis at earlier stages of ASD development. Re-test analyses as a measure of validity in independent samples showed an accuracy (proportion of observations that were correctly classified into patient or control group) of 73% in children aged ≤5 years. It has to be noted that the validation set only includes participants with an ASD diagnosis and so the validation can test for true positive and false negative ASD classifications.

The present study confirms that patients with ASD may show a distinct metabolic profile, demonstrating that this can be used to identify a subset of ASD patients with respect to TD at younger ages. We verified that in each age group, clinical variables such as cognitive levels (DQ/IQ) and autism severity (CSS) did not correlate with the discriminant metabolite levels. This implies that both clinical features were irrelevant to clinically discriminate the identified patient subset. It would be interesting to further investigate if individual component of behavioral scores instead of global scores and/or additional neurological features might be more helpful at the clinical level using larger samples that allow patient stratification (31).

The predictive metabolic profile identified in the present study is strongly supported by significant biological and experimental data associated with ASD:

(1) the present findings collectively suggest a reduced flux through the mitochondrial β-oxidation pathway in a subset of patients with ASD. The acyl-carnitine pattern found in ASD patients is not consistent with any known genetic disorders of fatty acid oxidation and organic acid metabolism, electron transport chain or urea cycle dysfunction, or other inherited metabolic diseases. Genetic defects of mitochondrial β-oxidation are a group of IEM caused by failure of a single mitochondrial enzyme of β-oxidation such as short chain acyl-CoA dehydrogenase

(SCAD), medium chain acyl-CoA dehydrogenase (MCAD), very long chain acyl-CoA dehydrogenase (VLCAD) or long chain 3-hydroxyacyl-CoA dehydrogenase (LCHAD). Mitochondrial β-oxidation defects may be secondary to dysfunction of dependent processes, such as deficiencies of the carnitine fatty acid transporter system, or mitochondrial electron transfer flavoprotein system (multiple acyl-CoA dehydrogenase deficiency) (40). The occurrence of developmental delay, autistic-like behavior or ASD in genetic defects of mitochondrial β-oxidation (41) particularly VLCAD (42) and LCHAD (43) suggests that impaired mitochondrial β-oxidation may contribute to dysfunctional energetic metabolism in subsets of patients with ASD. Deletion of the TMLHE gene, which is the first step in carnitine synthesis pathway and located on the X chromosome, is found more often in males with non-dysmorphic autism suggesting that TMLHE deficiency is a risk factor for autism, albeit with low penetrance (estimated at 2–4%) (44). Children with ASD, as a group, are deficient in Carnitine (45) with this deficiency potentially related to gastrointestinal symptom (46). Additionally, supplementing with Carnitine has been shown to improve core symptoms of ASD in two double-blind placebo controlled studies (47, 48).

(2) ASD features and ASD have been reported in patients with propionic acidemia (PA), a severe organic acidemia caused by propionic acid (PPA) accumulation due to propionyl-CoA carboxylase enzyme deficiency (49). Endogenous PPA derives from the catabolism of branched-chain amino acids and from odd-chain fatty acid catabolism. PPA is a fermentation product of many autism associated gut bacteria, and also a common food preservative (50). Intracerebral PPA injections in rodents induce behavioral, electrographic and biochemical changes consistent with rodent ASD model (PPA model) (51). Brain lipid analyses of PPA model show increase of short- and long-chain acyl-carnitines but not medium- chain acyl-carnitines (52). The acyl-carnitine profile of PPA model overlaps with those found in patients with ASD (32), also in the current study.

(3) Dysregulated cortical layer formation and layer-specific neuronal differentiation demonstrated in the neocortex of children with ASD, suggest possible defects in cell-cycle processes as well as in cell fate specification (53). The carnitine palmitoyl transferase (CPT) system, which mediates the entry of long-chain fatty acids into the mitochondria for ß-oxidation, operates in astrocytes (54, 55) and in embryonic and adult neural stem cells (NSC) (56, 57). Recent evidences show that fatty acids might represent an important oxidative fuel during embryonic and early postnatal development and a reduced flux through the mitochondrial fatty acid β-oxidation impairs NSC self-renewal in the mammalian embryonic brain and potentiates their transition to lineage-restricted cells (IPCs) (54–56). As a whole, experimental findings show a pivotal role for mitochondrial fatty acid β-oxidation in controlling NSC-to-IPC transition in mammalian embryonic and adult brain, and propose NSC self-renewal as a cellular mechanism underlying the association between disturbances of mitochondrial fatty acid oxidation and autism (56, 57).

We found a combined acyl-carnitine pattern in patients with ASD indicative of impaired mitochondrial fatty acid β-oxidation. The identified acyl-carnitine profile is characterized by a pattern of more elevated acyl-carnitine species in comparison with age-matched reference ranges. The presence of short-, medium-, and more elevated long-chain acyl-carnitine species, might reflect a mild generalized defect in FAO capacities, such as in FAO electron shuttle protein ETF (electron transferring factor), which is involved in the transfer of electrons coming from the short-chain, medium-chain and long-chain acyl-CoA dehydrogenases isoforms to the respiratory chain. Electrons from ETF feed the respiratory chain at the level of ETFDH (ETF dehydrogenase), a respiratory chain enzyme which transfers these electrons to coenzyme Q. Both inborn ETF and inborn ETFDH deficiency have been described in human, associated to a variety of phenotypes (58). The mechanisms responsible for expression of abnormal acyl-carnitine pattern in this subset of ASD patients cannot be inferred from the present study. Further studies are necessary to clarify if genetic variation of fatty acid oxidation and interaction with environmental factors including diet might account for acyl-carnitine accumulation. In view of the wide clinical features related to ASD we consecutively recruited patients with ASD diagnosis representing an heterogeneous ASD population: further studies are required to understand possible genetic and behavioral correlates of metabolic subtypes of ASD. One limitation of the present study is the lack of inclusion of a neurodevelopmental delay group to understand the performances of the algorithms for ASD vs. other developmental disabilities. Moreover, our study has been developed in a clinical sample. Similarly, classifiers have been applied to identify biomarkers of neurological and psychiatric diseases in clinical cohorts (28, 59). However, it has been recently highlighted that machine learning models should be adjusted to the epidemiological prevalence in the general population (60). Larger-scale studies or population analyses are therefore needed to assess performances in real life cohorts considering the actual prevalence rate. This will require resources for large-scale collaborative efforts worldwide (61).

CONCLUSION

The present study supports early recognition of a distinctive metabolic profile in DBS whose distinguishing features suggest a reduced flux through the mitochondrial fatty acid β-oxidation pathway and provides insight into concealed molecular mechanisms determining ASD. The results show higher classification performances in children with ASD younger than 5 years old suggesting a potential complementary and supportive ability to improve diagnosis at earlier stages of ASD development. The applied non-invasive methodology on DBS traditionally used for newborn screening is appropriate to evaluate metabolic profile changes across development. The present findings yield the evidence that metabolic biomarkers that identify subset of patients with ASD are helpful. Considering the heterogeneity of ASD, metabolic profiling may support the identification of phenotypes enabling individualized therapeutic approaches in children at risk of developing the disease.

AUTHOR CONTRIBUTIONS

RB and SA conceived the project with contributions by MM, AP, and AF. MM and ADP analyzed the clinical samples. MM, ADP and GT acquired the data and performed data analyses. RB, MG, FM, AGF, GR carried out participants' recruitment and clinical data analysis. SA, AP, AF performed statistical data analysis and computational analyses. RB and SA wrote the paper. RR, JB, RF performed critical revision of the manuscript for intellectual contents. All Authors read and approved the final manuscript.

MIMIC-AUTISM GROUP

List of coauthors included in MIMIC (Metabolism-Immunity-Metals Integrated Concepts), Autism project: a multilevel approach to understand and cure Autism Spectrum Disorders:

Prof. Agata Fiumara, Dr. Concetta Meli, Referral Centre for Inherited Metabolic Disorders,Department of Clinical and Experimental Medicine, University of Catania, Catania, Italy; **Dr. Mariangela Gulisano, Dr. Federica Maugeri, Dr. Adriana Prato**, Child Neurology and Psychiatry, Department of Clinical and Experimental Medicine, University of Catania, Catania, Italy; **Prof. Giovanna Russo**, Pediatric Hematology, Department of Clinical and Experimental Medicine, University of Catania, Catania, Italy; **Dr. Giovanni Tabbì**, Institute of Biostructures and Bioimaging (IBB), National Research Council (CNR), Catania, Italy.

ACKNOWLEDGMENTS

We would like to thank the children and families who participated in this study. Partial financial support from the University of Catania FIR-2014 ED99F1 MIMIC (Metabolism-Immunity-Metals Integrated Concepts) - Autism: a multilevel approach to understand and cure Autism Spectrum Disorders and from MIUR Fondo per le attività di base di ricerca to RB is gratefully acknowledged.

REFERENCES

1. Baio J, Wiggins L, Christensen DL, Maenner MJ, Daniels J, Warren Z, et al. Prevalence of autism spectrum disorder among children aged 8 years - autism and developmental disabilities monitoring network, 11 sites, United States, 2014. *MMWR Surveill Summ.* (2018) 67:1–23. doi: 10.15585/mmwr.ss6706a1
2. Narzisi A, Posada M, Barbieri F, Chericoni N, Ciuffolini D, Pinzino M, et al. Prevalence of autism spectrum disorder in a large italian catchment area: a school-based population study within the ASDEU project. *Epidemiol Psychiatr Sci.* (2018) 6:1–10. doi: 10.1017/S2045796018000483
3. American-Psychiatric-Association. *Diagnostic and Statistical Manual of Mental Disorders.* Washington, DC: American Psychiatric Publishing (2013).
4. Constantino JN, Charman T. Diagnosis of autism spectrum disorder: reconciling the syndrome, its diverse origins, and variation in expression. Lancet Neurol. (2016) 15:279–91. doi: 10.1016/S1474-4422(15)00151-9
5. Kiykim E, Zeybek CA, Zubarioglu T, Cansever S, Yalcinkaya C, Soyucen E, et al. Inherited metabolic disorders in Turkish patients with autism spectrum disorders. *Autism Res.* (2016) 9: 217–23. doi: 10.1002/aur.1507
6. Barone R, Sturiale L, Fiumara A, Palmigiano A, Bua RO, Rizzo R et al. CSF N-glycan profile reveals sialylation deficiency in a patient with GM2 gangliosidosis presenting as childhood disintegrative disorder. *Autism Res.* (2016) 9:423–8. doi: 10.1002/aur.1541
7. Wolfenden C, Wittkowski A, Hare DJ. Symptoms of autism spectrum disorder (ASD) in Individuals with Mucopolysaccharide Disease Type III (Sanfilippo Syndrome): a systematic review. *J Autism Dev Disord.* (2017) 47:3620–33. doi: 10.1007/s10803-017-3262-6
8. Rossignol DA, Frye RE. Mitochondrial dysfunction in autism spectrum disorders: a systematic review and meta-analysis. *Mol. Psychiatry* (2012) 17: 290–314. doi: 10.1038/mp.2010.136
9. Legido A, Jethva R, Goldenthal MJ. Mitochondrial dysfunction in autism. *Semin Pediatr Neurol.* (2013) 20:163–75. doi: 10.1016/j.spen.2013.10.008
10. Dawson G, Rogers S, Munson J, Smith M, Winter J, Greenson J, et al. Randomized, controlled trial of an intervention for toddlers with autism: the Early Start Denver Model. *Pediatrics* (2010) 125:e17–23. doi: 10.1542/peds.2009-0958
11. Yap IK, Angley M, Veselkov KA, Holmes E, Lindon JC, Nicholson JK. Urinary metabolic phenotyping differentiates children with autism from their unaffected siblings and age-matched controls. *J Proteome Res.* (2010) 9:2996–3004. doi: 10.1021/pr901188e
12. Ming X, Stein TP, Barnes V, Rhodes N, Guo L. Metabolic perturbance in autism spectrum disorders: a metabolomics study. *J Proteome Res.* (2012) 11:5856–62. doi: 10.1021/pr300910n
13. Emond P, Mavel S, Aidoud N, Nadal-Desbarats L, Montigny F, Bonnet-Brilhault F, et al. GC-MS-based urine metabolic profiling of autism spectrum disorders. *Anal Bioanal Chem.* (2013) 405:5291–300. doi: 10.1007/s00216-013-6934-x
14. Noto A, Fanos V, Barberini L, Grapov D, Fattuoni C, Zaffanello M, et al. The urinary metabolomics profile of an Italian autistic children population and their unaffected siblings. *J Matern Fetal Neonatal Med.* (2014) 2:46–52. doi: 10.3109/14767058.2014.954784
15. Diémé B, Mavel S, Blasco H, Tripi G, Bonnet-Brilhault F, Malvy J, et al. Metabolomics study of urine in autism spectrum disorders using a multiplatform analytical methodology. *J Proteome Res.* (2015) 14:5273–82. doi: 10.1186/s13229-016-0109-5
16. Gevi F, Zolla L, Gabriele S, Persico AM. Urinary metabolomics of young Italian autistic children supports abnormal tryptophan and purine metabolism. *Mol Autism* (2016) 24;7:47. doi: 10.1186/s13229-016-0109-5
17. West PR, Amaral DG, Bais P, Smith AM, Egnash LA, Ross ME, et al. Metabolomics as a tool for discovery of biomarkers of autism spectrum disorder in the blood plasma of children. *PLoS ONE* (2014) 9:e112445. doi: 10.1371/journal.pone.0112445
18. Wang H, Liang S, Wang M, Gao J, Sun C, Wang J, et al. Potential serum biomarkers from a metabolomics study of autism. *J. Psychiatry Neurosci.* (2016) 41: 27–37. doi: 10.1503/jpn.1 40009
19. Anwar A, Abruzzo P M, Pasha S, Rajpoot K, Bolotta A, Ghezzo A, et al. Advanced glycation endproducts, dityrosine and arginine transporter dysfunction in autism - a source of biomarkers for clinical diagnosis. *Mol Autism* (2018) 9:3. doi: 10.1186/s13229-017-0183-3
20. Wilcken B, Wiley V, Hammond J, Carpenter K. Wilcken B, Wiley V, et al. Screening newborns for inborn errors of metabolism by tandem mass spectrometry. *N Engl J Med.* (2003) 348:2304–12. doi: 10.1056/NEJMoa025225
21. Lord C, Rutter M, Le Couteur A. Autism diagnostic interview-revised: a revised version of a diagnostic interview for caregivers of individuals with possible pervasive developmental disorders. *J Autism Dev Disord.* (1994) 24:659–85. doi: 10.1007/BF02172145

22. Lord C, Risi S, Lambrecht L, Cook EH Jr, Leventhal BL, DiLavore PC, et al. The autism diagnostic observation schedule-generic: a standard measure of social and communication deficits associated with the spectrum of autism. *J Autism Dev Disord.* (2000) 30:205–23. doi: 10.1023/A:1005592401947
23. Gotham K, Pickles A, Lord C. Standardizing ADOS scores for a measure of severity in autism spectrum disorders. *J Autism Dev Disord.* (2009) 39:693–705. doi: 10.1007/s10803-008-0674-3
24. Rutter M, Bailey A, Lord C. *Social Communication Questionnaire.* Los Angeles, CA: Western Psychological Services (2003).
25. Iacobazzi V, Pasquali M, Singh R, Matern D, Rinaldo P, Amat di San Filippo C, et al. Response to therapy in carnitine/acylcarnitine translocase (CACT) deficiency due to a novel missense mutation. *Am J Med Genet A.* (2004) 126A:150–5. doi: 10.1002/ajmg.a.20573
26. Ritchie ME, Phipson B, Wu D, Hu Y, Law CW, Shi W, Smyth GK. limma powers differential expression analyses for RNA-sequencing and microarray studies. *Nucleic Acids Res.* (2015) 43:e47. doi: 10.1093/nar/gkv007
27. Benjamini, Y, Hochberg Y. Controlling the false discovery rate: a practical and powerful approach to multiple testing. *J R Stat Soc Ser B.* (1995) 57:289–300.
28. Howsmon DP, Vargason T, Rubin RA, Delhey L, Tippett M, Rose S, et al. Multivariate techniques enable a biochemical classification of children with autism spectrum disorder versus typically-developing peers: a comparison and validation study. *Bioeng Transl Med.* (2018) 3:156–65. doi: 10.1002/btm2.10095
29. Morava E, van den Heuvel L, Hol F, de Vries MC, Hogeveen M, Rodenburg RJ, et al. Mitochondrial disease criteria: diagnostic applications in children. *Neurology* (2006) 67:1823–26. doi: 10.1212/01.wnl.0000244435.27645.54
30. Rose S, Niyazov DM, Rossignol DA, Goldenthal M, Kahler SG, Frye RE. Clinical and molecular characteristics of mitochondrial dysfunction in autism spectrum disorder. *Mol Diagn Ther.* (2018) 22:571–593. doi: 10.1007/s40291-018-0352-x
31. Loth E, Murphy DG, Spooren W. Defining precision medicine approaches to autism spectrum disorders: concepts and challenges. *Front Psychiatry* (2016) 7:188. doi: 10.3389/fpsyt.2016.00188
32. Frye RE, Melnyk S, Macfabe DF. Unique acyl-carnitine profiles are potential biomarkers for acquired mitochondrial disease in autism spectrum disorder. *Transl Psychiatry* (2013) 3:e220. doi: 10.1038/tp.2012.143
33. Fragkos KC, Forbes A. Citrulline as a marker of intestinal function and absorption in clinical settings: a systematic review and meta-analysis. *United Eur Gastroenterol J.* (2018) 6:181–91. doi: 10.1177/2050640617737632
34. Waisbren SE, Cuthbertson D, Burgard P, Holbert A, McCarter R, Cederbaum S; Members of the urea cycle disorders consortium. Biochemical markers and neuropsychological functioning in distal urea cycle disorders. *J Inherit Metab Dis.* (2018) 41:657–67. doi: 10.1007/s10545-017-0132-5
35. Wang T, Shan L, Du L, Feng J, Xu Z, Staal WG, Jia F. Serum concentration of 25-hydroxyvitamin D in autism spectrum disorder: a systematic review and meta-analysis. *Eur Child Adolesc Psychiatry* (2016) 25:341–50. doi: 10.1007/s00787-015-0786-1
36. Dursun A, Aliefendioglu D, Ozkan B, Coşkun T. Carnitinuria in rickets due to vitamin D deficiency. *Turk J Pediatr.* (2000) 42:278–80.
37. Cavedon CT, Bourdoux P, Mertens K, Van Thi HV, Herremans N, de Laet C, Goyens P. Age-related variations in acylcarnitine and free carnitine concentrations measured by tandem mass spectrometry. *Clin Chem.* (2005) 51:745–52. doi: 10.1373/clinchem.2004.043646
38. Mandell DS, Novak MM, Zubritsky CD. Factors associated with age of diagnosis among children with autism spectrum disorders. *Pediatrics* (2005) 116:1480–6. doi: 10.1542/peds.2005-0185
39. Narzisi A, Costanza C, Ballottin U, Muratori F. Non-pharmacological treatments in autism spectrum disorders: an overview on early interventions for pre-schoolers. *Curr Clin Pharmacol.* (2014) 9:17–26. doi: 10.2174/15748847113086660071
40. Houten SM, Violante S, Ventura FV, Wanders RJ. The biochemistry and physiology of mitochondrial fatty acid β-oxidation and its genetic disorders. *Annu Rev Physiol.* (2016) 78:23–44. doi: 10.1146/annurev-physiol-021115-105045
41. Waisbren SE, Landau Y, Wilson J, Vockley J. Neuropsychological outcomes in fatty acid oxidation disorders: 85 cases detected by newborn screening. *Dev Disabil Res Rev.* (2013) 17:260–8. doi: 10.1002/ddrr.1119
42. Brown A, Crowe L, Andresen BS, Anderson V, Boneh A. Neurodevelopmental profiles of children with very long chain acyl-CoA dehydrogenase deficiency diagnosed by newborn screening. *Mol Genet Metab.* (2014) 113:278–82. doi: 10.1016/j.ymgme.2014.10.005
43. Strandqvist A, Haglind CB, Zetterström RH, Nemeth A, von Döbeln U, Stenlid MH, et al. Neuropsychological development in patients with long-chain 3-Hydroxyacyl-CoA dehydrogenase (LCHAD) deficiency. *JIMD Rep* (2016) 28:75–84. doi: 10.1007/8904_2015_505
44. Celestino-Soper PB1, Violante S, Crawford EL, Luo R, Lionel AC, Delaby E, et al. A common X-linked inborn error of carnitine biosynthesis may be a risk factor for non dysmorphic autism. *Proc. Natl. Acad. Sci. USA.* (2012) 109:7974–8. doi: 10.1073/pnas.1120210109
45. Filipek PA, Juranek J, Nguyen MT, Cummings C, Gargus JJ. Relative carnitine deficiency in autism. *J Autism Dev Disord.* (2004) 34:615–23. doi: 10.1007/s10803-004-5283-1
46. Mostafa GA, Al-Ayadhi LY. Reduced levels of plasma polyunsaturated fatty acids and serum carnitine in autistic children: relation to gastrointestinal manifestations. *Behav Brain Funct.* (2015) 11:4. doi: 10.1186/s12993-014-0048-2
47. Geier DA, Kern JK, Davis G, King PG, Adams JB, Young JL, Geier MR. A prospective double-blind, randomized clinical trial of levocarnitine to treat autism spectrum disorders. *Med Sci Monit.* (2011) 17:PI15–23. doi: 10.12659/MSM.881792
48. Fahmy SF, EL-hamamsy MH, Zaki OK, Badary OA. l-Carnitine supplementation improves the behavioral symptoms in autistic children. *Res Autism Spectr Disor.* (2013) 7:159–66. doi: 10.1016/j.rasd.2012.07.006
49. Witters P, Debbold E, Crivelly K, Vande Kerckhove K, Corthouts K, Debbold B, et al. Autism in patients with propionic acidemia. *Mol Genet Metab.* (2016) 119: 317–21. doi: 10.1016/j.ymgme.2016.10.009
50. MacFabe DF. Enteric short-chain fatty acids: microbial messengers of metabolism, mitochondria, and mind: implications in autism spectrum disorders. *Microb Ecol Health Dis.* (2015) 26:28177. doi: 10.3402/mehd.v26.28177
51. Shultz SR, MacFabe DF, Ossenkopp KP, Scratch S, Whelan J, Taylor R, et al. Intracerebroventricular injection of propionic acid, an enteric bacterial metabolic end-product, impairs social behavior in the rat: implications for an animal model of autism. *Neuropharmacology* (2008) 54:901–11. doi: 10.1016/j.neuropharm.2008.01.013
52. Thomas, R.H., Foley, K.A., Mepham, J.R., Tichenoff, L.J., Possmayer, F., MacFabe, D.F. Altered brain phospholipid and acylcarnitine profiles in propionic acid infused rodents: further development of a potential model of autism spectrum disorders. *J Neurochem.* (2010) 113:515–29. doi: 10.1111/j.1471-4159.2010.06614.x
53. Stoner R, Chow ML, Boyle MP, et al. Patches of disorganization in the neocortex of children with autism. *N Engl J Med.* (2014) 370:1209–19. doi: 10.1056/NEJMoa1307491
54. Panov A, Orynbayeva Z, Vavilin V, Lyakhovich V. Fatty acids in energy metabolism of the central nervous system. *Biomed Res Int.* (2014) 2014:472459. doi: 10.1155/2014/472459
55. Jernberg JN, Bowman CE, Wolfgang MJ, Scafidi S. Developmental regulation and localization of carnitine palmitoyltransferases (CPTs) in rat brain. *J Neurochem.* (2017) 142:407–19. doi: 10.1111/jnc.14072
56. Xie Z, Jones A, Deeney JT, Hur SK, Bankaitis VA. Inborn errors of long-chain fatty acid β-oxidation link neural stem cell self-renewal to autism. *Cell Rep.* (2016) 14:991–9. doi: 10.1016/j.celrep.2016.01.004
57. Knobloch M, Pilz GA, Ghesquière B, Kovacs WJ, Wegleiter T, Moore DL, et al. A fatty acid oxidation-dependent metabolic shift regulates adult neural stem cell activity. *Cell Rep.* (2017) 20:2144–55. doi: 10.1016/j.celrep.2017.08.029
58. Wanders RJ, Ruiter JP, IJLst L, Waterham HR, Houten SM. The enzymology of mitochondrial fatty acid beta-oxidation and its application to follow-up analysis of positive neonatal screening results. *J Inherit Metab Dis.* (2010) 33:479–94. doi: 10.1007/s10545-010-9104-8

59. Orrù G, Pettersson-Yeo W, Marquand AF, Sartori G, Mechelli A. Using support vector Machine to identify imaging biomarkers of neurological and psychiatric disease: a critical review. *Neurosci Biobehav Rev.* (2012) 36:1140–52. doi: 10.1016/j.neubiorev.2012.01.004
60. Abu-Akel A, Bousman C, Skafidas E, Pantelis C. Mind the prevalence rate: overestimating the clinical utility of psychiatric diagnostic classifiers. *Psychol Med.* (2018) 48:1225–7. doi: 10.1017/S00332917180 00673
61. Pratt J, Hall J. Biomarkers in neuropsychiatry: a prospect for the twenty-first Century? In: Geyer M, Ellenbroek B, Marsden C, editors. *Current Topics in Behavioral Neurosciences.* Berlin; Heidelberg : Springer (2018).

6

Neurobiology and Therapeutic Potential of Cyclooxygenase-2 (COX-2) Inhibitors for Inflammation in Neuropsychiatric Disorders

Rickinder Sethi[1], Nieves Gómez-Coronado[2], Adam J. Walker[3], Oliver D'Arcy Robertson[3,4], Bruno Agustini[3], Michael Berk[3,4,5,6,7] and Seetal Dodd[3,4,5,6]*

[1] Department of Psychiatry, Western University, London, ON, Canada, [2] Unidad de Gestión Clinica Salud Mental, Hospital Universitario Virgen del Rocio, Sevilla, Spain, [3] IMPACT Strategic Research Centre, Deakin University, Geelong, VIC, Australia, [4] University Hospital Geelong, Barwon Health, Geelong, VIC, Australia, [5] Department of Psychiatry, The University of Melbourne, Parkville, VIC, Australia, [6] Orygen, The National Centre of Excellence in Youth Mental Health, Parkville, VIC, Australia, [7] Department of Psychiatry, Florey Institute of Neuroscience and Mental Health, Parkville, VIC, Australia

***Correspondence:**
Michael Berk
michael.berk@barwonhealth.org.au

Neuropsychiatric disorders, such as depression, bipolar disorder, schizophrenia, obsessive-compulsive disorder, and neurodevelopmental disorders such as autism spectrum disorder, are associated with significant illness burden. Accumulating evidence supports an association between these disorders and inflammation. Consequently, anti-inflammatory agents, such as the cyclooxygenase-2 inhibitors, represent a novel avenue to prevent and treat neuropsychiatric illness. In this paper, we first review the role of inflammation in psychiatric pathophysiology including inflammatory cytokines' influence on neurotransmitters, the hypothalamic–pituitary–adrenal axis, and microglial mechanisms. We then discuss how cyclooxygenase-2-inhibitors influence these pathways with potential therapeutic benefit, with a focus on celecoxib, due to its superior safety profile. A search was conducted in PubMed, Embase, and PsychINFO databases, in addition to Clinicaltrials.gov and the Stanley Medical Research Institute trial registries. The results were presented as a narrative review. Currently available outcomes for randomized controlled trials up to November 2017 are also discussed. The evidence reviewed here suggests cyclooxygenase-2 inhibitors, and in particular celecoxib, may indeed assist in treating the symptoms of neuropsychiatric disorders; however, further studies are required to assess appropriate illness stage-related indication.

Keywords: depression, bipolar disorder, schizophrenia, obsessive compulsive disorder, autism spectrum disorder, psychiatry, inflammation, cyclooxygenase-2 inhibitors

INTRODUCTION

The immune system involves a complex array of cells, tissues, and organs working in concert to protect the body from foreign molecules at both the intracellular and extracellular level (1). Pro-inflammatory and anti-inflammatory cytokines, along with other mechanisms, balance the inflammatory response (1). External causes of inflammation include microbial or viral infections, cigarette smoking, poor dietary composition, air pollution, and trauma (both physical and psychological), among others (2). Internal causes may include ischemic events or malignancy (1).

In instances where inflammatory mediators are unable to inhibit the pro-inflammatory immune reaction, a chronic inflammatory state may ensue. Chronic activation of this system can lower the allostatic load threshold, contributing to the development of neuropsychiatric disorders (2).

While monoaminergic dysregulation remains a prevailing hypothesis regarding neuropsychiatric disorders, refractory illnesses remain a significant challenge in addition to a relative paucity of novel treatment options (3). In recent years, the inflammatory model has been revisited due to the fragmented efficacy of the current management approaches. As a result, more attention is being paid to pharmacotherapies that lay outside the traditional vault of psychotropic agents such as antidepressants and antipsychotics. Cyclooxygenase-2 inhibitors, best known for their role in acute pain management, are a potent example of this pharmacological appropriation. Celecoxib and rofecoxib—selective cyclooxygenase-2 inhibitors—have been investigated for their efficacy as both stand-alone therapies and augmentation agents in psychiatry.

The purpose of this paper is twofold: first, to review the relationship between inflammation and neuropsychiatric illnesses, and second, to provide a review of randomized control trials (RCTs) that investigate the use of cyclooxygenase-2 inhibitors for the treatment of select neuropsychiatric illnesses.

METHODS

A Boolean search was conducted for literature published up to November 19, 2017. We searched PubMed, Embase, and PsychINFO databases, and the Clinicaltrials.gov and The Stanley Medical Research Institute trial registries. Search terms included are attached in Appendix A. Articles were selected for human, randomized clinical trials and treatment efficacy. The search was augmented by manually searching the references of key papers and related literature. We adhered to PRISMA guidelines and flowsheet attached in Appendix A. **Table 1** contains a summary chart of the results. The results were presented as a narrative review format.

Abbreviations: 3MS-E, Modified Mini-Mental State Exam; AA, arachidonic acid; ABC-C, autism behavior checklist community edition; ACTH, adrenocorticotropic hormone; ASD, autism spectrum disorder; BDNF, brain derived neurotrophic factor; CCL2, C-C motif chemokine ligand 2; CGI-I, Clinical Global Impression: Improvement; CGI-S, Clinical Global Impression: Severity; CNS, central nervous system; COX, cyclooxygenase; CSF, cerebrospinal fluid; cPLA2, cytoplasmic phospholipase A2; CRH, corticotrophin releasing hormone; CRP, C-reactive protein; ECT, electroconvulsive therapy; ESRS, Extrapyramidal Symptoms Rating Scale; GDS, Geriatric Depression Scale; HAM-A, Hamilton Anxiety Rating Scale; HAM-D, Hamilton Depression Rating Scale; HDRS, Hamilton Depression Rating Scale; IDO, indolamine 2,3 dioxygenase; IL, interleukin; IL-1ra, interleukin-1 receptor antagonist; IFNα, interferon alpha; IFN-γ, interferon gamma; KA, kainic acid; LPS, lipopolysaccharide; MDD, major depressive disorder; mRNA, microribonucleic acid; NMDA, *N*-methyl-D-aspartate; NF, nuclear factor; OCD, obsessive compulsive disorder; PANS, pediatric acute-onset neuropsychiatric syndrome; PANDAS, pediatric autoimmune neuropsychiatric disorders associated with streptococcal; PANSS, Positive and Negative Syndrome Scale; PHQ-9, Patient Health Questionnaire-9; PGE2, prostaglandin E2; QUIN, quinolinic acid; RCT, randomized control trial; SANS, Scale for the Assessment of Negative Symptoms; SAS, Simpson–Angus Rating Scale of EPS; TAU, treatment as usual; TDO, tryptophan 2,3-dioxygenase; TNFα, tumor necrosis factor alpha

The Link Between Inflammatory System, the Brain, and Mental Illness

In 1927, Julius Wagner-Jauregg became the first and the only psychiatrist thus far to win a Nobel Prize in Medicine. His impactful discovery involved the association with inflammation *via* malaria inoculation to cure neuropsychiatric symptoms of syphilis (22). Unfortunately, this inflammatory etiological theory was set aside during the advent of the psychotropic revolution (23). While support for the monoamine hypothesis in neuropsychiatric disorders continued to gain traction in subsequent decades, a residual group of patients exhibited persistent treatment-refractory illnesses and chronic debilitating symptoms suggestive of alternate hypotheses for neuropsychiatric conditions (3).

Innate and Adaptive Immunity

Immune system responses are typically classified as either innate or adaptive. The innate immune system features elements that are both genetically heritable and evolutionarily ancient, found in all multicellular organisms (24, 25). The innate system's principal phagocytes include neutrophils, monocytes, and macrophages, which work in synergy to establish the first-line barrier of immunity (26). This line of defense is supplemented by the adaptive immune system, which includes specialized cells, B-lymphocytes and T-lymphocytes. Both response sectors produce a composite operation of moderating immunotransmitters, defined by cytokines. These immunomodulatory cytokines are typically categorized as pro-inflammatory or anti-inflammatory on the basis of their general effects. Pro-inflammatory cytokines such as tumor necrosis factor alpha (TNFα), interferon gamma (IFNγ), and interleukin (IL)-1 and IL-6 are primarily secreted by monocytes and macrophages, promoting additional complex inflammatory response systems, discussed in detail elsewhere [e.g., Ref. (27)]. Anti-inflammatory cytokines include IL-4, IL-10, IL-11, and IL-13 (26, 28). In simplistic terms, imbalanced pro-inflammatory over anti-inflammatory cytokine load will preferentially increase the throughput of pathological cellular pathways.

Central Nervous System Immunity

The blood–brain barrier is the brain's primary defense against chemical insult. During peripheral inflammatory activation, there is increased permeability of the blood–brain barrier (29, 30). Such increases in blood–brain permeability may exacerbate or possibly even initiate neuropsychiatric and neurological disorders [see Ref. (31) for a review]. Furthermore, recent identification of lymphatic vessels within the central nervous system (CNS) reveals an alternate route of communication with the immune system to the brain (32). Once activated, a host of cellular and chemical pathways within the brain can result in significant structural change.

Microglia are specialized macrophages localized to the CNS that also play an important regulatory role in inflammatory response. They secrete neurotrophic factors important for cellular repair and signal recruitment for immune cells (26, 33, 34). The role microglia play in inflammation-driven neuronal damage and degeneration is also well established (35). Microglia have been shown to express different phenotypes or polarizations,

TABLE 1 | Clinical trials investigating celecoxib in neuropsychiatric disorders.

Study	Sample	Study Design	Intervention and Dosage	Outcome Measures	Findings
Muller et al. (4)	Depression, *n* = 40	Double-blind, randomized, placebo-controlled add-on trial 6 weeks	Celecoxib 400 mg + Reboxetine VS Placebo + Reboxetine	HAM-D	Favor of adjuvant celecoxib
Akhondzadeh et al. (5)	Depression, *n* = 40	Double-blind, randomized, placebo-controlled add-on trial 6 weeks	Celecoxib 400 mg + fluoxetine VS Placebo + fluoxetine	HRDS	Favor of adjuvant celecoxib
Fields et al. (6)	Depression, *n* = 2,528 Elderly cohort	Double-blind, Multicenter, randomized, placebo-controlled add-on trial 6 weeks	Celecoxib 400 mg VS Naproxen 440 mg VS Placebo	GDS, Modified Mini-Mental State Exam (3MS-E)	Not in favor of celecoxib monotherapy
Abbasi et al. (7)	Depression, *n* = 40	Double-blind, randomized, placebo-controlled add-on trial 6 weeks	Celecoxib 400 mg + sertraline VS Placebo + sertraline	HAM-D	Favor of adjuvant celecoxib
Majd et al. (8)	Depression, *n* = 30	Double-blind, randomized, placebo-controlled add-on trial 8 weeks	Celecoxib 200 mg + sertraline VS Placebo + sertraline	HAM-D, HAM-A	Not in favor of celecoxib
Jafari et al. (9)	Depression, *n* = 40 Comorbid brucellosis	Double-blind, randomized, placebo-controlled add-on trial 8 weeks	Celecoxib 200 mg + antibiotics VS Placebo + antibiotics	HDRS	Favor of adjuvant celecoxib
Mohammad et al. (10)	Depression, *n* = 52 Comorbid breast cancer	Double-blind, randomized, placebo-controlled add-on trial 6 weeks	Celecoxib 400 mg VS diclofenac 100 mg	HDRS	Favor of celecoxib monotherapy
Alamdarsaravi et al. (11)	Depression, *n* = 40 Comorbid colorectal cancer	Double-blind, randomized, placebo-controlled add-on trial 6 weeks	Celecoxib 400 mg VS Placebo	HDRS	Favor of celecoxib monotherapy
Nery et al. (12)	Bipolar disorder–depression or mixed episode, *n* = 28	Double-blind, randomized, placebo-controlled add-on trial, 6 weeks	Celecoxib 400 mg + TAU VS Placebo + TAU	HDRS	Favor of adjuvant celecoxib
Kargar et al. (13)	Bipolar disorder–mania, *n* = 35	Double-blind, randomized, placebo-controlled add-on trial,	Celecoxib 400 mg + ECT VS Placebo + ECT	YMRS, BDNF serum levels	Not in favor of celecoxib
Arabzadeh et al. (14)	Bipolar disorder – mania, *n* = 46	Double-blind, randomized, placebo-controlled add-on trial, 6 weeks	Celecoxib 400 mg + Sodium Valproate VS Placebo + Sodium Valproate	YMRS, HDRS	Favor of adjuvant celecoxib
Shalbafan et al. (15)	OCD, *n* = 54	Double-blind, randomized, placebo-controlled add-on trial 10 weeks	Celecoxib 400 mg + Fluvoxamine 200 mg VS Placebo + Fluvoxamine 200 mg	Y-BOCS	Favor of adjuvant celecoxib
Sayyah et al. (16)	OCD, *n* = 56	Double-blind, randomized, placebo-controlled add-on trial 8 weeks	Celecoxib 400 mg + Fluoxetine VS Placebo + Fluoxetine	Y-BOCS	Favor of adjuvant celecoxib
Muller et al. (17)	Schizophrenia, *n* = 50	Double-blind, randomized, placebo-controlled add-on trial 5 weeks	Celecoxib 400 mg + Risperidone VS Placebo + Risperidone	PANSS, Simpson-Angus Rating Scale of EPS (SAS)	Favor of adjuvant celecoxib
Rapaport et al. (18)	Schizophrenia, *n* = 38	Double-blind, randomized, placebo-controlled add-on trial 9 weeks	Celecoxib 400 mg + TAU VS Placebo + TAU	PANSS, Scale for the Assessment of Negative Symptoms (SANS), CGI-S, Clinical Global Impression: Improvement (CGI-I), HAM-A	Not in favor of celecoxib
Akhondzadeh et al. (19)	Schizophrenia, *n* = 60	Double-blind, randomized, placebo-controlled add-on trial 8 weeks	Celecoxib 400 mg + Risperidone VS Placebo + Risperidone	PANSS, ESRS	Favor of adjuvant celecoxib
Muller et al. (20)	Schizophrenia, *n* = 49	Double-blind, randomized, placebo-controlled add-on trial 6 weeks	Celecoxib 400 mg+ Amisulpride 200–1,000 mg VS Placebo + Amisulpride 200–1,000 mg	PANSS, CGI	Favor of adjuvant celecoxib
Muller Trial ID: 01T-418 (yet to publish)	Schizophrenia, *n* = 40	Double-blind, randomized, placebo-controlled add-on trial 8 weeks	Celecoxib 400 mg + Risperidone VS Placebo + Risperidone	PANSS, SANS, CBI, ESRS, Barnes Akathisia QOL	Not in favor of celecoxib

(Continued)

TABLE 1 | Continued

Study	Sample	Study Design	Intervention and Dosage	Outcome Measures	Findings
Zhang Trial ID: 03T-459 (yet to publish)	Schizophrenia, *n* = 250	Double-blind, randomized, placebo-controlled add-on trial 12 weeks	Celecoxib 400 mg + Risperidone VS Placebo + Risperidone	PANSS, BPRS, SANS, ICG, WCST, N-back Test, WMS-R, CPT, WAIS-R, FSIQ, SAS, AIMS, MANOVAs	Favor of adjuvant celecoxib
Asadabadi et al. (21)	Autism, *n* = 40	Double-blind, randomized, placebo-controlled add-on trial	Celecoxib 300 mg BID + Risperidone VS Placebo + Risperidone	Autism Behaviour Checklist Community Edition (ABC-C)Rating Scale (Irritability subsection)	Favor of adjuvant celecoxib

classified as M1 and M2. M1 polarization is influenced by the pro-inflammatory state and acts in neuronal apoptosis, while the M2 polarization, in contrast, promotes neurogenesis (32, 36–39). Interferon alpha (IFNα) has been shown to induce a pro-inflammatory shift in microglial phenotype, from M2 to M1, resulting in depressive symptoms in mice (40, 41).

Inflammation and Neuropsychiatric Symptoms

When anti-inflammatory regulators are unable to balance pro-inflammatory reactions, inflammation can persist, in conjunction with sub-threshold neuropsychiatric symptoms (42). The following mechanisms describe the cytokine communication with neuropsychiatric symptoms and thus support the inflammatory hypothesis.

Pro-inflammatory markers have been associated with the development of neuropsychiatric symptoms (43). IL-6 activates the type 2 immune response, prompting the B-cell maturation pathway, consequently producing antibodies directed against extracellular pathogens. In addition, IL-6 activates the release of C-reactive protein (CRP) from the liver. Elevated levels of CRP and IL-6 in childhood were associated with an increased risk of developing depressive and psychotic symptoms in the future (44). Consistent with this, a significant association has been reported between CRP and several neuropsychiatric disorders, including depression, anxiety, and schizophrenia (45, 46). CRP is a well-established biomarker for an active inflammatory process and is a significant independent predictor of coronary heart disease risk (47–53). Furthermore, elevated CRP and IL-6 levels have also been associated with cognitive dysfunction (54). Studies have shown that biomarkers such as CRP and IL-6 may shed light on subtyping depression (55, 56). Several meta-analyses have demonstrated significant evidence of elevated pro-inflammatory cytokines in patients with depressive symptoms (43, 57, 58), bipolar disorder (58–60), schizophrenia (58, 61), obsessive compulsive disorder (OCD) (62), and autism spectrum disorders (ASDs) (63). These pro-inflammatory markers include CRP, IL-6, TNFα, and the IL-1 receptor antagonist (IL-1Ra) (43, 57–63). In addition, pro-inflammatory cytokines have been shown to trend toward normalization with symptom improvement indicating treatment response (64). Participation from microglia and peripheral macrophages are identified in activated inflammatory networks (65). An exaggerated immune response can be responsible for neuronal damage and decreased brain derived neurotrophic factor (BDNF), a protein integral to neuronal growth, plasticity, and survival (66–70). Excessive activation of the immune system may exacerbate mental illness in a subgroup of vulnerable individuals (71, 72). The inflammatory hypothesis suggests that hyperactivation of the immune system may produce nitro-oxidative stress and alterations of the kynurenine pathway, subsequently dysregulating monoamine levels and activating the glutamatergic system (2, 15, 73).

The evidence for cytokine-induced neuropsychiatric symptoms in healthy participants favors the inflammatory model. For example, healthy participants received an infusion of endotoxin to induce an inflammatory response, with resultant mood symptoms (74). Similarly, healthy individuals who received exogenous cytokines (IL-2, IFNα, and TNFα) also developed neuropsychiatric symptoms, including depression, mania, emotional dysregulation, cognitive impairment, and/or avolition (75). Elevated serum pro-inflammatory markers, TNFα, IL-6, and cortisol levels were observed by *Salmonella abortus equi* endotoxin injections (76). Subsequently, the subjects also exhibited neuropsychiatric symptoms of appetite changes, mood and anxiety symptoms, and cognitive decline without physical sickness symptoms (77). These findings were replicated with other vaccinations of healthy individuals (74, 78). Preclinical research has yielded similar findings, wherein lipopolysaccharide (LPS) and IL-1 injections in mice were found to result in sickness behavior, an analog to depressive symptoms (79).

Notably, pro-inflammatory agents such as recombinant IFNα and IL-2 have been used in the treatment of hepatitis C and carcinomas, respectively (80, 81). Interestingly, while effective for treating the targeted indication, IFNα was found to induce significant neuropsychiatric side effects with up to 80% of patients endorsing mild to moderate depressive symptoms (82–84). Grigoleit et al. (85) identified a positive dose-dependent association in IL-6, IL-10, TNFα, cortisol, and norepinephrine with neuropsychiatric symptoms. While some studies have reported that serum IL-6 and TNFα also appeared elevated in OCD patients compared to healthy controls [e.g., Ref. (86)], it should be noted that an earlier meta-analysis of OCD patients revealed no significant difference in TNFα or IL-6 (62). However, these authors did note a reduced level of pro-inflammatory IL-1β in OCD patients (62).

Autoimmune Conditions and Neuropsychiatric Disorders

Autoimmune and infectious conditions such as rheumatoid arthritis (87), type 1 diabetes (88), systemic lupus erythematosus (89), hepatitis, and sepsis (90) increase the risk of neuropsychiatric symptoms. An extensive Danish-based study found a 62% increased risk of mood disorders after infection-related hospitalizations (90). In patients who suffer from both Crohn's disease and depression, exacerbations of both physical and mental illnesses tend to occur at the same time (91). Patients experiencing psoriasis and anxiety symptoms were shown to benefit from treatment with cytokine inhibitors (92–94). In addition, a greater prevalence of autoimmune conditions such as pemphigus in bipolar disorder is observed (95). In a large epidemiological study, multiple infections and autoimmune disorders were associated with the increased lifetime prevalence of schizophrenia spectrum disorders (96).

In summary, multiple studies have indicated a positive association between inflammation and neuropsychiatric symptoms. Elevated pro-inflammatory markers are consistently associated with neuropsychiatric symptoms and reveal a bidirectional relationship.

Cyclooxygenase-2 (COX-2) Inhibitors

The COX pathway involves the precursor substrate of arachidonic acid (AA) to produce thromboxane, prostacyclin, and prostaglandins (PG) D2, E2, F2, and I2. AA is extracted from cell membranes by phospholipases, predominately cytoplasmic phospholipase A2 (cPLA2), and metabolized by the COX enzymes. The two rate-limiting enzymes within the COX pathways are COX-1 and COX-2. COX-1 is constitutionally expressed, and thus responsible for baseline prostaglandin levels, whereas COX-2 is inducible and expressed exclusively in the CNS, kidney, thymus, GI tract, and possibly in the female reproductive system (97–100). However, during inflammatory processes, COX-2 expression is promoted by and regulated by inflammatory stimuli, including lipopolysaccharide (LPS), IL-1, IL-6, TNF, IFNγ, and AA (101–108). The variability of isotype expressions COX-1 and COX-2 might be explained by the target tissue and type of insult (109, 110). The COX-2 enzyme produces prostaglandins, thromboxanes, prostacyclins, and leukotrienes downstream, which are suspected to be culprits for inflammation and neoplastic growth, in particular PGE_2 (111). Furthermore, COX-2 expression is supported by microglia (112) and is auto-regulated *via* its by-products, PGE_2 and $PGF_2\alpha$, perpetuating the inflammation process (113, 114). Additionally, PGE_2 promotes IL-6 production (115), subsequently reinforcing this positive inflammatory feedback loop (**Figure 1**). Notably, in COX-2 gene knockout mice, a decrease in PGE_2 and nuclear factor (NF)-κB activity was observed (114, 116, 117).

In 1995, the first generation of selective COX-2 inhibitors, celecoxib and rofecoxib, entered clinical trials (118). Over the next 4 years, numerous trials demonstrated selective COX-2 inhibitors could reduce pain and inflammation (119). From 2000 to 2004, larger trials such as CLASS, VIGOR, and TARGET identified the reduced gastrointestinal risks associated with COX-2 inhibitors, however, highlighted the increased cardiovascular risks leading

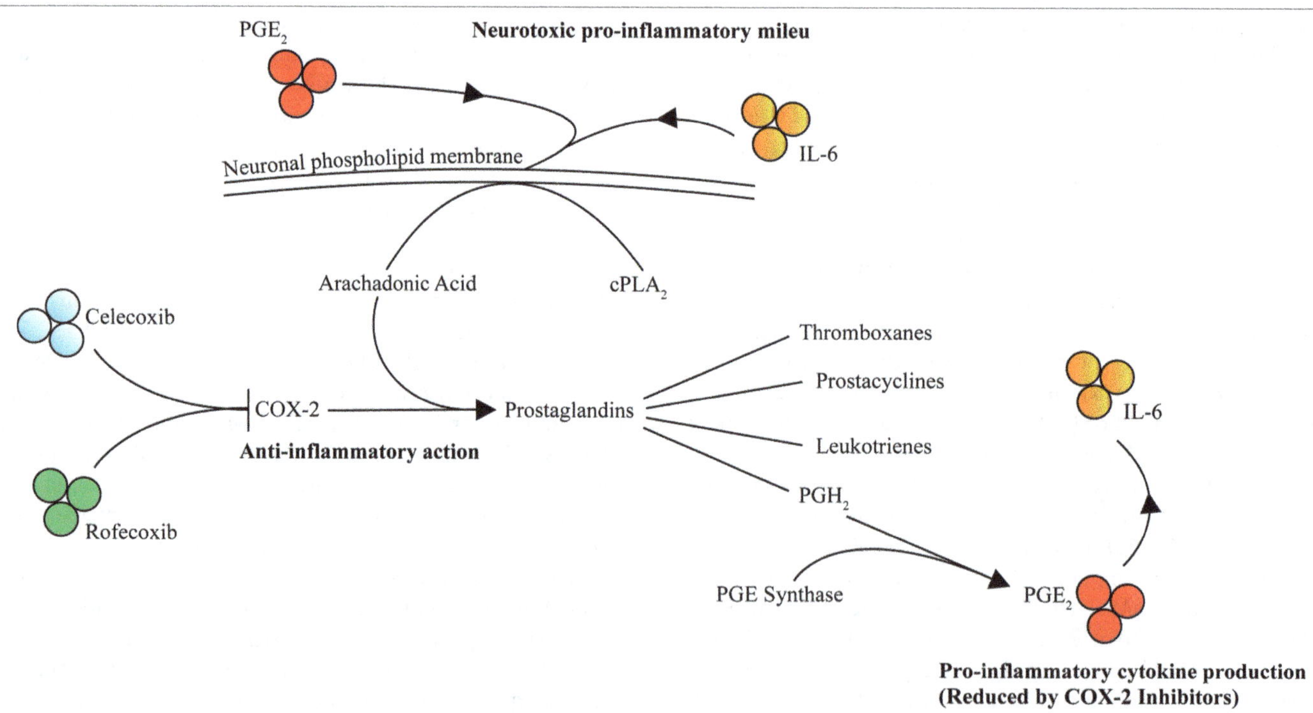

FIGURE 1 | COX-2 contributes to inflammation through PGE_2 and IL-6 and is selectively inhibited by celecoxib and rofecoxib. Activated by inflammatory cytokines including PGE_2 and IL-6, AA (the precursor substrate of the COX-2 pathway) is extracted from phospholipid membranes by phospholipases such as cPLA2. COX-2 then drives production of prostaglandins including prostaglandin H_2 (PGH_2), which in turn is converted to PGE_2 *via* PGE synthase. An accumulation of PGE_2 leads to increased IL-6 (along with other cytokines) contributing to the inflammatory milieu, further potentiation of the pathway and neurotoxicity contributing to psychopathology. Celecoxib and rofecoxib exert selective inhibition of COX-2 reducing this pathway's contribution to inflammation mediated neurotoxicity (→ = activates/increases, ⊥ = inhibits).

to rofecoxib being pulled from the market (120–123). In 2005, valdecoxib was also withdrawn from the market for similar concerns by the Food and Drug Administration (FDA). In 2011, celecoxib was withdrawn from the market for the indication of cancer prevention while still being indicated for rheumatoid arthritis, osteoarthritis, and acute pain. Subsequently, this led to cautious prescribing due to concerns of cardiovascular side effects (124).

Preclinical trials have shown that rofecoxib can increase serotonin levels in the frontal and temporoparietal cortex (125). In addition, celecoxib was shown to potentiate the effects of reboxetine and fluoxetine on cortical noradrenaline and serotonin output (126).

Although ubiquitously expressed, COX-1 is typically described as gastro-protective and neuroprotective (127, 128), and preclinical data reveal some contradictory evidence regarding the inflammatory classifications of the COX isoforms. COX-2 may have anti-inflammatory and neuroprotective properties, aiding in neurotransmitter release, long-term potentiation, blood flow regulation, and memory consolidation (129). It was reported that COX-2 gene knockout mice were susceptible to inflammation compared to healthy mice (130, 131). Deletion of the COX-2 gene causes increased permeability of the blood–brain barrier and leukocyte infiltration (132). Another study showed that maximal COX-2 expression coincided with inflammatory resolution and was associated with minimal PGE_2 synthesis (133).

Nevertheless, COX-2 inhibitors have proven to be beneficial in glutamate-mediated death prevention and suppression of pro-inflammatory cytokines (134, 135). Kainic acid (KA), a potent neurotoxin, elicits excitatory effects on *N*-methyl-D-aspartate (NMDA) receptors resulting in status epilepticus, neurodegeneration, and memory loss (134–138). KA has also been shown to increase COX-2 expression in the CNS (139); therefore, COX-2 inhibitors have been shown to prevent KA-induced neuronal death (140). There appears to be mounting evidence of therapeutic effect of COX-2 inhibitors in mediating glutamatergic processes (141–143). As well, there seems to be appropriate evidence for COX pathway in neuropsychiatric disorders.

Pathophysiology of Neuropsychiatric Disorders and the Efficacy of Cyclooxygenase-2 Inhibitors

We have now established there is substantive evidence for inflammation being a driver of neuropsychiatric symptoms by negatively impacting on neuronal proliferation, survival, and differentiation (144, 145). Furthermore, the COX pathway potentiates the inflammatory process and may exacerbate inflammation mediated neurodegeneration. COX-2 inhibition reduces this inflammatory load and thus the impact of these pathways on the brain.

In this section, we address the proposed mechanisms by which inflammatory states influence central monoamine effects, the hypothalamic–pituitary–adrenal (HPA) axis, and microglial activation, pathways at the center of neuropsychiatric pathogenesis. Discussion will focus on specific conditions including depression, bipolar disorder, schizophrenia, ASD, and OCD. Herein, a number of clinical trials investigating the efficacy of the cyclooxygenase-2 inhibitors for neuropsychiatric disorders are discussed, summarized in **Table 1**. Particular attention is being paid to the operative inflammatory pathways inherent to these conditions and the potential role for COX-2 inhibitors in their management.

Neurotransmitter Dysregulation Hypothesis

The dysregulation of the neurotransmitters such as serotonin, norepinephrine, dopamine, acetylcholine, and glutamate has been the foci of the biochemical etiology of neuropsychiatric illnesses. While treatment with antidepressants and neuroleptics aims to modulate monoamine signaling, there is a wealth of evidence supporting secondary mechanisms of action including effects on inflammatory pathways (27, 146). During inflammation, the pro-inflammatory cytokines IL-2 and IFNα have been shown to directly increase enzyme activity of the indoleamine-pyrrole 2,3-dioxygenase (IDO) enzyme of the kynurenine pathway, which promotes conversion of tryptophan to kynurenine, consequently depleting the antecedent supply to serotonin (147), in addition to direct catabolism of serotonin by IL-6 and IFNα (148, 149). This evidence supports the monoamine hypothesis regarding the hypoactive serotonin state featured in mood disorders (150–152). IFNα administration led to inflammation by increasing the concentration of kynurenine pathway metabolites in the CSF, namely kynurenine, kynurenic acid, and quinolinic acid (QUIN) (153). These metabolites have been presented as inducers of depressive and anxiety symptoms (154). Notably, QUIN can selectively activate NMDA receptors (155, 156) and has been associated with numerous neurological diseases, including: Alzheimer's disease, anxiety, depression, epilepsy, human immunodeficiency virus-associated neurocognitive disorders, and Huntington's disease (155, 157–161). QUIN has also been shown to cause neurodegeneration *via* multiple models (159).

HPA Axis Dysregulation

During a stress response, the HPA axis is activated (162). The hypothalamus secretes two hormones, corticotrophin releasing hormone (CRH) and arginine vasopressin, which act on the pituitary gland to increase adrenocorticotropic hormone (ACTH) release, subsequently accelerating the production of cortisol to aid in the homeostasis feedback loop (163). Studies have demonstrated an elevated inflammation state perpetuating cytokines such as IL-1, IL-6, TNFα, and IFNα; these in turn activate the HPA axis elevating levels of CRH, ACTH, and cortisol (162, 164–167). This relationship furthermore supports the feedback loop maintaining a hyperactive HPA system (163). Chronic elevation of endogenous glucocorticoids results in mood symptoms (163, 167). Additionally, it is proposed that cortisol increases the catabolizing enzyme tryptophan 2,3-dioxygenase (TDO) to deplete the precursor to serotonin implicating an association with the serotonin dysregulation (168, 169).

Contrary to advantageous effects of steroids in managing infections, there is evidence that glucocorticoid treatment duration for acute infections versus chronic infections results in changes of glucocorticoid receptor function and concentrations (170, 171). This subsequently influences HPA axis hyperactivity, which elevates cortisol and results in decreased function and quantity of glucocorticoid receptors resulting in impaired feedback and glucocorticoid resistance (170). Glucocorticoid resistance that is seen in depressed patients may also be a result of changes in expressed glucocorticoid receptors ratio *via* cellular phosphorylation (172–174). Patients with neuropsychiatric illnesses also exhibited heightened plasma, urine, and cerebrospinal fluid (CSF) levels of cortisol and anatomical changes in the pituitary and adrenal glands (175–178). Pavon et al. (179) reported elevated cortisol levels in depressed patients associated with elevated TNFα, in addition to decreased levels of IL-1β, suggesting that increased cortisol may influence inflammatory cytokines. However, it is important to bear in mind that while some subtypes of depression (namely melancholic or endogenous) are associated with hyperactive HPA axis, glucocorticoid resistance, and increased circulating cortisol levels, atypical and seasonal depression has been consistently reported to have normal or hypoactive HPA axis function (180, 181). Therefore, the hypothesis is supported regarding the impairment of the HPA axis through cellular mechanisms and dysfunctional feedback leading to HPA axis dysfunction, one of the most consistent findings in biological psychiatry, which is exhibited by patients with depression, bipolar disorder, and schizophrenia (169, 182).

Microglial Hyperactivation Hypothesis

Microglia function as macrophages of the CNS by clearing foreign particles and promoting healing after traumatic brain injury (183). They are also involved in the pruning process of neurons by tagging unutilized synapses for degradation to rebuild more active neurons during the maturation process (184). Pathological synaptic pruning may also contribute to prodromal, remittent and relapsing, and chronic stages of neuropsychiatric disorders (185–187). Prolonged microglial activation induces synaptic pruning subsequent to the accumulation of two pro-inflammatory cytokines, specifically TNFα and IL-1β, leading to neuronal apoptosis (188, 189). The subsequent dysfunctional neuronal pathways may be compensated by adaptive systems, which may resultantly produce and preserve maladaptive behaviors (190, 191). Individuals at an ultra-high risk for developing schizophrenia also appear to have significantly elevated activity of microglia (192). Histological changes in activated microglia have been observed in patients with schizophrenia who had committed suicide during an acute episode of psychosis (193). In contrast, conflicting data derived from post-mortem studies have reported reductions in microglial density and activation (194). These findings may indicate a difference of microglial activation depending on the stage of illness among other factors (194). Aberrant microglial activation is seen in other neuropsychiatric disorders including Alzheimer's dementia, Parkinson's disease, multiple sclerosis, herpes encephalitis, traumatic brain injury, and stroke (195, 196). Alterations in brain morphology have been described across the spectrum on neuropsychiatric conditions (197–201). Duration of mental illnesses also has evidence of significant brain morphologic changes (201). Mechanisms that may encourage these anatomical reductions include oxidative and nitrosative stress through activation of microglia (202).

Depression

Major depressive disorder (MDD) is highly prevalent throughout the world, and the prevalence has increased over time (73). The estimated lifetime prevalence of major depression and persistent depressive disorder in adults is 12% (203). In unipolar depression, inflammation and depressive symptoms share a bidirectional relationship. Immunological markers such as CRP, and cytokines IL-1, IL-6, and TNFα, are elevated in patients with depression (1, 204, 205). A recent meta-analysis comprised of 3,212 participants noted elevations in the concentrations of IL-6, TNFα, IL-10, the soluble IL-2 receptor, C-C chemokine ligand 2, IL-13, IL-18, IL-12, IL-1 receptor antagonist, and the soluble TNF receptor 2 in depression patients (1). Several groups of authors have reported that IL-6 may be a useful biomarker for predicting treatment response (115, 204–207). A prospective study revealed a correlation with elevated serum IL-6, as those with higher levels were more likely to be depressed by 18 years of age than individuals on the lower end levels (208). Pro-inflammatory cytokines have been shown to trend toward normalization with symptom improvement indicating treatment response (64).

Studies have shown biomarkers such as CRP and IL-6 may shed light on depression subtypes (55, 56). An interesting larger scale study, The Netherlands Study of Depression and Anxiety (NESDA), extrapolated gender variance while evaluating CRP and IL-6 (181). The authors described an increased level of CRP and IL-6 with normal levels of TNFα in male patients with depressive symptoms; however, there were no associations with the cytokines in women with depressive symptoms (209). Additionally, they noted a differential role of the HPA function, inflammatory markers, and metabolic variables between melancholic and atypical depression subtypes (181).

Elevated levels of kynurenine pathway toxic metabolites such as QUIN are also observed in patients with depression (210). Interestingly, in a 6-week RCT, Krause et al. (211) noted a correlation with kynurenine/tryptophan ratios that was predictive of celecoxib response to significant improvements in the Hamilton Depression Scale (HAMD-17) scores. Subsequently, the kynurenine/tryptophan ratio shows some promise as a potential biomarker for predicting response to COX-2 inhibitors.

Gałecki et al. (212) reported an increase of non-coding micro ribonucleic acid (mRNA) expression of the COX-2 enzyme in recurrent depression. COX-2 inhibitors decrease IDO activity, subsequently decreasing glutamatergic-active by-products such as QUIN, which may add in neuro-stabilizing effects (4, 213, 214). Higher concentrations of QUIN and 3-hydroxykynurenine have been reported in depression (210). Preclinical studies have shown that celecoxib administration in rats was associated with reductions in PGE_2 levels and a reversal of stress-induced depressive-like behaviors (215, 216). PGE_2 had been shown to contribute to monoamine imbalance with decreased norepinephrine central neuronal release and dysregulation of the HPA axis (217). Consequently, this alters cortisol synthesis and subsequently suppresses serotonin (215, 218–220). Consistent with this assertion, an animal-based model of depression in rats demonstrated that celecoxib independently enhances the release of serotonin in the brain (126).

Celecoxib has also been shown to attenuate pro-inflammatory cytokines IL-1β and TNFα and significantly increase IL-10 levels in animal models (109, 221). IL-1β has been identified as a modulator of BDNF (144). Some evidence exists indicating that elevated levels of IL-6 results in a reduction in BDNF, implicating in imbalanced neurogenesis, resulting in neural circuitry dysfunction in depressive symptomology (144). In a preclinical study with rats with a depression-like phenotype, augmentation with acetylsalicylic acid, a non-selective COX inhibitor, enhanced the efficacy of fluoxetine (222).

To date, several reviews have suggested that celecoxib may be efficacious for the management of depressive symptoms (1, 223, 224); however, some have suggested it is clinically inadequate (225). Abbasi et al. assigned adjuvant celecoxib to MDD patients on sertraline and measured IL-6 levels in samples of their serum. They reported a correlation between decreasing IL-6 concentrations and improvement in the Hamilton Depression Rating Scale (HDRS) scores as outlined in **Table 1,** along with the key findings of all clinical trials assessing celecoxib in neuropsychiatric disorders appearing in this review. In another RCT (8) assessing celecoxib augmentation with sertraline in the treatment of drug-naïve women with depression, the authors reported an improvement in HDRS and Hamilton Anxiety Rating Scale (HAM-A) scores compared to the placebo group after 4 weeks of treatment. However, there were no significant differences between both groups at the end of the 8-week trial. Interestingly, the remission rates in the celecoxib group were statistically higher in comparison to the placebo group. Subsequently, Akhondzadeh et al. assessed the HDRS in 40 individuals in a 6-week RCT receiving fluoxetine plus celecoxib versus fluoxetine alone. They demonstrated significant improvements in depressive symptoms, and response and remission rates in the celecoxib group (5). Another RCT found more significant improvements in depressive symptoms in the adjuvant celecoxib group with reboxetine compared to reboxetine alone (4). However, Fields commented that there were no significant changes in late-life depressive symptoms in patients prescribed either placebo, celecoxib, or naproxen (6). These discrepancies in the efficacy of COX-2 inhibitors for this indication might be explained by methodological heterogeneity and variance in target sample characteristics. For example, the Geriatric Depression Scale (GDS) was used for the geriatric patients with a yearly frequency, which may not be a specific tool for detecting variations in depression diagnosis (226). However, the study did have strength in having a large sample size and median follow-up of 2 years with patients.

Inflammation may be the primary mechanism of pathogenesis in brucellosis (227, 228). Therefore, Jafari et al. assessed 40 individuals with celecoxib for treatment of mild to moderate depression due to acute brucellosis. They reported an improvement of the HDRS in the 8-week trial with the celecoxib with antibiotics group than placebo with antibiotics (9).

In patients with comorbid osteoarthritis, pooled data from five post-approval trials, each at 6 weeks in length, participants were randomized in placebo, ibuprofen or naproxen, or celecoxib groups while assessing the Patient Health Questionnaire-9 (PHQ-9). The authors report a trend toward a reduction in PHQ-9 depression scores. However, this lack of robust data is possibly due to the lack of efficacious dosing of celecoxib of 200 mg (229).

Interestingly, celecoxib may exhibit benefits in patients with colorectal cancer. Investigations have illustrated that celecoxib initiation in the head, neck, and gastrointestinal cancer population is associated with improvements in biological symptoms of depression, including an increase in appetite, body mass index, and quality of life (230, 231). A 6-week RCT included 40 colon cancer participants randomly assigned to either celecoxib monotherapy or a placebo group, which resulted in significant improvements in the HDRS among the former group, starting as early as week 2 and was sustained until the end of the trial (11).

Another cancer trial consisted of 52 outpatients with breast cancer undergoing 6 weeks of treatment with either celecoxib or diclofenac for mild to moderate depression. The outcome measures were scored using the HDRS to compare the COX-2 inhibitor with an indiscriminate COX-inhibitor. They reported significant improvements in depressive symptoms in both groups by week 3 and significantly more considerable improvements with the celecoxib group compared to diclofenac by week 6. None of the participants experienced remission HDRS less than or equal to 7 (10). A meta-analysis demonstrated with 150 participants showed that the adjunctive celecoxib cohort had better response rates and remissions compared to placebo (224). In summary, interactions between the immune system and neurotransmitters, the tryptophan/kynurenine system, and the glutamatergic system provide links between the immune system and depression; furthermore, data are suggestive of a role for celecoxib in treatment of depressive symptoms (115).

Bipolar Disorder

The estimated lifetime prevalence of bipolar disorder among adults worldwide is 1% to 3% (232). For many, bipolar disorder is a chronic and debilitating illness, with patients often experiencing poor inter-episodic remission (233, 234). Pro-inflammatory markers, such as IL-4, TNFα, IL-1β, and CCL2 cytokine, which have an established role of inflammation in neuronal damage and degeneration, have been observed to be elevated in patients with bipolar disorder (35, 59, 233–236). Elevated CRP levels were also identified in a meta-analysis of 730 patients with bipolar disorder (237).

Interestingly, during the euthymic phase of bipolar disorder, IL-4 has been shown to return to baseline levels; this apparent relationship between inflammatory and mood states provides an avenue for prospective biomarker investigations (65, 238). Furthermore, accumulating evidence is suggestive of chronic low-grade inflammation in bipolar patients (239, 240). Scans employing positron emission tomography (PET) have supported neuroanatomical changes and hyperactive microglial state in bipolar disorder (241–244). Gray matter reduction was observed in the anterior limbic region (197, 198) including ventricular enlargement (245). Lithium, a well-established mood stabilizer, has been shown to reduce IL-2, IL-6, IL-10, and IFNα levels after long-term use, possibly inferring its nebulous mechanism of action through anti-inflammatory processes (246). In addition, lithium has some potential in neurogenesis, which may be linked with particular anti-inflammatory mechanisms (202).

Preclinical data also suggest that these mood stabilizing effects may downregulate the AA cascade, therefore decreasing COX-2 and prostaglandin levels (247–253).

A clinical trial investigated the efficacy of celecoxib in bipolar depression or mixed episode and found lower HAM-D scores initially after 1 week; however, no statistically significant difference was found at the end of the 6-week trial (12). In another study, celecoxib augmentation was trialed in individuals with acute mania without psychotic features alongside treatment-as-usual. This 6-week RCT demonstrated that adjuvant celecoxib with valproate was significantly effective for treatment in acute mania compared to valproate and placebo (14). The difference in trial outcomes may suggest greater inflammatory impact and therefore COX-2 inhibitor efficacy during the manic phase of illness, as opposed to the depressive phase; this is also supported by the relative increase in inflammatory markers in the former illness phase (66).

Electroconvulsive therapy (ECT) is an effective treatment modality for various phases of illness in bipolar disorder (254). ECT is reported to affect monoamines, hormones, in addition to the immune system, cytokines, ACTH, and cortisol (255–257). Immunomodulatory effects have also been reported, for example, effects on the kynurenine pathway *via* the decrease of QUIN concentrations in unipolar and bipolar depression (258, 259).

Kargar et al. (260) assessed cytokine and CRP changes in patients receiving both ECT and celecoxib, reporting a reduction in TNFα, but no significant changes in other inflammatory markers, such as IL-1β, IL-6, and CRP. However, they noted greater clinical improvement of depressive symptoms in the first week of celecoxib intervention but no persisting differences thereafter (260). Notably, the authors hypothesized that immunomodulatory effects associated with ECT might explain the baseline return of TNFα concentrations; however, no significant cytokine changes were observed. This may also be due to the post-ECT acute induction of cytokines hindering statistical significance (255, 261). Another RCT with 35 ECT participants with focus on BDNF levels in patients with mania concluded no statistical difference in BDNF levels or treatment efficacy with adjuvant celecoxib (13). The authors of this study suggested these effects were nearing statistical significance, and that their BDNF sampling protocol may have been a confounding factor (13). A longer multicenter trial has been proposed to assess augmentation with celecoxib and/or minocycline alongside treatment as usual (TAU) in bipolar I or bipolar II patients in depressive state; however, these results are yet to be published (262). Bipolar disorder has significant associations with inflammatory modulation resulting in aberrant brain changes that warrant further investigation of the roles of anti-inflammatory agents. In particular, celecoxib shows some promise requiring further investigation, particularly during a set phase of the bipolar illness.

Schizophrenia

Schizophrenia is a severe, chronic, and among the most disabling and economically catastrophic medical disorders. The World Health Organization ranks schizophrenia as one of the top 10 illnesses contributing to the global burden of disease (263). The dysregulation of dopamine and glutamatergic pathways in various brain regions are implicated in the positive, negative, and cognitive symptom domains of schizophrenia (264). Pro-inflammatory cytokines such as IL-1β and IL-6 can influence neuronal development, specifically on the dopaminergic and serotonergic systems (265–268). IL-1β administration after birth can influence the dopamine system in adulthood, which has been associated in dopaminergic and serotonergic neuronal moderation in rat models (266). In schizophrenia, elevated serum and CSF concentrations of kynurenine were reported (269). Developing findings are suggesting that infectious exposure during the prenatal period may contribute to the pathogenesis of schizophrenia (270). Raised maternal levels of IL-8 during pregnancy are associated with an increased risk for schizophrenia in offspring, in addition to decreased brain volumes, independent of the inflammatory etiology (271). Maternal immune activation in animal models generated oxidative stress in the fetus (264). Observed infectious agents including *Toxoplasma gondii*, Chlamydia, bornavirus cytomegalovirus, and influenza seem to increase the risk of schizophrenia. This may, however, occur as a result of the immune response rather than an infectious etiology (270). Several epidemiological studies have observed an elevated prevalence of schizophrenia in cohorts born during influenza epidemics (272) and significant association with immunological disorders (273). There is a higher prevalence of schizophrenia in individuals with celiac disease, bullous pemphigoid, interstitial cystitis, thyrotoxicosis, and acquired hemolytic anemia (273, 274). Surprisingly, rheumatoid arthritis reveals lower rates of co-morbid schizophrenia compared to the general population (275).

Post-mortem brain studies from schizophrenia patients have revealed significant inflammatory processes (276). In addition, PET imaging has signified microglial activation resulting in brain morphological changes in first-episode and chronic psychosis (277–280). These morphological changes have been expressed during prodromal phases of first-episode psychosis (281–283), suggestive of neurotoxic processes resulting in poor prognosis (281, 284). Moreover, some authors have shown a relationship between brain volume, IL-1, and IL-6 (285–287). Collectin inflammatory markers have also been implicated in patients with schizophrenia, C4A in particular, whose role is to influence microglial hyperactivity, neurodegeneration, and subsequent brain cortical volume reductions (288, 289). These microglial changes may derive from established elevations in serum pro-inflammatory factors, such as PGE_2, CRP, IL-1β, IL-6, IL-8, and TNFα (290–292). In addition, cytokines have shown some correlation with negative symptoms, cognitive deficits, and psychomotor retardation (293–295).

Positive correlations with cognitive severity and inflammatory markers have also been highlighted (296–298). In the first-episode and acutely relapsed patients with psychosis, an elevated level of pro-inflammatory cytokines, IL-6, TNFα, TGF-β, and IFNγ, was observed (61). In addition, IL-10 concentrations were decreased in acutely relapsed patients compared to controls (61). Cytokine concentrations at different stages of the disease and variable treatment agents may alter neuroprogression (115, 299).

Further support is provided from studies suggesting antipsychotics may exhibit immune-modulatory properties (264); however, there remains evidence that is contrary to this notion (300, 301). Patients undergoing long-term treatment with antipsychotics exhibit reduced pro-inflammatory cytokine levels (IL-1β, IL-6, sIL-6R, and TNFα) (302–304) and elevated anti-inflammatory markers (sIL-1RA, sIL-2R, and IL-10) (305–307). Second-generation antipsychotics may elicit more potent anti-inflammatory effects than to first-generation agents (303, 308).

Dysregulation of the tryptophan metabolism has been implicated with notable elevations of kynurenic acid in patients with schizophrenia (309). Furthermore, long-term antipsychotic treatments have an impact on kynurenic acid concentrations in rodent models (310). Preclinical studies suggest that COX-2 inhibitors protect against glutamate-mediated neurotoxicity, which may highlight an application to mediate neurodegeneration in kynurenine system (18, 135, 311).

One of the first RCTs evaluating the use of COX inhibitors for schizophrenia indication consisted of 50 patients with acute exacerbation of psychosis who were admitted and treated with risperidone with one group augmented with celecoxib versus placebo for 5 weeks (17). The celecoxib group revealed significant positive effects on the Positive and Negative Syndrome Scale (PANSS) (17). *Post hoc* analyses indicated an improvement in cognition parameters with augmentation of celecoxib in schizophrenia in this trial (312).

In contrast, Rapaport and colleagues assessed outpatients with schizophrenia on stable psychotropic regimens of olanzapine or risperidone, finding no significant changes with celecoxib augmentation in several of the psychometric parameters (18). This finding could be explained by differences in the study cohorts, given the participants in Müller's study were acutely psychotic, whereas Rapaport's sample consisted of patients in more stabilized psychotic states.

During an 8-week RCT, the treatment of 60 acutely psychotic patients was augmented with celecoxib (19). The risperidone and celecoxib combination was superior in the improvement of PANSS total scores over risperidone alone (19). Also, the Extrapyramidal Symptoms Rating Scale (ESRS) scores for the placebo group were higher than in the celecoxib group over the trial but not statistically significant (18). Müller et al. (20) completed a 6-week, RCT of 49 patients during their first-episode of schizophrenia. They were treated with amisulpride with random assignment of celecoxib or placebo (20). There was an improvement in the PANSS in the adjunct celecoxib group compared to the placebo group (20). The adjunct celecoxib group in this study also showed a significant improvement on the clinical global impression (CGI) scale (20). Overall, a superior therapeutic effect with augmentation with celecoxib was found, in particular a trend for improvement in negative symptoms.

A recent meta-analysis, including the above RCTs in addition to two inaccessible RCTs, revealed that adjunctive celecoxib did not prove efficacy over placebo in overall samples (313). However, with the sub-analysis, they discovered superior efficacy with celecoxib to placebo in first-episode patients (313). This may be explained by data from preclinical studies suggesting celecoxib's effects on cytokines and behavioral symptoms are dependent on the stage of illness and time of intervention (217).

It is important to note the comorbid conditions that may contribute to inflammation and confound interpretation of outcomes, including trauma, stress, smoking, metabolic syndrome, diet, exercise, and poor dental hygiene (2). Nonetheless, there is an apparent association between inflammation and schizophrenia, with celecoxib demonstrating promise possibly during early disease onset.

Autism Spectrum Disorder

ASD is a neurodevelopmental disorder defined by impairments in two domains: 1) shortages in social communication and social interaction and 2) restricted repetitive patterns of behavior, interests, and activities (314). The prevalence of ASD in Western countries appears to have increased, possibly as a result of definition changes and heightened awareness. The pathogenesis of ASD remains idiopathic, although the consensus points to altered brain development leading to impairment in social and communication maturation, therefore resulting in restricted interests and repetitive behaviors (315). These brain morphologic aberrations appear to be a result of neural pruning processes and neuroinflammation (316–319).

An association with ASD and inflammatory response through the measles, mumps, and rubella (MMR) vaccine and enterocolitis were reported first in 1998 (320) and subsequently retracted. However, controversy still exists among these allegations in select groups, despite it being established that there is no causal association between MMR vaccine and ASD (320–324).

Similar to discussions in Schizophrenia section with respect to schizophrenia, prenatal infections during early development may also be associated with the development of ASD (325–327). Moreover, there seem to be shared immune-related genetic abnormalities between the two disorders (325, 328). Aberrant activity of the glutamatergic system might play a role in neurotoxicity of both disorders. Kynurenine pathway abnormalities may also be linked to 16p11.2 mutations in ASD resulting in glutamatergic activity (329).

Associations with changes in the immunomodulatory system of ASD patients have been identified. Disruption in immunomodulatory proponents such as T-cells and monocytes have been noted (316, 330), in addition to changes in the concentration of immunoglobulins (331) and autoantibodies production (332). Furthermore, polymorphisms identified in macrophage migration inhibitory factor (MIF), seen in ASD-related abnormalities, seem to also activate the COX-2 system in microglia (333, 334).

Post-mortem studies revealed greater microglial densities in the visual cortex, cerebellum, anterior cingulate gyri, and dorsolateral prefrontal cortex (DLPFC) of ASD patients (335–338). Some studies have also shown elevated TNFα, IFNγ, IL-1, IL-6, IL-8, IL-12, CCL2, CCL5, and CCL11 in plasma and CSF of autistic subjects (317, 318, 338–340).

A study showed that repurposed anti-inflammatory agents such as pioglitazone resulted in moderation of irritability, lethargy, stereotypy, and hyperactivity symptoms in ASD (341). The pioglitazone class of drugs has been shown to inhibit COX-2 in LPS-stimulated microglia and neurons (342, 343). Celecoxib in the rat model has shown to also inhibit LPS-induced neuronal toxicity (344).

Our search yielded only one randomized, double-blind placebo-controlled trial of celecoxib combination with risperidone. Asadabadi et al. (21) assessed 40 patients diagnosed with ASD in a 10-week trial with the aberrant behavior checklist-community edition (ABC-C), which showed superior efficacy of adjuvant celecoxib with risperidone in the domains of irritability, social withdrawal, and stereotypy in children with ASD.

Paucity of evidence is opportune for further investigations with COX-2 inhibitors in neurodevelopmental disorders such as ASD as seen by preclinical and limited clinical data.

Obsessive-Compulsive Disorder

Obsessive-compulsive disorder (OCD) is a relatively common neuropsychiatric disorder with a reported lifetime prevalence of 1–3% in the general population (345, 346). At least one-third of individuals with OCD fail to adequately respond to current pharmacological treatment (347, 348). The cortico-striatal-thalamo-cortical (CSTC) circuit dysfunction is implicated in the pathophysiology of OCD (349).

There is evidence of early childhood infections, pediatric acute-onset neuropsychiatric syndrome (PANS), which encompasses pediatric autoimmune neuropsychiatric disorders associated with streptococcal (PANDAS), evoking OCD-like neuropsychiatric symptoms (15). This is suggestive of an inflammatory etiology to a subsect of this illness. Furthermore, immunomodulation treatment resulted in improvement of OCD-like neuropsychiatric symptoms (350).

Although the minority of cases of OCD results from PANS, it is speculated that the active inflammatory model may be relevant for the progression of OCD. As well, brain morphological changes have also been noted in OCD indicating progression in the neurodegenerative process (351). Rodent models exposed to LPS-induced inflammation exhibited increased anxiety with reduced exploration in the open field test (352, 353). The inducible chemokine, CXCL12, resulted in anxiety-like features in rat models (353), further supporting the role of inflammation in neuropsychiatric symptoms in anxiety disorders.

Animal models are suggestive of alternative microglial phenotypes, resulting in OCD-like behavior (354). Translocator protein distribution volume, a marker of increased microglial activation and thus neuroinflammation (355–358), was investigated after a prior study found increased expression in PANDAS patients (359). Kumar et al. discovered an increased translocator protein density in the CSTC circuit compared to healthy controls. Interestingly, this circuit involves multiple neuropsychiatric disorders aforementioned such as Huntington disease, cerebral vascular disease, Tourette disorders, and Sydenham chorea (360, 361). Repurposed microglial modulators such as minocycline have shown a reduction in the Yale-Brown Obsessive-Compulsive Scale (Y-BOCS) scores in a recent RCT in combination with fluvoxamine (362).

Most recently, Konuk et al. (86) reported significantly elevated levels of both IL-6 and TNFα in OCD patients compared to healthy controls. Furthermore, a correlation between elevated TNFα and onset with minimal association between IL-6 levels and duration of illness (86). A meta-analysis revealed no significant findings in TNFα and IL-6 plasma levels in OCD patients relative to controls; however, the authors did note reduced IL-1β in OCD patients (62). As celecoxib is shown to reduce levels of both IL-6 and TNFα, support for improving clinical symptoms of OCD is plausible (6).

Sayyah et al. (16) noted an improvement in the Y-BOCS for OCD patients with the augmentation of celecoxib with fluoxetine compared to fluoxetine alone. In addition, another recent RCT utilizing fluvoxamine with celecoxib augmentation compared to fluvoxamine alone noted an improvement in the celecoxib group (15). It is proposed that the notable efficacy in OCD, in addition to the microglial mechanisms, results from increased monoamines such as norepinephrine and serotonin *via* inhibition of prostaglandin synthesis by celecoxib (5, 306). However, further studies with larger sample sizes, longer duration, and measurements of pro-inflammatory markers may provide more robust evidence.

CONCLUSION

Evidence for the inflammatory hypothesis and the role of anti-inflammatory agents continues to accumulate suggesting etiological impact on the development of neuropsychiatric conditions, such as depression, bipolar disorder, schizophrenia, ASD, and OCD. A promising body of evidence suggests a role for COX-2 inhibition, in particular celecoxib, for phase-related interventions in bipolar disorder, schizophrenia, and possibly depression, ASD, and OCD. Despite the paucity of data for COX-2 inhibitors and investigated agents, including aspirin, minocycline, and statins, with purported pleiotropic anti-inflammatory mechanisms, further research is necessary to clarify the role of immunomodulation therapies and their comparative efficacies for integration of the psychiatric professions' current paradigm of treatment modalities (146, 363).

AUTHOR CONTRIBUTIONS

RS was the primary author of this manuscript, conducted initial literature search, review and synthesis of first draft and subsequent revisions. NG-C contributed to literature search and revisions. AW contributed to synthesis initial draft and revisions. OR contributed to manuscript draft, revisions and created figure. BA contributed to drafting and revision process. MB and SD were lead investigators providing initial concept and ongoing guidance throughout.

FUNDING

Berk A is supported by Stanley Medical Research Foundation NIH, MBF, NHMRC, NHMRC Senior Principal Research Fellowship (APP1059660 and APP1156072), Cooperative Research Centre, Simons Autism Foundation, Cancer Council of Victoria,

MBF, Rotary Health, Meat and Livestock Board Woolworths, BeyondBlue, Geelong Medical Research Foundation Bristol Myers Squibb, Eli Lilly, Glaxo SmithKline, Organon, Novartis, Mayne Pharma, Servier. Berk is the speaker in Astra Zeneca, Bristol Myers Squibb Eli Lilly, Glaxo SmithKline Lundbeck, Pfizer, Sanofi Synthelabo Servier, Solvay, Wyeth; and consultant in AstraZeneca, Bristol Myers Squibb Eli Lilly, Bioadvantex, Merck, Glaxo SmithKline Lundbeck, Janssen Cilag Servier. Berk is a co-inventor of two provisional patents regarding the use of NAC and related compounds for psychiatric indications, which, while assigned to the Mental Health Research Institute, could lead to personal remuneration upon a commercialisation event. Walker A is supported by the Trisno Family Fellowship.

ACKNOWLEDGMENTS

The team would like to thank the IMPACT Strategic Research Centre for their support in providing work spaces and accommodation for our international team during the initial stages of this manuscript. Without their support this work would not have been achievable and their generosity should not go without thanks.

REFERENCES

1. Kohler CA, Freitas TH, Maes M, de Andrade NQ, Liu CS, Fernandes BS, et al. Peripheral cytokine and chemokine alterations in depression: a meta-analysis of 82 studies. *Acta Psychiatr Scand* (2017) 135(5):373–87. doi: 10.1111/acps.12698
2. Berk M, Williams LJ, Jacka FN, O'Neil A, Pasco JA, Moylan S, et al. So depression is an inflammatory disease, but where does the inflammation come from? *BMC Med* (2013) 11(1):200. doi: 10.1186/1741-7015-11-200
3. Huynh NN, McIntyre RS. What are the implications of the STAR*D trial for primary care? A review and synthesis. *Prim Care Companion J Clin Psychiatry* (2008) 10(2):91–6. doi: 10.4088/PCC.v10n0201
4. Muller N, Schwarz MJ, Dehning S, Douhe A, Cerovecki A, Goldstein-Muller B, et al. The cyclooxygenase-2 inhibitor celecoxib has therapeutic effects in major depression: results of a double-blind, randomized, placebo controlled, add-on pilot study to reboxetine. *Mol Psychiatry* (2006) 11(7):680–4. doi: 10.1038/sj.mp.4001805
5. Akhondzadeh S, Jafari S, Raisi F, Nasehi AA, Ghoreishi A, Salehi B, et al. Clinical trial of adjunctive celecoxib treatment in patients with major depression: a double blind and placebo controlled trial. *Depress Anxiety* (2009) 26(7):607–11. doi: 10.1002/da.20589
6. Fields C, Drye L, Vaidya V, Lyketsos C. Celecoxib or naproxen treatment does not benefit depressive symptoms in persons age 70 and older: findings from a randomized controlled trial. *Am J Geriatr Psychiatry* (2012) 20(6):505–13. doi: 10.1097/JGP.0b013e318227f4da
7. Abbasi SH, Hosseini F, Modabbernia A, Ashrafi M, Akhondzadeh S. Effect of celecoxib add-on treatment on symptoms and serum IL-6 concentrations in patients with major depressive disorder: randomized double-blind placebo-controlled study. *J Affect Disord* (2012) 141(2–3):308–14. doi: 10.1016/j.jad.2012.03.033
8. Majd M, Hashemian F, Hosseini SM, Vahdat Shariatpanahi M and Sharifi A. A randomized, double-blind, placebo-controlled trial of celecoxib uugmentation of sertraline in treatment of drug-naive depressed women: a pilot study. *IJPR* (2015) 14(3):891–9.
9. Jafari S, Ashrafizadeh SG, Zeinoddini A, Rasoulinejad M, Entezari P, Seddighi S, et al. Celecoxib for the treatment of mild-to-moderate depression due to acute brucellosis: a double-blind, placebo-controlled, randomized trial. *J Clin Pharm Ther* (2015) 40(4):441–6. doi: 10.1111/jcpt.12287
10. Mohammadinejad P, Arya P, Esfandbod M, Kaviani A, Najafi M, Kashani L, et al. Celecoxib versus diclofenac in mild to moderate depression management among breast cancer patients: a double-blind, placebo-controlled, randomized trial. *Ann Pharmacother* (2015) 49(9):953–61. doi: 10.1177/1060028015592215
11. Alamdarsaravi M, Ghajar A, Noorbala A-A, Arbabi M, Emami A, Shahei F, et al. Efficacy and safety of celecoxib monotherapy for mild to moderate depression in patients with colorectal cancer: a randomized double-blind, placebo controlled trial. *Psychiatry Res* (2017) 255:59–65. doi: 10.1016/j.psychres.2017.05.029
12. Nery FG, Monkul ES, Hatch JP, Fonseca M, Zunta-Soares GB, Frey BN, et al. Celecoxib as an adjunct in the treatment of depressive or mixed episodes of bipolar disorder: a double-blind, randomized, placebo-controlled study. *Hum Psychopharmacol* (2008) 23(2):87–94. doi: 10.1002/hup.912
13. Kargar M, Yoosefi A, Akhondzadeh S, Artonian V, Ashouri A, Ghaeli P. Effect of adjunctive celecoxib on BDNF in manic patients undergoing electroconvulsive therapy: a randomized double blind controlled trial. *Pharmacopsychiatry* (2015) 48(7):268–73. doi: 10.1055/s-0035-1559667
14. Arabzadeh S, Ameli N, Zeinoddini A, Rezaei F, Farokhnia M, Mohammadinejad P, et al. Celecoxib adjunctive therapy for acute bipolar mania: a randomized, double-blind, placebo-controlled trial. *Bipolar Disord* (2015) 17(6):606–14. doi: 10.1111/bdi.12324
15. Shalbafan M, Mohammadinejad P, Shariat SV, Alavi K, Zeinoddini A, Salehi M, et al. Celecoxib as an adjuvant to fluvoxamine in moderate to severe obsessive-compulsive disorder: a double-blind, placebo-controlled, randomized trial. *Pharmacopsychiatry* (2015) 48(4–5):136–40. doi: 10.1055/s-0035-1549929
16. Sayyah M, Boostani H, Pakseresht S, Malayeri A. A preliminary randomized double-blind clinical trial on the efficacy of celecoxib as an adjunct in the treatment of obsessive-compulsive disorder. *Psychiatry Res* (2011) 189(3):403–6. doi: 10.1016/j.psychres.2011.01.019
17. Muller N, Riedel M, Scheppach C, Brandstatter B, Sokullu S, Krampe K, et al. Beneficial antipsychotic effects of celecoxib add-on therapy compared to risperidone alone in schizophrenia. *Am J Psychiatry* (2002) 159(6):1029–34. doi: 10.1176/appi.ajp.159.6.1029
18. Rapaport MH, Delrahim KK, Bresee CJ, Maddux RE, Ahmadpour O, Dolnak D. Celecoxib augmentation of continuously ill patients with schizophrenia. *Biol Psychiatry* (2005) 57(12):1594–6. doi: 10.1016/j.biopsych.2005.02.024
19. Akhondzadeh S, Tabatabaee M, Amini H, Ahmadi Abhari SA, Abbasi SH, Behnam B. Celecoxib as adjunctive therapy in schizophrenia: a double-blind, randomized and placebo-controlled trial. *Schizophr Res* (2007) 90(1–3):179–85. doi: 10.1016/j.schres.2006.11.016
20. Müller N, Krause D, Dehning S, Musil R, Schennach-Wolff R, Obermeier M, et al. Celecoxib treatment in an early stage of schizophrenia: results of a randomized, double-blind, placebo-controlled trial of celecoxib augmentation of amisulpride treatment. *Schizophr Res* (2010) 121(1–3):118–24. doi: 10.1016/j.schres.2010.04.015
21. Asadabadi M, Mohammadi MR, Ghanizadeh A, Modabbernia A, Ashrafi M, Hassanzadeh E, et al. Celecoxib as adjunctive treatment to risperidone in children with autistic disorder: a randomized, double-blind, placebo-controlled trial. *Psychopharmacology* (2013) 225(1):51–9. doi: 10.1007/s00213-012-2796-8
22. Raju TN. Hot brains: manipulating body heat to save the brain. *Pediatrics* (2006) 117(2):e320–1. doi: 10.1542/peds.2005-1934
23. Lopez-Munoz F, Alamo C. Monoaminergic neurotransmission: the history of the discovery of antidepressants from 1950s until today. *Curr Pharm Des* (2009) 15(14):1563–86. doi: 10.2174/138161209788168001
24. Chaplin DD. Overview of the immune response. *J Allergy Clin Immunol* (2010) 125(2 Suppl 2):S3–23. doi: 10.1016/j.jaci.2009.12.980
25. Simon AK, Hollander GA, McMichael A. Evolution of the immune system in humans from infancy to old age. *Proc R Soc B: Biol Sci* (2015) 282(1821):20143085. doi: 10.1098/rspb.2014.3085

26. Jiang Z, Jiang JX, Zhang GX. Macrophages: a double-edged sword in experimental autoimmune encephalomyelitis. *Immunol Lett* (2014) 160(1):17–22. doi: 10.1016/j.imlet.2014.03.006
27. McNamara RK, Lotrich FE. Elevated immune-inflammatory signaling in mood disorders: a new therapeutic target? *Expert Rev Neurother* (2012) 12(9):1143–61. doi: 10.1586/ern.12.98
28. Kronfol Z, Remick DG. Cytokines and the brain: implications for clinical psychiatry. *Am J Psychiatry* (2000) 157(5):683–94. doi: 10.1176/appi.ajp.157.5.683
29. Banks WA, Kastin AJ, Broadwell RD. Passage of cytokines across the blood-brain barrier. *Neuroimmunomodulation* (1995) 2(4):241–8. doi: 10.1159/000097202
30. Quan N, Whiteside M, Herkenham M. Time course and localization patterns of interleukin-1beta messenger RNA expression in brain and pituitary after peripheral administration of lipopolysaccharide. *Neuroscience* (1998) 83(1):281–93. doi: 10.1016/S0306-4522(97)00350-3
31. Morris G, Fernandes BS, Berk M. Leaky brain in neurological and psychiatric disorders: drivers and consequences. *Aust N Z J Psychiatry* (2018) 52(10):92448. doi: 10.1177/0004867418796955
32. Haroon E, Raison CL, Miller AH. Psychoneuroimmunology meets neuropsychopharmacology: translational implications of the impact of inflammation on behavior. *Neuropsychopharmacology* (2012) 37(1):137–62. doi: 10.1038/npp.2011.205
33. Bentivoglio M, Mariotti R, Bertini G. Neuroinflammation and brain infections: historical context and current perspectives. *Brain Res Rev* (2011) 66(1-2):152–73. doi: 10.1016/j.brainresrev.2010.09.008
34. Block ML, Zecca L, Hong JS. Microglia-mediated neurotoxicity: uncovering the molecular mechanisms. *Nat Rev Neurosci* (2007) 8(1):57–69. doi: 10.1038/nrn2038
35. Goldstein BI, Kemp DE, Soczynska JK, McIntyre RS. Inflammation and the phenomenology, pathophysiology, comorbidity, and treatment of bipolar disorder: a systematic review of the literature. *J Clin Psychiatry* (2009) 70(8):1078–90. doi: 10.4088/JCP.08r04505
36. Najjar S, Pearlman DM, Alper K, Najjar A, Devinsky O. Neuroinflammation and psychiatric illness. *J Neuroinflammation* (2013) 10:43. doi: 10.1186/1742-2094-10-43
37. Orihuela R, McPherson CA, Harry GJ. Microglial M1/M2 polarization and metabolic states. *Br J Pharmacol* (2016) 173(4):649–65. doi: 10.1111/bph.13139
38. Schwartz M, Butovsky O, Bruck W, Hanisch UK. Microglial phenotype: is the commitment reversible? *Trends Neurosci* (2006) 29(2):68–74. doi: 10.1016/j.tins.2005.12.005
39. van Kesteren CF, Gremmels H, de Witte LD, Hol EM, Van Gool AR, Falkai PG, et al. Immune involvement in the pathogenesis of schizophrenia: a meta-analysis on postmortem brain studies. *Transl Psychiatry* (2017) 7(3):e1075. doi: 10.1038/tp.2017.4
40. Cherry JD, Olschowka JA, O'Banion MK. Neuroinflammation and M2 microglia: the good, the bad, and the inflamed. *J Neuroinflammation* (2014) 11(1):98. doi: 10.1186/1742-2094-11-98
41. Wachholz S, Esslinger M, Plumper J, Manitz MP, Juckel G, Friebe A. Microglia activation is associated with IFN-alpha induced depressive-like behavior. *Brain Behav Immun* (2016) 55:105–13. doi: 10.1016/j.bbi.2015.09.016
42. Sokol CL, Luster AD. The chemokine system in innate immunity. *Cold Spring Harb Perspect Biol* (2015) 7(5):a016303. doi: 10.1101/cshperspect.a016303
43. Kohler O, Krogh J, Mors O, Benros ME. Inflammation in depression and the potential for anti-inflammatory treatment. *Curr Neuropharmacol* (2016) 14(7):732–42. doi: 10.2174/1570159X14666151208113700
44. Kohler-Forsberg O, Buttenschon HN, Tansey KE, Maier W, Hauser J, Dernovsek MZ, et al. Association between C-reactive protein (CRP) with depression symptom severity and specific depressive symptoms in major depression. *Brain Behav Immun* (2017) 62:344–50. doi: 10.1016/j.bbi.2017.02.020
45. Inoshita M, Numata S, Tajima A, Kinoshita M, Umehara H, Nakataki M, et al. A significant causal association between C-reactive protein levels and schizophrenia. *Sci Rep* (2016) 6:26105. doi: 10.1038/srep26105
46. Wium-Andersen MK, Orsted DD, Nielsen SF, Nordestgaard BG. Elevated C-reactive protein levels, psychological distress, and depression in 73, 131 individuals. *JAMA Psychiatry* (2013) 70(2):176–84. doi: 10.1001/2013.jamapsychiatry.102
47. Danesh J, Wheeler JG, Hirschfield GM, Eda S, Eiriksdottir G, Rumley A, et al. C-reactive protein and other circulating markers of inflammation in the prediction of coronary heart disease. *N Engl J Med* (2004) 350(14):1387–97. doi: 10.1056/NEJMoa032804
48. Koenig W, Sund M, Frohlich M, Fischer HG, Lowel H, Doring A, et al. C-Reactive protein, a sensitive marker of inflammation, predicts future risk of coronary heart disease in initially healthy middle-aged men: results from the MONICA (Monitoring Trends and Determinants in Cardiovascular Disease) Augsburg Cohort Study, 1984 to 1992. *Circulation* (1999) 99(2):237–42. doi: 10.1161/01.CIR.99.2.237
49. Lindahl B, Toss H, Siegbahn A, Venge P, Wallentin L. Markers of myocardial damage and inflammation in relation to long-term mortality in unstable coronary artery disease. *N Engl J Med* (2000) 343(16):1139–47. doi: 10.1056/NEJM200010193431602
50. Nordestgaard BG, Chapman MJ, Humphries SE, Ginsberg HN, Masana L, Descamps OS, et al. Familial hypercholesterolaemia is underdiagnosed and undertreated in the general population: guidance for clinicians to prevent coronary heart disease: Consensus Statement of the European Atherosclerosis Society. *Eur Heart J* (2013) 34(45):3478–90. doi: 10.1093/eurheartj/eht273
51. Pepys MB, Hirschfield GM. C-reactive protein: a critical update. *J Clin Invest* (2003) 111(12):1805–12. doi: 10.1172/JCI200318921
52. Ridker PM, Hennekens CH, Buring JE, Rifai N. C-reactive protein and other markers of inflammation in the prediction of cardiovascular disease in women. *N Engl J Med* (2000) 342(12):836–43. doi: 10.1056/NEJM200003233421202
53. Tracy RP, Lemaitre RN, Psaty BM, Ives DG, Evans RW, Cushman M, et al. Relationship of C-reactive protein to risk of cardiovascular disease in the elderly. Results from the Cardiovascular Health Study and the Rural Health Promotion Project. *Arterioscler Thromb Vasc Biol* (1997) 17(6):1121–7. doi: 10.1161/01.ATV.17.6.1121
54. Krogh J, Benros ME, Jorgensen MB, Vesterager L, Elfving B, Nordentoft M. The association between depressive symptoms, cognitive function, and inflammation in major depression. *Brain Behav Immun* (2014) 35:70–6. doi: 10.1016/j.bbi.2013.08.014
55. Furtado M, Katzman MA. Examining the role of neuroinflammation in major depression. *Psychiatry Res* (2015) 229(1–2):27–36. doi: 10.1016/j.psychres.2015.06.009
56. Karlovic D, Serretti A, Vrkic N, Martinac M, Marcinko D. Serum concentrations of CRP, IL-6, TNF-alpha and cortisol in major depressive disorder with melancholic or atypical features. *Psychiatry Res* (2012) 198(1):74–80. doi: 10.1016/j.psychres.2011.12.007
57. Felger JC, Lotrich FE. Inflammatory cytokines in depression: neurobiological mechanisms and therapeutic implications. *Neuroscience* (2013) 246:199–229. doi: 10.1016/j.neuroscience.2013.04.060
58. Goldsmith DR, Rapaport MH, Miller BJ. A meta-analysis of blood cytokine network alterations in psychiatric patients: comparisons between schizophrenia, bipolar disorder and depression. *Mol Psychiatry* (2016) 21(12):1696–709. doi: 10.1038/mp.2016.3
59. Modabbernia A, Taslimi S, Brietzke E, Ashrafi M. Cytokine alterations in bipolar disorder: a meta-analysis of 30 studies. *Biol Psychiatry* (2013) 74(1):15–25. doi: 10.1016/j.biopsych.2013.01.007
60. Munkholm K, Vinberg M, Vedel Kessing L. Cytokines in bipolar disorder: a systematic review and meta-analysis. *J Affect Disord* (2013b) 144(1–2):16–27. doi: 10.1016/j.jad.2012.06.010
61. Miller BJ, Buckley P, Seabolt W, Mellor A, Kirkpatrick B. Meta-analysis of cytokine alterations in schizophrenia: clinical status and antipsychotic effects. *Biol Psychiatry* (2011b) 70(7):663–71. doi: 10.1016/j.biopsych.2011.04.013
62. Gray SM, Bloch MH. Systematic review of proinflammatory cytokines in obsessive-compulsive disorder. *Curr Psychiatry Rep* (2012) 14(3):220–8. doi: 10.1007/s11920-012-0272-0
63. Masi A, Quintana DS, Glozier N, Lloyd AR, Hickie IB, Guastella AJ. Cytokine aberrations in autism spectrum disorder: a systematic review and meta-analysis. *Mol Psychiatry* (2015) 20(4):440–6. doi: 10.1038/mp.2014.59
64. Hannestad J, DellaGioia N, Bloch M. The effect of antidepressant medication treatment on serum levels of inflammatory cytokines: a meta-analysis. *Neuropsychopharmacology* (2011) 36(12):2452–9. doi: 10.1038/npp.2011.132

65. Licinio J, Wong ML. Pathways and mechanisms for cytokine signaling of the central nervous system. *J Clin Invest* (1997) 100(12):2941–7. doi: 10.1172/JCI119846
66. Brietzke E, Stertz L, Fernandes BS, Kauer-Sant'anna M, Mascarenhas M, Escosteguy Vargas A, et al. Comparison of cytokine levels in depressed, manic and euthymic patients with bipolar disorder. *J Affect Disord* (2009) 116(3):214–7. doi: 10.1016/j.jad.2008.12.001
67. de Oliveira GS, Cereser KM, Fernandes BS, Kauer-Sant'Anna M, Fries GR, Stertz L, et al. Decreased brain-derived neurotrophic factor in medicated and drug-free bipolar patients. *J Psychiatr Res* (2009) 43(14):1171–4. doi: 10.1016/j.jpsychires.2009.04.002
68. Fernandes BS, Molendijk ML, Kohler CA, Soares JC, Leite CM, Machado-Vieira R, et al. Peripheral brain-derived neurotrophic factor (BDNF) as a biomarker in bipolar disorder: a meta-analysis of 52 studies. *BMC Med* (2015a) 13:289. doi: 10.1186/s12916-015-0529-7
69. Fernandes BS, Berk M, Turck CW, Steiner J, Goncalves CA. Decreased peripheral brain-derived neurotrophic factor levels are a biomarker of disease activity in major psychiatric disorders: a comparative meta-analysis. *Mol Psychiatry* (2014) 19(7):750–1. doi: 10.1038/mp.2013.172
70. Fernandes BS, Steiner J, Berk M, Molendijk ML, Gonzalez-Pinto A, Turck CW, et al. Peripheral brain-derived neurotrophic factor in schizophrenia and the role of antipsychotics: meta-analysis and implications. *Mol Psychiatry* (2015b) 20(9):1108–19. doi: 10.1038/mp.2014.117
71. Dantzer R, O'Connor JC, Freund GG, Johnson RW, Kelley KW. From inflammation to sickness and depression: when the immune system subjugates the brain. *Nat Rev Neurosci* (2008) 9(1):46–56. doi: 10.1038/nrn2297
72. Leonard BE. The concept of depression as a dysfunction of the immune system. *Curr Immunol Rev* (2010) 6(3):205–12. doi: 10.2174/157339510791823835
73. Andrade L, Caraveo-Anduaga JJ, Berglund P, Bijl RV, De Graaf R, Vollebergh W, et al. The epidemiology of major depressive episodes: results from the International Consortium of Psychiatric Epidemiology (ICPE) Surveys. *Int J Methods Psychiatr Res* (2003) 12(1):3–21. doi: 10.1002/mpr.138
74. Wright CE, Strike PC, Brydon L, Steptoe A. Acute inflammation and negative mood: mediation by cytokine activation. *Brain Behav Immun* (2005) 19(4):345–50. doi: 10.1016/j.bbi.2004.10.003
75. O'Connor J, Lawson M, André C, Moreau M, Lestage J, Castanon N, et al. 'Lipopolysaccharide-induced depressive-like behavior is mediated by indoleamine 2,3-dioxygenase activation in mice. *Mol Psychiatry* (2009) 14(5):511–22. doi: 10.1038/sj.mp.4002148
76. Reichenberg A, Yirmiya R, Schuld A, Kraus T, Haack M, Morag A, et al. Cytokine-associated emotional and cognitive disturbances in humans. *Arch Gen Psychiatry* (2001) 58(5):445–52. doi: 10.1001/archpsyc.58.5.445
77. Euteneuer F, Schwarz MJ, Hennings A, Riemer S, Stapf T, Selberdinger V, et al. Depression, cytokines and experimental pain: evidence for sex-related association patterns. *J Affect Disord* (2010) 131(1):143–9. doi: 10.1016/j.jad.2010.11.017
78. Brydon L, Walker C, Wawrzyniak A, Whitehead D, Okamura H, Yajima J, et al. Synergistic effects of psychological and immune stressors on inflammatory cytokine and sickness responses in humans. *Brain Behav Immun* (2009) 23(2):217–24. doi: 10.1016/j.bbi.2008.09.007
79. Dunn AJ, Swiergiel AH. Effects of interleukin-1 and endotoxin in the forced swim and tail suspension tests in mice. *Pharmacol Biochem Behav* (2005) 81(3):688–93. doi: 10.1016/j.pbb.2005.04.019
80. Eggermont AM, Suciu S, Santinami M, Testori A, Kruit WH, Marsden J, et al. Adjuvant therapy with pegylated interferon alfa-2b versus observation alone in resected stage III melanoma: final results of EORTC 18991, a randomised phase III trial. *Lancet* (2008) 372(9633):117–26. doi: 10.1016/S0140-6736(08)61033-8
81. Liang TJ, Ghany MG. Current and future therapies for hepatitis C virus infection. *N Engl J Med* (2013) 368(20):1907–17. doi: 10.1056/NEJMra1213651
82. Friebe A, Horn M, Schmidt F, Janssen G, Schmid-Wendtner MH, Volkenandt M, et al. Dose-dependent development of depressive symptoms during adjuvant interferon-{alpha} treatment of patients with malignant melanoma. *Psychosomatics* (2010) 51(6):466–73. doi: 10.1176/appi.psy.51.6.466
83. Reichenberg A, Gorman JM, Dieterich DT. Interferon-induced depression and cognitive impairment in hepatitis C virus patients: a 72 week prospective study. *Aids* (2005) 19 Suppl 3:S174–8. doi: 10.1097/01.aids.0000192087.64432.ae
84. Udina M, Castellvi P, Moreno-Espana J, Navines R, Valdes M, Forns X, et al. Interferon-induced depression in chronic hepatitis C: a systematic review and meta-analysis. *J Clin Psychiatry* (2012) 73(8):1128–38. doi: 10.4088/JCP.12r07694
85. Grigoleit J-S, Kullmann JS, Wolf OT, Hammes F, Wegner A, Jablonowski S, et al. Dose-dependent effects of endotoxin on neurobehavioral functions in humans. *PLoS One* (2011) 6(12):e28330. doi: 10.1371/journal.pone.0028330
86. Konuk N, Tekın IO, Ozturk U, Atik L, Atasoy N, Bektas S, et al. Plasma levels of tumor necrosis factor-alpha and interleukin-6 in obsessive compulsive disorder. *Mediators Inflamm* (2007) 2007:65704. doi: 10.1155/2007/65704
87. Dickens C, McGowan L, Clark-Carter D, Creed F. Depression in rheumatoid arthritis: a systematic review of the literature with meta-analysis. *Psychosom Med* (2002) 64(1):52–60. doi: 10.1097/00006842-200201000-00008
88. Korczak DJ, Pereira S, Koulajian K, Matejcek A, Giacca A. Type 1 diabetes mellitus and major depressive disorder: evidence for a biological link. *Diabetologia* (2011) 54(10):2483–93. doi: 10.1007/s00125-011-2240-3
89. Zhang L, Fu T, Yin R, Zhang Q, Shen B. Prevalence of depression and anxiety in systemic lupus erythematosus: a systematic review and meta-analysis. *BMC Psychiatry* (2017) 17(1):70. doi: 10.1186/s12888-017-1234-1
90. Benros ME, Waltoft BL, Nordentoft M, Ostergaard SD, Eaton WW, Krogh J, et al. Autoimmune diseases and severe infections as risk factors for mood disorders: a nationwide study. *JAMA Psychiatry* (2013) 70(8):812–20. doi: 10.1001/jamapsychiatry.2013.1111
91. Mardini HE, Kip KE, Wilson JW. Crohn's disease: a two-year prospective study of the association between psychological distress and disease activity. *Dig Dis Sci* (2004) 49(3):492–7. doi: 10.1023/B:DDAS.0000020509.23162.cc
92. Langley RG, Feldman SR, Han C, Schenkel B, Szapary P, Hsu MC, et al. Ustekinumab significantly improves symptoms of anxiety, depression, and skin-related quality of life in patients with moderate-to-severe psoriasis: results from a randomized, double-blind, placebo-controlled phase III trial. *J Am Acad Dermatol* (2010) 63(3):457–65. doi: 10.1016/j.jaad.2009.09.014
93. Menter A, Augustin M, Signorovitch J, Yu AP, Wu EQ, Gupta SR, et al. The effect of adalimumab on reducing depression symptoms in patients with moderate to severe psoriasis: a randomized clinical trial. *J Am Acad Dermatol* (2010) 62(5):812–8. doi: 10.1016/j.jaad.2009.07.022
94. Tyring S, Gottlieb A, Papp K, Gordon K, Leonardi C, Wang A, et al. Etanercept and clinical outcomes, fatigue, and depression in psoriasis: double-blind placebo-controlled randomised phase III trial. *Lancet* (2006) 367(9504):29–35. doi: 10.1016/S0140-6736(05)67763-X
95. Kridin K, Zelber-Sagi S, Comaneshter D, Cohen AD. Bipolar disorder associated with another autoimmune disease-pemphigus: a population-based study. *Can J Psychiatry* (2017) 63(7):474–80. doi: 10.1177/0706743717740344
96. Benros ME, Nielsen PR, Nordentoft M, Eaton WW, Dalton SO, Mortensen PB. Autoimmune diseases and severe infections as risk factors for schizophrenia: a 30-year population-based register study. *Am J Psychiatry* (2011) 168(12):1303–10. doi: 10.1176/appi.ajp.2011.11030516
97. Harris RC, McKanna JA, Akai Y, Jacobson HR, Dubois RN, Breyer MD. Cyclooxygenase-2 is associated with the macula densa of rat kidney and increases with salt restriction. *J Clin Invest* (1994) 94(6):2504–10. doi: 10.1172/JCI117620
98. Hirst JJ, Teixeira FJ, Zakar T, Olson DM. Prostaglandin endoperoxide-H synthase-1 and -2 messenger ribonucleic acid levels in human amnion with spontaneous labor onset. *J Clin Endocrinol Metab* (1995) 80(2):517–23. doi: 10.1210/jc.80.2.517
99. Kirkby NS, Zaiss AK, Urquhart P, Jiao J, Austin PJ, Al-Yamani M, et al. LC-MS/MS confirms that COX-1 drives vascular prostacyclin whilst gene expression pattern reveals non-vascular sites of COX-2 expression. *PLoS One* (2013) 8(7):e69524. doi: 10.1371/journal.pone.0069524
100. Williams CS, Mann M, DuBois RN. The role of cyclooxygenases in inflammation, cancer, and development. *Oncogene* (1999) 18:7908. doi: 10.1038/sj.onc.1203286
101. Coyne DW, Nickols M, Bertrand W, Morrison AR. Regulation of mesangial cell cyclooxygenase synthesis by cytokines and glucocorticoids. *Am J Physiol* (1992) 263(1 Pt 2):F97–102. doi: 10.1152/ajprenal.1992.263.1.F97

102. DeWitt DL, Meade EA, Smith WL. PGH synthase isoenzyme selectivity: the potential for safer nonsteroidal antiinflammatory drugs. *Am J Med* (1993) 95(2a):40s–4s. doi: 10.1016/0002-9343(93)90396-7
103. Fu JY, Masferrer JL, Seibert K, Raz A, Needleman P. The induction and suppression of prostaglandin H2 synthase (cyclooxygenase) in human monocytes. *J Biol Chem* (1990) 265(28):16737–40.
104. Geng Y, Blanco FJ, Cornelisson M, Lotz M. Regulation of cyclooxygenase-2 expression in normal human articular chondrocytes. *J Immunol* (1995) 155(2):796–801.
105. Jones DA, Carlton DP, McIntyre TM, Zimmerman GA, Prescott SM. Molecular cloning of human prostaglandin endoperoxide synthase type II and demonstration of expression in response to cytokines. *J Biol Chem* (1993) 268(12):9049–54.
106. Lee SH, Soyoola E, Chanmugam P, Hart S, Sun W, Zhong H, et al. Selective expression of mitogen-inducible cyclooxygenase in macrophages stimulated with lipopolysaccharide. *J Biol Chem* (1992) 267(36):25934–8.
107. O'Sullivan MG, Huggins EM, Jr., Meade EA, DeWitt DL, McCall CE. Lipopolysaccharide induces prostaglandin H synthase-2 in alveolar macrophages. *Biochem Biophys Res Commun* (1992) 187(2):1123–7. doi: 10.1016/0006-291X(92)91313-F
108. Riese J, Hoff T, Nordhoff A, DeWitt DL, Resch K, Kaever V. Transient expression of prostaglandin endoperoxide synthase-2 during mouse macrophage activation. *J Leukoc Biol* (1994) 55(4):476–82. doi: 10.1002/jlb.55.4.476
109. Maes M. Targeting cyclooxygenase-2 in depression is not a viable therapeutic approach and may even aggravate the pathophysiology underpinning depression. *Metab Brain Dis* (2012) 27(4):405–13. doi: 10.1007/s11011-012-9326-6
110. Minghetti L, Greco A, Potenza RL, Pezzola A, Blum D, Bantubungi K, et al. Effects of the adenosine A2A receptor antagonist SCH 58621 on cyclooxygenase-2 expression, glial activation, and brain-derived neurotrophic factor availability in a rat model of striatal neurodegeneration. *J Neuropathol Exp Neurol* (2007) 66(5):363–71. doi: 10.1097/nen.0b013e3180517477
111. Song C, Lin A, Bonaccorso S, Heide C, Verkerk R, Kenis G, et al. The inflammatory response system and the availability of plasma tryptophan in patients with primary sleep disorders and major depression. *J Affect Disord* (1998) 49(3):211–9. doi: 10.1016/S0165-0327(98)00025-1
112. Rapoport SI. Lithium and the other mood stabilizers effective in bipolar disorder target the rat brain arachidonic acid cascade. *ACS Chem Neurosci* (2014) 5(6):459–67. doi: 10.1021/cn500058v
113. Inoue H, Tanabe T, Umesono K. Feedback control of cyclooxygenase-2 expression through PPARgamma. *J Biol Chem* (2000) 275(36):28028–32. doi: 10.1074/jbc.M001387200
114. Sales KJ, Grant V, Jabbour HN. Prostaglandin E2 and F2alpha activate the FP receptor and up-regulate cyclooxygenase-2 expression *via* the cyclic AMP response element. *Mol Cell Endocrinol* (2008) 285(1–2):51–61. doi: 10.1016/j.mce.2008.01.016
115. Müller N. Immunological aspects of the treatment of depression and schizophrenia. *Dialogues Clin Neurosci* (2017) 19(1):55–63.
116. Choi SH, Langenbach R, Bosetti F. Cyclooxygenase-1 and -2 enzymes differentially regulate the brain upstream NF-kappa B pathway and downstream enzymes involved in prostaglandin biosynthesis. *J Neurochem* (2006) 98(3):801–11. doi: 10.1111/j.1471-4159.2006.03926.x
117. Rao JS, Langenbach R, Bosetti F. Down-regulation of brain nuclear factor-kappa B pathway in the cyclooxygenase-2 knockout mouse. *Brain Res Mol Brain Res* (2005) 139(2):217–24. doi: 10.1016/j.molbrainres.2005.05.008
118. Hawkey CJ. COX-2 chronology. *Gut* (2005) 54(11):1509. doi: 10.1136/gut.2005.065003
119. FitzGerald GA, Patrono C. The coxibs, selective inhibitors of cyclooxygenase-2. *N Engl J Med* (2001) 345(6):433–42. doi: 10.1056/NEJM200108093450607
120. Bombardier C, Laine L, Reicin A, Shapiro D, Burgos-Vargas R, Davis B, et al. Comparison of upper gastrointestinal toxicity of rofecoxib and naproxen in patients with rheumatoid arthritis. *N Engl J Med* (2000) 343(21):1520–8. doi: 10.1056/NEJM200011233432103
121. Bresalier RS, Sandler RS, Quan H, Bolognese JA, Oxenius B, Horgan K, et al. Cardiovascular events associated with rofecoxib in a colorectal adenoma chemoprevention trial. *N Engl J Med* (2005) 352(11):1092–102. doi: 10.1056/NEJMoa050493
122. Farkouh ME, Kirshner H, Harrington RA, Ruland S, Verheugt FW, Schnitzer TJ, et al. 'Comparison of lumiracoxib with naproxen and ibuprofen in the Therapeutic Arthritis Research and Gastrointestinal Event Trial (TARGET), cardiovascular outcomes: randomised controlled trial. *Lancet* (2004) 364(9435):675–84. doi: 10.1016/S0140-6736(04)16894-3
123. Schnitzer TJ, Burmester GR, Mysler E, Hochberg MC, Doherty M, Ehrsam E, et al. Comparison of lumiracoxib with naproxen and ibuprofen in the Therapeutic Arthritis Research and Gastrointestinal Event Trial (TARGET), reduction in ulcer complications: randomised controlled trial. *Lancet* (2004) 364(9435):665–74. doi: 10.1016/S0140-6736(04)16893-1
124. Scarpignato C, Lanas A, Blandizzi C, Lems WF, Hermann M, Hunt RH. Safe prescribing of non-steroidal anti-inflammatory drugs in patients with osteoarthritis—an expert consensus addressing benefits as well as gastrointestinal and cardiovascular risks. *BMC Med* (2015) 13:55. doi: 10.1186/s12916-015-0285-8
125. Sandrini M, Vitale G, Pini LA. Effect of rofecoxib on nociception and the serotonin system in the rat brain. *Inflamm Res* (2002) 51(3):154–9. doi: 10.1007/PL00000287
126. Johansson D, Falk A, Marcus MM, Svensson TH. Celecoxib enhances the effect of reboxetine and fluoxetine on cortical noradrenaline and serotonin output in the rat. *Prog Neuropsychopharmacol Biol Psychiatry* (2012) 39(1):143–8. doi: 10.1016/j.pnpbp.2012.06.003
127. Choi S-H, Aid S, Bosetti F. The distinct roles of cyclooxygenase-1 and -2 in neuroinflammation: implications for translational research. *Trends Pharmacol Sci* (2009) 30(4):174–81. doi: 10.1016/j.tips.2009.01.002
128. Minghetti L, Pocchiari M. Cyclooxygenase-2, prostaglandin E2, and microglial activation in prion diseases. *Int Rev Neurobiol* (2007) 82:265–75. doi: 10.1016/S0074-7742(07)82014-9
129. Gilroy DW, Stables M, Newson J. *In vivo* models to study cyclooxygenase products in health and disease: introduction to part III. *Methods Mol Biol* (2010) 644:181–8. doi: 10.1007/978-1-59745-364-6_15
130. Dinchuk JE, Car BD, Focht RJ, Johnston JJ, Jaffee BD, Covington MB, et al. Renal abnormalities and an altered inflammatory response in mice lacking cyclooxygenase II. *Nature* (1995) 378(6555):406–9. doi: 10.1038/378406a0
131. Morham SG, Langenbach R, Loftin CD, Tiano HF, Vouloumanos N, Jennette JC, et al. Prostaglandin synthase 2 gene disruption causes severe renal pathology in the mouse. *Cell* (1995) 83(3):473–82. doi: 10.1016/0092-8674(95)90125-6
132. Aid S, Silva AC, Candelario-Jalil E, Choi SH, Rosenberg GA, Bosetti F. Cyclooxygenase-1 and -2 differentially modulate lipopolysaccharide-induced blood–brain barrier disruption through matrix metalloproteinase activity. *J Cereb Blood Flow Metab* (2010) 30(2):370–80. doi: 10.1038/jcbfm.2009.223
133. Gilroy DW, Colville-Nash PR, Willis D, Chivers J, Paul-Clark MJ, Willoughby DA. Inducible cyclooxygenase may have anti-inflammatory properties. *Nat Med* (1999) 5(6):698–701. doi: 10.1038/9550
134. Kimura T, Iwase M, Kondo G, Watanabe H, Ohashi M, Ito D, et al. Suppressive effect of selective cyclooxygenase-2 inhibitor on cytokine release in human neutrophils. *Int Immunopharmacol* (2003) 3(10–11):1519–28. doi: 10.1016/S1567-5769(03)00179-6
135. Strauss KI, Marini AM. Cyclooxygenase-2 inhibition protects cultured cerebellar granule neurons from glutamate-mediated cell death. *J Neurotrauma* (2002) 19(5):627–38. doi: 10.1089/089771502753754091
136. Izquierdo LA, Barros DM, Ardenghi PG, Pereira P, Rodrigues C, Choi H, et al. Different hippocampal molecular requirements for short- and long-term retrieval of one-trial avoidance learning. *Behav Brain Res* (2000) 111(1–2):93–8. doi: 10.1016/S0166-4328(00)00137-6
137. Zagulska-Szymczak S, Filipkowski RK, Kaczmarek L. Kainate-induced genes in the hippocampus: lessons from expression patterns. *Neurochem Int* (2001) 38(6):485–501. doi: 10.1016/S0197-0186(00)00101-7
138. Zheng X-Y, Zhang H-L, Luo Q, Zhu J. Kainic acid-induced neurodegenerative model: potentials and limitations. *J Biomed Biotechnol* (2011) 2011:457079. doi: 10.1155/2011/457079
139. Ciceri P, Zhang Y, Shaffer AF, Leahy KM, Woerner MB, Smith WG, et al. Pharmacology of celecoxib in rat brain after kainate administration. *J Pharmacol Exp Ther* (2002) 302(3):846. doi: 10.1124/jpet.302.3.846
140. Byun J-S, Cho S-Y, Kim S-I, Kwon Y-S, Jeon S-H, Kim M-J, et al. Celecoxib attenuates kainic acid-induced neuronal cell death through suppression of

microglial c-Jun N-terminal kinase phosphorylation. *Exp Neurobiol* (2009) 18(1):13–8. doi: 10.5607/en.2009.18.1.13

141. Baik EJ, Kim EJ, Lee SH, Moon C-H. Cyclooxygenase-2 selective inhibitors aggravate kainic acid induced seizure and neuronal cell death in the hippocampus. *Brain Res* (1999) 843(1):118–29. doi: 10.1016/S0006-8993(99)01797-7
142. Nogawa S, Zhang F, Ross ME, Iadecola C. Cyclo-oxygenase-2 gene expression in neurons contributes to ischemic brain damage. *J Neurosci* (1997) 17(8):2746–55. doi: 10.1523/JNEUROSCI.17-08-02746.1997
143. Tian J, Kim SF, Hester L, Snyder SH. S-nitrosylation/activation of COX-2 mediates NMDA neurotoxicity. *Proc Natl Acad Sci U S A* (2008) 105(30):10537–40. doi: 10.1073/pnas.0804852105
144. Calabrese F, Rossetti AC, Racagni G, Gass P, Riva MA, Molteni R. Brain-derived neurotrophic factor: a bridge between inflammation and neuroplasticity. *Front Cell Neurosci* (2014) 8:430. doi: 10.3389/fncel.2014.00430
145. Hayley S. The neuroimmune-neuroplasticity interface and brain pathology. *Front Cell Neurosci* (2014) 8:419. doi: 10.3389/fncel.2014.00419
146. Robertson, OD, Coronado, NG, Sethi, R, Berk, M, Dodd, S. Putative neuroprotective pharmacotherapies to target the staged progression of mental illness. *Early Intervention in Psychiatry* (2019) 1–18. doi: 10.1111/eip.12775
147. Capuron L, Miller AH. Immune system to brain signaling: neuropsychopharmacological implications. *Pharmacol Ther* (2011) 130(2): 226–38. doi: 10.1016/j.pharmthera.2011.01.014
148. Miller AH, Haroon E, Raison CL, Felger JC. Cytokine targets in the brain: impact on neurotransmitters and neurocircuits. *Depress Anxiety* (2013) 30(4):297–306. doi: 10.1002/da.22084
149. Peters JC. Tryptophan nutrition and metabolism: an overview. *Adv Exp Med Biol* (1991) 294:345–58. doi: 10.1007/978-1-4684-5952-4_32
150. Hirschfeld RM. History and evolution of the monoamine hypothesis of depression. *J Clin Psychiatry* (2000) 61(Suppl 6):4–6.
151. Maes M. The cytokine hypothesis of depression: inflammation, oxidative & nitrosative stress (IO&NS) and leaky gut as new targets for adjunctive treatments in depression. *Neuro Endocrinol Lett* (2008) 29(3):287–91.
152. Wang J, Dunn AJ. Mouse interleukin-6 stimulates the HPA axis and increases brain tryptophan and serotonin metabolism. *Neurochem Int* (1998) 33(2):143–54. doi: 10.1016/S0197-0186(98)00016-3
153. Raison CL, Dantzer R, Kelley KW, Lawson MA, Woolwine BJ, Vogt G, et al. CSF concentrations of brain tryptophan and kynurenines during immune stimulation with IFN-alpha: relationship to CNS immune responses and depression. *Mol Psychiatry* (2010) 15(4):393–403. doi: 10.1038/mp.2009.116
154. Steiner J, Walter M, Gos T, Guillemin GJ, Bernstein H-G, Sarnyai Z, et al. Severe depression is associated with increased microglial quinolinic acid in subregions of the anterior cingulate gyrus: evidence for an immune-modulated glutamatergic neurotransmission? *J Neuroinflammation* (2011) 8(1):94. doi: 10.1186/1742-2094-8-94
155. Stone TW, Darlington LG. Endogenous kynurenines as targets for drug discovery and development. *Nat Rev Drug Discov* (2002) 1(8):609–20. doi: 10.1038/nrd870
156. Stone TW, Stoy N, Darlington LG. An expanding range of targets for kynurenine metabolites of tryptophan. *Trends Pharmacol Sci* (2013) 34(2):136–43. doi: 10.1016/j.tips.2012.09.006
157. Beal MF, Matson WR, Swartz KJ, Gamache PH, Bird ED. Kynurenine pathway measurements in Huntington's disease striatum: evidence for reduced formation of kynurenic acid. *J Neurochem* (1990) 55(4):1327–39. doi: 10.1111/j.1471-4159.1990.tb03143.x
158. Irwin MR, Miller AH. Depressive disorders and immunity: 20 years of progress and discovery. *Brain Behav Immun* (2007) 21(4):374–83. doi: 10.1016/j.bbi.2007.01.010
159. Lugo-Huitrón R, Muñiz U,P, Pineda B, Pedraza-Chaverrí J, Ríos C, Pérez-de la Cruz V. Quinolinic acid: an endogenous neurotoxin with multiple targets. *Oxid Med Cell Longev* (2013) 2013:14. doi: 10.1155/2013/104024
160. Miller AH. Conceptual confluence: the kynurenine pathway as a common target for ketamine and the convergence of the inflammation and glutamate hypotheses of depression. *Neuropsychopharmacology* (2013) 38(9):1607–8. doi: 10.1038/npp.2013.140
161. Schwarcz R. 'The kynurenine pathway of tryptophan degradation as a drug target. *Curr Opin Pharmacol* (2004) 4(1):12–7. doi: 10.1016/j.coph.2003.10.006
162. Herman JP, McKlveen JM, Ghosal S, Kopp B, Wulsin A, Makinson R, et al. Regulation of the hypothalamic–pituitary–adrenocortical stress response. *Compr Physiol* (2016) 6(2):603–21. doi: 10.1002/cphy.c150015
163. McKay MS, Zakzanis KK. The impact of treatment on HPA axis activity in unipolar major depression. *J Psychiatr Res* (2010) 44(3):183–92. doi: 10.1016/j.jpsychires.2009.07.012
164. Beishuizen A, Thijs LG. Endotoxin and the hypothalamo-pituitary-adrenal (HPA) axis. *J Endotoxin Res* (2003) 9(1):3–24. doi: 10.1179/096805103125001298
165. Dunn AJ. Cytokine activation of the HPA axis. *Ann N Y Acad Sci* (2000) 917:608–17. doi: 10.1111/j.1749-6632.2000.tb05426.x
166. Silverman MN, Pearce BD, Biron CA, Miller AH. Immune modulation of the hypothalamic–pituitary–adrenal (HPA) axis during viral infection. *Viral Immunol* (2005) 18(1):41–78. doi: 10.1089/vim.2005.18.41
167. Silverman MN, Sternberg EM. Glucocorticoid regulation of inflammation and its behavioral and metabolic correlates: from HPA axis to glucocorticoid receptor dysfunction. *Ann N Y Acad Sci* (2012) 1261:55–63. doi: 10.1111/j.1749-6632.2012.06633.x
168. Oxenkrug GF. Tryptophan–kynurenine metabolism as a common mediator of genetic and environmental impacts in major depressive disorder: the serotonin hypothesis revisited 40 years later. *Isr J Psychiatry Relat Sci* (2010) 47(1):56–63.
169. Rosenblat JD, Cha DS, Mansur RB, McIntyre RS. 'Inflamed moods: a review of the interactions between inflammation and mood disorders. *Prog Neuropsychopharmacol Biol Psychiatry* (2014) 53:23–34. doi: 10.1016/j.pnpbp.2014.01.013
170. McQuade R, Young AH. Future therapeutic targets in mood disorders: the glucocorticoid receptor. *Br J Psychiatry* (2000) 177:390–5. doi: 10.1192/bjp.177.5.390
171. Raison CL, Miller AH. When not enough is too much: the role of insufficient glucocorticoid signaling in the pathophysiology of stress-related disorders. *Am J Psychiatry* (2003) 160(9):1554–65. doi: 10.1176/appi.ajp.160.9.1554
172. Adzic M, Djordjevic J, Djordjevic A, Niciforovic A, Demonacos C, Radojcic M, et al. Acute or chronic stress induce cell compartment-specific phosphorylation of glucocorticoid receptor and alter its transcriptional activity in Wistar rat brain. *J Endocrinol* (2009) 202(1):87–97. doi: 10.1677/JOE-08-0509
173. Anacker C, Zunszain PA, Carvalho LA, Pariante CM. The glucocorticoid receptor: pivot of depression and of antidepressant treatment? *Psychoneuroendocrinology* (2011) 36(3):415–25. doi: 10.1016/j.psyneuen.2010.03.007
174. Pariante CM. Risk factors for development of depression and psychosis. Glucocorticoid receptors and pituitary implications for treatment with antidepressant and glucocorticoids. *Ann N Y Acad Sci* (2009) 1179:144–52. doi: 10.1111/j.1749-6632.2009.04978.x
175. Atmaca M, Yildirim H, Ozler S, Koc M, Kara B, Sec S. Smaller pituitary volume in adult patients with obsessive-compulsive disorder. *Psychiatry Clin Neurosci* (2009) 63(4):516–20. doi: 10.1111/j.1440-1819.2009.01981.x
176. Clark IA, Mackay CE, Goodwin GM. 'Pituitary gland volumes in bipolar disorder. *J Affect Disord* (2014) 169:197–202. doi: 10.1016/j.jad.2014.08.022
177. Nemeroff CB, Vale WW. The neurobiology of depression: inroads to treatment and new drug discovery. *J Clin Psychiatry* (2005) 66(Suppl 7):5–13.
178. Nordholm D, Krogh J, Mondelli V, Dazzan P, Pariante C, Nordentoft M. Pituitary gland volume in patients with schizophrenia, subjects at ultra high-risk of developing psychosis and healthy controls: a systematic review and meta-analysis. *Psychoneuroendocrinology* (2013) 38(11):2394–404. doi: 10.1016/j.psyneuen.2013.06.030
179. Pavon L, Sandoval-Lopez G, Eugenia Hernandez M, Loria F, Estrada I, Perez M, et al. Th2 cytokine response in major depressive disorder patients before treatment. *J Neuroimmunol* (2006) 172(1–2):156–65. doi: 10.1016/j.jneuroim.2005.08.014
180. Bocharova M, Agustini B, Young A, Juruena MF. HPA axis function as biomarker for atypical and melancholic depression. *Front Psychiatry* (2019). doi: 10.3389/conf.fpsyt.2017.48.00006
181 Lamers F, Vogelzangs N, Merikangas KR, de Jonge P, Beekman AT, Penninx BW. Evidence for a differential role of HPA-axis function, inflammation and metabolic syndrome in melancholic versus atypical depression. *Mol Psychiatry* (2013) 18(6):692–9. doi: 10.1038/mp.2012.144

182. Girshkin L, Matheson SL, Shepherd AM, Green MJ. Morning cortisol levels in schizophrenia and bipolar disorder: a meta-analysis. *Psychoneuroendocrinology* (2014) 49:187–206. doi: 10.1016/j.psyneuen.2014.07.013
183. Russo MV, McGavern DB. Inflammatory neuroprotection following traumatic brain injury. *Science* (2016) 353(6301):783–5. doi: 10.1126/science.aaf6260
184. Paolicelli RC, Bolasco G, Pagani F, Maggi L, Scianni M, Panzanelli P, et al. Synaptic pruning by microglia is necessary for normal brain development. *Science* (2011) 333(6048):1456–8. doi: 10.1126/science.1202529
185. Keshavan MS, Anderson S, Pettergrew JW. Is Schizophrenia due to excessive synaptic pruning in the prefrontal cortex? The Feinberg hypothesis revisited. *J Psychiatr Res* (1994) 28(3):239–65. doi: 10.1016/0022-3956(94)90009-4
186. Kim HJ, Cho MH, Shim WH, Kim JK, Jeon EY, Kim DH, et al. Deficient autophagy in microglia impairs synaptic pruning and causes social behavioral defects. *Mol Psychiatry* (2016) 22:1576. doi: 10.1038/mp.2016.103
187. Stertz L, Magalhaes PV, Kapczinski F. Is bipolar disorder an inflammatory condition? The relevance of microglial activation. *Curr Opin Psychiatry* (2013) 26(1):19–26. doi: 10.1097/YCO.0b013e32835aa4b4
188. Ekdahl CT. Microglial activation—tuning and pruning adult neurogenesis. *Front Pharmacol* (2012) 3:41. doi: 10.3389/fphar.2012.00041
189. Kraft AD, Harry GJ. Features of microglia and neuroinflammation relevant to environmental exposure and neurotoxicity. *Int J Environ Res Public Health* (2011) 8(7):2980–3018. doi: 10.3390/ijerph8072980
190. Paradise MB, Naismith SL, Norrie LM, Graeber MB, Hickie IB. The role of glia in late-life depression. *Int Psychogeriatr* (2012) 24(12):1878–90. doi: 10.1017/S1041610212000828
191. Park KM, Bowers WJ. Tumor necrosis factor-alpha mediated signaling in neuronal homeostasis and dysfunction. *Cell Signal* (2010) 22(7):977–83. doi: 10.1016/j.cellsig.2010.01.010
192. Bloomfield PS, Selvaraj S, Veronese M, Rizzo G, Bertoldo A, Owen DR, et al. Microglial activity in people at ultra high risk of psychosis and in schizophrenia; an [(11)C]PBR28 PET brain imaging study. *Am J Psychiatry* (2016) 173(1):44–52. doi: 10.1176/appi.ajp.2015.14101358
193. Laskaris LE, Di Biase MA, Everall I, Chana G, Christopoulos A, Skafidas E, et al. Microglial activation and progressive brain changes in schizophrenia. *Br J Pharmacol* (2016) 173(4):666–80. doi: 10.1111/bph.13364
194. Trépanier MO, Hopperton KE, Mizrahi R, Mechawar N, Bazinet RP. Postmortem evidence of cerebral inflammation in schizophrenia: a systematic review. *Mol Psychiatry* (2016) 21:1009. doi: 10.1038/mp.2016.90
195. Katsumoto A, Lu H, Miranda AS, Ransohoff RM. Ontogeny and functions of central nervous system macrophages. *J Immunol* (2014) 193(6):2615–21. doi: 10.4049/jimmunol.1400716
196. Ransohoff RM, Brown MA. Innate immunity in the central nervous system. *J Clin Invest* (2012) 122(4):1164–71. doi: 10.1172/JCI58644
197. Bora E, Fornito A, Pantelis C, Yucel M. Gray matter abnormalities in major depressive disorder: a meta-analysis of voxel based morphometry studies. *J Affect Disord* (2012a) 138(1–2):9–18. doi: 10.1016/j.jad.2011.03.049
198. Bora E, Fornito A, Yucel M, Pantelis C. Voxelwise meta-analysis of gray matter abnormalities in bipolar disorder. *Biol Psychiatry* (2010) 67(11):1097–105. doi: 10.1016/j.biopsych.2010.01.020
199. Bora E, Harrison BJ, Davey CG, Yucel M, Pantelis C. Meta-analysis of volumetric abnormalities in cortico-striatal-pallidal-thalamic circuits in major depressive disorder. *Psychol Med* (2012b) 42(4):671–81. doi: 10.1017/S0033291711001668
200. Goodkind M, Eickhoff SB, Oathes DJ, Jiang Y, Chang A, Jones-Hagata LB, et al. Identification of a common neurobiological substrate for mental illness. *JAMA Psychiatry* (2015) 72(4):305–15. doi: 10.1001/jamapsychiatry.2014.2206
201. Takahashi T, Yucel M, Lorenzetti V, Nakamura K, Whittle S, Walterfang M, et al. Midline brain structures in patients with current and remitted major depression. *Prog Neuropsychopharmacol Biol Psychiatry* (2009) 33(6):1058–63. doi: 10.1016/j.pnpbp.2009.05.020
202. Dodd S, Maes M, Anderson G, Dean OM, Moylan S, Berk M. Putative neuroprotective agents in neuropsychiatric disorders. *Prog Neuropsychopharmacol Biol Psychiatry* (2013) 42:135–45. doi: 10.1016/j.pnpbp.2012.11.007
203. Kessler RC, Ormel J, Petukhova M, McLaughlin KA, Green JG, Russo LJ, et al. Development of lifetime comorbidity in the World Health Organization world mental health surveys. *Arch Gen Psychiatry* (2011) 68(1):90–100. doi: 10.1001/archgenpsychiatry.2010.180
204. Dowlati Y, Herrmann N, Swardfager W, Liu H, Sham L, Reim EK, et al. A meta-analysis of cytokines in major depression. *Biol Psychiatry* (2010) 67(5):446–57. doi: 10.1016/j.biopsych.2009.09.033
205. Howren MB, Lamkin DM, Suls J. Associations of depression with C-reactive protein, IL-1, and IL-6: a meta-analysis. *Psychosom Med* (2009) 71(2):171–86. doi: 10.1097/PSY.0b013e3181907c1b
206. Lanquillon S, Krieg JC, Bening-Abu-Shach U, Vedder H. Cytokine production and treatment response in major depressive disorder. *Neuropsychopharmacology* (2000) 22(4):370–9. doi: 10.1016/S0893-133X(99)00134-7
207. O'Brien SM, Scully P, Fitzgerald P, Scott LV, Dinan TG. Plasma cytokine profiles in depressed patients who fail to respond to selective serotonin reuptake inhibitor therapy. *J Psychiatr Res* (2007) 41(3–4):326–31. doi: 10.1016/j.jpsychires.2006.05.013
208. Khandaker GM, Pearson RM, Zammit S, Lewis G, Jones PB. Association of serum interleukin 6 and C-reactive protein in childhood with depression and psychosis in young adult life: a population-based longitudinal study. *JAMA Psychiatry* (2014) 71(10):1121–8. doi: 10.1001/jamapsychiatry.2014.1332
209. Penninx BW, Beekman AT, Smit JH, Zitman FG, Nolen WA, Spinhoven P, et al. The Netherlands Study of Depression and Anxiety (NESDA): rationale, objectives and methods. *Int J Methods Psychiatr Res* (2008) 17(3):121–40. doi: 10.1002/mpr.256
210. Savitz J, Drevets WC, Wurfel BE, Ford BN, Bellgowan PS, Victor TA, et al. Reduction of kynurenic acid to quinolinic acid ratio in both the depressed and remitted phases of major depressive disorder. *Brain Behav Immun* (2015) 46:55–9. doi: 10.1016/j.bbi.2015.02.007
211. Krause D, Myint AM, Schuett C, Musil R, Dehning S, Cerovecki A, et al. High kynurenine (a tryptophan metabolite) predicts remission in patients with major depression to add-on treatment with celecoxib. *Front Psychiatry* (2017) 8:16. doi: 10.3389/fpsyt.2017.00016
212. Gałecki P, Galecka E, Maes M, Chamielec M, Orzechowska A, Bobinska K, et al. The expression of genes encoding for COX-2, MPO, iNOS, and sPLA2-IIA in patients with recurrent depressive disorder. *J Affect Disord* (2012) 138(3):360–6. doi: 10.1016/j.jad.2012.01.016
213. Lee SY, Choi HK, Lee KJ, Jung JY, Hur GY, Jung KH, et al. The immune tolerance of cancer is mediated by IDO that is inhibited by COX-2 inhibitors through regulatory T cells. *J Immunother* (2009) 32(1):22–8. doi: 10.1097/CJI.0b013e31818ac2f7
214. Miller AH, Maletic V, Raison CL. Inflammation and its discontents: the role of cytokines in the pathophysiology of major depression. *Biol Psychiatry* (2009) 65(9):732–41. doi: 10.1016/j.biopsych.2008.11.029
215. Hu F, Wang X, Pace TWW, Wu H, Miller AH. Inhibition of COX-2 by celecoxib enhances glucocorticoid receptor function. *Mol Psychiatry* (2005) 10(5):426–8. doi: 10.1038/sj.mp.4001644
216. Song C, Zhang XY, Manku M. Increased phospholipase A2 activity and inflammatory response but decreased nerve growth factor expression in the olfactory bulbectomized rat model of depression: effects of chronic ethyl-eicosapentaenoate treatment. *J Neurosci* (2009a) 29(1):14–22. doi: 10.1523/JNEUROSCI.3569-08.2009
217. Hillier K, Templeton WW. Regulation of noradrenaline overflow in rat cerebral cortex by prostaglandin E2. *Br J Pharmacol* (1980) 70(3):469–73. doi: 10.1111/j.1476-5381.1980.tb08725.x
218. Casolini P, Catalani A, Zuena AR, Angelucci L. Inhibition of COX-2 reduces the age-dependent increase of hippocampal inflammatory markers, corticosterone secretion, and behavioral impairments in the rat. *J Neurosci Res* (2002) 68(3):337–43. doi: 10.1002/jnr.10192
219. Konsman JP, Parnet P, Dantzer R. Cytokine-induced sickness behaviour: mechanisms and implications. *Trends Neurosci* (2002) 25(3):154–9. doi: 10.1016/S0166-2236(00)02088-9
220. Schiepers OJ, Wichers MC, Maes M. Cytokines and major depression. *Prog Neuropsychopharmacol Biol Psychiatry* (2005) 29(2):201–17. doi: 10.1016/j.pnpbp.2004.11.003
221. Myint AM, Kim YK, Verkerk R, Scharpe S, Steinbusch H, Leonard B. Kynurenine pathway in major depression: evidence of impaired neuroprotection. *J Affect Disord* (2007) 98(1–2):143–51. doi: 10.1016/j.jad.2006.07.013
222. Brunello N, Alboni S, Capone G, Benatti C, Blom JM, Tascedda F, et al. Acetylsalicylic acid accelerates the antidepressant effect of fluoxetine in the

chronic escape deficit model of depression. *Int Clin Psychopharmacol* (2006) 21(4):219–25. doi: 10.1097/00004850-200607000-00004

223. Kohler O, Benros ME, Nordentoft M, Farkouh ME, Iyengar RL, Mors O, et al. Effect of anti-inflammatory treatment on depression, depressive symptoms, and adverse effects: a systematic review and meta-analysis of randomized clinical trials. *JAMA Psychiatry* (2014) 71(12):1381–91. doi: 10.1001/jamapsychiatry.2014.1611
224. Na KS, Lee KJ, Lee JS, Cho YS, Jung HY. Efficacy of adjunctive celecoxib treatment for patients with major depressive disorder: a meta-analysis. *Prog Neuropsychopharmacol Biol Psychiatry* (2014) 48:79–85. doi: 10.1016/j.pnpbp.2013.09.006
225. Eyre HA, Air T, Pradhan A, Johnston J, Lavretsky H, Stuart MJ, et al. A meta-analysis of chemokines in major depression. *Prog Neuropsychopharmacol Biol Psychiatry* (2016) 68:1–8. doi: 10.1016/j.pnpbp.2016.02.006
226. Kim JY, Park JH, Lee JJ, Huh Y, Lee SB, Han SK, et al. Standardization of the Korean version of the Geriatric Depression Scale: reliability, validity, and factor structure. *Psychiatry Investig* (2008) 5(4):232–8. doi: 10.4306/pi.2008.5.4.232
227. Baldi PC, Giambartolomei GH. Immunopathology of Brucella infection. *Recent Pat Antiinfect Drug Discov* (2013a) 8(1):18–26. doi: 10.2174/1574891X11308010005
228. Baldi PC, Giambartolomei GH. Pathogenesis and pathobiology of zoonotic brucellosis in humans. *Rev Sci Tech* (2013b) 32(1):117–25. doi: 10.20506/rst.32.1.2192
229. Iyengar RL, Gandhi S, Aneja A, Thorpe K, Razzouk L, Greenberg J, et al. NSAIDs are associated with lower depression scores in patients with osteoarthritis. *Am J Med* (2013) 126(11):1017.e11–8. doi: 10.1016/j.amjmed.2013.02.037
230. Lai V, George J, Richey L, Kim HJ, Cannon T, Shores C, et al. Results of a pilot study of the effects of celecoxib on cancer cachexia in patients with cancer of the head, neck, and gastrointestinal tract. *Head Neck* (2008) 30(1):67–74. doi: 10.1002/hed.20662
231. Lundholm K, Daneryd P, Korner U, Hyltander A, Bosaeus I. Evidence that long-term COX-treatment improves energy homeostasis and body composition in cancer patients with progressive cachexia. *Int J Oncol* (2004) 24(3):505–12. doi: 10.3892/ijo.24.3.505
232. Pedersen CB, Mors O, Bertelsen A, Waltoft BL, Agerbo E, McGrath JJ, et al. A comprehensive nationwide study of the incidence rate and lifetime risk for treated mental disorders. *JAMA Psychiatry* (2014) 71(5):573–81. doi: 10.1001/jamapsychiatry.2014.16
233. Malhi GS, Ivanovski B, Hadzi-Pavlovic D, Mitchell PB, Vieta E, Sachdev P. Neuropsychological deficits and functional impairment in bipolar depression, hypomania and euthymia. *Bipolar Disord* (2007) 9(1–2):114–25. doi: 10.1111/j.1399-5618.2007.00324.x
234. Marotta A, Chiaie RD, Spagna A, Bernabei L, Sciarretta M, Roca J, et al. Impaired conflict resolution and vigilance in euthymic bipolar disorder. *Psychiatry Res* (2015) 229(1–2):490–6. doi: 10.1016/j.psychres.2015.06.026
235. Baumeister D, Russell A, Pariante CM, Mondelli V. Inflammatory biomarker profiles of mental disorders and their relation to clinical, social and lifestyle factors. *Soc Psychiatry Psychiatr Epidemiol* (2014) 49(6):841–9. doi: 10.1007/s00127-014-0887-z
236. Drexhage RC, van der Heul-Nieuwenhuijsen L, Padmos RC, van Beveren N, Cohen D, Versnel MA, et al. Inflammatory gene expression in monocytes of patients with schizophrenia: overlap and difference with bipolar disorder. A study in naturalistically treated patients. *Int J Neuropsychopharmacol* (2010b) 13(10):1369–81. doi: 10.1017/S1461145710000799
237. Dargel AA, Godin O, Kapczinski F, Kupfer DJ, Leboyer M. C-reactive protein alterations in bipolar disorder: a meta-analysis. *J Clin Psychiatry* (2015) 76(2):142–50. doi: 10.4088/JCP.14r09007
238. Munkholm K, Brauner JV, Kessing LV, Vinberg M. 'Cytokines in bipolar disorder vs. healthy control subjects: a systematic review and meta-analysis. *J Psychiatr Res* (2013a) 47(9):1119–33. doi: 10.1016/j.jpsychires.2013.05.018
239. Barbosa IG, Bauer ME, Machado-Vieira R, Teixeira AL. Cytokines in bipolar disorder: paving the way for neuroprogression. *Neural Plast* (2014a) 2014:360481. doi: 10.1155/2014/360481
240. Barbosa IG, Machado-Vieira R, Soares JC, Teixeira AL. The immunology of bipolar disorder. *Neuroimmunomodulation* (2014b) 21(2-3):117–22. doi: 10.1159/000356539
241. Haarman BC, Riemersma-Van der Lek RF, de Groot JC, Ruhe HG, Klein HC, Zandstra TE, et al. Neuroinflammation in bipolar disorder - A [(11) C]-(R)-PK11195 positron emission tomography study. *Brain Behav Immun* (2014) 40:219–25. doi: 10.1016/j.bbi.2014.03.016
242. Jakobsson J, Bjerke M, Sahebi S, Isgren A, Ekman CJ, Sellgren C, et al. Monocyte and microglial activation in patients with mood-stabilized bipolar disorder. *J Psychiatry Neurosci* (2015) 40(4):250–8. doi: 10.1503/jpn.140183
243. Rao JS, Harry GJ, Rapoport SI, Kim HW. Increased excitotoxicity and neuroinflammatory markers in postmortem frontal cortex from bipolar disorder patients. *Mol Psychiatry* (2010) 15(4):384–92. doi: 10.1038/mp.2009.47
244. Schneider MR, DelBello MP, McNamara RK, Strakowski SM, Adler CM. Neuroprogression in bipolar disorder. *Bipolar Disord* (2012) 14(4):356–74. doi: 10.1111/j.1399-5618.2012.01024.x
245. Strakowski SM, Adler CM, Almeida J, Altshuler LL, Blumberg HP, Chang KD, et al. The functional neuroanatomy of bipolar disorder: a consensus model. *Bipolar Disord* (2012) 14(4):313–25. doi: 10.1111/j.1399-5618.2012.01022.x
246. Boufidou F, Nikolaou C, Alevizos B, Liappas IA, Christodoulou GN. Cytokine production in bipolar affective disorder patients under lithium treatment. *J Affect Disord* (2004) 82(2):309–13. doi: 10.1016/j.jad.2004.01.007
247. Basselin M, Kim H-W, Chen M, Ma K, Rapoport SI, Murphy RC, et al. Lithium modifies brain arachidonic and docosahexaenoic metabolism in rat lipopolysaccharide model of neuroinflammation. *J Lipid Res* (2010) 51(5):1049–56. doi: 10.1194/jlr.M002469
248. Breunis MN, Kupka RW, Nolen WA, Suppes T, Denicoff KD, Leverich GS, et al. High numbers of circulating activated T cells and raised levels of serum IL-2 receptor in bipolar disorder. *Biol Psychiatry* (2003) 53(2):157–65. doi: 10.1016/S0006-3223(02)01452-X
249. Chiu CT, Wang Z, Hunsberger JG, Chuang DM. Therapeutic potential of mood stabilizers lithium and valproic acid: beyond bipolar disorder. *Pharmacol Rev* (2013) 65(1):105–42. doi: 10.1124/pr.111.005512
250. Knijff EM, Breunis MN, Kupka RW, de Wit HJ, Ruwhof C, Akkerhuis GW, et al. An imbalance in the production of IL-1beta and IL-6 by monocytes of bipolar patients: restoration by lithium treatment. *Bipolar Disord* (2007) 9(7):743–53. doi: 10.1111/j.1399-5618.2007.00444.x
251. Lee HJ, Rao JS, Rapoport SI, Bazinet RP. Antimanic therapies target brain arachidonic acid signaling: lessons learned about the regulation of brain fatty acid metabolism. *Prostaglandins Leukot Essent Fatty Acids* (2007) 77(5–6):239–46. doi: 10.1016/j.plefa.2007.10.018
252. O'Brien SM, Scully P, Scott LV, Dinan TG. Cytokine profiles in bipolar affective disorder: focus on acutely ill patients. *J Affect Disord* (2006) 90(2–3):263–7. doi: 10.1016/j.jad.2005.11.015
253. Rapoport SI, Bosetti F. Do lithium and anticonvulsants target the brain arachidonic acid cascade in bipolar disorder? *Arch Gen Psychiatry* (2002) 59(7):592–6. doi: 10.1001/archpsyc.59.7.592
254. Perugi G, Medda P, Toni C, Mariani MG, Socci C, Mauri M. The role of electroconvulsive therapy (ect) in bipolar disorder: effectiveness in 522 patients with bipolar depression, mixed-state, mania and catatonic features. *Curr Neuropharmacol* (2017) 15(3):359–71. doi: 10.2174/1570159X14666161017233642
255. Fluitman SB, Heijnen CJ, Denys DA, Nolen WA, Balk FJ, Westenberg HG. Electroconvulsive therapy has acute immunological and neuroendocrine effects in patients with major depressive disorder. *J Affect Disord* (2011) 131(1–3):388–92. doi: 10.1016/j.jad.2010.11.035
256. Hestad KA, Tonseth S, Stoen CD, Ueland T, Aukrust P. Raised plasma levels of tumor necrosis factor alpha in patients with depression: normalization during electroconvulsive therapy. *J ECT* (2003) 19(4):183–8. doi: 10.1097/00124509-200312000-00002
257. Taylor S. Electroconvulsive therapy: a review of history, patient selection, technique, and medication management. *South Med J* (2007) 100(5):494–8. doi: 10.1097/SMJ.0b013e318038fce0
258. Guloksuz S, Arts B, Walter S, Drukker M, Rodriguez L, Myint AM, et al. The impact of electroconvulsive therapy on the tryptophan–kynurenine metabolic pathway. *Brain Behav Immun* (2015) 48:48–52. doi: 10.1016/j.bbi.2015.02.029
259. Schwieler L, Samuelsson M, Frye MA, Bhat M, Schuppe-Koistinen I, Jungholm O, et al. Electroconvulsive therapy suppresses the neurotoxic branch of the kynurenine pathway in treatment-resistant depressed patients. *J Neuroinflammation* (2016) 13(1):51. doi: 10.1186/s12974-016-0517-7
260. Kargar M, Yousefi A, Mojtahedzadeh M, Akhondzadeh S, Artounian V, Abdollahi A, et al. Effects of celecoxib on inflammatory markers in bipolar

patients undergoing electroconvulsive therapy: a placebo-controlled, double-blind, randomised study. Swiss Med Wkly (2014) 144:w13880. doi: 10.4414/smw.2014.13880

261. Lehtimaki K, Keranen T, Huuhka M, Palmio J, Hurme M, Leinonen E, et al. Increase in plasma proinflammatory cytokines after electroconvulsive therapy in patients with depressive disorder. *J ECT* (2008) 24(1):88–91. doi: 10.1097/YCT.0b013e3181571abb
262. Husain MI, Chaudhry IB, Hamirani MM, Minhas FA, Kazmi A, Hodsoll J, et al. Minocycline and celecoxib as adjunctive treatments for bipolar depression: a study protocol for a multicenter factorial design randomized controlled trial. *Neuropsychiatr Dis Treat* (2016) 13:1–8. doi: 10.2147/NDT.S115002
263. van Os J, Kapur S. Schizophrenia. *Lancet* (2009) 374(9690):635–45. doi: 10.1016/S0140-6736(09)60995-8
264. Marini S, De Berardis D, Vellante F, Santacroce R, Orsolini L, Valchera A, et al. Celecoxib adjunctive treatment to antipsychotics in schizophrenia: a review of randomized clinical add-on trials. *Mediators Inflamm* (2016) 2016:3476240. doi: 10.1155/2016/3476240
265. Jarskog LF, Xiao H, Wilkie MB, Lauder JM, Gilmore JH. Cytokine regulation of embryonic rat dopamine and serotonin neuronal survival *in vitro*. *Int J Dev Neurosci* (1997) 15(6):711–6. doi: 10.1016/S0736-5748(97)00029-4
266. Kabiersch A, Furukawa H, del Rey A, Besedovsky HO. Administration of interleukin-1 at birth affects dopaminergic neurons in adult mice. *Ann N Y Acad Sci* (1998) 840:123–7. doi: 10.1111/j.1749-6632.1998.tb09556.x
267. Ling ZD, Potter ED, Lipton JW, Carvey PM. Differentiation of mesencephalic progenitor cells into dopaminergic neurons by cytokines. *Exp Neurol* (1998) 149(2):411–23. doi: 10.1006/exnr.1998.6715
268. Potter ED, Ling ZD, Carvey PM. Cytokine-induced conversion of mesencephalic-derived progenitor cells into dopamine neurons. *Cell Tissue Res* (1999) 296(2):235–46. doi: 10.1007/s004410051285
269. Kegel ME, Bhat M, Skogh E, Samuelsson M, Lundberg K, Dahl ML, et al. Imbalanced kynurenine pathway in schizophrenia. *Int J Tryptophan Res* (2014) 7:15–22. doi: 10.4137/IJTR.S16800
270. Zuckerman L, Weiner I. Maternal immune activation leads to behavioral and pharmacological changes in the adult offspring. *J Psychiatr Res* (2005) 39(3):311–23. doi: 10.1016/j.jpsychires.2004.08.008
271. Brown AS. Prenatal infection as a risk factor for schizophrenia. *Schizophr Bull* (2006) 32(2):200–2. doi: 10.1093/schbul/sbj052
272. Brown AS, Derkits EJ. Prenatal infection and schizophrenia: a review of epidemiologic and translational studies. *Am J Psychiatry* (2010) 167(3):261–80. doi: 10.1176/appi.ajp.2009.09030361
273. Eaton WW, Byrne M, Ewald H, Mors O, Chen CY, Agerbo E, et al. Association of schizophrenia and autoimmune diseases: linkage of Danish national registers. *Am J Psychiatry* (2006) 163(3):521–8. doi: 10.1176/appi.ajp.163.3.521
274. Chen YJ, Wu CY, Lin MW, Chen TJ, Liao KK, Chen YC, et al. Comorbidity profiles among patients with bullous pemphigoid: a nationwide population-based study. *Br J Dermatol* (2011) 165(3):593–9. doi: 10.1111/j.1365-2133.2011.10386.x
275. Eaton WW, Hayward C, Ram R. Schizophrenia and rheumatoid arthritis: a review. *Schizophr Res* (1992) 6(3):181–92. doi: 10.1016/0920-9964(92)90001-L
276. Korschenhausen DA, Hampel HJ, Ackenheil M, Penning R, Muller N. Fibrin degradation products in post mortem brain tissue of schizophrenics: a possible marker for underlying inflammatory processes. *Schizophr Res* (1996) 19(2–3):103–9. doi: 10.1016/0920-9964(95)00073-9
277. Doorduin J, de Vries EF, Willemsen AT, de Groot JC, Dierckx RA, Klein HC. Neuroinflammation in schizophrenia-related psychosis: a PET study. *J Nucl Med* (2009) 50(11):1801–7. doi: 10.2967/jnumed.109.066647
278. Monji A, Kato T, Kanba S. Cytokines and schizophrenia: microglia hypothesis of schizophrenia. *Psychiatry Clin Neurosci* (2009) 63(3):257–65. doi: 10.1111/j.1440-1819.2009.01945.x
279. Takano A, Arakawa R, Ito H, Tateno A, Takahashi H, Matsumoto R, et al. Peripheral benzodiazepine receptors in patients with chronic schizophrenia: a PET study with [11C]DAA1106. *Int J Neuropsychopharmacol* (2010) 13(7):943–50. doi: 10.1017/S1461145710000313
280. van Berckel BN, Bossong MG, Boellaard R, Kloet R, Schuitemaker A, Caspers E, et al. Microglia activation in recent-onset schizophrenia: a quantitative (R)-[11C]PK11195 positron emission tomography study. *Biol Psychiatry* (2008) 64(9):820–2. doi: 10.1016/j.biopsych.2008.04.025
281. Arango C, Rapado-Castro M, Reig S, Castro-Fornieles J, Gonzalez-Pinto A, Otero S, et al. Progressive brain changes in children and adolescents with first-episode psychosis. *Arch Gen Psychiatry* (2012) 69(1):16–26. doi: 10.1001/archgenpsychiatry.2011.150
282. DeLisi LE, Szulc KU, Bertisch HC, Majcher M, Brown K. Understanding structural brain changes in schizophrenia. *Dialogues Clin Neurosci* (2006) 8(1):71–8.
283. Steen RG, Mull C, McClure R, Hamer RM, Lieberman JA. Brain volume in first-episode schizophrenia: systematic review and meta-analysis of magnetic resonance imaging studies. *Br J Psychiatry* (2006) 188:510–8. doi: 10.1192/bjp.188.6.510
284. Kahn RS, Sommer IE. The neurobiology and treatment of first-episode schizophrenia. *Mol Psychiatry* (2015) 20(1):84–97. doi: 10.1038/mp.2014.66
285. Fillman SG, Cloonan N, Miller LC, Weickert CS. Markers of inflammation in the prefrontal cortex of individuals with schizophrenia. *Mol Psychiatry* (2013) 18(2):133. doi: 10.1038/mp.2012.199
286. Garver DL, Tamas RL, Holcomb JA. Elevated interleukin-6 in the cerebrospinal fluid of a previously delineated schizophrenia subtype. *Neuropsychopharmacology* (2003) 28(8):1515–20. doi: 10.1038/sj.npp.1300217
287. Meisenzahl EM, Rujescu D, Kirner A, Giegling I, Kathmann N, Leinsinger G, et al. Association of an interleukin-1beta genetic polymorphism with altered brain structure in patients with schizophrenia. *Am J Psychiatry* (2001) 158(8):1316–9. doi: 10.1176/appi.ajp.158.8.1316
288. Cannon TD, Chung Y, He G, Sun D, Jacobson A, van Erp TG, et al. Progressive reduction in cortical thickness as psychosis develops: a multisite longitudinal neuroimaging study of youth at elevated clinical risk. *Biol Psychiatry* (2015) 77(2):147–57. doi: 10.1016/j.biopsych.2014.05.023
289. Sekar A, Bialas AR, de Rivera H, Davis A, Hammond TR, Kamitaki N, et al. Schizophrenia risk from complex variation of complement component 4. *Nature* (2016) 530(7589):177–83. doi: 10.1038/nature16549
290. Drexhage RC, Knijff EM, Padmos RC, Heul-Nieuwenhuijzen L, Beumer W, Versnel MA, et al. The mononuclear phagocyte system and its cytokine inflammatory networks in schizophrenia and bipolar disorder. *Expert Rev Neurother* (2010a) 10(1):59–76. doi: 10.1586/ern.09.144
291. Fan X, Goff DC, Henderson DC. Inflammation and schizophrenia. *Expert Rev Neurother* (2007) 7(7):789–96. doi: 10.1586/14737175.7.7.789
292. Potvin S, Stip E, Sepehry AA, Gendron A, Bah R, Kouassi E. Inflammatory cytokine alterations in schizophrenia: a systematic quantitative review. *Biol Psychiatry* (2008) 63(8):801–8. doi: 10.1016/j.biopsych.2007.09.024
293. Holden JM, Meyers-Manor JE, Overmier JB, Gahtan E, Sweeney W, Miller H. Lipopolysaccharide-induced immune activation impairs attention but has little effect on short-term working memory. *Behav Brain Res* (2008) 194(2):138–45. doi: 10.1016/j.bbr.2008.06.032
294. Moller HJ. Clinical evaluation of negative symptoms in schizophrenia. *Eur Psychiatry* (2007) 22(6):380–6. doi: 10.1016/j.eurpsy.2007.03.010
295. Tandon R, Nasrallah HA, Keshavan MS. Schizophrenia, "just the facts" 4. Clinical features and conceptualization. *Schizophr Res* (2009) 110(1–3):1–23. doi: 10.1016/j.schres.2009.03.005
296. Dickerson F, Stallings C, Origoni A, Boronow J, Yolken R. C-reactive protein is associated with the severity of cognitive impairment but not of psychiatric symptoms in individuals with schizophrenia. *Schizophr Res* (2007) 93(1–3):261–5. doi: 10.1016/j.schres.2007.03.022
297. Liu L, Jia F, Yuan G, Chen Z, Yao J, Li H, et al. Tyrosine hydroxylase, interleukin-1beta and tumor necrosis factor-alpha are overexpressed in peripheral blood mononuclear cells from schizophrenia patients as determined by semi-quantitative analysis. *Psychiatry Res* (2010) 176(1):1–7. doi: 10.1016/j.psychres.2008.10.024
298. Pedersen A, Diedrich M, Kaestner F, Koelkebeck K, Ohrmann P, Ponath G, et al. Memory impairment correlates with increased S100B serum concentrations in patients with chronic schizophrenia. *Prog Neuropsychopharmacol Biol Psychiatry* (2008) 32(8):1789–92. doi: 10.1016/j.pnpbp.2008.07.017
299. Miller B, Buckley PF, Mellor A, Kirkpatrick BW. Meta-analysis of cytokine alterations in schizophrenia: clinical status, symptoms, and antipsychotic effects. *Schizophr Bull* (2011a) 37:57.
300. Baumeister D, Ciufolini S, Mondelli V. Effects of psychotropic drugs on inflammation: consequence or mediator of therapeutic effects in psychiatric

treatment? *Psychopharmacology (Berl)* (2016) 233(9):1575–89. doi: 10.1007/s00213-015-4044-5

301. Fernandes BS, Steiner J, Bernstein HG, Dodd S, Pasco JA, Dean OM, et al. C-reactive protein is increased in schizophrenia but is not altered by antipsychotics: meta-analysis and implications. *Mol Psychiatry* (2016) 21(4):554–64. doi: 10.1038/mp.2015.87
302. Kim YK, Myint AM, Verkerk R, Scharpe S, Steinbusch H, Leonard B. Cytokine changes and tryptophan metabolites in medication-naive and medication-free schizophrenic patients. *Neuropsychobiology* (2009) 59(2):123–9. doi: 10.1159/000213565
303. Pollmacher T, Haack M, Schuld A, Kraus T, Hinze-Selch D. Effects of antipsychotic drugs on cytokine networks. *J Psychiatr Res* (2000) 34(6):369–82. doi: 10.1016/S0022-3956(00)00032-7
304. Song XQ, Lv LX, Li WQ, Hao YH, Zhao JP. The interaction of nuclear factor-kappa B and cytokines is associated with schizophrenia. *Biol Psychiatry* (2009b) 65(6):481–8. doi: 10.1016/j.biopsych.2008.10.018
305. Cazzullo CL, Sacchetti E, Galluzzo A, Panariello A, Adorni A, Pegoraro M, et al. Cytokine profiles in schizophrenic patients treated with risperidone: a 3-month follow-up study. *Prog Neuropsychopharmacol Biol Psychiatry* (2002) 26(1):33–9. doi: 10.1016/S0278-5846(01)00221-4
306. Maes M, Bosmans E, Kenis G, De Jong R, Smith RS, Meltzer HY. In vivo immunomodulatory effects of clozapine in schizophrenia. *Schizophr Res* (1997) 26(2–3):221–5. doi: 10.1016/S0920-9964(97)00057-1
307. Song C, Lin A, Kenis G, Bosmans E, Maes M. Immunosuppressive effects of clozapine and haloperidol: enhanced production of the interleukin-1 receptor antagonist. *Schizophr Res* (2000) 42(2):157–64. doi: 10.1016/S0920-9964(99)00116-4
308. Drzyzga L, Obuchowicz E, Marcinowska A, Herman ZS. Cytokines in schizophrenia and the effects of antipsychotic drugs. *Brain Behav Immun* (2006) 20(6):532–45. doi: 10.1016/j.bbi.2006.02.002
309. Plitman E, Iwata Y, Caravaggio F, Nakajima S, Chung JK, Gerretsen P, et al. Kynurenic acid in schizophrenia: a systematic review and meta-analysis. *Schizophr Bull* (2017) 43(4):764–77. doi: 10.1093/schbul/sbw221
310. Ceresoli-Borroni G, Rassoulpour A, Wu HQ, Guidetti P, Schwarcz R. Chronic neuroleptic treatment reduces endogenous kynurenic acid levels in rat brain. *J Neural Transm (Vienna)* (2006) 113(10):1355–65. doi: 10.1007/s00702-005-0432-z
311. Mirjany M, Ho L, Pasinetti GM. Role of cyclooxygenase-2 in neuronal cell cycle activity and glutamate-mediated excitotoxicity. *J Pharmacol Exp Ther* (2002) 301(2):494–500. doi: 10.1124/jpet.301.2.494
312. Muller N, Riedel M, Schwarz MJ, Engel RR. Clinical effects of COX-2 inhibitors on cognition in schizophrenia. *Eur Arch Psychiatry Clin Neurosci* (2005) 255(2):149–51. doi: 10.1007/s00406-004-0548-4
313. Zheng W, Cai DB, Yang XH, Ungvari GS, Ng CH, Muller N, et al. Adjunctive celecoxib for schizophrenia: a meta-analysis of randomized, double-blind, placebo-controlled trials. *J Psychiatr Res* (2017) 92:139–46. doi: 10.1016/j.jpsychires.2017.04.004
314. Diagnostic and statistical manual of mental disorders: DSM-5. 2013, American Psychiatric Association, Arlington, VA.
315. Muhle R, Trentacoste SV, Rapin I. The genetics of autism. *Pediatrics* (2004) 113(5):e472–86. doi: 10.1542/peds.113.5.e472
316. Goines P, Van de Water J. The immune system's role in the biology of autism. *Curr Opin Neurol* (2010) 23(2):111–7. doi: 10.1097/WCO.0b013e3283373514
317. Nakagawa Y, Chiba K. Involvement of neuroinflammation during brain development in social cognitive deficits in autism spectrum disorder and schizophrenia. *J Pharmacol Exp Ther* (2016) 358(3):504. doi: 10.1124/jpet.116.234476
318. Onore C, Careaga M, Ashwood P. The role of immune dysfunction in the pathophysiology of autism. *Brain Behav Immun* (2012) 26(3):383–92. doi: 10.1016/j.bbi.2011.08.007
319. Petrelli F, Pucci L, Bezzi P. Astrocytes and microglia and their potential link with autism spectrum disorders. *Front Cell Neurosci* (2016) 10:21. doi: 10.3389/fncel.2016.00021
320. Wakefield AJ, Murch SH, Anthony A, Linnell J, Casson DM, Malik M, et al. Ileal-lymphoid-nodular hyperplasia, non-specific colitis, and pervasive developmental disorder in children. *Lancet* (1998) 351(9103):637–41. doi: 10.1016/S0140-6736(97)11096-0
321. Fombonne E, Chakrabarti S. No evidence for a new variant of measles-mumps-rubella-induced autism. *Pediatrics* (2001) 108(4):E58. doi: 10.1542/peds.108.4.e58
322. Gerber JS, Offit PA. Vaccines and autism: a tale of shifting hypotheses. *Clin Infect Dis* (2009) 48(4):456–61. doi: 10.1086/596476
323. Offit PA, Coffin SE. Communicating science to the public: MMR vaccine and autism. *Vaccine* (2003) 22(1):1–6. doi: 10.1016/S0264-410X(03)00532-2
324. Taylor B, Miller E, Lingam R, Andrews N, Simmons A, Stowe J. Measles, mumps, and rubella vaccination and bowel problems or developmental regression in children with autism: population study. *BMJ* (2002) 324(7334):393–6. doi: 10.1136/bmj.324.7334.393
325. Brown AS. Epidemiologic studies of exposure to prenatal infection and risk of schizophrenia and autism. *Dev Neurobiol* (2012) 72(10):1272–6. doi: 10.1002/dneu.22024
326. Fang SY, Wang S, Huang N, Yeh HH, Chen CY. Prenatal Infection and autism spectrum disorders in childhood: a population-based case-control study in Taiwan. *Paediatr Perinat Epidemiol* (2015) 29(4):307–16. doi: 10.1111/ppe.12194
327. Jiang HY, Xu LL, Shao L, Xia RM, Yu ZH, Ling ZX, et al. Maternal infection during pregnancy and risk of autism spectrum disorders: A systematic review and meta-analysis. *Brain Behav Immun* (2016) 58:165–72. doi: 10.1016/j.bbi.2016.06.005
328. Ziats MN, Rennert OM. Expression profiling of autism candidate genes during human brain development implicates central immune signaling pathways. *PLoS One* (2011) 6(9):e24691. doi: 10.1371/journal.pone.0024691
329. Lim CK, Essa MM, de Paula Martins R, Lovejoy DB, Bilgin AA, Waly MI, et al. Altered kynurenine pathway metabolism in autism: Implication for immune-induced glutamatergic activity. *Autism Res* (2016) 9(6):621–31. doi: 10.1002/aur.1565
330. Ashwood P, Krakowiak P, Hertz-Picciotto I, Hansen R, Pessah I, Van de Water J. Elevated plasma cytokines in autism spectrum disorders provide evidence of immune dysfunction and are associated with impaired behavioral outcome. *Brain Behav Immun* (2011) 25(1):40–5. doi: 10.1016/j.bbi.2010.08.003
331. Heuer L, Ashwood P, Schauer J, Goines P, Krakowiak P, Hertz-Picciotto I, et al. Reduced levels of immunoglobulin in children with autism correlates with behavioral symptoms. *Autism Res* (2008) 1(5):275–83. doi: 10.1002/aur.42
332. Wills S, Cabanlit M, Bennett J, Ashwood P, Amaral D, Van de Water J. Autoantibodies in autism spectrum disorders (ASD). *Ann N Y Acad Sci* (2007) 1107:79–91. doi: 10.1196/annals.1381.009
333. Grigorenko EL, Han SS, Yrigollen CM, Leng L, Mizue Y, Anderson GM, et al. Macrophage migration inhibitory factor and autism spectrum disorders. *Pediatrics* (2008) 122(2):e438–45. doi: 10.1542/peds.2007-3604
334. Wang F, Wu H, Xu S, Guo X, Yang J, Shen X. Macrophage migration inhibitory factor activates cyclooxygenase 2-prostaglandin E2 in cultured spinal microglia. *Neurosci Res* (2011) 71(3):210–8. doi: 10.1016/j.neures.2011.07.1821
335. Blaylock RL, Strunecka A. Immune-glutamatergic dysfunction as a central mechanism of the autism spectrum disorders. *Curr Med Chem* (2009) 16(2):157–70. doi: 10.2174/092986709787002745
336. Morgan JT, Chana G, Pardo CA, Achim C, Semendeferi K, Buckwalter J, et al. Microglial activation and increased microglial density observed in the dorsolateral prefrontal cortex in autism. *Biol Psychiatry* (2010) 68(4):368–76. doi: 10.1016/j.biopsych.2010.05.024
337. Tetreault NA, Hakeem AY, Jiang S, Williams BA, Allman E, Wold BJ, et al. Microglia in the cerebral cortex in autism. *J Autism Dev Disord* (2012) 42(12):2569–84. doi: 10.1007/s10803-012-1513-0
338. Vargas DL, Nascimbene C, Krishnan C, Zimmerman AW, Pardo CA. Neuroglial activation and neuroinflammation in the brain of patients with autism. *Ann Neurol* (2005) 57(1):67–81. doi: 10.1002/ana.20315
339. Careaga M, Schwartzer J, Ashwood P. Inflammatory profiles in the BTBR mouse: how relevant are they to autism spectrum disorders? *Brain Behav Immun* (2015) 43:11–6. doi: 10.1016/j.bbi.2014.06.006
340. El-Ansary A, Al-Ayadhi L. Neuroinflammation in autism spectrum disorders. *J Neuroinflammation* (2012) 9:265. doi: 10.1186/1742-2094-9-265
341. Boris M, Kaiser CC, Goldblatt A, Elice MW, Edelson SM, Adams JB, et al. Effect of pioglitazone treatment on behavioral symptoms in autistic children. *J Neuroinflammation* (2007) 4:3. doi: 10.1186/1742-2094-4-3

342. Kim EJ, Kwon KJ, Park JY, Lee SH, Moon CH, Baik EJ. Effects of peroxisome proliferator-activated receptor agonists on LPS-induced neuronal death in mixed cortical neurons: associated with iNOS and COX-2. *Brain Res* (2002) 941(1–2):1–10. doi: 10.1016/S0006-8993(02)02480-0
343. Sepanjnia K, Modabbernia A, Ashrafi M, Modabbernia MJ, Akhondzadeh S. Pioglitazone adjunctive therapy for moderate-to-severe major depressive disorder: randomized double-blind placebo-controlled trial. *Neuropsychopharmacology* (2012) 37(9):2093–100. doi: 10.1038/npp.2012.58
344. Kaizaki A, Tien L-T, Pang Y, Cai Z, Tanaka S, Numazawa S, et al. Celecoxib reduces brain dopaminergic neuronal dysfunction, and improves sensorimotor behavioral performance in neonatal rats exposed to systemic lipopolysaccharide. *J Neuroinflammation* (2013) 10(1):818. doi: 10.1186/1742-2094-10-45
345. de Mathis MA, Diniz JB, Hounie AG, Shavitt RG, Fossaluza V, Ferrao Y, et al. Trajectory in obsessive-compulsive disorder comorbidities. *Eur Neuropsychopharmacol* (2013) 23(7):594–601. doi: 10.1016/j.euroneuro.2012.08.006
346. Heidari M, Zarei M, Hosseini SM, Taghvaei R, Maleki H, Tabrizi M, et al. Ondansetron or placebo in the augmentation of fluvoxamine response over 8 weeks in obsessive-compulsive disorder. *Int Clin Psychopharmacol* (2014) 29(6):344–50. doi: 10.1097/YIC.0000000000000043
347. Askari N, Moin M, Sanati M, Tajdini M, Hosseini SM, Modabbernia A, et al. Granisetron adjunct to fluvoxamine for moderate to severe obsessive-compulsive disorder: a randomized, double-blind, placebo-controlled trial. *CNS Drugs* (2012) 26(10):883–92. doi: 10.2165/11635850-000000000-00000
348. Erzegovesi S, Cavallini MC, Cavedini P, Diaferia G, Locatelli M, Bellodi L. Clinical predictors of drug response in obsessive-compulsive disorder. *J Clin Psychopharmacol* (2001) 21(5):488–92. doi: 10.1097/00004714-200110000-00006
349. Milad MR, Rauch SL. Obsessive-compulsive disorder: beyond segregated cortico-striatal pathways. *Trends Cogn Sci* (2012) 16(1):43–51. doi: 10.1016/j.tics.2011.11.003
350. Perlmutter SJ, Leitman SF, Garvey MA, Hamburger S, Feldman E, Leonard HL, et al. Therapeutic plasma exchange and intravenous immunoglobulin for obsessive-compulsive disorder and tic disorders in childhood. *Lancet* (1999) 354(9185):1153–8. doi: 10.1016/S0140-6736(98)12297-3
351. Boedhoe PS, Schmaal L, Abe Y, Ameis SH, Arnold PD, Batistuzzo MC, et al. Distinct subcortical volume alterations in pediatric and adult OCD: a worldwide meta- and mega-analysis. *Am J Psychiatry* (2017) 174(1):60–9.
352. Salazar A, Gonzalez-Rivera BL, Redus L, Parrott JM, O'Connor JC. Indoleamine 2,3-dioxygenase mediates anhedonia and anxiety-like behaviors caused by peripheral lipopolysaccharide immune challenge. *Horm Behav* (2012) 62(3):202–9. doi: 10.1016/j.yhbeh.2012.03.010
353. Yang L, Wang M, Guo YY, Sun T, Li YJ, Yang Q, et al. Systemic inflammation induces anxiety disorder through CXCL12/CXCR4 pathway. *Brain Behav Immun* (2016) 56:352–62. doi: 10.1016/j.bbi.2016.03.001
354. Antony JM. Grooming and Growing with Microglia. *Sci Signal* (2010) 3(147):jc8. doi: 10.1126/scisignal.3147jc8
355. Banati RB, Myers R, Kreutzberg GW. PK ('peripheral benzodiazepine')—binding sites in the CNS indicate early and discrete brain lesions: microautoradiographic detection of [3H]PK11195 binding to activated microglia. *J Neurocytol* (1997) 26(2):77–82. doi: 10.1023/A:1018567510105
356. Hannestad J, DellaGioia N, Gallezot JD, Lim K, Nabulsi N, Esterlis I, et al. The neuroinflammation marker translocator protein is not elevated in individuals with mild-to-moderate depression: a [(1)(1)C]PBR28 PET study. *Brain Behav Immun* (2013) 33:131–8. doi: 10.1016/j.bbi.2013.06.010
357. Kreutzberg GW. Microglia: a sensor for pathological events in the CNS. *Trends Neurosci* (1996) 19(8):312–8. doi: 10.1016/0166-2236(96)10049-7
358. Martin A, Boisgard R, Theze B, Van Camp N, Kuhnast B, Damont A, et al. Evaluation of the PBR/TSPO radioligand [(18)F]DPA-714 in a rat model of focal cerebral ischemia. *J Cereb Blood Flow Metab* (2010) 30(1):230–41. doi: 10.1038/jcbfm.2009.205
359. Kumar A, Williams MT, Chugani HT. Evaluation of basal ganglia and thalamic inflammation in children with pediatric autoimmune neuropsychiatric disorders associated with streptococcal infection and Tourette syndrome: a positron emission tomographic (PET) study using 11C-[R]-PK11195. *J Child Neurol* (2015) 30(6):749–56. doi: 10.1177/0883073814543303
360. Fettes P, Schulze L, Downar J. Cortico-striatal-thalamic loop circuits of the orbitofrontal cortex: promising therapeutic targets in psychiatric illness. *Front Syst Neurosci* (2017) 11:25. doi: 10.3389/fnsys.2017.00025
361. Peters SK, Dunlop K, Downar J. Cortico-striatal-thalamic loop circuits of the salience network: a central pathway in psychiatric disease and treatment. *Front Syst Neurosci* (2016) 10:104. doi: 10.3389/fnsys.2016.00104
362. Esalatmanesh S, Abrishami Z, Zeinoddini A, Rahiminejad F, Sadeghi M, Najarzadegan MR, et al. Minocycline combination therapy with fluvoxamine in moderate-to-severe obsessive-compulsive disorder: a placebo-controlled, double-blind, randomized trial. *Psychiatry Clin Neurosci* (2016) 70(11):517–26. doi: 10.1111/pcn.12430
363. Miller AH, Raison CL. Are anti-inflammatory therapies viable treatments for psychiatric disorders? where the rubber meets the road. *JAMA Psychiatry* (2015) 6:527–8. doi: 10.1001/jamapsychiatry.2015.22

7

Genetic Variants of the Brain-Derived Neurotrophic Factor and Metabolic Indices in Veterans with Posttraumatic Stress Disorder

Lucija Tudor[1], Marcela Konjevod[1], Matea Nikolac Perkovic[1], Dubravka Svob Strac[1], Gordana Nedic Erjavec[1], Suzana Uzun[2,3], Oliver Kozumplik[2,3], Marina Sagud[4,5], Zrnka Kovacic Petrovic[2,6] and Nela Pivac[1*]

[1] Laboratory for Molecular Neuropsychiatry, Division of Molecular Medicine, Rudjer Boskovic Institute, Zagreb, Croatia, [2] Department of Biological Psychiatry and Psychogeriatry, University Psychiatric Hospital Vrapce, Zagreb, Croatia, [3] Faculty of Medicine, Josip Juraj Strossmayer University of Osijek, Osijek, Croatia, [4] School of Medicine, University of Zagreb, Zagreb, Croatia, [5] Department of Psychiatry, University Hospital Centre Zagreb, Zagreb, Croatia, [6] Department of Psychopharmacology, Croatian Institute for Brain Research, School of Medicine, University of Zagreb, Zagreb, Croatia

***Correspondence:**
Nela Pivac
npivac@irb.hr

Posttraumatic stress disorder (PTSD) is a trauma and stressor related disorder that may develop after exposure to an event that involved the actual or possible threat of death, violence or serious injury. Its molecular underpinning is still not clear. Brain-derived neurotrophic factor (BDNF) modulates neuronal processes such as the response to stress, but also weight control, energy and glucose homeostasis. Plasma BDNF levels and a functional *BDNF* Val66Met (rs6265) polymorphism were reported to be associated with PTSD, as well as with increased body mass index (BMI) and dyslipidaemia in healthy subjects and patients with cardio-metabolic diseases, but these results are controversial. The other frequently studied *BDNF* polymorphism, C270T (rs56164415), has been associated with the development of different neuropsychiatric symptoms/disorders. As far as we are aware, there are no data on the association of *BDNF* Val66Met and C270T polymorphisms with metabolic indices in PTSD. Due to high rates of obesity and dyslipidaemia in PTSD, the aim of this study was to elucidate the association of *BDNF* Val66Met and C270T polymorphisms with BMI and lipid levels in veterans with PTSD. We hypothesized that *BDNF* variants contribute to susceptibility to metabolic disturbances in PTSD. The study included 333 Caucasian males with combat related PTSD, diagnosed according to DSM-5 criteria. Genotyping of the *BDNF* Val66Met and C270T polymorphisms was performed using the real-time PCR method. Results were analyzed using hierarchical multiple linear regression and the Mann–Whitney test, with *p*-value corrected to 0.005. The results showed that *BDNF* Val66Met and *BDNF* C270T polymorphisms were not significantly associated with BMI, total cholesterol, LDL-cholesterol, HDL-cholesterol or triglycerides. Although the *BDNF* C270T polymorphism was nominally associated only with HDL-cholesterol in veterans with PTSD, this significance disappeared after controlling for the effect of age. Namely, slightly higher plasma HDL values in T allele carriers, compared to CC homozygotes, were associated with differences in age. Our results, controlled for the critical covariates, revealed that *BDNF* Val66Met and C270T were not significantly associated with metabolic indices in veterans with PTSD and that these genetic variants do not contribute to susceptibility to metabolic disturbances in PTSD.

Keywords: *BDNF*, Val66Met, C270T, BMI, plasma lipid levels, metabolic indices, PTSD

INTRODUCTION

Posttraumatic Stress Disorder

Posttraumatic stress disorder (PTSD) is a trauma- and stressor-related disorder (1) that develops in some, but not all individuals exposed to death, threatened death, actual or threatened serious injury, or actual or threatened sexual violence. Its molecular underpinning is still not clear. Various potential stressful events or traumas happen to people during their lifetime, but different populations vary in their exposure to traumatic events (2, 3). PTSD commonly co-occurs with different somatic disorders (4), such as cardiovascular, metabolic, dermatological, musculoskeletal, and pulmonary diseases (5).

Metabolic Disturbances in PTSD

Metabolic complications and components of the metabolic syndrome are associated with increased body mass index (BMI) values or weight gain, and with other clusters of physiological, biochemical, clinical, and metabolic factors that strongly increase the risk of type 2 diabetes and different cardiovascular diseases (6). These metabolic abnormalities include central obesity measured as waist circumference, dyslipidaemia (reduced HDL levels and increased triglyceride levels), high blood pressure, insulin resistance, as well as raised fasting plasma glucose. People with a sedentary life style, who do not exercise, consume a high fat diet and develop these metabolic abnormalities, have increased risk for cardiovascular and metabolic disorders (6).

Metabolic syndrome is frequent in PTSD (7–14). Metabolic complications include insulin resistance (15), higher mean triglycerides, higher blood pressure and fasting glucose levels, and lower HDL values in individuals with PTSD than in subjects from the general population (8). Young US veterans with PTSD had BMI values in the overweight range, higher than controls (15). Similarly, Croatian veterans with combat related PTSD had more frequently comorbid cardiometabolic disorders than control subjects (5), and this population had a high prevalence of obesity (16). Therefore, there is an urgent need for establishing the potential biomarkers of metabolic disturbances in PTSD (17).

Brain-Derived Neurotrophic Factor

The most abundant neurotrophin in the central nervous system is brain-derived neurotrophic factor (BDNF) and it modulates neuronal differentiation, synapse formation, survival, support and function of neurons, brain neurotransmission, proliferation, long-term potentiation, and synaptic growth in the central nervous system (18). Due to its localization and expression in the limbic system, brain regions that are involved in the regulation of fear and stress responses, and its modulatory role in dopaminergic, serotonergic and glutamatergic synthesis, metabolism, neuronal activity and release (18, 19), it is not surprising that BDNF is involved in the development of different neuropsychiatric disorders, including PTSD (19–21).

BDNF Genetic Variants

In humans, BDNF is encoded by the *BDNF* gene which extends over 70 kb, located on chromosome 11, region p13–14 (22). There are hundreds of polymorphisms in the *BDNF* gene, however, the most frequently studied functional polymorphisms include the Val66Met single-nucleotide polymorphism (rs6265) in the coding exon (23), and the C270T single-nucleotide polymorphism (rs56164415), in the 5′-untranslated region (UTR) of the *BDNF* gene (24). The A (Met) allele, compared to the G (Val) allele, of the *BDNF* Val66Met is associated with disrupted cellular processing, trafficking and intracellular packaging of the pro-BDNF and reduced activity-dependent secretion of the mature BDNF (23, 25). The other polymorphism, *BDNF* C270T, in the *BDNF* 5'-non-coding region (26), may affect *BDNF* expression (27) and might lead to regionally specific quantitative BDNF disbalance in the brain (24). Consequently, both BDNF polymorphisms, *BDNF* Val66Met (19, 28) and *BDNF* C270T (24, 29) have been associated with different neuropsychiatric disorders.

BDNF and PTSD

In patients with PTSD, inconsistent findings were reported regarding peripheral BDNF levels: blood levels were reported to be decreased (30), unchanged (31, 32), or increased (15, 33, 34). However, a meta-analysis did not confirm a significant association between BDNF levels and PTSD (35), which is in line with no significant relationship between cerebrospinal fluid BDNF levels and PTSD (36). There are conflicting findings on the relationship between *BDNF* genetic variants and PTSD (21, 37–40). The association between *BDNF* Val66Met and PTSD was confirmed in only one study (40), while other studies failed to detect a significant association (41–45). The association between PTSD and the other C270T polymorphism in the *BDNF* gene was investigated in two individual case-control studies, producing opposite results: positive (46) as well as no (45) association.

BDNF and Metabolic Complications

The localization of BDNF in the hippocampus and the hypothalamus explains its moderating effects on energy metabolism, homeostasis, metabolic regulation (47, 48), weight control, fasting and feeding (49, 50). BDNF is located also in lungs, heart, spleen, gastrointestinal tract and liver, and it is involved in the development of cardiovascular and metabolic disorders, metabolic syndrome (51), and body weight gain (52, 53). In the blood, BDNF is stored mainly in platelets and released into plasma (54), but it is also synthesized and released from different cell types including cells from the cardiovascular system (55, 56), pancreatic beta cells, as well as cells from adipose tissue (57). BDNF exhibits an anorexigenic effect and suppresses food intake (48). A sedentary life style, overweight, obesity and lack of exercise are related to reduced BDNF signaling and increased activity of the sympathetic nervous system, decreased activity of the parasympathetic outflow, increased heart rate, blood pressure, elevated inflammation, and reduced gut motility (49).

There are conflicting data regarding an association of plasma or serum BDNF levels and metabolic indices. Reduced BDNF levels were detected in patients with type 2 diabetes (58), metabolic or coronary syndromes (57, 59, 60), non-obese and non-diabetic subjects with acute coronary syndrome (60), and in patients with angina pectoris (61). Increased BDNF levels were found in a population based study showing a positive association with increased risk for obesity, metabolic syndrome and coronary disease (51, 62). In contrast, in another study, subjects with or without metabolic syndrome had similar serum BDNF levels (63). A recent meta-analysis found lower BDNF levels associated with the presence of metabolic syndrome in healthy adult subjects (64). On the other hand, a longitudinal study including a large community-based cohort (65) detected higher serum BDNF levels significantly associated with lower risk of cardiovascular diseases and mortality, independent of markers of low-grade inflammation, BMI, physical activity, and depression.

BDNF gene variants were studied as risk factors for metabolic complications, such as BMI, dyslipidaemia, obesity, insulin resistance (66–68) and eating disorders (19). The A allele of the *BDNF* Val66Met polymorphism has been associated with higher BMI in adult women (69) and in young preschool children (70), but not in older healthy individuals (71). When these adult healthy groups were enlarged, a significant association was found between BMI categories and *BDNF* Val66Met (52, 72), since the A allele was more frequently found in the group with normal weight (52, 72–74). In conformation, obese subjects more frequently had the G allele of the *BDNF* Val66Met (73, 75). As far as we are aware, the reports on the association between the *BDNF* C270T polymorphism and BMI or plasma lipid levels in humans have not been studied.

In addition, to the best of our knowledge, there are no data on the association of *BDNF* Val66Met and *BDNF* C270T polymorphisms with metabolic indices in PTSD. Due to the high rates of both obesity and dyslipidaemia in PTSD, the aim of this study was to elucidate the association of *BDNF* Val66Met and *BDNF* C270T polymorphisms with BMI and lipid levels in veterans with PTSD. We hypothesized that *BDNF* variants might contribute to susceptibility to metabolic disturbances in PTSD and that these *BDNF* metabolic-risk variants might be more frequently present in patients with PTSD in comparison to healthy subjects or other diagnostic categories.

METHODS

Participants

The study included 333 male veterans with combat related PTSD, with median Clinician Administered PTSD Scale (CAPS) scores of 86 (range 68–102). They were all unrelated Caucasian subjects of Croatian origin. The diagnosis of current and chronic PTSD was done using SCID based on DSM-5 criteria (1). Participants were sampled consecutively in the University Psychiatric Hospital Vrapce, Zagreb, from September 2015 to June 2017. They were exposed to similar potentially traumatic events during the Homeland war in Croatia. Inclusion criteria were in- and out-patients aged 38–77 years. Exclusion criteria were: drug abuse, alcohol dependence or pathophysiological changes in the liver, such as fibrosis, sclerosis, cirrhosis and malignant liver disease [alcoholic liver cirrhosis (K70.3), alcoholic liver fibrosis and sclerosis (K70.2) and hepatocellular carcinoma (C22.0), according to ICD-10], schizophrenia, bipolar disorder, adult ADHD, Alzheimer's disease (according to DSM-5 criteria), current or recent (previous 3 months) use of lipid-lowering agents, antihypertensive and antidiabetic medication. The study was approved by the Ethics Committee of the University Psychiatric Hospital Vrapce, Zagreb, Croatia, and was carried out in accordance with the Helsinki declaration (1975), as revised in 1983. All patients have signed informed consent prior to study procedures.

Anthropological Measures

Height of subjects wearing no shoes was measured with a meter to the nearest 0.5 cm; whereas body weight of subjects was measured with a digital scale to the nearest 0.1 kg. BMI was calculated as ratio of weight (kg) over height (m^2).

Measurements of the Metabolic Indices

Blood samples were collected between 7:30 a.m. and 8:00 a.m. after overnight fasting. Total cholesterol (normal values <5 mmol/l) was determined with cholesterol oxidase-phenol aminophenazone method and the absorbance read on a Siemens Dimension Xpand analyser. Triglycerides (normal values <1.7 mmol/l), LDL (normal values <3 mmol/l), and HDL (normal values >1.2 mmol/L) were determined using the enzymatic-colorimetric assay and were analyzed with Siemens Dimension Xpand analyser.

Genotyping

Genomic DNA was isolated from peripheral blood using a salting out method (76). *BDNF* Val66Met (rs6265) and C270T (rs56164415) were determined with TaqMan® Genotyping Assays (Applied Biosystems, Foster City, CA, USA) following the manufacturer's protocol on an Applied Biosystems® 7300 Real-Time PCR System apparatus. The 10 μL reaction volume contained around 20 ng of DNA. Assay IDs were C_11592758_10 for rs6265 and C_89097201_10 for rs56164415. Around 10% of randomly selected samples were genotyped again as a quality control for genotyping assays.

Minor allele frequency (MAF) for *BDNF* Val66Met in our sample was 19% (A allele), which is in accordance with the MAF of 20% (A allele) in the European population (77). In our

European sample, MAF for *BDNF* C270T was 17% (T allele), while 1000 Genomes reports much smaller frequency of T allele (6%) in this population.

Since there were only 6 AA genotype carriers (of the *BDNF* Val66Met) and 3 TT genotype carriers (of the *BDNF* C270T) in the whole sample, we assessed only the dominant model for the *BDNF* Val66Met: A carriers (AA + AG) vs. GG homozygous genotype, and the dominant model for the *BDNF* C270T: T carriers (TT + TC) vs. CC homozygous genotype (78, 79).

Statistical Analysis

All data regarding lipid levels, BMI and age failed to reach normal distribution (Kolmogorov-Smirnov test). The data were expressed as median, 25th (Q1) and 75th (Q3) percentile after excluding outliers. Outliers were determined as values that lie below Q1–1.5 interquartile range (IQR) or above Q3+1.5 IQR. Hierarchical multiple linear regression was used to determine possible effect of age, smoking, BMI, *BDNF* Val66Met, and *BDNF* C270T on each metabolic parameter after excluding outliers. The data were evaluated with the non-parametric Mann-Whitney test for each metabolic parameter using Sigma Stat 3.5 (Jandell Scientific Corp. San Raphael, California, USA). For determination of the linkage disequilibrium (LD) between *BDNF* Val66Met and C270T loci, we used Haploview software v. 4.2 (80). Loci are considered to be in high LD if the D' coefficient is >0.80 and logarithm of odds (LOD) ≥ 2 (80, 81). In our study these two loci were not in high LD since the D′ coefficient was <0.80 (D′ = 0.36; LOD = 0.32). Therefore, we did not perform haplotype analysis. Due to multiple ($N = 10$) comparisons (testing the association of 2 single nucleotide polymorphisms (SNPs) with 5 metabolic indices=10), a Bonferroni correction was performed and p-value was set to $p = 0.005$. Before the study G*Power 3 Software (82) was used to determine the required sample size and actual statistical power. For hierarchical multiple linear regression, with $p = 0.005$; medium effect size = 0.25; and power $(1 - \beta) = 0.800$; number of predictors = 5; the required sample size was 142. For the Mann–Whitney test, with $p = 0.005$; medium effect size = 0.15; and power $(1 - \beta) = 0.800$; the required sample size was 217. Since the study included 333 participants in the beginning, and 294–311 participants after the removal of outliers, it had adequate sample size and statistical power to detect significant differences among the groups.

RESULTS

Clinical Data

Demographic and clinical data, including age, levels of total, HDL and LDL cholesterol, triglyceride levels, and BMI, of veterans with PTSD are presented in **Table 1**. Initially, the study enrolled 333 subjects. However, after removal of the outliers for each metabolic parameter (values that were lower than Q1–1.5 IQR or higher Q3+1.5 IQR in our sample), there were $N = 294$ participants for HDL (removed HDL values ≤0.5 and HDL ≥ 2.0), $N = 316$ for BMI (removed BMI values ≤19); $N = 315$ for cholesterol (removed cholesterol values ≥8.4), $N = 311$ for LDL (removed LDL values ≥5.7 and LDL ≤0.2) and $N = 303$ for triglycerides (removed triglyceride values ≥3.8), respectively.

TABLE 1 | Demographic and clinical data of veterans with PTSD.

	N	Median (25th; 75th)	Min–Max
Age (years)	333	56 (51; 63)	38–77
TC (mmol/L)	315	5.20 (4.50; 6.00)	2.90–8.10
HDL (mmol/L)	294	1.20 (1.10; 1.40)	0.80–1.80
LDL (mmol/L)	311	2.80 (2.40; 3.60)	0.90–5.60
TG (mmol/L)	303	1.60 (1.30; 2.20)	0.60–3.70
BMI (kg/m^2)	316	28.03 (25.85; 30.45)	20.32–35.92

Results are presented as median and 25th (Q1) and 75th (Q3) percentiles. N is number of subjects after removing outliers. PTSD, posttraumatic stress disorder; TC, total cholesterol; HDL, high density lipoprotein cholesterol; LDL, low density lipoprotein cholesterol; TG, triglycerides; BMI, body mass index.

The Effect of Age, Smoking, BMI, and *BDNF* Polymorphisms on Metabolic Parameters

Hierarchical multiple linear regression was performed in order to assess the influence of various independent variables, such as age, smoking, BMI, and *BDNF* Val66Met and *BDNF* C270T on different metabolic parameters (dependent variables) (**Table 2**). It was designed in the following way: for all metabolic indices, except BMI, the first step included age, BMI, and smoking status as dependent variables, and the second step *BDNF* Val66Met genotype (dominant model) and *BDNF* C2790T genotype (dominant model). For BMI, age, and smoking were entered as dependent variables in the first step, while both genotypes were added in the second one. Hierarchical multiple regression revealed age as the only significant ($p < 0.001$) variable influencing HDL and triglycerides, while other variables were not significantly associated with metabolic indices due to Bonferroni corrected significance ($p = 0.005$).

BDNF Val66Met and *BDNF* C270T Polymorphisms and Metabolic Indices

Table 3 shows that metabolic parameters did not differ significantly between individuals with PTSD subdivided into A carriers (AA+AG) vs. homozygous GG genotype carriers of *BDNF* Val66Met, as well as between T carriers (TT+CT) vs. CC genotype carriers of the *BDNF* C270T. Namely, no significant differences between A carriers and GG homozygotes of the *BDNF* Val66Met polymorphism, were detected in the BMI values ($p = 0.979$), plasma concentrations of total ($p = 0.933$), HDL ($p = 0.829$), and LDL (p=0.146) cholesterol, as well as triglycerides ($p = 0.409$). In the case of the *BDNF* C270T polymorphism, similar results were observed. The Mann Whitney test revealed that BMI ($p = 0.822$), plasma concentrations of total ($p = 0.738$) and LDL ($p = 0.290$) cholesterol, as well as triglyceride ($p = 0.092$) levels were similar in T carriers and CC homozygotes. However, HDL levels differed nominally ($p = 0.006$) between T carriers and CC homozygotes of the *BDNF* C270T polymorphism. Since this association was not confirmed using hierarchical multiple linear regression, the observed difference in HDL levels was

TABLE 2 | Hierarchical multiple linear regression showing variables influencing different metabolic parameters.

		TC	HDL	LDL	TG	BMI
Step 1	Model summary	adjR^2 = −0.006; ΔR^2 = 0.005; F = 0.449; p = 0.718	adjR^2 = 0.065; ΔR^2 = 0.076; F = 7.355; p < 0.001;	adjR^2 = −0.004; ΔR^2 = 0.006; F = 0.621; p = 0.602;	adjR^2 = 0.042; ΔR^2 = 0.052; F = 5.057; p = 0.002;	adjR^2 = −0.003; ΔR^2 = 0.004; F = 0.577; p = 0.652;
	Age	β = −0.051; p = 0.387	β = −0.246; p < 0.001	β = 0.039; p = 0.508	β = 3.406; p = 0.001	β = 0.015; p = 0.804
	BMI	β = 0.034; p = 0.564	β = 0.129; p = 0.029	β = −0.070; p = 0.237	β = −0.012; p = 0.835	-
	Smoking	β = 0.032; p = 0.583	β = 0.008; p = 0.896	β = −0.015; p = 0.798	β = 0.116; p = 0.050	β = −0.061; p = 0.299
Step 2	Model summary	adjR^2 = −0.006; ΔR^2 = 0.006; F = 0.637; p = 0.672;	adjR^2 = 0.065; ΔR^2 = 0.007; F = 4.820; p < 0.001;	adjR^2 = −0.008; ΔR^2 = 0.003; F = 0.537; p = 0.746;	adjR^2 = 0.040; ΔR^2 = 0.005; F = 3.337; p = 0.006;	adjR^2 = −0.010; ΔR^2 = 0.000; F = 0.300; p = 0.878;
	Age	β = −0.023; p = 0.714	β = −0.216; p = 0.001	β = 0.037; p = 0.552	β = 2.922; p = 0.004	β = 0.014; p = 0.820
	BMI	β = 0.033; p = 0.573	β = 0.128; p = 0.030	β = −0.070; p = 0.209	β = −0.012; p = 0.842	-
	Smoking	b = 0.035; p = 0.557	β = 0.009; p = 0.877	β = −0.015; p = 0.806	β = 0.113; p = 0.055	β = −0.061; p = 0.302
	BDNF Val66Met	β = −0.020; p = 0.735	β = 0.007; p = 0.908	β = −0.050; p = 0.398	β = 0.062; p = 0.298	β = −0.013; p = 0.828
	BDNF C270T	β = −0.084; p = 0.180	β = −0.088; p = 0.162	β = 0.016; p = 0.803	β = 0.048; p = 0.434	b = −0.004; p = 0.953

A carriers (AA + AG) combined genotypes of the BDNF Val66Met; T carriers (TT + TC) combined genotypes of the BDNF C270T; BDNF, brain derived neurotrophic factor; BMI, body mass index; TC, total cholesterol; HDL: high density lipoprotein cholesterol; LDL, low density lipoprotein cholesterol; TG, triglycerides.

presumably associated with the age differences between these groups.

Therefore, as age was a significant ($p < 0.001$) variable that affects HDL and triglycerides in the regression model, and HDL levels were nominally ($p = 0.006$) different between T carriers and CC homozygotes, to further evaluate this age-related, but also *BDNF* C270T -related influence, patients were additionally subdivided into 3 age groups. Since the age range of the patients was 38–77, we subdivided participants into approximately 13-year age groups, i.e., into individuals between the ages of 38 and 51 ($N = 76$ for HDL, and $N = 74$ for triglycerides after removing outliers), ages 52–65 ($N = 162$ for HDL, $N = 171$ for triglycerides), and ages 66–77 ($N = 56$ for HDL and $N = 58$ for triglycerides). The Mann-Whitney test demonstrated no significant ($p > 0.005$) differences between *BDNF* Val66Met A vs. GG genotype carriers, and between *BDNF* C270T T vs. CC genotype carriers in HDL and triglyceride levels (**Table 4**) in each age group. These results revealed that these two polymorphisms were not significantly associated with HDL and triglyceride levels in any of the age groups. Nevertheless, median HDL values (**Table 4**) showed a decline (as evidenced by the multiple linear regression analysis: $\beta = -0.243$) with increased age in both T and CC genotype carriers.

DISCUSSION

The results of this study revealed that in a homogeneous sample of middle-aged Caucasian (Croatian origin) veterans with combat related PTSD: (1) *BDNF* Val66Met and *BDNF* C270T polymorphisms were not significantly associated with BMI or plasma lipid levels; (2) the presence of one or two T alleles of *BDNF* C270T polymorphism was related to slightly (nominally) higher HDL cholesterol values; but this association disappeared after controlling for the influence of age.

In the present study, veterans had chronic and current PTSD, and moderate PTSD symptoms, as revealed by their mean CAPS scores of 86 (range 68–102) (83). Their lipid levels were either slightly higher (total cholesterol and triglycerides) or within the normal laboratory range (i.e., for HDL and LDL cholesterol levels). Data from the literature regarding lipid levels in PTSD are inconsistent (84). Similar HDL and LDL cholesterol levels were found in different groups of Caucasian veterans with PTSD of the same origin (85), or in Japanese civilians with PTSD, who were victims of sarin poisoning (86). Further, HDL levels did not differ between civilian participants with and without PTSD (87, 88). Similarly, PTSD was associated with unchanged LDL cholesterol levels (89, 90). Other studies found dyslipidaemia, i.e., increased cholesterol, triglyceride, and LDL cholesterol levels in PTSD (88, 91–93). In contrast to our data, some studies have detected lower HDL cholesterol levels in PTSD (89, 90, 94), or similar triglyceride levels in large groups of community-living adults with or without PTSD (87). Further, cholesterol, LDL cholesterol and triglyceride levels did not differ between participants with PTSD compared to non-PTSD individuals (94). Dyslipidaemia and increased BMI are risk factors for various cardiovascular diseases and myocardial

TABLE 3 | The metabolic parameters of veterans with PTSD subdivided according to the *BDNF* Val66Met and *BDNF* C270T genetic variants.

	SNP	*BDNF* Val66Met		*BDNF* C270T	
	Genotype	**A carriers**	**GG carriers**	**T carriers**	**CC carriers**
BMI (kg/m^2)	Median	27.75	27.91	27.77	28.06
	Percentile 25th; 75th	26.26; 30.11	25.69; 30.47	25.86; 30.47	26.03; 30.45
	Min; Max	20.32; 35.92	20.76; 35.71	20.76; 33.91	21.26; 35.92
	Statistics	$U = 10581.00$; $p = 0.979$		$U = 10743.50$; $p = 0.822$	
TC (mmol/L)	Median	5.20	5.20	5.20	4.90
	Percentile 5th; 75th	4.50; 5.70	4.50; 6.10	4.50; 6.10	4.50; 6.00
	Min; Max	2.90; 8.10	2.90; 7.90	3.00; 8.10	2.90; 7.90
	Statistics	$U = 10485.00$; $p = 0.933$		$U = 10555.00$; $p = 0.738$	
HDL (mmol/L)	Median	1.20	1.20	1.20	1.20
	Percentile 25th; 75th	1.10; 1.40	1.10; 1.40	1.10; 1.50	1.10; 1.30
	Min; Max	0.80; 1.80	0.80; 1.80	0.80; 1.80	0.80; 1.80
	Statistics	$U = 9065.50$; $p = 0.829$		$U = 7561.50$; $p = 0.006$	
LDL (mmol/L)	Median	3.00	2.80	2.80	2.90
	Percentile 25th; 75th	2.40; 3.60	2.30; 3.50	2.20; 3.60	2.40; 3.60
	Min; Max	0.90; 5.40	0.90; 5.60	0.90; 5.60	0.90; 5.40
	Statistics	$U = 9157.00$; $p = 0.146$		$U = 9658.00$; $p = 0.290$	
TG (mmol/L)	Median	1.60	1.60	1.55	1.60
	Percentile 25th; 75th	1.30; 2.10	1.30; 2.20	1.20; 2.10	1.30; 2.30
	Min; Max	0.60; 3.70	0.60; 3.70	0.60; 3.70	0.60; 3.70
	Statistics	$U = 9165.50$; $p = 0.409$		$U = 8637.00$; $p = 0.092$	

Results are presented as median and 25th (Q1) and 75th (Q3) percentiles after excluding outliers. A carriers (AA + AG) of the BDNF Val66Met; GG (GG homozygous genotype) carriers of the BDNF Val66Met; T carriers (TT + TC) of the BDNF C270T; CC carriers (CC homozygous genotype) of the BDNF C270T; BDNF: brain derived neurotrophic factor; BMI, Body mass index; HDL, high density lipoprotein cholesterol; LDL, low density lipoprotein cholesterol; PTSD, posttraumatic stress disorder; TC, total cholesterol; TG, triglycerides.

infarction in all subjects (6), especially individuals with PTSD (4, 8, 10, 13). Therefore, careful monitoring of these patients is warranted to prevent development of cardiometabolic disorders. The current investigation included patients with PTSD without cardiovascular diseases and the exclusion criteria included taking cardiovascular drugs or statins, but their mean BMI values of almost 28 suggest that the majority of participants were overweight. This is in line with data obtained with the different groups of Croatian veterans with PTSD (16) but also with data from a Croatian population sample (16), and with findings from young military US veterans with PTSD, who were all overweight (15). All these findings suggest that overweight, obesity and dyslipidaemia are becoming health risks in PTSD, but also global health problems in the general population. Various risk factors such as different diagnoses and sizes of the groups, civilian or military individuals, diet, food, sedentary life style and physical activity, age, exercise, alcohol dependence, and smoking might affect BMI and lipid levels. As this study did not intend to compare BMI and lipid levels between individuals with PTSD and control subjects, we may conclude that our results on the lipid levels and BMI are in line with most of the cited data.

There was one study showing positive association (40) and others reporting no associations (41–45) between *BDNF* Val66Met and PTSD. In our previous study that included different groups of war veterans (42), the frequency of the *BDNF* Val66Met genotypes did not differ between veterans with or without PTSD. Therefore, the present study with other groups of veterans with PTSD did not evaluate this possible association and did not include control subjects. The explanation for these inconsistent findings might be sought in the frequency of trauma exposure, traumatic load, early traumatic experience and stressful life events, age, and other study conditions among the participants (21).

We did not confirm our hypothesis that *BDNF* variants contributed to susceptibility to metabolic disturbances in PTSD. In our study *BDNF* Val66Met polymorphism was not

TABLE 4 | The HDL and TG values in different age groups of veterans with PTSD subdivided according to the *BDNF* Val66Met and *BDNF* C270T genetic variants.

	Age group	**38–51 years**		**52–65 years**		**66–77 years**	
***BDNF* Val66Met**	**Genotype**	**A carriers ($N = 32$)**	**GG carriers ($N = 44$)**	**A carriers ($N = 56$)**	**GG carriers ($N = 106$)**	**A carriers ($N = 15$)**	**GG carriers ($N = 41$)**
HDL (mmol/L)	Median	1.30	1.30	1.20	1.20	1.20	1.10
	Percentile 25th; 75th	1.10; 1.50	1.10; 1.50	1.00; 1.30	1.10; 1.30	1.10; 1.20	1.00; 1.20
	Min; Max	0.80; 1.80	0.80; 1.80	0.80; 1.80	0.80; 1.80	0.90; 1.40	0.80; 1.80
	Statistics	$U = 690.00$; $p = 0.754$		$U = 2740.50$; $p = 0.660$		$U = 161.50$; $p = 0.149$	
***BDNF* Val66Met**	**Genotype**	**A carriers ($N = 32$)**	**GG carriers ($N = 42$)**	**A carriers ($N = 58$)**	**GG carriers ($N = 113$)**	**A carriers ($N = 15$)**	**GG carriers ($N = 43$)**
TG (mmol/L)	Median	1.50	1.60	1.60	1.60	1.50	2.20
	Percentile 25th; 75th	1.30; 1.80	1.20; 1.80	1.30; 2.20	1.20; 2.20	0.90; 2.20	1.50; 3.20
	Min; Max	0.60; 2.70	0.60; 3.70	0.60; 3.70	0.60; 3.70	0.70; 3.70	0.70; 3.70
	Statistics	$U = 639.50$; $p = 0.721$		$U = 3135.50$; $p = 0.790$		$U = 139.00$; $p = 0.042$	
***BDNF* C270T**	**Genotype**	**T carriers ($N = 38$)**	**CC carriers ($N = 38$)**	**T carriers ($N = 52$)**	**CC carriers ($N = 110$)**	**T carriers ($N = 4$)**	**CC carriers ($N = 52$)**
HDL (mmol/L)	Median	1.30	1.30	1.20	1.20	1.10	1.10
	Percentile 25th; 75th	1.10; 1.50	1.10; 1.50	1.10; 1.50	1.10; 1.20	1.00; 1.45	1.00; 1.20
	Min; Max	0.80; 1.80	0.80; 1.80	0.80; 1.80	0.80; 1.80	0.90; 1.80	0.80; 1.80
	Statistics	$U = 723.00$; $p = 0.992$		$U = 2333.00$; $p = 0.054$		$U = 106.00$; $p = 0.963$	
***BDNF* C270T**	**Genotype**	**T carriers ($N = 34$)**	**CC carriers ($N = 40$)**	**T carriers ($N = 56$)**	**CC carriers ($N = 115$)**	**T carriers ($N = 4$)**	**CC carriers ($N = 54$)**
TG (mmol/L)	Median	1.55	1.50	1.55	1.60	1.55	2.20
	Percentile 25th; 75th	1.30; 1.80	1.20; 1.80	1.20; 2.00	1.30; 2.30	1.35; 1.90	1.50; 2.70
	Min; Max	0.80; 3.70	0.60; 3.40	0.60; 3.60	0.60; 3.70	1.20; 2.20	0.70; 3.70
	Statistics	$U = 632.00$; $p = 0.463$		$U = 2945.50$; $p = 0.365$		$U = 66.50$; $p = 0.212$	

Results are presented as median and 25th (Q1) and 75th (Q3) percentiles after excluding outliers. A carriers (AA + AG) of the BDNF Val66Met (rs6265); GG (GG homozygous genotype) carriers of the BDNF Val66Met; T carriers (TT + TC) of the BDNF C270T; CC carriers (CC homozygous genotype) of the BDNF C270T; BDNF, brain derived neurotrophic factor; HDL, high density lipoprotein cholesterol; PTSD, posttraumatic stress disorder; TG, triglycerides.

significantly associated with metabolic indices in Caucasian veterans with PTSD. Namely, BMI values, as well as plasma total cholesterol, triglycerides, HDL and LDL cholesterol levels did not differ significantly in veterans with PTSD subdivided into carriers of the A allele (AA+AG) or the GG homozygous genotype of *BDNF* Val66Met polymorphism. As there are no such data in the literature, we might presume that this study is the first to show no association of *BDNF* Val66Met variants with BMI in combat veterans with PTSD. In line with our data, BMI was not significantly different in A carriers compared to GG genotype carriers of the *BDNF* Val66Met in elderly healthy Chinese subjects (95), or in elderly healthy individuals who were followed longitudinally (71). However, there are conflicting results in the literature regarding this polymorphism and BMI in control subjects. Opposing data were reported showing that the A allele was associated with higher BMI in healthy adult subjects (96), adult women (69), and in young preschool children (70). On the other hand, there are also data showing that A carriers were more frequently found in the group with lower BMI in a large Korean epidemiological cohort (74), in a large cohort of male Boston Puerto Rican subjects (67), adult healthy Caucasian women (73, 75), healthy control male and female subjects from the same population of Caucasian subjects of Croatian origin (52, 72), or in children and adolescents (97). A recent meta-analysis confirmed only one *BDNF* SNP, rs925946, significantly related to obesity and BMI in large groups of healthy subjects (98). Discrepancies in the results could be explained by the different diagnostic groups (PTSD vs. controls), ethnic background (19, 99, 100), age, gender, living environment, diet, lifestyle, and smoking (95). Since recently a strong LD between

BDNF rs6265 and rs10501087 was reported, suggesting that these two SNPs are dependent genetic markers associated with BMI (98), in future studies this *BDNF* SNP, rs10501087, should be also evaluated.

Our study did not detect any significant association between *BDNF* Val66Met and lipid levels in PTSD. There are no findings in the literature regarding the association between *BDNF* Val66Met and lipid levels in PTSD. However, in volunteers without kidney and cardiovascular diseases, no association was found between *BDNF* Val66Met polymorphism and serum TG and HDL cholesterol levels (63). This finding agrees with the results from our study, since our veterans with PTSD, who did not have any cardiovascular or metabolic diseases, had similar plasma lipid levels when subdivided into carriers of different *BDNF* Val66Met variants. In children and adolescents from the general population, the *BDNF* Val66Met polymorphism was not associated with any of the lipid indices (97). In contrast to our study and cited (63, 97) findings, the presence of one or two A alleles of the *BDNF* Val66Met was significantly associated with lower HDL cholesterol levels and higher risk for obesity in old and very old Chinese healthy subjects (95). In that particular study subjects carrying the A allele had elevated triglyceride levels, but reduced HDL cholesterol levels compared to the GG genotype carriers (95). The differences between studies are in the diagnosis (PTSD vs. normal controls) and in the age of included subjects (i.e., Peng's study included three groups: age ≥90; age 60–77; and age 60–75, while our veterans were on average 56 years old). To control for the effect of age, in our study participants with PTSD were subdivided into different age groups (age range 38–51, 52–65, and 66–77 years), and their plasma HDL and triglyceride levels (that were significantly affected by age in the hierarchical regression analysis) did not differ between *BDNF* Val66Met A vs. GG genotype carriers and between *BDNF* C270T T vs. CC genotype carriers. In addition, the observed differences between studies might be due to ethnicity (Chinese vs. Caucasian subjects), since there were significant ethnic related differences in the frequency of the *BDNF* Val66Met genotypes, especially the frequency of the AA genotype, between Asian and Caucasian subjects (100).

Unlike *BDNF* Val66Met, the *BDNF* C270T polymorphism has only recently gained attention in studies of neuropsychiatric disorders (101). The T allele of the *BDNF* C270T polymorphism was reported to be a risk factor for PTSD (46), schizophrenia (29), bulimia nervosa (102), and amyotrophic lateral sclerosis (24), but not for Alzheimer's disease (78). The T allele prevalence in our study was 17% and it was the same as the T allele frequency in a Chinese sample with PTSD (46). This frequency differs significantly from the T allele frequency in our healthy Caucasian subjects (6%, unpublished data) and in the general East Asian population [6%, (77)] or in other diagnostic groups. Namely, in Caucasian patients with schizophrenia this frequency was around 8% (29), while in Caucasian patients with bulimia nervosa and control subjects it was around 5% (102). Higher prevalence of the T allele in our Caucasian subjects and in Chinese subjects with PTSD (46) compared to control subjects (102) and patients with schizophrenia (29) or bulimia (102), might be an outcome of different clinical diagnoses (PTSD vs. schizophrenia vs. bulimia nervosa/controls). This is also supported by the fact that no obvious ethnic differences in *BDNF* C270T genotype frequency were found in a recent meta-analysis (78) and reported by The 1000 Genomes Project Consortium (77), with the exception of South Asian populations (India, Bangladesh, Pakistan) where the T allele is present in 29% of population.

The *BDNF* C270T polymorphism was related to PTSD in one study, since the T allele frequency was significantly higher in a group with sporadic PTSD compared to a control group (46). Another study did not find a significant association, but this trial comprised only 96 subjects with PTSD (45). Since in our study we have not compared the frequency of the *BDNF* C270T genotypes in PTSD vs. controls, we cannot confirm or reject this finding.

This investigation has not found a significant association between *BDNF* C270T and BMI, total cholesterol, LDL cholesterol and triglyceride levels in veterans with PTSD. A slight association between *BDNF* C270T and HDL cholesterol in veterans with PTSD was detected, as carriers of the T alleles had nominally higher HDL cholesterol levels than CC carriers. This significance did not survive a Bonferroni correction, and was not confirmed by hierarchical multiple regression and further testing. Only HDL and triglyceride levels were affected by age. Other metabolic indices were not associated with age, smoking, *BDNF* Val66Met or *BDNF* C270T polymorphisms. To further evaluate these findings, HDL and triglyceride levels were evaluated in participants subdivided into 13-year age groups, i.e., into individuals in the age range from 38 to 51, from 52 to 65, and from 66 to 77 years, although we are aware of the limited power due to the stratification of data into smaller groups. HDL and triglyceride levels did not differ between *BDNF* Val66Met A allele carriers vs. GG genotype carriers, and between *BDNF* C270T T allele carriers vs. CC genotype carriers. As both *BDNF* C270T T allele carriers and CC genotype carriers showed reduced median HDL values in older age, these results confirmed that HDL was affected by age and not by the presence of the T allele.

There are no other data on the association of this *BDNF* C270T polymorphism and HDL cholesterol in PTSD, and there are no data showing either a positive association or no association between *BDNF* C270T polymorphism and BMI, total cholesterol, LDL cholesterol and triglyceride levels in PTSD. Although this was the first study to evaluate a link between BDNF C270T and metabolic indices in PTSD, no associations were found between either of the variants and these metabolic indices. One study reported that *BDNF* C270T polymorphism was not associated with BMI in patients with anorexia nervosa and bulimia nervosa (103), while another found a significant association between the T allele of the *BDNF* C270T polymorphism and lower BMI in bulimia nervosa (102). The discrepancies between these and our study might be explained by the differences in diagnoses (PTSD vs. eating disorders).

Our results did not confirm our hypothesis that *BDNF* Val66Met and C270T variants contribute to susceptibility to metabolic disturbances in PTSD. Lower HDL cholesterol values were detected in older individuals with PTSD, but were not associated with any of the *BDNF* Val66Met and C270T genotypes. Routine monitoring of individuals with PTSD, in terms of HDL cholesterol levels, might prevent possible cardiovascular events including myocardial infarction, that are frequent in PTSD (5, 17, 84).

Some limitations need to be considered in interpreting these results: the study included only Caucasian PTSD veterans, and all participants were males. Therefore, we could not compare our data with those in control subjects, and we could not evaluate possible ethnic and gender related differences. In this study we included only the two SNPs (*BDNF* Val66Met and C270T polymorphisms), so additional *BDNF* gene polymorphisms should be included in future studies, such as those evaluated in healthy control subjects: *BDNF* rs12291063 polymorphism associated with BMI and obesity (104), *BDNF* rs10767664 polymorphism associated with BMI, weight, fat mass, waist circumference, LDL cholesterol and total cholesterol (105), or *BDNF* rs925946 polymorphism associated with BMI (98), or GWAS data. Data on physical activity and eating habits were not collected. A significant limitation of this study is a lack of replication sample.

Advantages of the present study are the use of a fairly large group of veterans with PTSD, sampled from the same center, and in the fact that diagnosis and screening for PTSD was done by psychiatrists using SCID and CAPS. We also took into account alcohol dependence and use of statins and cardiovascular drugs, we removed outliers, carefully monitored the confounders by a hierarchical multiple linear regression, used a homogeneous group of Caucasians of Croatian origin with similar combat trauma exposure and ensured that the study had the required sample size and statistical power.

CONCLUSION

This is a first report showing that variants of the *BDNF* Val66Met and *BDNF* C270T polymorphisms were not associated with BMI or plasma lipid levels in veterans with PTSD. Our findings suggest that *BDNF* Val66Met and C270T variants do not contribute to susceptibility to metabolic disturbances in PTSD. Other metabolic indices and other *BDNF* and other gene variants should be evaluated as metabolic risk factors in PTSD in further larger multi-ethnic studies, including females, larger sample-sizes, with well-matched controls.

AUTHOR CONTRIBUTIONS

NP developed the original idea. LT, MK, MNP, DSS, and GNE managed the experimental work, collected blood samples, isolated DNA and did the BDNF rs6265 and rs56164415 genotyping, and processed data for analysis. LT performed the statistical analysis. SU, OK, and ZKP explained the research goals and described protocol in details to the patients; explained the inclusion/exclusion criteria, insured participant adherence for the participation in the study, motivated, selected, diagnosed, evaluated and sampled patients with PTSD. NP did the data analysis and interpretation. NP and MS wrote the first and the final draft of the article. DSS wrote part of the article and revised the article. MNP and DSS did the proof reading of the manuscript. All authors contributed to the final version of the manuscript. All authors have revised the article and approved the final article.

FUNDING

This work has been supported by the Croatian Science Foundation, project No. IP-2014-09-4289 Glycogene-PTSD: Genomic and glycomic biomarkers for PTSD; PI: NP.

ACKNOWLEDGMENTS

The authors thank Marija-Mary Sopta, Ph.D., Senior Research Associate, from Division of Molecular Biology, Rudjer Boskovic Institute, Zagreb, Croatia, for the English corrections and proofreading of the manuscript.

REFERENCES

1. American Psychiatric Association. *Diagnostic and Statistical Manual of Mental disorders - DSM-5.* Washington, DC: American Psychiatric Association (2013).
2. Kessler RC, Aguilar-Gaxiola S, Alonso J, Benjet C, Bromet EJ, Cardoso G, et al. Trauma and PTSD in the WHO World Mental Health Surveys, Eur. *J Psychotraumatol.* (2017) 8:1353383. doi: 10.1080/20008198.2017
3. Liu H, Petukhova MV, Sampson NA, Aguilar-Gaxiola S, Alonso J, Andrade LH. Association of DSM-IV posttraumatic stress disorder with traumatic experience type and history in the World Health Organization World Mental Health Surveys. *JAMA Psychiatry* (2017) 74:270–81. doi: 10.1001/jamapsychiatry.2016.3783
4. Mellon SH, Gautam A, Hammamieh R, Jett M, Wolkowitz OM. Metabolism, metabolomics, and inflammation in post-traumatic stress disorder. *Biol Psychiatry* (2018) 83:866–75. doi: 10.1016/j.biopsych.2018.02.007
5. Britvic D, Anticevic V, Kaliterna M, Lusic L, Beg A, Brajevic-Gizdic I, et al. Comorbidities with PTSD among combat veterans; 15 years postwar analysis. *Int J Clin Health Psychol.* (2015) 15:81–92. doi: 10.1016/j.ijchp.2014.11.002
6. Kaur J. A comprehensive review on metabolic syndrome. *Cardiol. Res. Pract.* (2014) 2014:1–21, doi: 10.1155/2014/943162
7. Bartoli F, Carrà G, Crocamo C, Carretta D, Clerici M. Metabolic syndrome in people suffering from Posttraumatic Stress Disorder: a systematic review and meta-analysis. *Metab Syndr Relat Disord.* (2013) 11:301–8. doi: 10.1089/met.2013.0010
8. Heppner PS, Crawford EF, Haji UA, Afari N, Hauger RL, Dashevsky BA, et al. The association of posttraumatic stress disorder and metabolic syndrome: a study of increased health risk in veterans. *BMC Med.* (2009) 7:1. doi: 10.1186/1741-7015-7-1
9. Jakovljevic M, Babić D, Crncević Z, Martinac M, Maslov B, Topić R. Metabolic syndrome and depression in war veterans with post-traumatic stress disorder. *Psychiatr Danub.* (2008) 20:406–10.
10. Michopoulos V, Vester A, Neigh G. Posttraumatic stress disorder: a metabolic disorder in disguise?. *Exp Neurol.* (2016) 284:220–9. doi: 10.1016/j.expneurol.2016.05.038
11. Rosenbaum S, Stubbs B, Ward PB, Steel Z, Lederman O, Vancampfort D. The prevalence and risk of metabolic syndrome and its components among people with posttraumatic stress disorder: a systematic review and meta-analysis. *Metabolism* (2015) 64:926–33. doi: 10.1016/j.metabol.2015.04.009

12. Weiss T, Skelton K, Phifer J, Jovanovic T, Gillespie CF, Smith A, et al. posttraumatic stress disorder is a risk factor for metabolic syndrome in an impoverished urban population. *Gen Hosp Psychiatry* (2011) 33:135–42. doi: 10.1016/j.genhosppsych.2011.01.002
13. Wolf EJ, Bovin MJ, Green JD, Mitchell KS, Stoop TB, Barretto KM, et al. Longitudinal associations between posttraumatic stress disorder and metabolic syndrome severity. *Psychol Med.* (2016) 46:2215–26. doi: 10.1017/S0033291716000817
14. Wolf EJ, Miller DR, Logue MW, Sumner J, Stoop TB, Leritz EC, et al. Contributions of polygenic risk for obesity to PTSD-related metabolic syndrome and cortical thickness. *Brain Behav Immun.* (2017) 65:328–36. doi: 10.1016/j.bbi.2017.06.001
15. Blessing EM, Reus V, Mellon SH, Wolkowitz OM, Flory JD, Bierer L, et al. Biological predictors of insulin resistance associated with posttraumatic stress disorder in young military veterans. *Psychoneuroendocrinology* (2017) 82:91–7. doi: 10.1016/j.psyneuen.2017.04.016
16. Kozaric-Kovacic D, Ilic MG, Romic Z, Vidovic A, Jendricko T, Pivac N. Body mass index in male caucasian veterans with or without posttraumatic stress disorder. *Prog Neuropsychopharmacol Biol Psychiatry* (2009) 33:1447–50. doi: 10.1016/j.pnpbp.2009.07.026
17. Sagud M, Jaksic N, Vuksan-Cusa B, Loncar M, Loncar I, Mihaljevic Peles A, et al. Cardiovascular disease risk factors in patients with posttraumatic stress disorder (ptsd): a narrative review. *Psychiatr Danub.* (2017) 29:421–30. doi: 10.24869/psyd.2017.421
18. Russo-Neustadt A. Brain-derived neurotrophic factor, behavior, and new directions for the treatment of mental disorders. *Semin Clin Neuropsychiatry* (2003) 8:109–18. doi: 10.1053/scnp.2003.50014
19. Gratacos M, Gonzalez JR, Mercader JM, De Cid R, Urretavizcaya M, Estivill X. Brain-Derived Neurotrophic Factor Val66Met and psychiatric disorders: meta-analysis of case-control studies confirm association to substance-related disorders, eating disorders, and schizophrenia. *Biol Psychiatry* (2007) 61:911–22. doi: 10.1016/j.biopsych.2006.08.025
20. Hong CJ, Liou YJ, Tsai SJ. Effects of BDNF polymorphisms on brain function and behavior in health and disease. *Brain Res Bull.* (2011) 86:287–97. doi: 10.1016/j.brainresbull.2011.08.019
21. Zhang L, Li XX, Hu XZ. Post-traumatic stress disorder risk and brain-derived neurotrophic factor Val66Met. *World J Psychiatry* (2016) 6:1–6. doi: 10.5498/wjp.v6.i1.1
22. Cattaneo A, Cattane N, Begni V, Pariante CM, Riva MA. The human BDNF gene: peripheral gene expression and protein levels as biomarkers for psychiatric disorders. *Transl Psychiatry* (2016) 6:958. doi: 10.1038/tp.2016.214
23. Chen ZY, Patel PD, Sant G, Meng CX, Teng KK, Hempstead BL, et al. Variant brain-derived neurotrophic factor (BDNF) (Met66) alters the intracellular trafficking and activity-dependent secretion of wild-type BDNF in neurosecretory cells and cortical neurons. *J Neurosci.* (2004) 24:4401–11. doi: 10.1523/jneurosci.0348-04.2004
24. Xu L, Tian D, Li J, Chen L, Tang L, Fan D. The analysis of two BDNF polymorphisms G196A/C270T in Chinese sporadic amyotrophic lateral sclerosis. *Front Aging Neurosci.* (2017) 10:135. doi: 10.3389/fnagi.2017.00135
25. Egan MF, Kojima M, Callicott JH, Goldberg TE, Kolachana BS, Bertolino A, et al. The BDNF Val66Met polymorphism affects activity-dependent secretion of BDNF and human memory and hippocampal function. *Cell* (2003) 112:257–69. doi: 10.1016/S0092-8674(03)00035-7
26. Kunugi H, Ueki A, Otsuka M, Isse K, Hirasawa H, Kato N, et al. A novel polymorphism of the brain-derived neurotrophic factor (BDNF) gene associated with late-onset Alzheimer's disease. *Mol Psychiatry* (2001) 6:83–6. doi: 10.1038/sj.mp.4000792
27. Nagata T, Shinagawa S, Nukariya K, Ochiai Y, Kawamura S, Agawa-Ohta M, et. al. Association between brain-derived neurotrophic factor (BDNF) gene polymorphisms and executive function in japanese patients with Alzheimer's Disease. *Psychogeriatrics* (2011) 11:141–9. doi: 10.1111/j.1479-8301.2011.00364.x
28. Notaras M, Hill R, van den Buuse M. The BDNF gene Val66Met polymorphism as a modifier of psychiatric disorder susceptibility: progress and controversy. *Mol Psychiatry* (2015) 20:916–30. doi: 10.1038/mp.2015.27
29. Watanabe Y, Nunokawa A, Someya T. Association of the BDNF C270T polymorphism with schizophrenia: updated meta-analysis. *Psychiatry Clin Neurosci.* (2013) 67:123–5. doi: 10.1111/pcn.12018
30. Dell'Osso L, Carmassi C, Del Debbio A, Dell'Osso MC, Bianchi C, da Pozzo E, et al. Brain Derived Neurotrophic Factor plasma levels in patients suffering from post-traumatic stress disorder. *Prog Neuro-Psychopharmacol Biol Psychiatry* (2009). 33:899–902. doi: 10.1016/j.pnpbp.2009.04.018
31. Su S, Xiao Z, Lin Z, Qiu Y, Jin Y, Wang Z. Plasma brain-derived neurotrophic factor levels in patients suffering from post-traumatic stress disorder. *Psychiatry Res.* (2015) 229:365–9. doi: 10.1016/j.psychres.2015.06.038
32. van den Heuvel L, Suliman S, Malan-Müller S, Hemmings S, Seedat S. Brain-derived neurotrophic factor (BDNF) Val66Met polymorphism and plasma levels in road traffic accident survivors. *Anxiety Stress Coping* (2016) 5806:1–33. doi: 10.1080/10615806.2016.1163545
33. Matsuoka Y, Nishi D, Noguchi H, Kim Y, Hashimoto K. Longitudinal changes in serum brain-derived neurotrophic factor in accident survivors with posttraumatic stress disorder. *Neuropsychobiology* (2013) 68:44–50. doi: 10.1159/000350950
34. Hauck S, Kapczinski F, Roesler R, de Moura Silveira E, Magalhães PV, Kruel LRP, et al. Serum brain-derived neurotrophic factor in patients with trauma psychopathology. *Prog Neuro-Psychopharmacol Biol Psychiatry* (2010) 34:459–62. doi: 10.1016/j.pnpbp.2010.01.010
35. Suliman S, Hemmings SM, Seedat S. Brain-derived neurotrophic factor (BDNF) protein levels in anxiety disorders: systematic review and meta-regression analysis. *Front Integr Neurosci.* (2013) 7:55. doi: 10.3389/fnint.2013.00055
36. Bonne O, Gill JM, Luckenbaugh DA, Collins C, Owens MJ, Alesci S, et al. Corticotropin-releasing factor, interleukin-6, brain derived neurotrophic factor, insulin-like growth factor-1, and substance p in the cerebrospinal fluid of civilians with posttraumatic stress disorder before and after treatment with paroxetine. *J Clin Psychiatry* (2011) 72:1124–8. doi: 10.4088/JCP.09m05106blu
37. Bountress KE, Bacanu SA, Tomko RL, Korte KJ, Hicks T, Sheerin C, et al. The effects of a BDNF Val66Met polymorphism on posttraumatic stress disorder: a meta-analysis. *Neuropsychobiology* (2018) 6:1–7. doi: 10.1159/000489407
38. Bruenig D, Lurie J, Morris CP, Harvey W, Lawford B, Young R, et al. A case-control study and meta-analysis reveal BDNF Val66Met is a possible risk factor for PTSD. *Neural Plast.* (2016) 2016:6979435. doi: 10.1155/2016/6979435
39. Wang Y, Zhang H, Li Y, Wang Z, Fan Q, Yu S, et al. BDNF Val66Met polymorphism and plasma levels in chinese han population with obsessive-compulsive disorder and generalized anxiety disorder. *J Affect Disord.* (2015) 186:7–12. doi: 10.1016/j.jad.2015.07.023
40. Zhang L, Benedek DM, Fullerton CS, Forsten RD, Naifeh JA, Li XX, et al. PTSD risk is associated with BDNF Val66Met and BDNF overexpression. *Mol Psychiatry* (2014) 19:8–10. doi: 10.1038/mp.2012.180
41. Lee HJ, Kang RH, Lim SW, Paik JW, Choi MJ, Lee MS. No association between the brain-derived neurotrophic factor gene Val66Met polymorphism and post-traumatic stress disorder. *Stress Health* (2006) 22:115–9. doi: 10.1002/ajmg.b.32122
42. Pivac N, Kozarić-Kovačić D, Grubišić-Ilić M, Nedić G, Rakoš I, Nikolac M, et al. The association between brain-derived neurotrophic factor Val66Met variants and psychotic symptoms in posttraumatic stress disorder. *World J Biol Psychiatry* (2012) 13:306–11. doi: 10.3109/15622975.2011.582883
43. Valente NLM, Vallada H, Cordeiro Q, Miguita K, Bressan RA, Andreoli SB, et al. Candidate-gene approach in posttraumatic stress disorder after urban violence: association analysis of the genes encoding serotonin transporter, dopamine transporter, and BDNF. *J Mol Neurosci.* (2011) 44:59–67. doi: 10.1007/s12031-011-9513-7
44. Wang T. Does BDNF Val66Met polymorphism confer risk for posttraumatic stress disorder? *Neuropsychobiology* (2015) 71:149–53. doi: 10.1159/000381352
45. Zhang H, Ozbay F, Lappalainen J, Kranzler HR, van Dyck CH, Charney DS, et al. Brain Derived Neurotrophic Factor (BDNF) gene variants and Alzheimer's disease, affective disorders, posttraumatic stress disorder, schizophrenia, and substance dependence. *Am J Med Genet B Neuropsychiatr Genet.* (2006) 141:387–93. doi: 10.1002/ajmg.b.30332

46. Guo JC, Yang YJ, Guo M, Wang XD, Juan Y, Gao YS, et al. Correlations of four genetic single nucleotide polymorphisms in brain-derived neurotrophic factor with posttraumatic stress disorder. *Psychiatry Invest.* (2018) 15:407–12. doi: 10.30773/pi.2017.06.17.1
47. Gómez-Pinilla F. Brain foods: the effects of nutrients on brain function. *Nat Rev Neurosci.* (2008) 9:568–78. doi: 10.1038/nrn2421
48. Rios M. BDNF and the central control of feeding: accidental bystander or essential player? *Trends Neurosci.* (2013) 36:83–90. doi: 10.1016/j.tins.2012.12.009
49. Marosi K, Mattson MP. BDNF mediates adaptive brain and body responses to energetic challenges. *Trends Endocrinol Metab.* (2014) 25:89–98. doi: 10.1016/j.tem.2013.10.006
50. Lebrun B, Bariohay B, Moyse E, Jean A. Brain-derived neurotrophic factor (BDNF) and food intake regulation: a minireview. *Auton Neurosci.* (2006) 126–127:30–38. doi: 10.1016/j.autneu.2006.02.027
51. Golden E, Emiliano A, Maudsley S, Windham BG, Carlson OD, Egan JM, et al. Circulating Brain-Derived Neurotrophic Factor and indices of metabolic and cardiovascular health: data from the baltimore longitudinal study of aging. *PLoS ONE* (2010) 5:e10099. doi: 10.1371/journal.pone.0010099
52. Svob Strac D, Nikolac Perkovic M, Nedic Erjavec G, Uzun S, Sagud M, Zivkovic M, et al. The role of brain-derived neurotrophic factor (BDNF) in cognition and treatment response. In: Bennet C, editor. *Brain-Derived Neurotrophic Factor (BDNF): Therapeutic Approaches, Role in Neuronal Development and Effects on Cognitive Health* (New York, NY: Nova Sci. Publ.) (2015). p. 67–146.
53. Briana DD, Malamitsi-Puchner A. Developmental origins of adult health and disease: the metabolic role of BDNF from early life to adulthood. *Metab Clin Exp.* (2018) 81:45–51. doi: 10.1016/j.metabol.2017.11.019
54. Fujimura H, Altar CA, Chen R, Nakamura T, Nakahashi T, Kambayashi J, et al. Brain-Derived Neurotrophic Factor is stored in human platelets and released by agonist stimulation. *Thromb Haemost.* (2002) 87:728–34. doi: 10.1055/s-0037-1613072
55. Cai D, Holm JM, Duignan IJ, Zheng J, Xaymardan M, Chin A, et al. BDNF-mediated enhancement of inflammation and injury in the aging heart. *Physiol Genom.* (2006) 24:191–7. doi: 10.1152/physiolgenomics.00165.2005
56. Tasci I, Kabul HK, Aydogdu A. Brain derived neurotrophic factor (BDNF) in cardiometabolic physiology and diseases. *Anadolu Kardiyol Der.* (2012) 12:684–8. doi: 10.5152/akd.2012.221
57. Yanev S, Aloe L, Fiore F, Chaldakov GN. Neurotrophic and metabotrophic potential of nerve growth factor and brain-derived neurotrophic factor: linking cardiometabolic and neuropsychiatric diseases. *World J Pharmacol.* (2013) 2:92–9. doi: 10.5497/wjp.v2.i4.92
58. Krabbe KS1, Nielsen AR, Krogh-Madsen R, Plomgaard P, Rasmussen P, Erikstrup C, et al. Brain-derived neurotrophic factor (BDNF) and type 2 diabetes. *Diabetologia* (2007) 50:431–8. doi: 10.1007/s00125-006-0537-4
59. Chaldakov GN, Fiore M, Stankulov IS, Hristova M, Antonelli A, Manni L, et al. NGF, BDNF, leptin, and mast cells in human coronary atherosclerosis and metabolic syndrome. *Arch Physiol Biochem.* (2001) 109:357–60. doi: 10.1076/apab.109.4.357.4249
60. Manni L, Nikolova V, Vyagova D, Chaldakov GN, Aloe L. Reduced plasma levels of NGF and BDNF in patients with acute coronary syndromes. *Int J Cardiol.* (2005) 102:169–71. doi: 10.1016/j.ijcard.2004.10.041
61. Jiang H, Liu Y, Zhang Y, Chen ZY. Association of plasma brain-derived neurotrophic factor and cardiovascular risk factors and prognosis in angina pectoris. *Biochem Biophys Res Commun.* (2011) 415:99–103. doi: 10.1016/j.bbrc.2011.10.020
62. Jung SH, Kim J, Davis JM, Blair SN, Cho HC. Association among basal serum bdnf, cardiorespiratory fitness and cardiovascular disease risk factors in untrained healthy Korean men. *Eur J Appl Physiol.* (2011) 111:303–11. doi: 10.1007/s00421-010-1658-5
63. Suriyaprom K, Tungtrongchitr R, Thawnasom K. Measurement of the levels of leptin, BDNF associated with polymorphisms LEP G2548A, LEPR Gln223Arg and BDNF Val66Met in Thai with metabolic syndrome. *Diabetol Metab Syndr.* (2014) 6:6. doi: 10.1186/1758-5996-6-6
64. Kavya K, Arul Kumaran KSG, Thomas A, Rao NV, Mathews KA, Mangathayaru K. A study of the association between brain derived neurotrophic factor and metabolic syndrome: a preliminary systematic review and meta-analysis of case-control studies. *Sri Ramachandra J Med.* 8:1.
65. Kaess BM, Preis SR, Lieb W, Beiser AS, Yang Q, Chen TC, et al. Circulating brain-derived neurotrophic factor concentrations and the risk of cardiovascular disease in the community. *J Am Heart Assoc.* (2015) 4:3. doi: 10.1161/JAHA.114.001544
66. Friedel S, Horro FF, Wermter AK, Geller F, Dempfle AK, Reichwald J, et al. Mutation screen of the brain derived neurotrophic factor gene (BDNF): identification of several genetic variants and association studies in patients with obesity, eating disorders, and attention-deficit/hyperactivity disorder. *Am J Med Genet B Neuropsychiatr Genet.* (2005) 132:96–9. doi: 10.1002/ajmg.b.30090
67. Ma XY, Qiu WQ, Smith CE, Parnell LD, Jiang ZY, Ordovas JM, et al. Association between BDNF rs6265 and obesity in the Boston Puerto Rican Health Study. *J Obes.* (2012) 2012:102942. doi: 10.1155/2012/102942
68. Wu L, Xi B, Zhang M, Shen Y, Zhao X, Cheng H, et al. Associations of six single nucleotide polymorphisms in obesity-related genes with BMI and risk of obesity in chinese children. *Diabetes* (2010) 59:3085–9. doi: 10.2337/db10-0273
69. Beckers S, Peeters A, Zegers D, Mertens I, Van Gaal L, Van Hul W. Association of the BDNF Val66Met variation with obesity in women. *Mol Genet Metab.* (2008) 95:110–2. doi: 10.1016/j.ymgme.2008.06.008
70. Skledar M, Nikolac M, Dodig-Curkovic K, Curkovic M, Borovecki F, Pivac N. Association between brain-derived neurotrophic factor Val66Met and obesity in children and adolescents. *Progr Neuro-Psychopharmacol Biol Psychiatry* (2012) 36:136–40. doi: 10.1016/j.pnpbp.2011.08.003
71. Nikolac Perkovic M, Mustapic M, Pavlovic M, Uzun S, Kozumplik O, Barisic I, et al. Lack of association between brain-derived neurotrophic factor val66met polymorphism and body mass index change over time in healthy adults. *Neurosci Lett.* (2013) 545:127–31. doi: 10.1016/j.neulet.2013.04.036
72. Sustar A, Nikolac Perkovic M, Nedic Erjavec G, Svob Strac D, Pivac N. A protective effect of the BDNF Met/Met genotype in obesity in healthy caucasian subjects but not in patients with coronary heart disease. *Eur Rev Med Pharmacol Sci.* (2016) 20:3417–26.
73. Gunstad J, Schofield P, Paul RH, Spitznagel MB, Cohen RA, Williams LM, et al. BDNF Val66Met polymorphism is associated with body mass index in healthy adults. *Neuropsychobiology* (2006) 53:153–6. doi: 10.1159/000093341
74. Hong KW, Lim JE, Go MJ, Shin Cho Y, Ahn Y, Han BG, et al. Recapitulation of the association of the Val66Met polymorphism of BDNF gene with BMI in Koreans. *Obesity* (2012) 20:1871–5. doi: 10.1038/oby.2011.352
75. Shugart YY, Chen L, Day IN, Lewis SJ, Timpson NJ, Yuan W, et al. Two british women studies replicated the association between the Val66Met polymorphism in the brain-derived neurotrophic factor (BDNF) and BMI, Eur. *J Hum Genet.* (2009) 17:1050–5. doi: 10.1038/ejhg.2008.272
76. Miller SA, Dykes DD, Polesky HF. A simple salting out procedure for extracting DNA from human nucleated cells. *Nucleic Acids Res.* (1988) 16:1215. doi: 10.1093/nar/16.3.1215
77. The 1000 Genomes Project Consortium. (2015). A global reference for human genetic variation, *Nature* 526:68–74 doi: 10.1038/nature15393
78. Shovit R, Praveen KS. Association of brain-derived neurotrophic factor (BDNF) gene SNPs G196A and C270T with Alzheimer's Disease: a meta-analysis. *J Alzheimers Dis Parkinson* (2017) 7:323. doi: 10.4172/2161-0460.1000323
79. Shovit R, Praveen KS. Association of Brain-derived Neurotrophic Factor (BDNF) gene SNPs G196A and C270T with Parkinson's disease: a meta-analysis. *Biomed J Sci Tech Res.* (2018) 6:2018. doi: 10.26717/BJSTR.2018.06.001314
80. Barrett JC, Fry B, Maller J, Daly MJ. Haploview: analysis and visualization of LD and Haplotype Maps. *Bioinformatics* (2005) 21:263–5. doi: 10.1093/bioinformatics/bth457
81. Gabriel SB, Schaffner SF, Nguyen H, Moore JM, Roy J, Blumenstiel B, et al. The structure of haplotype blocks in the human genome. *Science* (2002) 296:2225–9. doi: 10.1126/science.1069424
82. Faul F, Erdfelder E, Buchner A, Lang AG. Statistical power analyses using G*Power 3.1: tests for correlation and regression analyses. *Behav Res Methods* (2009) 41:1149–60. doi: 10.3758/BRM.41.4.1149

83. Weathers FW, Blake DD, Schnurr PP, Kaloupek DG, Marx BP, Keane TM. *The Clinician-Administered PTSD Scale for DSM-5 (CAPS-5)*. National Center for PTSD (2013). Available online at: www.ptsd.va.gov
84. Von Känel R, Kraemer B, Saner H, Schmid JP, Abbas CC, and Begré S. (2010). Posttraumatic stress disorder and dyslipidemia: previous research and novel findings from patients with PTSD caused by myocardial infarction. *World J Biol Psychiatry* 11:141–7. doi: 10.3109/15622970903449846
85. Jendricko T, Vidovic A, Grubisic-Ilic M, Romic Z, Kovacic Z, Kozaric-Kovacic D. Homocysteine and serum lipids concentration in male war veterans with posttraumatic stress disorder. *Prog Neuro-Psychopharmacol Biol Psychiatry* (2009) 33:134–40. doi: 10.1016/j.pnpbp.2008.11.002
86. Tochigi M, Umekage T, Otani T, Kato T, Iwanami A, Asukai N, et al. Serum cholesterol, uric acid and cholinesterase in victims of the Tokyo subway sarin poisoning: a relation with post-traumatic stress disorder. *Neurosci Res.* (2002) 44:267–72. doi: 10.1016/S0168-0102(02)00146-3
87. Spitzer C, Barnow S, Volzke H, Wallaschofski H, John U, Freyberger HJ, et al. Association of posttraumatic stress disorder with low-grade elevation of c reactive protein: evidence from the general population. *J Psychiatr Res.* (2010) 44:15–21. doi: 10.1016/j.jpsychires.2009.06.002
88. Talbot LS, Rao MN, Cohen BE, Richards A, Inslicht SS, O'Donovan A, et al. Metabolic risk factors and posttraumatic stress disorder: the role of sleep in young, healthy adults. *Psychosom Med.* (2015) 77:383–91. doi: 10.1097/PSY.0000000000000176
89. Dennis PA, Ulmer CS, Calhoun PS, Sherwood A, Watkins LL, Dennis MF, et al. Behavioral health mediators of the link between posttraumatic stress disorder and dyslipidemia. *J Psychosom Res.* (2014) 77:45–50. doi: 10.1016/j.jpsychores.2014.05.001
90. Hamazaki K, Nishi D, Yonemoto N, Noguchi H, Kim Y, Matsuoka Y. The role of high-density lipoprotein cholesterol in risk for posttraumatic stress disorder: taking a nutritional approach toward universal prevention. *Eur Psychiatry* (2014) 29:408–13. doi: 10.1016/j.eurpsy.2014.05.002
91. Kagan BL, Leskin G, Haas B, Wilkins J, Foy D. Elevated lipid levels in vietnam veterans with chronic posttraumatic stress disorder. *Biol Psychiatry* (1999) 45:374–7. doi: 10.1016/S0006-3223(98)00059-6
92. Karlovic D, Buljan D, Martinac M, Marcinko D. Serum lipid concentrations in croatian veterans with post-traumatic stress disorder, post-traumatic stress disorder comorbid with major depressive disorder, or major depressive disorder. *J Korean Med Sci.* (2004) 19:431–6. doi: 10.3346/jkms.2004.1 9.3.431
93. Dzubur Kulenovic A, Kucukalic A, Malec D. Changes in plasma lipid concentrations and risk of coronary artery disease in army veterans suffering from chronic posttraumatic stress disorder. *Croat Med J.* (2008) 49:506–14. doi: 10.3325/cmj.2008.4.506
94. Tae H, Huh HJ, Hwang J, Chae JH. Relationship between serum lipid concentrations and posttraumatic stress symptoms in the bereaved after the Sewol ferry disaster: a prospective cohort study. *Psychiatry Res.* (2018) 266:132–7. doi: 10.1016/j.psychres.2018.04.058
95. Peng JH, Liu CW, Pan SL, Wu HY, Liang QH, Gan RJ, et al. Potential unfavorable impacts of BDNF Val66Met polymorphisms on metabolic risks in average population in a longevous area. *BMC Geriatr.* (2017) 17:4. doi: 10.1186/s12877-016-0393-0
96. Thorleifsson G, Walters GB, Gudbjartsson DF, Steinthorsdottir V, Sulem P, Helgadottir A, et al Genome-wide association yields new sequence variants at seven loci that associate with measures of obesity. *Nat Genet.* (2009) 41:18–24. doi: 10.1038/ng.274
97. Kalenda A, Landgraf K, Löffler D, Kovacs P, Kiess W, Körner A. The BDNF Val66Met polymorphism is associated with lower BMI, lower postprandial glucose levels and elevated carbohydrate intake in children and adolescents. *Pediatr Obes.* (2018) 13:159–67. doi: 10.1111/ijpo.12238
98. Akbarian SA, Salehi-Abargouei A, Pourmasoumi M, Kelishadi R, Nikpour P, Heidari-Beni M. Association of Brain-Derived Neurotrophic Factor gene polymorphisms with body mass index: a systematic review and meta-analysis. *Adv Med Sci.* (2018) 63:43–56. doi: 10.1016/j.advms.2017.07.002
99. Petryshen TL, Sabeti PC, Aldinger KA, Fry B, Fan JB, Schaffner SF, et al. Population genetic study of the brain-derived neurotrophic factor (BDNF) gene. *Mol Psychiatry* (2010) 15:810–5. doi: 10.1038/mp.2009.24
100. Pivac N, Kim B, Nedic G, Joo YH, Kozaric-Kovacic D, Hong JP, et al. Ethnic differences in the brain-derived neurotrophic factor Val66Met polymorphism in Croatian and Korean healthy subjects. *Croat Med J.* (2009) 50:43–8. doi: 10.3325/cmj.2009.50.43
101. Autry AE, Monteggia LM. Brain-derived neurotrophic factor and neuropsychiatric disorders. *Pharmacol Rev.* (2012) 64:238–58. doi: 10.1124/pr.111.005108
102. Ribases M, Gratacòs M, Fernández-Aranda F, Bellodi L, Boni C, Anderluh M, et al. Association of BDNF with anorexia, bulimia and age of onset of weight loss in six European populations. *Hum Mol Genet.* (2004) 13:1205–12. doi: 10.1093/hmg/ddh137
103. Yilmaz Z, Kaplan AS, Tiwari AK, Levitan RD, Piran S, Bergen AW, et al. The Role of leptin, melanocortin, and neurotrophin system genes on body weight in anorexia nervosa and bulimia nervosa. *J Psychiatr Res.* (2014) 55:77–86. doi: 10.1016/j.jpsychires.2014.04.005
104. Mou Z, Hyde TM, Lipska BK, Martinowich K, Wei P, Ong CJ, et al. Human obesity associated with an intronic SNP in the brain-derived neurotrophic factor locus. *Cell Rep.* (2015) 13:1073–80. doi: 10.1016/j.celrep.2015.09.065
105. de Luis DA, Romero E, Izaola O, Primo D, Aller R. Cardiovascular risk factors and insulin resistance after two hypocaloric diets with different fat distribution in obese subjects: effect of the rs10767664 gene variant in brain-derived neurotrophic factor. *J Nutrigenet Nutrigenom.* (2017) 10:163–71. doi: 10.1159/000485248

8

Mitochondrial Dysfunction is Inducible in Lymphoblastoid Cell Lines from Children with Autism and May Involve the TORC1 Pathway

*Sirish C. Bennuri[1], Shannon Rose[1] and Richard E. Frye[2,3]**

[1] Arkansas Children's Research Institute and Department of Pediatrics, University of Arkansas for Medical Sciences, Little Rock, AR, United States, [2] Barrow Neurologic Institute at Phoenix Children's Hospital, Phoenix, AZ, United States, [3] Department of Child Health, University of Arizona College of Medicine—Phoenix, Phoenix, AZ, United States

Correspondence:
Richard E. Frye
rfrye@phoenixchildrens.com

We previously developed a lymphoblastoid cell line (LCL) model of mitochondrial dysfunction in autism spectrum disorder (ASD); some individuals with ASD showed mitochondrial dysfunction (AD-A) while other individuals (AD-N) demonstrated mitochondrial respiration similar to controls (CNT). To test the hypothesis that mitochondrial dysfunction could be a consequence of environmental exposures through chronic elevations in reactive oxygen species (ROS), we exposed LCLs to prolonged ROS. We also examined expression of metabolic regulatory genes and the modulating effect of the mechanistic target of rapamycin (mTOR) pathway. Prolonged ROS exposure induced or worsened mitochondrial dysfunction in all LCL groups. Expression of genes associated with ROS protection was elevated in both AD-N and AD-A LCLs, but mitochondrial fission/fusion and mitoplasticity gene expression was only increased in AD-N LCLs. Partial least squares discriminant analysis showed that mTOR, UCP2 (uncoupling protein 2), SIRT1 (sirtuin 1), and MFN2 (mitofusin-2) gene expression differentiated LCL groups. Low-dose rapamycin (0.1 nM) normalized respiration with the magnitude of this normalization greater for AD-A LCLs, suggesting that the mammalian target of rapamycin complex 1 (mTORC1) pathway may have a different dynamic range for regulating mitochondrial activity in individuals with ASD with and without mitochondrial dysfunction, potentially related to S6K1 (S6 kinase beta-1) regulation. Understanding pathways that underlie mitochondrial dysfunction in ASD may lead to novel treatments.

Keywords: autism, mitochondria, mitoplasticity, mechanistic target of rapamycin, reactive oxygen species

INTRODUCTION

Mitochondria are involved in many essential cellular functions; besides production of adenosine triphosphate (ATP), mitochondria are essential for calcium buffering, redox regulation, apoptosis, and inflammation. Classic mitochondrial diseases are rare, but novel forms of mitochondrial dysfunction are believed to be associated with more common diseases, particularly those where the environment contributes to the etiology. Mitochondrial dysfunction is documented in psychiatric diseases (1–4), neurodegenerative disorders (5), persistent systemic inflammation (6), cardiac disease (7), cancer (8), and diabetes (9). Mitochondrial dysfunction is also closely associated with neurodevelopmental disorders, particularly autism spectrum disorder (ASD) (10, 11) and genetic syndromes closely associated with ASD including mechanistic target of rapamycin (mTOR) (12–15); phosphatase and tensin homolog (PTEN) (16) and WDR45 (17) mutations; Rett (18–20), Phelan–McDermid (21), Angelman (22), and Down (23, 24) syndromes; as well as 15q11-q13 duplication (25, 26) and septo-optic dysplasia (27).

Mitochondrial dysfunction in ASD is unique. First, the great majority (~75%) of those with both ASD and mitochondrial disease *do not* show mitochondrial or nuclear genetic abnormalities, suggesting that the changes in mitochondrial function are either secondary to alterations in nonmitochondrial metabolic or regulatory pathways and/or due to changes in nonmitochondrial genes or epigenetic changes (11). Second, unlike classic mitochondrial disease, where mitochondrial activity is depressed, electron transport chain (ETC) activity in individuals with ASD has been reported to be elevated significantly above normal in muscle (28, 29), skin (30), gut mucosa (31), buccal epithelium (32–34), and brain (35).

In a series of studies, the authors have described and validated a lymphoblastoid cell line (LCL) model of mitochondrial dysfunction in samples obtained from individuals with ASD (36–42). In this model, about one-third of individuals with ASD (called AD-A) have LCLs with respiratory rates twice that of LCLs from control (CNT) individuals, while the remainder of the individuals with ASD (called AD-N) have LCLs with respiratory rates equivalent to LCLs from CNT individuals. Using the Mitochondrial Oxidative Stress Test (MOST) (43), we systematically increased reactive oxygen species (ROS) *in vitro* to demonstrate that AD-A LCLs are sensitive to physiological stress as they consistently show a depletion in reserve capacity (RC) as ROS is increased (36–42). In addition, we have demonstrated that mitochondrial respiration of AD-A LCLs responds differently to environmental toxicants (38, 40) and enteric short-chain fatty acids (39, 42) as compared to mitochondrial function in AD-N and CNT LCLs. In addition, we have linked this atypical mitochondrial function seen in AD-A LCLs to ASD behaviors; indeed, higher respiratory rates in the ASD LCLs were found to be associated with more severe repetitive behaviors measured on the gold-standard diagnostic tool for ASD, the Autism Diagnostic Observation Schedule (ADOS) (41).

The reason for the abnormal mitochondrial function in the AD-A LCLs is not obvious; we previously hypothesized that this elevation in mitochondrial respiration was an adaptive response that developed as a consequence of previous exposure(s) to chronic extrinsic and/or intrinsic stressors (37), a hypothesis that this paper is designed to test. Since many environmental stressors may have their biological effect through increases in ROS (21, 44–46) and since ROS is elevated in many ASD-derived tissues (45), including LCLs (37) and brain (47, 48), we hypothesized that prolonged environmental exposures, potentially through prolonged exposure to ROS, would alter long-term mitochondrial function by increasing respiratory rates. Since this hypothesis has never been tested directly, we will test this hypothesis in this paper by exposing ASD and CNT LCLs to prolonged ROS.

Thus, in this study, we determine whether prolonged exposure to ROS will increase mitochondrial respiratory rates in our LCL model so that LCLs with normal mitochondrial respiration (i.e., AD-N, CNT) will demonstrate increases in mitochondrial respiration and LCLs with increased respiration (i.e., AD-A) will further demonstrate increases in mitochondrial respiration. Showing that such a change can be induced would support the hypothesis that this change in mitochondrial respiration is inducible.

We also examined changes in molecular pathways associated with mitochondrial dysfunction by measuring the expression of genes, including those involved in regulating redox metabolism (uncoupling protein 2, UCP2; mitochondrial superoxide dismutase 2, SOD2) (49–51), mitochondrial response to stress (sirtuin 1, SIRT1; sirtuin 3, SIRT3; hypoxia-inducible factor 1-alpha, HIF1α; peroxisome proliferator-activated receptor gamma coactivator 1-alpha, PGC1α) (52–54), mitophagy (PTEN-induced putative kinase 1; PINK1), mitochondrial fusion (mitofusin-2, MFN2), mitochondrial fission (dynamin-1-like protein, DRP1), and those that can modulate cellular metabolism (AMP-activated protein kinase, AMPK; RAC-alpha serine/threonine-protein kinase, AKT1) and are associated with ASD (PTEN; mTOR) (55). We examined both the average expression across groups and the relationship between expressions of genes in various pathways.

Lastly, we examined the relationship of bioenergetic abnormalities found in ASD LCLs to the mTOR pathway for several reasons. First, abnormalities in mTOR complex 1 (mTORC1) signaling occurs in approximately 25% of individuals with nonsyndromic autism (56), which is a similar proportion of ASD LCLs with atypical bioenergetics (36, 37) (i.e., AD-A) in our model. Second, mTOR can influence mitochondrial function through several molecular pathways: mTORC1 inhibits eukaryotic translation initiation factor 4E-binding proteins (4EBP) that in turn releases inhibition of eIF4E and promotes translation of nuclear-encoded mitochondria-related messenger ribonucleic acids (mRNAs) and an increase in ETC activity (57) and mTORC1 positively influences ribosomal protein S6 kinase beta-1 (S6K1), which negatively regulates mitochondrial function through inhibition of the expression of such genes as UCP2, PGC1α, and DRP1 (58). Activation of S6K1 by mTORC1 is inhibited by low-dose rapamycin while high-dose rapamycin inhibits both S6K1 and 4EBP (59). Thus, as an additional experiment, we examined the effect of mTORC1 by determining whether low-dose rapamycin modulates mitochondrial respiration and whether such changes are more significant in the LCLs with higher respiratory rates (i.e., AD-A LCLs).

METHODS

Lymphoblastoid Cell Lines and Culture Conditions

LCLs derived from white males diagnosed with autistic disorder (AD) were chosen from pedigrees with at least one other affected male sibling (i.e., multiplex family) [mean (SD) age, 8.5 (3.0) years]. These LCLs were obtained from the Autism Genetic Resource Exchange (Los Angeles, CA, USA) and the National

Institute of Mental Health (Bethesda, MD, USA) center for collaborative genomic studies on mental disorders. All relevant guidelines and regulations were followed. These deidentified human samples were determined to be exempt from institutional review board (IRB) review by the University of Arkansas for Medical Science IRB. Donors were diagnosed using the ADOS or the Autism Diagnostic Interview–Revised (ADI-R), both gold-standard instruments.

In our previous studies (36–42), these LCLs were categorized into two different types: ones with atypical mitochondrial respiration (AD-A) and those with typical respiration (AD-N). These metabolic groupings are repeatable across several studies (36–42). All respiratory parameters were reviewed to ensure that the Seahorse runs for each LCL were consistent with their assigned group. Only one case was found where the Seahorse respiratory measurements of an LCL was not consistent with the expected group. One AD-N LCL (02C10618) demonstrated baseline respiratory parameters more consistent with AD-A LCLs in the rapamycin experiment, so it was excluded from the analysis.

CNT LCLs were derived from healthy white boys with no documented behavioral or neurological disorder and without any first-degree relative suffering from a medical disorder that might involve mitochondrial dysfunction [mean (SD) age, 8.5 (2.8) years]. CNT LCLs came from Coriell Cell Repository (Camden, NJ, USA).

The average cell passage was 12, with a maximum passage of 15, since genomic stability is very high at this low passage number. Cells were maintained in Roswell Park Memorial Institute (RPMI) 1640 culture medium with 15% fetal bovine serum and 1% penicillin/streptomycin (Invitrogen, Grand Island, NY, USA) in a humidified incubator at 37°C with 5% CO_2.

Seahorse Assay

A Seahorse Extracellular Flux (XF) 96 Analyzer (Agilent Technologies, Santa Clara, CA, USA) measured oxygen consumption rate (OCR), an indicator of mitochondrial respiration, in live intact LCLs in real time. Each run (each line of **Supplementary Tables 1** and **2**) examined matched LCL groups (CNT, AD-N, AD-A) on the same plate to control for experimental variation in mitochondrial activity measurement. The assay (**Figure 1A**), which has been described previously (36–42), provides measures of *ATP-linked respiration (ALR), proton leak respiration (PLR), maximal respiratory capacity (MRC), and reserve capacity (RC).*

Mitochondrial Oxidative Stress Test

To determine the vulnerability of the mitochondria to acute ROS exposure, we developed the Mitochondrial Oxidative Stress Test (MOST) in our previous studies (43). We examined the sensitivity of LCLs to various increasing levels of ROS by systematically exposing LCLs to increasing concentrations of 2,3-dimethoxy-1,4-napthoquinone (DMNQ; Sigma-Aldrich, St. Louis, MO, USA) for 1 h prior to the Seahorse assay. LCLs were exposed to 0 μM (control no exposure), 5 μM, 10 μM, and 15 μM DMNQ since these concentrations of DMNQ provide a full range of ROS challenge such that the highest concentration (15 μM DMNQ) significantly reduced RC to its minimum in almost every LCL type. A 5 mg/mL DMNQ solution was diluted in DMEM XF assay media into a 10X stock and added to cells in an XF-PS plate in a non-CO_2 incubator at 37°C 1 h prior to the Seahorse assay.

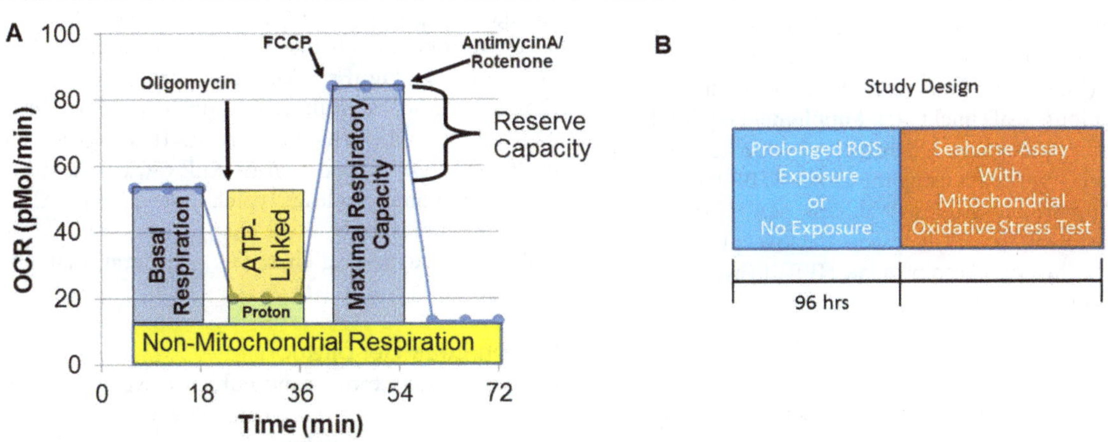

FIGURE 1 | Seahorse assay and outline of the prolonged reactive oxygen species (ROS) exposure experiment. **(A)** Mitochondrial respiration is inferred by measuring oxygen consumption rate (OCR). OCR is measured three times over 18 min at each measurement phase. Initially, basal respiration is measured. The complex V inhibitor oligomycin is then used to determine how much of basal respiration is *ATP-linked respiration* and *proton leak respiration.* Then, a protonophore, carbonyl cyanide-*p*-trifluoromethoxyphenyl-hydrazon (FCCP) is used to drive the respiratory chain to its maximal rate by collapsing the inner membrane gradient, allowing *maximal respiratory capacity* to be determined. To determine non-mitochondrial respiration, antimycin A and rotenone, Complex III and I inhibitors, are added to stop the respiratory chain. *Reserve capacity* is calculated as the difference between basal respiration and maximal respiratory capacity. **(B)** Prolonged exposure (96 h) to a low concentration of DMNQ is used to simulate chronic exposure to a low level of ROS while other cells had no exposure to DMNQ as a control.

Prolonged Low-Concentration Reactive Oxygen Species Exposure

To simulate prolonged exposure to low concentrations of ROS, 13 sets of LCLs (**Supplementary Table 1**) were cultured in 1 μM DMNQ for 96 h prior to the Seahorse assay or left untreated (0 μM) (**Figure 1B**). Thirteen pairs of AD-N and AD-A LCLs were matched with an age-matched male CNT LCL. Due to the low availability of CNT LCLs that fit our criteria, a single CNT LCL was matched with two ASD LCLs in two cases. Also, three AD-A LCLs were matched twice with AD-N LCLs. Matching was done to control for variations in measurement of mitochondrial function.

Rapamycin Exposure

To determine the influence of the mTOR pathway, we first used both low (0.01 nM and 0.1 nM) and high (1 nM and 10 nM) concentrations of rapamycin with both 1 h and 2 h exposure times on one set of AD-A and AD-N LCLs to determine if there was a differential effect of low-dose rapamycin between the two cell lines and, if so, the optimal rapamycin concentration and exposure time. As a result of this titration, eight pairs of AD-A and AD-N LCLs (**Supplementary Table 2**) were exposed to 0.1 nM of rapamycin for 2 h prior to the Seahorse assay or left untreated (0 nM). Rapamycin was used as it preferentially inhibits the effect of mTORC1 (60), particularly on S6K1 at low dose (59).

Gene Expression

Total RNA was isolated from 2 million CNT, AD-N, and AD-A LCLs (**Supplementary Table 3**) using the RNeasy mini kit (Qiagen, Hilden, Germany) following the manufacturer's protocol. Complementary deoxyribonucleic acid (cDNA) synthesis (2 μg per 20-μL reaction mix) was performed using the High-Capacity cDNA Reverse Transcription Kit (Applied Biosystems, Waltham, MA, USA) as indicated by the manufacturer. Primers were designed using the online real-time polymerase chain reaction (PCR) tool from IDT DNA (www.idtdna.com/scitools/Applications/RealTimePCR/). **Supplementary Table S4** outlines the primer sequences. Quantitative PCR reactions were performed for all target genes using the Power SYBR Green PCR Master Mix (Applied Biosystems, Waltham, MA, USA) on an ABI 7900HT Fast Real Time PCR system. Relative quantification was performed to the housekeeping gene, HPRT1 (hypoxanthine phosphoribosyltransferase 1).

Analytic Approach

To analyze group effects, a mixed-model regression was conducted *via* SAS version 9.3 (Cary, NC, USA) "glmmix" procedure. The mixed model allows matched samples on each Seahorse plate to be compared to one another while controlling for any variation associated with the Seahorse assay itself. The mitochondrial parameters were response variables with a between-group effect of LCL group (e.g., AD-N v AD-A v CNT) and within-group repeated factors of prolonged ROS exposure (exposed vs. nonexposed) and DMNQ concentration as well as the interaction between these effects. DMNQ concentration was a continuous variable. For all models, random effects included the intercept. F tests evaluated significance. Planned *post hoc* orthogonal contrasts, which are t-distributed, examined significant group effects. Data were normally distributed and variation was similar across groups. Graphs show standard error bars. Gene expression was similarly analyzed, although without the DMNQ concentration variable. Rapamycin exposure data were similarly analyzed, although the exposure variable was with rapamycin. We also performed partial least squares discriminant analysis (PLSDA) using R version 3.5.0 mixOmics Omics Data Integration Project version 6.3.2.

RESULTS

Prolonged Exposure to Reactive Oxygen Species: Mitochondrial Function

To determine if prolonged exposure to low concentrations of ROS can alter mitochondrial function, potentially producing the atypical patterns of respiration seen in the AD-A LCLs, we exposed the three types of LCLs (CNT, AD-N, and AD-A) to a low concentration of DMNQ for 96 h or cultured normally (control). We then conducted the Seahorse assay including the MOST. This allowed us to determine if prolonged ROS exposure changed overall average respiration and/or the susceptibility of the mitochondria to acute ROS increases. Thus, we report the change in overall average respiration and the change in respiration with ROS challenge (as part of the MOST) as a result of prolonged (96 h) exposure to low levels of ROS.

Adenosine Triphosphate–Linked Respiration

Prolonged ROS exposure increased overall ALR [$F(1,1144) = 4.71, p < 0.05$], with this effect not significantly different across LCL groups. The change in ALR with increasing DMNQ was changed by prolonged ROS exposure [$F(1,1144) = 5.07, p < 0.01$] without this change being significantly different across LCL groups (**Figure 2A**). Thus, prolonged ROS exposure changed mitochondrial respiration to have a higher baseline ALR and a greater change in ALR. This suggests that indeed prolonged ROS exposure shifts ALR toward the mitochondrial dysfunction abnormalities typically seen in the AD-A LCLs at baseline. Interestingly, these changes seem to be similar across LCL types, suggesting that it is a general adaptation of the mitochondria.

Proton Leak Respiration

Prolonged ROS exposure did influence overall PLR [$F(1,1144) = 52.02, p < 0.001$], but this change was not significantly different across LCL groups. The typical increase in PLR that occurs with redox challenge was amplified after prolonged ROS exposure [$F(1,1144) = 3.95, p < 0.01$] but this change was not significantly different across LCL groups (**Figure 2B**). Thus, prolonged ROS exposure changed mitochondrial respiration to have a greater change in PLR. This suggests that indeed prolonged ROS exposure shifts PLR toward the mitochondrial abnormalities seen in the AD-A LCLs at baseline.

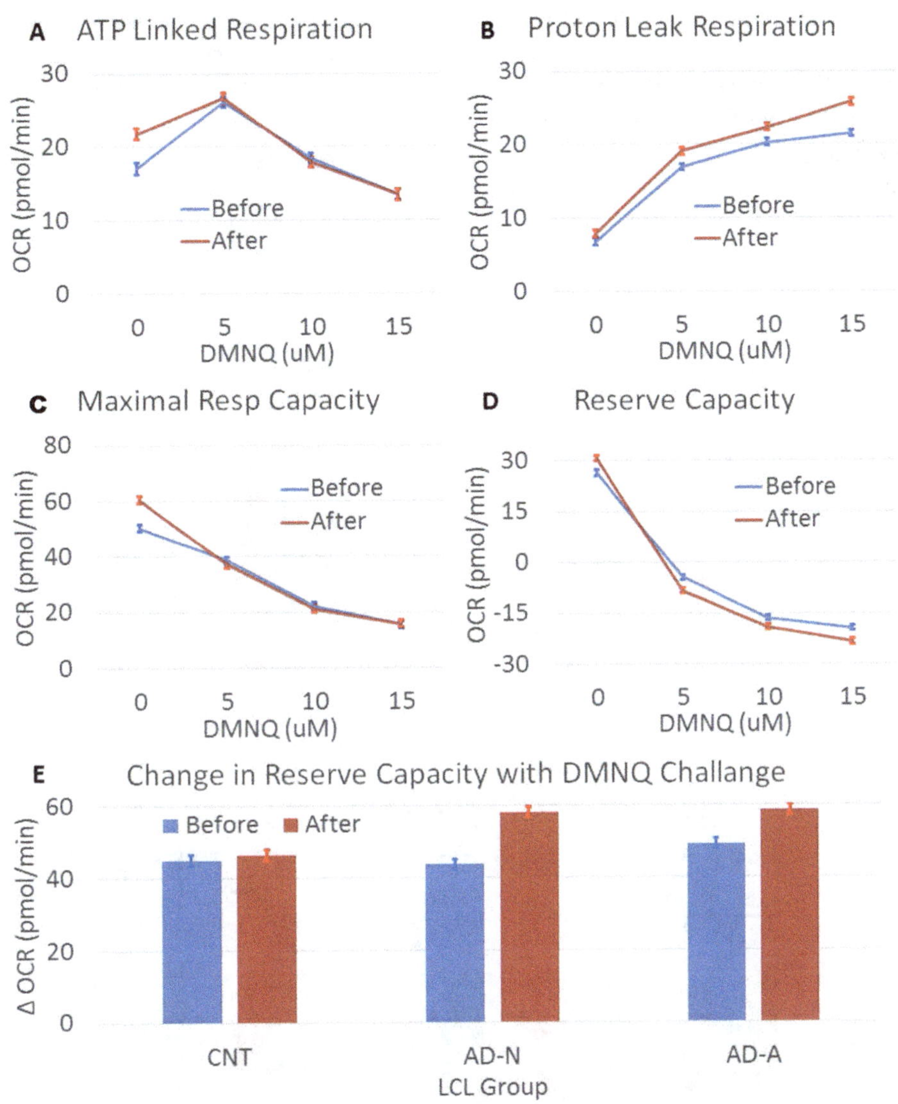

FIGURE 2 | The effect of prolonged (96 h) ROS exposure on mitochondrial function in lymphobastoid cell lines (LCLs). In these expierments, 2,3-dimethoxy-1,4-napthoquinone (DMNQ) was used to increase ROS *in vitro* both during the prolonged incubation and 1 h prior to the mitochondrial measurements in order to determine the effect of acute increases in ROS on the LCLs. Prolonged ROS exposure (red) shifted mitochondrial function toward an atypical pattern that has been reported in a subset of LCLs derived from children with autistic disorder (AD). This includes increasing **(A)** ATP-linked respiration, **(B)** proton leak respiration, **(C)** maximal respiratory capacity, and **(D)** reserve capacity, along with a greater drop in reserve capacity when challanged with an acute increase in ROS. **(E)** The change in reserve capacity with increasing acute DMNQ concetration was different across the LCL groups, so the difference between the lowest (0 μM) and highest (15 μM) DMNQ concentrations is depicted in the bottom graph to demonstrate the interaction.

Maximal Respiratory Capacity

Prolonged ROS exposure increased overall MRC [$F(1,1144) = 4.97, p < 0.05$], with this change not significantly different across LCL groups. The change (decrease) in MRC was accentuated after prolonged ROS exposure [$F(1,1144) = 9.37, p < 0.0001$], with this effect not significantly different across LCL groups (**Figure 2C**). Thus, prolonged ROS exposure changed mitochondrial respiration to increase overall MRC and cause a greater change in MRC. This suggests that indeed prolonged ROS exposure shifts MRC toward abnormalities seen in the AD-A LCLs at baseline.

Reserve Capacity

Prolonged ROS exposure increased overall RC [$F(1,1144) = 7.81, p < 0.01$], with this effect not significantly different across LCL groups. Prolonged ROS exposure also augmented the change (decrease) in RC [$F(1,1144) = 11.55, p < 0.0001$] (**Figure 2D**), with this effect significantly different across LCL groups [$F(6,1144) = 2.37, p < 0.05$] (**Figure 2E**). As can be seen in **Figure 2E**, the change in RC with the acute ROS challenge is greater for the AD groups than the CNT group. Thus, prolonged ROS exposure changed mitochondrial respiration to have a higher overall RC and greater change in RC, with some of these effects more prominent in the

ASD LCLs. This suggests that indeed prolonged ROS exposure shifts RC toward abnormalities seen in the AD-A LCLs at baseline.

Gene Expression Differences Across Lymphoblastoid Cell Line Groups: Statistical Differences

To understand differences in molecular pathway regulation of mitochondrial and redox homeostasis across LCL groups, expression of key genes was examined (**Figure 3**). Gene expression was averaged across ROS exposure since differences in gene expression between AD and CNT LCL groups were independent of the ROS effect except for one gene.

No Differences

There were no differences in PTEN and AKT1 expression between LCL groups.

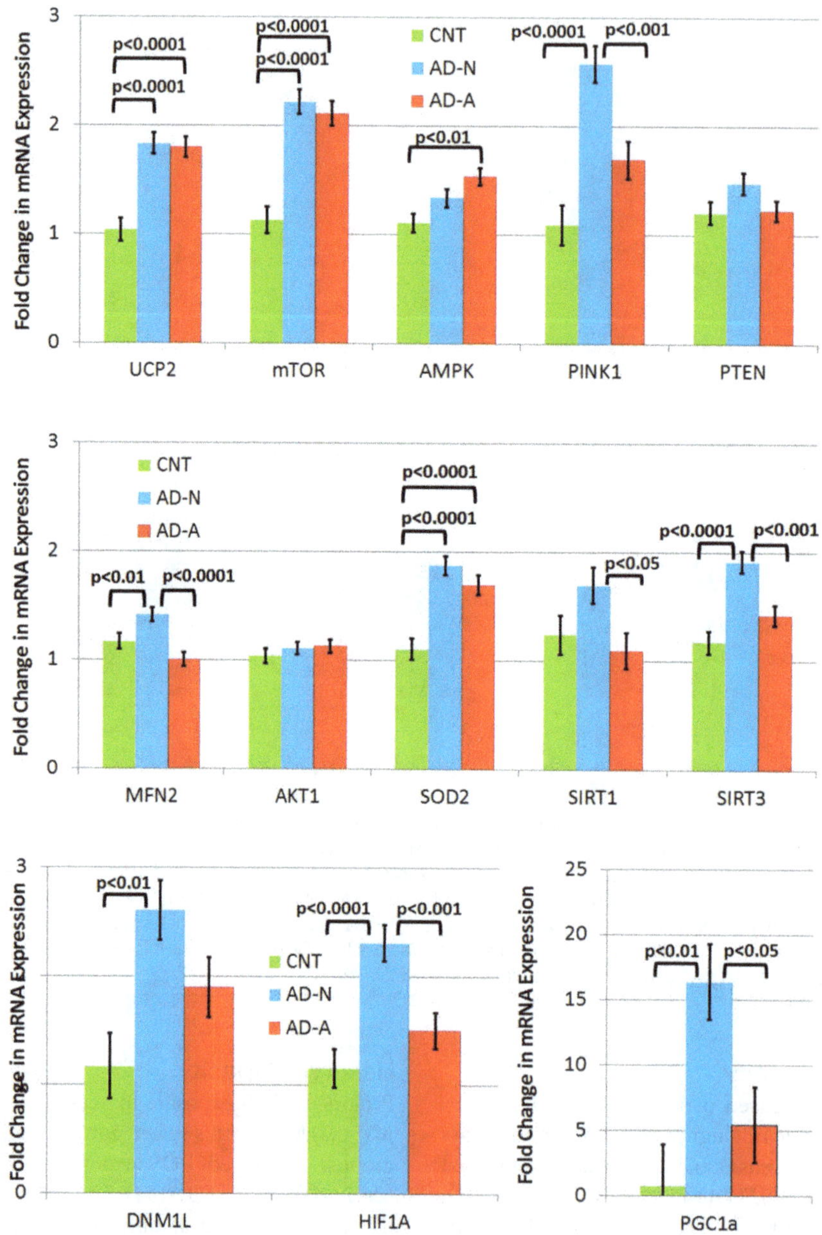

FIGURE 3 | Gene expression in three different types of lymphobastoid cell lines (LCLs) collapsed across the prolonged (96 h) ROS exposure condition. While LCLs derived from individuals with autistic disorder (AD) demonstrated increases in expression in several genes, including UCP2, mTOR, and SOD2, in comparison to controls (CNT), most of the elevation in gene expression related to the genes involved in response to physiological stress was seen only one AD LCL group (i.e., AD-N).

Gene Expression Elevated in Autistic Disorder Lymphoblastoid Cell Lines Compared to Control Lymphoblastoid Cell Lines

UCP2 expression was significantly different across LCL groups [$F(2,44) = 19.12$, $p < 0.0001$] due to higher expression in AD-N [$t(44) = 5.54$, $p < 0.0001$] and AD-A [$t(44) = 5.31$, $p < 0.0001$] LCLs as compared to CNT LCLs. SOD2 expression was significantly different across LCL groups [$F(2,44) = 19.78$, $p < 0.0001$] due to higher expression in AD-N [$t(44) = 6.07$, $p < 0.0001$] and AD-A [$t(44) = 4.68$, $p < 0.0001$] LCLs as compared to CNT LCLs. mTOR expression was significantly different across LCL groups [$F(2,44) = 26.04$, $p < 0.0001$] due to higher expression in AD-N [$t(44) = 6.63$, $p < 0.0001$] and AD-A [$t(44) = 5.99$, $p < 0.0001$] LCLs as compared to CNT LCLs.

Gene Expression Elevated in AD-A Lymphoblastoid Cell Lines

AMPK expression was significantly different across LCL groups [$F(2,44) = 6.53$, $p < 0.005$] due to higher expression in the AD-A LCL as compared to CNT LCLs [$t(44) = 3.61$, $p < 0.005$].

Gene Expression Elevated in AD-N Lymphoblastoid Cell Lines

PINK1 expression was significantly different across LCL groups [$F(2,44) = 19.78$, $p < 0.0001$] due to higher expression in AD-N LCLs as compared to CNT [$t(44) = 6.20$, $p < 0.0001$] and AD-A [$t(44) = 3.89$, $p < 0.0005$] LCLs. HIF1α expression was significantly different across LCL groups [$F(2,44) = 11.99$, $p < 0.0001$] due to higher expression in AD-N LCLs as compared to CNT [$t(44) = 4.71$, $p < 0.0001$] and AD-A [$t(44) = 3.42$, $p = 0.001$] LCLs. SIRT3 expression was significantly different across LCL groups [$F(2,44) = 14.08$, $p < 0.0001$] due to higher expression in AD-N LCLs as compared to CNT [$t(44) = 5.16$, $p < 0.0001$] and AD-A [$t(44) = 3.56$, $p < 0.001$] LCLs. PCG1α expression was significantly different across LCL groups [$F(2,44) = 7.42$, $p = 0.01$] due to higher expression in AD-N LCLs as compared to CNT [$t(44) = 3.70$, $p < 0.005$] and AD-A [$t(44) = 2.73$, $p < 0.05$] LCLs. MFN2 expression was significantly different across LCL groups [$F(2,44) = 10.66$, $p < 0.0005$] due to higher expression in AD-N LCLs as compared to CNT [$t(44) = 2.60$, $p = 0.01$] and AD-A [$t(44) = 4.60$, $p < 0.0001$] LCLs. SIRT1 expression was significantly different across LCL groups [$F(2,44) = 3.58$, $p < 0.05$] due to higher expression in AD-N LCLs as compared to AD-A [$t(44) = 2.58$, $p < 0.05$] LCLs. DNM1L was significantly different across LCL groups [$F(2,44) = 6.18$, $p < 0.005$] due to higher expression in AD-N LCLs as compared to CNT [$t(44) = 3.51$, $p < 0.005$] LCLs.

Gene Expression Changes Resulting From Prolonged Reactive Oxygen Species Exposure

There was also an LCL group by prolonged ROS exposure interaction [$F(2,44) = 3.24$, $p = 0.05$] driven by the fact that MFN2 (fusion) expression decreased in the AD-N LCLs while it increased in the CNT [$t(44) = 2.27$, $p < 0.05$] and AD-A [$t(44) = 2.10$, $p < 0.05$] LCLs following prolonged ROS exposure.

Gene Expression Patterns Differentiate Lymphoblastoid Cell Line Groups: Visual Analysis

To better understand gene expression that differentiates LCL groups, particularly LCLs with and without mitochondrial dysfunction, the statistical differences found above were displayed in a functional diagram representing pathway interconnections (**Figure 4**). This diagram shows that ASD

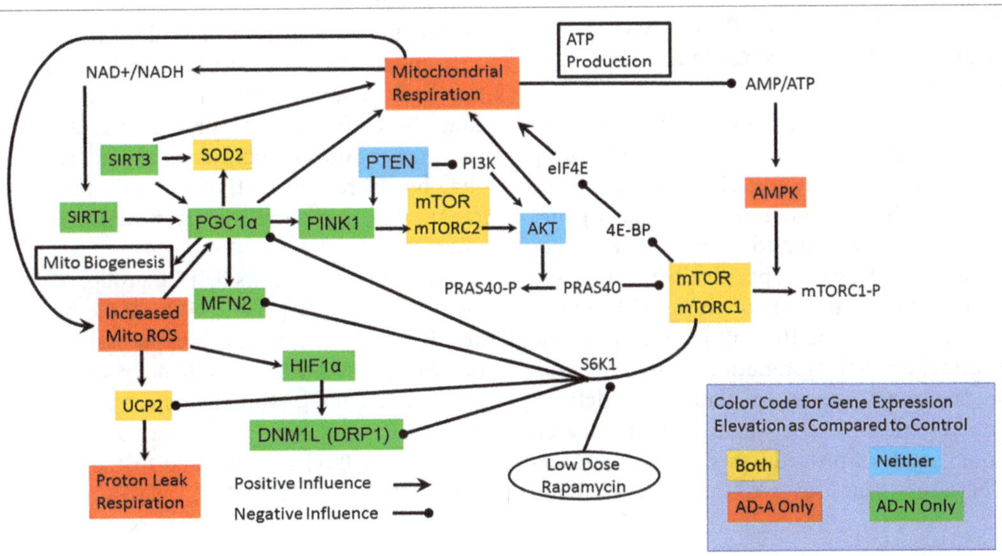

FIGURE 4 | Interconnection of the pathways studied, the genes in which we have measured expression and connection to mitochondrial respiration. The colors represent the groups that have elevations in the expression of specific genes. Most notable are the two pathways by which mTOR can influence mitochondrial function. S6K1 pathway inhibits many of the pathways involved in mitochondrial maintainance and response to stress while the 4E-BP/eIF4E pathway more directly can increase mitochondrial function.

LCLs, both AD-A and AD-N LCLs, demonstrate an increase in SOD and UCP2, as would be expected for LCLs under chronic oxidative stress, as has been shown for ASD LCLs previously in several studies (37, 41, 61). One pattern that differentiates AD-A from AD-N is that many genes associated with mitochondrial maintenance (DRP1, MFN2) and response to physiological stress (PCG1α) are only elevated for AD-N LCLs but not AD-A LCLs. This is surprising, as the mitochondria with more abnormal respiratory rates would be expected to be under greater physiological stress.

For both types of ASD LCLs, mTOR is increased, which could represent either the mTORC1 or mTORC2 complex, but here we concentrate on mTORC1 because of its interactions with other pathways. The S6K1 pathway can be promoted by mTORC1. Since S6K1 inhibits many of the pathways involved in mitochondrial maintenance and response to stress, an increase in S6K1 pathway in the AD-A LCLs could explain why expression of many of the genes responsible for mitochondrial maintenance and response to stress are not elevated. The effect of S6K1 specific to mitochondrial dysfunction in the AD-A LCLs will be tested in the rapamycin experiment below. Why activation of the S6K1 pathway would be greater in the AD-A LCLs than in the AD-N LCLs is not immediately obvious, but this may be due to the differences in the dynamics of mTOR in the two ASD LCL subsets. Indeed, AMPK elevation appears to be specific for AD-A LCLs and would result in a greater phosphorylation and inactivation of mTORC1. Higher AMPK levels could explain the increase in mTOR expression for the AD-A LCLs since greater inactivation of mTORC1 could drive greater production of unphosphorylated mTORC1. The elevation in mTOR expression in AD-N LCLs could be driven by PINK1, but we would expect AKT1 to also be increased in expression.

Gene Expression Patterns Differentiate Lymphoblastoid Cell Line Groups: Discriminant Analysis

To complement the qualitative description of the different patterns that differentiate the LCL groups, a machine learning technique was used to independently verify patterns unique to the LCL groups. Since the expression between many genes are interdependent, PLSDA was used to select the key genes that differentiate LCL characteristics, specifically whether the LCLs came from individuals with ASD or those with typical development, and whether or not the mitochondria in the LCLs manifested mitochondrial dysfunction. Thus, we used PLSDA to extract the most important genes that defined these specific characteristics. PLSDA was used as compared to other discriminant analysis procedures since it considers the relationship between genes as well as their absolute expression levels.

Autism vs. Nonautism

Overall accuracy of the canonical discriminant function was 97% using two components that accounted for 56% and 13% of the variance. The most significant component loadings were represented by six genes: mTOR, UCP2, PTEN, AKT1, SIRT1, and MFN2.

Mitochondrial Dysfunction vs. Normal Mitochondrial Function

Overall accuracy of the canonical discriminant function was 84% using two components that accounted for 51% and 11% of the variance. The most significant component loadings were represented by six genes: mTOR, UCP2, DRP1, AMPK, SIRT1, and MFN2.

Thus, the PLSDA demonstrated that several common genes differentiated the bioenergetic and clinical characteristics of the cells, specifically mTOR, UCP2, SIRT1, and MFN2. Two genes were more specific to the clinical characteristics of the patients from which the LCLs were derived, specifically PTEN and AKT1, and two genes where more specific for the bioenergetic characteristics of the LCLs, specifically AMPK and DRP1.

Changes in Mitochondrial Respiration With Rapamycin Treatment

In order to determine if modulation of S6K1 could affect mitochondrial function, we investigated whether low-dose rapamycin did indeed differentiate the two ASD LCL groups. First, we did a titration experiment to find the optimal low dose of rapamycin and to confirm that low-dose but not high-dose rapamycin differentially influenced the two ASD groups. As seen in **Figure 5**, low-dose rapamycin markedly reduced the respiratory indexes in the AD-A LCLs but not the AD-N LCLs as expected. From these experiments, we selected the optimal low dose to examine this effect on a larger number of LCL pairs.

Mitochondrial function was measured in eight pairs of LCLs from the two AD LCL groups (AD-N and AD-A) with and without exposure to low-dose (0.1 nM) rapamycin since this concentration of rapamycin has a more selective effect on the regulation of S6K1 by mTOR (59). We hypothesized that the activation of S6K1 by mTORC1 suppresses genes for mitochondrial maintenance and response to stress and that by decreasing activity of this pathway using low-dose rapamycin, mitochondrial dysfunction in the AD-A LCLs will normalize.

Analyzing the results by LCL group, rapamycin was found to decrease PLR [$F(1,13) = 7.37, p < 0.05$] but not ALR (**Figure 6A** and **B**). Consistent with our hypothesis, rapamycin significantly decreased MRC [$F(1,13) = 20.06, p < 0.001$] and RC [$F(1,13) = 23.41, p < 0.001$], with this effect significantly greater for the AD-A LCLs [MRC: $F(1,13) = 12.07, p < 0.005$; RC: $F(1,13) = 23.05, p < 0.001$] as compared to the AD-N LCLs (**Figure 6C** and **D**). In fact, for AD-A LCLs, MRC and RC decreased toward the AD-N respiratory parameters indicating normalization to these respiratory parameters.

We then determined if the effect of low-dose rapamycin was dependent on baseline mitochondrial respiration independent of the LCL grouping, by examining the relationship between the baseline respiratory parameters and the change in the

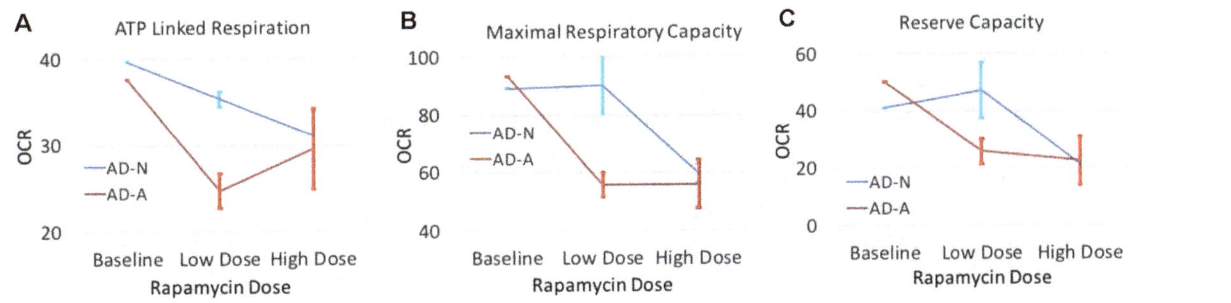

FIGURE 5 | The effect of both low-dose and high-dose rapamycin on one pair of ASD LCLs. LCLs were exposed to low dose (0.01 nM and 0.1 nM) or high dose (1 nM and 10 nM) for either 1 h or 2 h followed by the Seahorse assay. For presentation purposes, both low doses at both time points were combined into one average data point and both high doses at both time points were combined into one data point. Standard error bars are also shown. Respiratory parameters including **(A)** ATP Linked Respiration, **(B)** Maximal Respiratory Capacity and **(C)** Reserve Capacity are shown.

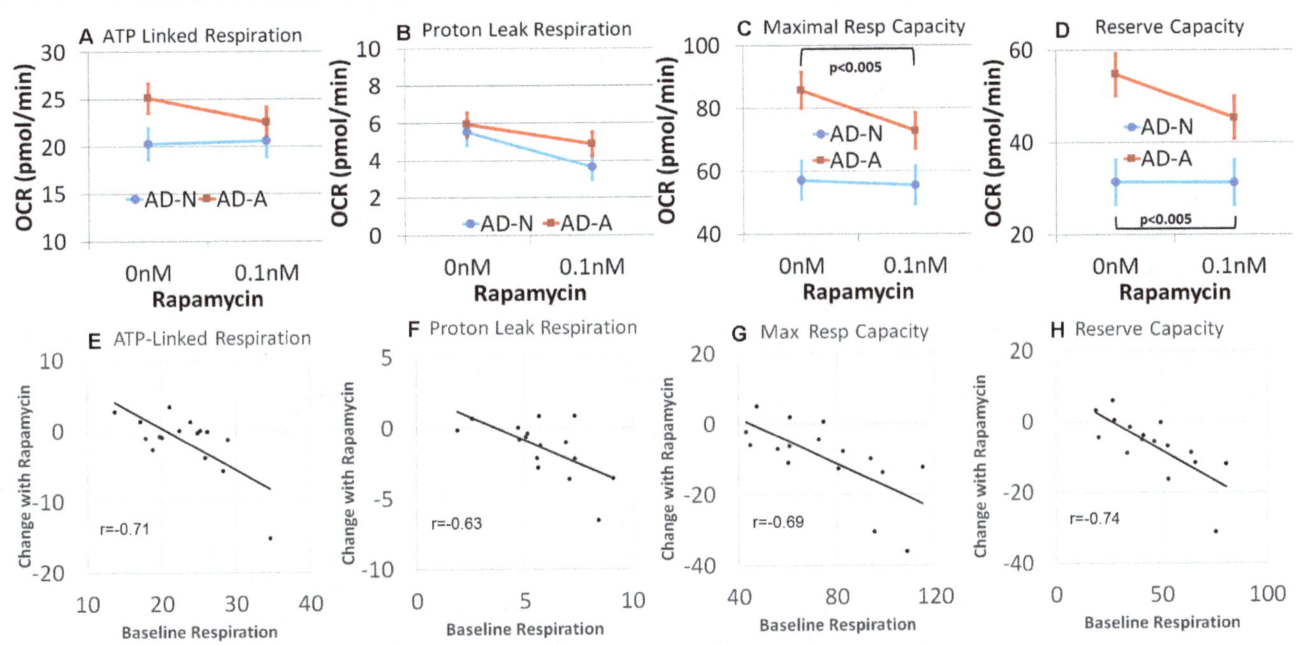

FIGURE 6 | Rapamycin modulates mitochondrial function differently depending on the underlying baseline repiratory rate in lymphobastoid cell lines (LCLs) derived from children with autistic disorder (AD). **(A–D)** Group differences in the effect of rapamycin. The AD-N LCLs demonstrate more typical mitochondrial function and have less influence from rapamycin while the AD-A LCLs, which demonstrate elevated mitochondrial function, are more influenced by rapamycin. **(E–H)** The linear relationship between the underlying baseline respiratory rate and the change in respirataory rate for both groups of LCLs. The higher the baseline respiratory rate, the greater the effect of rapamycin.

respiratory parameter with rapamycin exposure. A significant relationship between the baseline respiratory parameter and change in the respiratory parameter with rapamycin treatment was found for all respiratory parameters [ALR: $F(1,12) = 7.85$, $p < 0.05$, $r = -0.71$; PLR: $F(1,12) = 14.35$, $p < 0.005$, $r = -0.63$; MRC: $F(1,12) = 8.20$, $p = 0.01$, $r = -0.69$; RC: $F(1,12) = 12.77$, $p < 0.005$, $r = -0.74$; **Figure 6E–H**]. In general, rapamycin had a greater effect on reducing mitochondrial respiration for those LCLs with higher respiratory rates at baseline. All correlation coefficients were significant, and these relationships were not significantly different across AD groups. Thus, in general, it appeared that rapamycin had a greater effect on reducing mitochondrial respiration when mitochondrial respiratory rates were higher.

DISCUSSION

This study examines important aspects of mitochondrial function and the origins of atypical mitochondrial respiration previously observed in a subset of ASD LCL in at least seven independent studies (36–42). In our previous studies, we hypothesized that

ASD LCLs with atypical mitochondrial respiration, called AD-A LCLs, developed atypical mitochondrial respiration as an adaptation to previous environmental exposures, potentially through prolonged exposure to ROS since oxidative stress is a common mechanism in which environmental agents perturb cellular physiology.

In this study, we conducted three experiments: 1) we examined the effect of prolonged exposure to ROS on mitochondrial respiration; 2) we examined differences in the expression of genes important for mitochondrial respiration, particularly those involved in allowing the mitochondria to adapt to adverse physiological conditions, across different clinical types (ASD vs. typical developing) and physiological types (atypical vs. normal mitochondrial function); and 3) we also examined the effect of low-dose rapamycin on mitochondrial function, to determine whether a specific regulatory pathway (S6K1) may be involved in maintaining atypical mitochondrial function in the AD-A LCLs.

First, we examined the effect of prolonged exposure to low concentrations of an agent (DMNQ) that increased intracellular ROS to alter baseline mitochondrial respiration. We examined this in three types of LCLs, those derived from typically developing children (CNT) and two types from children with ASD. One of the subsets of LCLs derived from children with ASD are known to have atypical mitochondrial respiration (AD-A), which has been hypothesized to be an adaptive response to previous exposures to environmental stressors involving ROS. The prolonged exposure to ROS did result in changes in mitochondrial respiration, some of which were more significant and marked in the AD LCLs, but, overall, did influence the CNT LCLs also. These changes were similar to the differences seen in the AD-A LCLs at baseline, suggesting that the pattern of mitochondrial dysfunction displayed in the AD-A LCLs may have arisen from previous prolonged exposure to ROS.

Interestingly, the analysis of changes in gene expression with prolonged exposure to ROS found that MFN2 (fusion) gene expression changed, although in different directions for the different LCLs groups. While MFN2 expression decreased for AD-N LCLs and increased for both AD-A and CNT LCLs, it needs to be noted that the AD-N LCLs showed a higher expression of this gene at baseline. What is also potentially significant is that MFN2 appears to be significant in differentiating both clinical groups and bioenergetic characteristics of the LCLs, pointing to the potential importance of the maintenance of optimal mitochondria function in ASD. It is also of interest that the AD-A LCLs demonstrated significantly lower MFN2 at baseline as compared to the AD-N LCLs. Thus, in lowering MFN2 expression for AD-N LCLs, prolonged ROS exposure did alter MFN2 toward the baseline expression of the AD-A LCLs, suggesting that this difference in MFN2 expression may be an integral part of the regulation and maintenance of the atypical mitochondrial activity.

Second, we examined gene expression in three types of LCLs that have different intrinsic mitochondrial function and underlying intracellular ROS profiles. Both types of ASD LCLs demonstrated increased expression of UCP2, SOD2, and mTOR. As both types of ASD LCLs are known to have increased intracellular ROS, it is not surprising that UCP2 and SOD2 were increased, although our previous study suggested that UCP2 was higher in AD-A as compared to AD-N LCL when the protein content was measured (37). Further, since glutathionylation (62) activates UCP2, relative changes in glutathione in the ASD LCLs also likely modulate UCP2 function. Thus, UCP2 gene expression between ASD LCLs only provides one aspect of its function in LCLs under chronic ROS.

The AD-N LCLs clearly demonstrated an increase in several genes involved in mitochondrial response to stress and mitochondrial dynamics aimed at improving mitochondrial fidelity. Previous studies have demonstrated that overexpression of PCG1α in ASD LCLs results in upregulation of mitochondrial ETC Complex I and III as well as reduces mitochondrial ROS (54). Thus, AD-N LCLs appear to have pathways for supporting mitochondrial response to stress even without an exogenous ROS challenge. The fact that the AD-A LCLs did not demonstrate an increase in these genes was surprising and may suggest that their abnormal mitochondrial function is an alternative adaptation to the chronic intracellular ROS. Visual analysis of pathways suggested that the S6K1 pathway, which is activated by mTORC1, could suppress these pathways and account for a suppression of pathways important for mitochondrial response to stress and maintenance. Our third experiment tests this hypothesis.

The AD-A LCLs also demonstrated an increase in AMPK expression, which is unexpected as AMPK is inhibited by elevation in intracellular ATP, and from our previous studies, the AD-A appears to be overproducing ATP. This result would appear to suggest that despite increased production of ATP, AD-A LCLs remain at an overall ATP deficit or, alternatively, an upstream signal is activating AMPK. Either way, this elevation in AMPK can significantly affect mTORC1 levels in the LCLs as higher AMPK will enhance the phosphorylation of mTORC1, thereby inactivating its influences on downstream signals. This could explain the increase in mTOR expression for the AD-A LCLs as more mTOR would need to be produced to maintain an active mTORC1 complex.

Third, we examined the effect of low-dose rapamycin on parameters of mitochondrial respiration. We found that overall rapamycin decreased MRC and RC, with this decrease much greater in the LCLs with higher respiration, the AD-A LCLs, as compared to those with lower respiratory rates, the AD-N LCLs. We also found that the effect of low-dose rapamycin in decreasing respiratory parameters was proportional to the amount they were increased at baseline, so that the higher the baseline respiratory parameter value, the more low-dose rapamycin decreased the parameter. This appears to be consistent across the four respiratory parameters measured. Others have found that low-dose rapamycin modulates the effect of mTOR on S6K1. S6K1 inhibits several of the genes that are elevated in the AD-N but not the AD-A LCLs. Thus, by decreasing the positive influence of mTOR on S6K1, the inhibitory effect on genes associated with mitochondrial response to stress and mitochondria maintenance could be uninhibited. If these mitochondrial regulatory pathways were responsible for maintaining normal mitochondrial respiration in the context of chronic oxidative stress, uninhibiting them could normalize mitochondrial function in the AD-A LCLs. This is exactly what was found. However, the effect of normalizing mitochondrial respiration was proportional to the abnormal elevation in mitochondrial respiration regardless of whether the LCLs were in the AD-A or AD-N group. Thus, this does suggest that the abnormalities in mitochondrial respiration may be on a continuum. Such a notion would be consistent with the fact that chronic exposure to ROS can change the respiratory characteristics of LCLs toward this atypical pattern with the magnitude of this change different for the different LCL groups.

mTORC1 is known to stimulate mitochondrial ATP production (57, 63), but both ASD LCLs demonstrate similar mTOR gene expression. The AD-A LCLs demonstrate elevated expression of AMPK that phosphorylates regulatory-associated protein of mTOR (RAPTOR), inhibiting its activity. This would be expected to decrease the activity of the mTOR pathway. However, the rapamycin experiments suggest that the mTOR pathway is relevant to mitochondrial function in AD-A LCLs. It is possible that the increased sensitivity to rapamycin and the preferential activation of the S6K1 pathways as compared to the 4E-BP pathway by mTORC1 in AD-A LCLs are due to the fact that it has a more narrow range of activation because it is chronically inhibited by a chronic increase in AMPK.

The Role of Mitochondrial Dysfunction in Neurodevelopmental Disorders

Interestingly, the pattern of a significant elevation in mitochondrial respiratory activity found in the AD-A LCLs is not unprecedented and has been associated with genetic syndromes and models of ASD resulting from environmental influences. For example, genetic syndromes associated with ASD, including patients with Phelan–McDermid syndrome (33), WDR45 (17), 22q13 duplication (21), and Rett syndrome (18), as well as the PTEN haploinsufficient mouse model of ASD (16) have demonstrated significant elevations in ETC function. Also, brain tissue from the maternal immune activation (MIA) mouse, a model of ASD induced by prenatal environmental stress, has overactivity in Complex I and IV (64). This abnormal pattern of mitochondrial function has also been associated with other disorders. For example, ETC Complex IV underactivity is found in chronic multiple sclerosis lesions during inflammation but ETC Complex IV has been found to be overactive in these lesions once inflammation has resolved, suggesting that inflammation had a long-term effect on mitochondrial activity (65, 66). Significantly, this "hyperactive" state of ETC Complex IV has been described during reperfusion following ischemia and is believed to contribute to the increased production of ROS during reperfusion (67). Thus, a better understanding of this atypical increase in respiratory rate and its role in disease may have significant consequences.

The Link Between Environmental Factors and Mitochondrial Function

Interestingly, consistent with the chronic ROS exposure experiment, we have found that environmental influences associated with ASD can alter mitochondrial function in CNT LCLs to make them more like AD-A LCLs, thereby supporting our original hypothesis. For example, in a recent study, we demonstrated that prolonged exposure to trichloroacetaldehyde hydrate, the active metabolite of an environmental toxicant associated with ASD, can alter CNT LCLs to have mitochondrial function like AD-A LCLs and that AD-A LCLs are more resilient to the detrimental effect of trichloroacetaldehyde hydrate on the mitochondria as compared to AD-N LCLs (40). In addition, further studies have implicated the enteric microbiome-derived short-chain fatty acids butyrate (42) and propionic acid (39) in increasing respiratory rates of mitochondria in LCLs from children with ASD.

Overall, we believe that the experiments reported in this manuscript may provide insight into adaptive changes in mitochondrial function that are only starting to be recognized. We believe that these changes may be caused by environmental influences in many cases and the information uncovered may be helpful in understanding environmentally induced diseases in greater depth. In addition, it appears that the mTOR pathway may have a role in modulating changes in mitochondrial function in the context of these atypical changes in mitochondrial function and may have a role in developing novel treatments.

AUTHOR CONTRIBUTIONS

All authors were involved in the design and conceptualization of the experiments. Laboratory experiments were conducted by SB and SR. Data were analyzed by all authors. All authors were involved in drafting, editing, and finalizing the manuscript. All authors approved the final manuscript.

ACKNOWLEDGMENTS

We thank the families and individuals with ASD that participated in the Autism Genetic Research Exchange and the studies at the National Institute of Mental Health for providing cell lines for research. We would like to thank the supporters of our research studies, including the Arkansas Biosciences Institute (Little Rock, AR), the Jonty Foundation (St. Paul, MN), the Autism Research Institute (San Diego, CA), the Gupta Family Foundation (Atherton, CA), the Jane Botsford Johnson Foundation (New York, NY), the Jager Family Foundation (Chicago, IL), and the Phoenix Children's Hospital Foundation (Phoenix, AZ).

REFERENCES

1. Scaglia F. The role of mitochondrial dysfunction in psychiatric disease. *Dev Disabil Res Rev* (2010) 16(2):136–43. doi: 10.1002/ddrr.115
2. Clay HB, Sillivan S, Konradi C. Mitochondrial dysfunction and pathology in bipolar disorder and schizophrenia. *Int J Dev Neurosci* (2011) 29(3):311–24. doi: 10.1016/j.ijdevneu.2010.08.007
3. Kato M, Nakamura M, Ichiba M, Tomiyasu A, Shimo H, Higuchi I, et al. Mitochondrial DNA deletion mutations in patients with neuropsychiatric symptoms. *Neurosci Res* (2011) 69(4):331–6. doi: 10.1016/j.neures.2010.12.013
4. Verge B, Alonso Y, Valero J, Miralles C, Vilella E, Martorell L. Mitochondrial DNA (mtDNA) and schizophrenia. *Eur Psychiatry* (2011) 26(1):45–56. doi: 10.1016/j.eurpsy.2010.08.008
5. Federico A, Cardaioli E, Da Pozzo P, Formichi P, Gallus GN, Radi E. Mitochondria, oxidative stress and neurodegeneration. *J Neurol Sci* (2012) 322(1–2):254–62. doi: 10.1016/j.jns.2012.05.030
6. Cox CE. Persistent systemic inflammation in chronic critical illness. *Respir Care* (2012) 57(6):859–64; discussion 864-856. doi: 10.4187/respcare.01719
7. Dai DF, Rabinovitch PS, Ungvari Z. Mitochondria and cardiovascular aging. *Circ Res* (2012) 110(8):1109–24. doi: 10.1161/CIRCRESAHA.111.246140
8. Formentini L, Martinez-Reyes I, Cuezva JM. The mitochondrial bioenergetic capacity of carcinomas. *IUBMB Life* (2010) 62(7):554–60. doi: 10.1002/iub.352
9. Naudi A, Jove M, Ayala V, Cassanye A, Serrano J, Gonzalo H, et al. Cellular dysfunction in diabetes as maladaptive response to mitochondrial oxidative stress. *Exp Diabetes Res* (2012) 2012:696215. doi: 10.1155/2012/696215
10. Gimsa U, Kanitz E, Otten W, Aheng C, Tuchscherer M, Ricquier D, et al. Alterations in anxiety-like behavior following knockout of the uncoupling protein 2 (ucp2) gene in mice. *Life Sci* (2011) 89(19–20):677–84. doi: 10.1016/j.lfs.2011.08.009
11. Rossignol DA, Frye RE. Mitochondrial dysfunction in autism spectrum disorders: a systematic review and meta-analysis. *Mol Psychiatry* (2012a) 17(3):290–314. doi: 10.1038/mp.2010.136
12. Goto J, Talos DM, Klein P, Qin W, Chekaluk YI, Anderl S, et al. Regulable neural progenitor-specific Tsc1 loss yields giant cells with organellar dysfunction in a model of tuberous sclerosis complex. *Proc Natl Acad Sci U S A* (2011) 108(45):E1070–9. doi: 10.1073/pnas.1106454108
13. Yui K, Sato A, Imataka G. Mitochondrial dysfunction and its relationship with mTOR signaling and oxidative damage in autism spectrum disorders. *Mini Rev Med Chem* (2015) 15(5):373–89. doi: 10.2174/1389557515666150324122930
14. Ebrahimi-Fakhari D, Saffari A, Wahlster L, Di Nardo A, Turner D, Lewis TL, Jr., et al. Impaired mitochondrial dynamics and mitophagy in neuronal models of tuberous sclerosis complex. *Cell Rep* (2016) 17(4):1053–70. doi: 10.1016/j.celrep.2016.09.054
15. Ebrahimi-Fakhari D, Saffari A, Wahlster L, Sahin M. Using tuberous sclerosis complex to understand the impact of MTORC1 signaling on mitochondrial dynamics and mitophagy in neurons. *Autophagy* (2017) 13(4):754–6. doi: 10.1080/15548627.2016.1277310
16. Napoli E, Ross-Inta C, Wong S, Hung C, Fujisawa Y, Sakaguchi D, et al. Mitochondrial dysfunction in Pten haplo-insufficient mice with social deficits and repetitive behavior: interplay between Pten and p53. *PLoS One* (2012) 7(8):e42504. doi: 10.1371/journal.pone.0042504
17. Burger BJ, Rose S, Bennuri SC, Gill PS, Tippett ML, Delhey L, et al. Autistic siblings with novel mutations in two different genes: insight for genetic workups of autistic siblings and connection to mitochondrial dysfunction. *Front Pediatr* (2017) 5:219. doi: 10.3389/fped.2017.00219
18. Condie J, Goldstein J, Wainwright MS. Acquired microcephaly, regression of milestones, mitochondrial dysfunction, and episodic rigidity in a 46,XY male with a *de novo* MECP2 gene mutation. *J Child Neurol* (2010) 25(5): 633–6. doi: 10.1177/0883073809342004
19. Gibson JH, Slobedman B, Harikrishnan, KN, Williamson SL, Minchenko D, et al. Downstream targets of methyl CpG binding protein 2 and their abnormal expression in the frontal cortex of the human Rett syndrome brain. *BMC Neurosci* (2010) 11:53. doi: 10.1186/1471-2202-11-53
20. Grosser E, Hirt U, Janc OA, Menzfeld C, Fischer M, Kempkes B, et al. Oxidative burden and mitochondrial dysfunction in a mouse model of Rett syndrome. *Neurobiol Dis* (2012) 48(1):102–14. doi: 10.1016/j.nbd.2012.06.007
21. Frye RE. Biomarkers of abnormal energy metabolism in children with autism spectrum disorder. *N A J Med Sci* (2012a) 5(3):141–7. doi: 10.7156/v5i3p141
22. Su H, Fan W, Coskun PE, Vesa J, Gold JA, Jiang YH, et al. Mitochondrial dysfunction in CA1 hippocampal neurons of the UBE3A deficient mouse model for Angelman syndrome. *Neurosci Lett* (2011) 487(2):129–33. doi: 10.1016/j.neulet.2009.06.079
23. Pallardo FV, Lloret A, Lebel M, d'Ischia M, Cogger VC, Le Couteur DG, et al. Mitochondrial dysfunction in some oxidative stress-related genetic diseases: ataxia–telangiectasia, Down syndrome, Fanconi anaemia and Werner syndrome. *Biogerontology* (2010) 11(4):401–19. doi: 10.1007/s10522-010-9269-4
24. Pagano G, Castello G. Oxidative stress and mitochondrial dysfunction in Down syndrome. *Adv Exp Med Biol* (2012) 724:291–9. doi: 10.1007/978-1-4614-0653-2_22
25. Filipek PA, Juranek J, Smith M, Mays LZ, Ramos ER, Bocian M, et al. Mitochondrial dysfunction in autistic patients with 15q inverted duplication. *Ann Neurol* (2003) 53(6):801–4. doi: 10.1002/ana.10596
26. Frye RE. 15q11.2-13 duplication, mitochondrial dysfunction, and developmental disorders. *J Child Neurol* (2009) 24(10):1316–20. doi: 10.1177/0883073809333531
27. Schuelke M, Krude H, Finckh B, Mayatepek E, Janssen A, Schmelz M, et al. Septo-optic dysplasia associated with new mitochondrial cytochrome b mutation. *Ann Neurol* (2002) 51(3):388–92. doi: 10.1002/ana.10151
28. Frye RE, Naviaux RK. Autistic disorder with complex IV overactivity: a new mitochondrial syndrome. *J Pediatr Neurol* (2011) 9:427–34. doi: 10.3233/JPN-2011-0507
29. Frye RE. Novel cytochrome B gene mutations causing mitochondrial disease in autism. *J Pediatr Neurol* (2012b) 10:35–40. doi: 10.3233/JPN-2012-0530
30. Frye RE, Melnyk S, Macfabe DF. Unique acyl-carnitine profiles are potential biomarkers for acquired mitochondrial disease in autism spectrum disorder. *Transl Psychiatry* (2013) 3:e220. doi: 10.1038/tp.2012.143
31. Rose S, Bennuri SC, Murray KF, Buie T, Winter H, Frye RE. Mitochondrial dysfunction in the gastrointestinal mucosa of children with autism: a blinded case–control study. *PLoS One* (2017a) 12(10):e0186377. doi: 10.1371/journal.pone.0186377
32. Goldenthal MJ, Damle S, Sheth S, Shah N, Melvin J, Jethva R, et al. Mitochondrial enzyme dysfunction in autism spectrum disorders; a novel biomarker revealed from buccal swab analysis. *Biomark Med* (2015) 9(10):957–65. doi: 10.2217/bmm.15.72
33. Frye RE, Cox D, Slattery J, Tippett M, Kahler S, Granpeesheh D, et al. Mitochondrial dysfunction may explain symptom variation in Phelan–McDermid syndrome. *Sci Rep* (2016a) 6:19544. doi: 10.1038/srep19544
34. Delhey L, Kilinc EN, Yin L, Slattery J, Tippett M, Wynne R, et al. Bioenergetic variation is related to autism symptomatology. *Metab Brain Dis* (2017) 32(6):2021–31. doi: 10.1007/s11011-017-0087-0
35. Palmieri L, Papaleo V, Porcelli V, Scarcia P, Gaita L, Sacco R, et al. Altered calcium homeostasis in autism-spectrum disorders: evidence from biochemical and genetic studies of the mitochondrial aspartate/glutamate carrier AGC1. *Mol Psychiatry* (2010) 15(1):38–52. doi: 10.1038/mp.2008.63
36. Rose S, Frye RE, Slattery J, Wynne R, Tippett M, Melnyk S, et al. Oxidative stress induces mitochondrial dysfunction in a subset of autistic lymphoblastoid cell lines. *Transl Psychiatry* (2014a) 4:e377. doi: 10.1038/tp.2014.15
37. Rose S, Frye RE, Slattery J, Wynne R, Tippett M, Pavliv O, et al. Oxidative stress induces mitochondrial dysfunction in a subset of autism lymphoblastoid cell lines in a well-matched case control cohort. *PLoS One* (2014b) 9(1):e85436. doi: 10.1371/journal.pone.0085436
38. Rose S, Wynne R, Frye RE, Melnyk S, James SJ. Increased susceptibility to ethylmercury-induced mitochondrial dysfunction in a subset of autism lymphoblastoid cell lines. *J Toxicol* (2015) 2015:573701. doi: 10.1155/2015/573701
39. Frye RE, Rose S, Chacko J, Wynne R, Bennuri SC, Slattery JC, et al. Modulation of mitochondrial function by the microbiome metabolite propionic acid in autism and control cell lines. *Transl Psychiatry* (2016b) 6(10):e927. doi: 10.1038/tp.2016.189

40. Frye RE, Rose S, Wynne R, Bennuri SC, Blossom S, Gilbert KM, et al. Oxidative stress challenge uncovers trichloroacetaldehyde hydrate-induced mitoplasticity in autistic and control lymphoblastoid cell lines. *Sci Rep* (2017) 7(1):4478. doi: 10.1038/s41598-017-04821-3
41. Rose S, Bennuri SC, Wynne R, Melnyk S, James SJ, Frye RE. Mitochondrial and redox abnormalities in autism lymphoblastoid cells: A sibling control study. *FASEB J* (2017b) 31(3):904–9. doi: 10.1096/fj.201601004R
42. Rose S, Bennuri SC, Davis JE, Wynne R, Slattery JC, Tippett M, et al. Butyrate enhances mitochondrial function during oxidative stress in cell lines from boys with autism. *Transl Psychiatry* (2018a) 8(1):42. doi: 10.1038/s41398-017-0089-z
43. Rose S, Niyazov DM, Rossignol DA, Goldenthal M, Kahler SG, Frye RE. Clinical and molecular characteristics of mitochondrial dysfunction in autism spectrum disorder. *Mol Diagn Ther* (2018b) 22(5):571–93. doi: 10.1007/s40291-018-0352-x
44. Rossignol DA, Frye RE. A review of research trends in physiological abnormalities in autism spectrum disorders: immune dysregulation, inflammation, oxidative stress, mitochondrial dysfunction and environmental toxicant exposures. *Mol Psychiatry* (2012b) 17(4):389–401. doi: 10.1038/mp.2011.165
45. Frye RE, James SJ. Metabolic pathology of autism in relation to redox metabolism. *Biomark Med* (2014) 8(3):321–30. doi: 10.2217/bmm.13.158
46. Rossignol DA, Genuis SJ, Frye RE. Environmental toxicants and autism spectrum disorders: a systematic review. *Transl Psychiatry* (2014) 4:e360. doi: 10.1038/tp.2014.4
47. Rose S, Melnyk S, Pavliv O, Bai S, Nick TG, Frye RE, et al. Evidence of oxidative damage and inflammation associated with low glutathione redox status in the autism brain. *Transl Psychiatry* (2012) 2:e134. doi: 10.1038/tp.2012.61
48. Rossignol DA, Frye RE. Evidence linking oxidative stress, mitochondrial dysfunction, and inflammation in the brain of individuals with autism. *Front Physiol* (2014) 5:150. doi: 10.3389/fphys.2014.00150
49. Andrews ZB. Uncoupling protein-2 and the potential link between metabolism and longevity. *Curr Aging Sci* (2010) 3(2):102–12. doi: 10.2174/1874609811003020102
50. Jastroch M, Divakaruni AS, Mookerjee S, Treberg JR, Brand MD. Mitochondrial proton and electron leaks. *Essays Biochem* (2010) 47:53–67. doi: 10.1042/bse0470053
51. Indo HP, Yen HC, Nakanishi I, Matsumoto K, Tamura M, Nagano Y, et al. A mitochondrial superoxide theory for oxidative stress diseases and aging. *J Clin Biochem Nutr* (2015) 56(1):1–7. doi: 10.3164/jcbn.14-42
52. Wang CH, Wu SB, Wu YT, Wei YH. Oxidative stress response elicited by mitochondrial dysfunction: implication in the pathophysiology of aging. *Exp Biol Med (Maywood)* (2013) 238(5):450–60. doi: 10.1177/1535370213493069
53. Shaughnessy DT, McAllister K, Worth L, Haugen AC, Meyer JN, Domann FE, et al. Mitochondria, energetics, epigenetics, and cellular responses to stress. *Environ Health Perspect* (2014) 122(12):1271–8. doi: 10.1289/ehp.1408418
54. Bu XS, Wu D, Lu XM, Yang L, Xu XY, Wang J, et al. Role of SIRT1/PGC-1alpha in mitochondrial oxidative stress in autistic spectrum disorder. *Neuropsychiatr Dis Treat* (2017) 13:1633–45. doi: 10.2147/NDT.S129081
55. Lipton JO, Sahin M. The neurology of mTOR. *Neuron* (2014) 84(2):275–91. doi: 10.1016/j.neuron.2014.09.034
56. Suzuki AM, Griesi-Oliveira K, de Oliveira Freitas Machado C, Vadasz E, Zachi EC, et al. Altered mTORC1 signaling in multipotent stem cells from nearly 25% of patients with nonsyndromic autism spectrum disorders. *Mol Psychiatry* (2015) 20(5):551–2. doi: 10.1038/mp.2014.175
57. Morita M, Gravel SP, Chenard V, Sikstrom K, Zheng L, Alain T, et al. mTORC1 controls mitochondrial activity and biogenesis through 4E-BP-dependent translational regulation. *Cell Metab* (2013) 18(5):698–711. doi: 10.1016/j.cmet.2013.10.001
58. Park J, Tran Q, Mun K, Masuda K, Kwon SH, Kim SH, et al. Involvement of S6K1 in mitochondria function and structure in HeLa cells. *Cell Signal* (2016) 28(12):1904–15. doi: 10.1016/j.cellsig.2016.09.003
59. Mukhopadhyay S, Frias MA, Chatterjee A, Yellen P, Foster DA. The enigma of rapamycin dosage. *Mol Cancer Ther* (2016) 15(3):347–53. doi: 10.1158/1535-7163.MCT-15-0720
60. McCubrey JA, Steelman LS, Chappell WH, Abrams SL, Franklin RA, Montalto G, et al. Ras/Raf/MEK/ERK and PI3K/PTEN/Akt/mTOR cascade inhibitors: How mutations can result in therapy resistance and how to overcome resistance. *Oncotarget* (2012) 3(10):1068–111. doi: 10.18632/oncotarget.659
61. James SJ, Rose S, Melnyk S, Jernigan S, Blossom S, Pavliv O, et al. Cellular and mitochondrial glutathione redox imbalance in lymphoblastoid cells derived from children with autism. *Faseb J* (2009) 23(8):2374–83. doi: 10.1096/fj.08-128926
62. Mailloux RJ, Seifert EL, Bouillaud F, Aguer C, Collins S, Harper ME. Glutathionylation acts as a control switch for uncoupling proteins UCP2 and UCP3. *J Biol Chem* (2011) 286(24):21865–75. doi: 10.1074/jbc.M111.240242
63. Morita M, Gravel SP, Hulea L, Larsson O, Pollak M, St-Pierre J, et al. mTOR coordinates protein synthesis, mitochondrial activity and proliferation. *Cell Cycle* (2015) 14(4):473–80. doi: 10.4161/15384101.2014.991572
64. Naviaux RK, Zolkipli Z, Wang L, Nakayama T, Naviaux JC, Le TP, et al. Antipurinergic therapy corrects the autism-like features in the poly(IC) mouse model. *PLoS One* (2013) 8(3):e57380. doi: 10.1371/journal.pone.0057380
65. Lu F, Selak M, O'Connor J, Croul S, Lorenzana C, Butunoi C, et al. Oxidative damage to mitochondrial DNA and activity of mitochondrial enzymes in chronic active lesions of multiple sclerosis. *J Neurol Sci* (2000) 177(2):95–103. doi: 10.1016/S0022-510X(00)00343-9
66. Mahad DJ, Ziabreva I, Campbell G, Lax N, White K, Hanson PS, et al. Mitochondrial changes within axons in multiple sclerosis. *Brain* (2009) 132(Pt 5):1161–74. doi: 10.1093/brain/awp046
67. Huttemann M, Helling S, Sanderson TH, Sinkler C, Samavati L, Mahapatra G, et al. Regulation of mitochondrial respiration and apoptosis through cell signaling: cytochrome c oxidase and cytochrome c in ischemia/reperfusion injury and inflammation. *Biochim Biophys Acta* (2012) 1817(4):598–609. doi: 10.1016/j.bbabio.2011.07.001

9

The Role of Neuroinflammation in Postoperative Cognitive Dysfunction: Moving from Hypothesis to Treatment

Seyed A. Safavynia[1] and Peter A. Goldstein[1,2,3]*

[1] Department of Anesthesiology, Weill Cornell Medical College, New York, NY, United States, [2] Department of Medicine, Weill Cornell Medical College, New York, NY, United States, [3] Neuroscience Graduate Program, Weill Cornell Medical College, New York, NY, United States

***Correspondence:**
Seyed A. Safavynia
sas9204@med.cornell.edu

Postoperative cognitive dysfunction (POCD) is a common complication of the surgical experience and is common in the elderly and patients with preexisting neurocognitive disorders. Animal and human studies suggest that neuroinflammation from either surgery or anesthesia is a major contributor to the development of POCD. Moreover, a large and growing body of literature has focused on identifying potential risk factors for the development of POCD, as well as identifying candidate treatments based on the neuroinflammatory hypothesis. However, variability in animal models and clinical cohorts makes it difficult to interpret the results of such studies, and represents a barrier for the development of treatment options for POCD. Here, we present a broad topical review of the literature supporting the role of neuroinflammation in POCD. We provide an overview of the cellular and molecular mechanisms underlying the pathogenesis of POCD from pre-clinical and human studies. We offer a brief discussion of the ongoing debate on the root cause of POCD. We conclude with a list of current and hypothesized treatments for POCD, with a focus on recent and current human randomized clinical trials.

Keywords: postoperative cognitive dysfunction, cognitive decline, neuroinflammation, central nervous system, microglia, anesthesia

INTRODUCTION

Disordered neurocognitive function following surgery is a heterogenous set of conditions, which includes both the fluctuating and typically transient postoperative delirium and the more protracted problem of postoperative cognitive dysfunction (POCD). POCD is a well-known risk of the surgical experience, having been described as a consequence of anesthesia as early as 1887 (1), and a common complication of cardiac surgery since the 1950's (2). More than 60 years following its modern description, it is only just now that clearly articulated guidelines have been suggested for identifying POCD (3). POCD has been loosely defined as a significant reduction in cognitive performance from baseline following surgery, and diagnosed as subtle deficits in multiple core neurocognitive domains, including executive function, attention, verbal memory, psychomotor speed, and visuospatial abstraction (4, 5). Given that the literature thus far has used the term POCD to describe these deficits, we will also use the term here, but recognize going forward the nomenclature will likely evolve so as to conform with new guidelines (3). Since the 1950's, advanced age has been shown to be one of the strongest associations for development of POCD: the incidence of POCD is reported to be anywhere between 9 and 54% 1 week after surgery in adults over age 65 (6), with no difference in rates based on the type of surgery and/or anesthetic (7). POCD itself can persist long after surgery, with an incidence between 10 and 17% at 3 months following surgery (7, 8) and 3% at 12 months following surgery (9). Moreover, POCD can contribute to severe cognitive deficits over the long term, affecting overall morbidity and mortality, with increased hospital costs (10, 11). The health and economic burdens of POCD are likely to increase over the next several years: Life expectancy is increasing, and more than 30% of individuals over age 65 have surgery annually (12).

At the epidemiological level, a handful of risk factors for the development of POCD have emerged from population studies; controversy exists, however, in the interpretation of these data and their clinical implications. Risk factors for POCD were initially identified in patients undergoing cardiac surgery, and included advanced age, aortic valve replacement, and prolonged (mean 70 min) cardiopulmonary bypass (CPB) time (13). While advanced age (>65 years) has been consistently identified as a risk factor for POCD (8, 14), the evidence is less convincing with other potential risk factors due to differences in populations and neurocognitive testing modalities (4, 7). For example, it has long been thought that preexisting frailty in general (15–20), and neurocognitive frailty in particular (9, 21, 22) may be a risk factor for POCD as these patients may be vulnerable to cognitive insults at baseline. Indeed, observational studies have shown that surgery may precipitate further cognitive decline in patients with neurodegenerative disorders such as Alzheimer's disease (AD) (23), and biomarkers of AD such as the apolipoprotein E4 (APOE-4) genotype have also been associated with development of POCD in elderly patients (24, 25). However, a long-term retrospective analysis did not show an accelerated progression to dementia in patients with AD after non-cardiac surgery (26). More recent data in humans show that while the CSF tau/β-amyloid ratio increases following surgery, the increase is independent of the type of anesthetic (i.e., propofol vs. isoflurane) (27), further calling into question the predictive value of these biomarker studies. These discrepancies may be in part due to confounders such as temperature regulation; hypothermia rather than anesthesia *per se* seems to be the driver behind the observed tauopathy (28, 29), with dexmedetomidine as a possible exception (30). Chronic inflammatory states such as diabetes, metabolic syndrome, and atherosclerosis have all been proposed as potential risk factors for POCD (31–33), while pro-cognitive activities such as sleep, exercise, and level of education seem to be protective (34). Despite these data, the heterogeneous populations and study paradigms used inherently limit the clinical interpretation of these risk factors.

At the cellular level, data from animal and human studies suggest that neuroinflammation from either surgery or anesthesia is a major contributor to the development of POCD, yet the specific relationship between inflammation and POCD remains unknown. Multiple rodent models of surgery have shown upregulation of pro-inflammatory cytokines and inflammatory mediators in both peripheral tissues and the central nervous system (CNS) (35, 36). Similarly in rats, inflammation in the form of prior infection can also increase the incidence and severity of POCD (37, 38). In human studies, patients who develop POCD also show increases in serum and cerebrospinal fluid (CSF) pro-inflammatory cytokines, irrespective of the type of surgery (39–42), which has been corroborated in meta-analyses (43, 44). However, there seems to be little relationship between the magnitude of the neuroinflammation and the development of POCD. For example, while CPB was thought to be a strong initiator of peripheral and subsequent neuroinflammation (45), the rates of POCD in cardiac and non-cardiac surgery are similar (7), as well as in pulsatile vs. non-pulsatile CPB (46) and on-pump and off-pump cardiac surgery (45). Meta-regressions show a slight relationship with plasma levels of interleukin-6 (IL-6) and S100 calcium-binding protein β (S100β) and POCD, but no other cytokines studied have shown any correlation (43). While inflammation always occurs with surgery, POCD does not, and it remains unclear what specific risk factors and triggers are responsible for this conversion.

Despite the advances in research, fundamental barriers exist to understanding POCD in a generalized context, limiting the ability to predict patients at risk for POCD and develop appropriate therapies for such patients. Firstly, POCD has been broadly defined, with no historical formal clinical definition (5, 47, 48). Similarly, animal models of POCD are defined using a variety of metrics, each testing different cognitive domains as a proxy for POCD (49). Without a formal definition, it is difficult to accurately and consistently identify patients with POCD and construct appropriate animal models, thereby limiting a generalized understanding of the epidemiology and pathogenesis of the disorder. Secondly, determining the root causes of POCD is difficult as surgery and anesthesia occur almost invariably in tandem (48), with larger and more high-risk surgery often necessitating longer anesthetic times. Thirdly, proposed treatments showing promise in animal studies are often not as effective when tested in clinical trials, revealing a need for a more nuanced understanding of POCD.

We present a broad topical overview of the current state of the literature regarding the effects of neuroinflammation on the development of POCD. We will review the proposed cellular mechanisms underlying the pathogenesis of POCD in pre-clinical and human studies. We will present the evidence underlying the debate on the etiologic contributions of neuroinflammation and POCD in both animal models and human studies, whether surgical, anesthetic, or both. Lastly, we will discuss proposed treatments for POCD, with a focus on recent and current human randomized clinical trials.

While POCD is often grouped with postoperative delirium (POD) in the literature, we limit the discussion in this review to POCD and not POD. POD and POCD are distinct disorders: Delirium is defined in the fifth edition of the Diagnostic and Statistical Manual of Mental Disorders (DSM-5) as a disorder of reduced attention and orientation to the environment, accompanied by cognitive disturbances in an acute and fluctuating course with lucid intervals (50). By contrast, POCD is described as an objectively measured decline in cognition in the postoperative state compared to the preoperative state (48). Unlike delirium, the time course of POCD does not fluctuate with lucid intervals, and some patients never recover from the initial insult (51, 52). Nevertheless, there is a growing body of evidence suggesting that neuroinflammation contributes to POD; for a detailed review on the role of neuroinflammation on POD, please see Maldonado (53).

PROPOSED MECHANISMS FOR PATHOGENESIS OF POCD

Taken together, data from animal and human studies have fueled the ***hypothesis** that peripheral surgical trauma causes CNS inflammation via disruption of the blood-brain barrier (BBB), which then causes a functional disruption in neural activity, leading to POCD.* Each component of this hypothesis is regulated by a variety of inflammatory mediators discussed below. This sequence of events can persist long after surgery and resolution of neuroinflammation, and can accelerate neurocognitive decline in neurocognitively frail populations.

Peripheral Initiation of Inflammation

It is well-known that aseptic surgical trauma causes inflammation at the surgical site, which is amplified *via* peripheral pro-inflammatory cytokines. In response to surgical trauma, damaged cells at the site of injury passively release small biomolecules known as damage-associated molecular patterns (or danger-associated molecular patterns; DAMPs) (4, 54). In particular, the DAMP known as high molecular group box 1 protein (HMGB1) is released following surgical trauma and binds to Toll-like receptors (TLRs) and the receptor for advanced glycosylation end products (RAGE) on the cell membrane of peripherally circulating bone marrow derived monocytes (BMDMs) (55) (**Figure 1**). In rats, surgery and anesthesia have been associated with increased hippocampal HMGB1 expression (56); similarly, human studies have shown that plasma HMGB1 levels are correlated with the level of inflammation in both non-cardiac surgery and non-surgical inflammatory states (57). In rodents, elevations of HMGB1 are associated with cognitive deficits (58), which can be mitigated in the presence of HMGB1 inhibitors (4, 59). These results are corroborated by evidence that HMGB1 levels are elevated in patients with POCD following gastrointestinal surgery (60).

When bound by HMGB1, both TLR-4 and RAGE activate nuclear factor kappa B (NF-κB), a transcription factor which regulates the expression of pro-inflammatory cytokines (**Figure 1**). Normally, cytosolic NF-κB is bound to the NF-κB inhibitor IκB in an inactive state; however, when IκB is phosphorylated by IκB kinase (IKK), NF-κB is released and enters the nucleus, causing pro-inflammatory cytokine upregulation (55). Once activated by NF-κB, the pro-inflammatory cytokines interleukin-1 beta (IL-1β), IL-6, and tumor necrosis factor alpha (TNFα) cause further release of HMGB1 in a positive feedback loop, amplifying the inflammatory response (57). Additionally, IL-1 and TNFα can cause further activation of NF-κB, resulting in cyclooxygenase 2 isozyme (COX-2) upregulation (34). There is a strong association between elevations in serum pro-inflammatory cytokines and POCD in both animal models (61, 62) and human studies (41, 44). Moreover, in rats, inhibition of NF-κB and pro-inflammatory cytokines has been associated with a reduction in POCD using various metrics (including Morris water maze, elevated plus maze, fear conditioning, and passive avoidance test) (63–65).

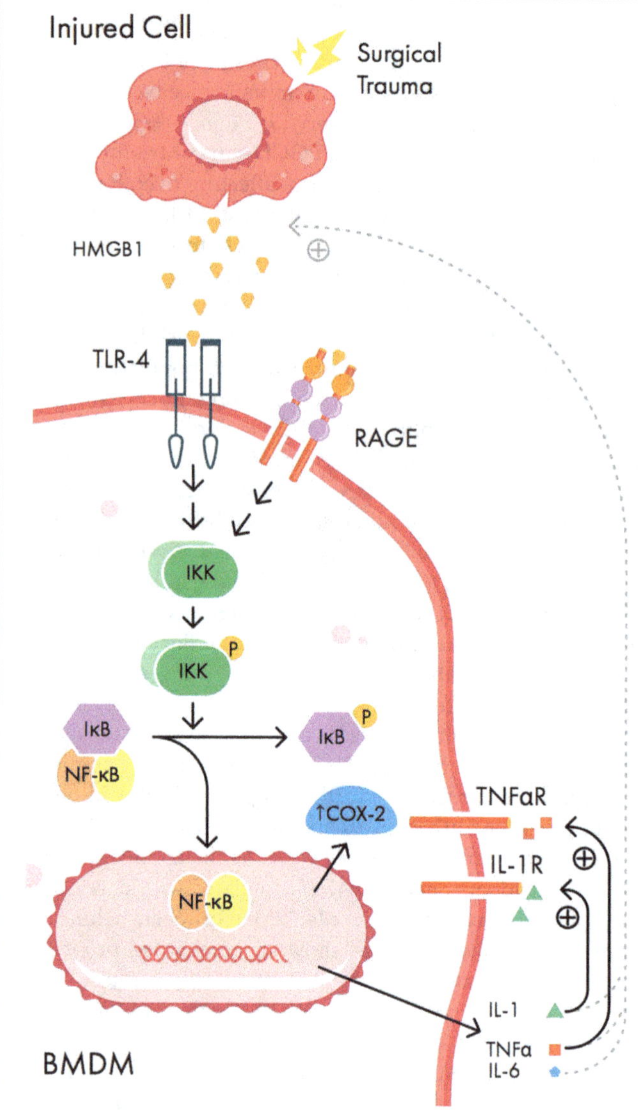

FIGURE 1 | Signaling pathways involved in peripheral initiation of inflammation. Injured cells release damage-associated molecular patterns (DAMPs) including high mobility group box-1 protein (HMGB1) in response to surgical trauma. HMGB1 activates nuclear factor-kappa B (NF-κB) signaling pathways in bone marrow derived monocytes (BMDMs), causing nuclear translocation of NF-κB, increased expression of cyclooxygenase 2 isozyme (COX-2) upregulation, and expression of pro-inflammatory cytokines interleukin-1 beta (IL-1β), interleukin 6 (IL-6), and tumor necrosis factor alpha (TNFα). These pro-inflammatory cytokines can act back on BMDMs in positive feedback loops (solid curved lines) as well as promote further release of HMGB1 from injured cells by unknown mechanisms (dashed curved lines). IKK, IκB kinase; IL-6R, IL-6 receptor; P, phosphate group; RAGE, receptor for advanced glycosylation end products; TLR-4, Toll-like receptor 4; TNFαR, TNFα receptor.

Blood-Brain Barrier Breakdown

Peripheral pro-inflammatory cytokines disrupt BBB permeability *via* COX-2 upregulation and matrix metalloproteinases (MMPs), allowing pro-inflammatory cytokines to enter the CNS

(**Figure 2**). Normally, the BBB is made up of tight junctions held together by transmembrane proteins (i.e., occludins, claudins, junctional adhesion molecules) between neurovascular endothelial cells (66). This structure only allows for the passive diffusion of water, gases, and small lipid-soluble molecules (67). However, pro-inflammatory cytokines IL-1 and TNFα can upregulate COX-2 in neurovascular endothelial cells, which promotes local prostaglandin synthesis (68) and disrupts BBB permeability (69) (**Figure 2**). TNFα, IL-1β, and IL-6 have all been found in hippocampal tissue in rats (69–71) and in human CSF (42, 72) following surgical trauma, suggestive of a breakdown in the BBB. Cytokine elevation in the CNS has also been associated with memory dysfunction in mice (73) and cognitive dysfunction (measured by different neurocognitive metrics—see **Table 2**) in humans (41, 42). These data suggest that BBB breakdown is associated with cytokine influx and cognitive impairment, however this evidence does not rule out the possibility that the cytokine elevation may be generated locally within the CNS. More convincingly, immunoglobulin G (IgG), which is not present normally in the brain, has also been identified in hippocampal slices in rats following surgery (56, 74). Similarly, CNS-specific proteins such as S100β and neuron-specific enolase (NSE) are found in plasma following cardiac and non-cardiac surgery in patients with POCD (43, 75, 76). TNFα can also upregulate transcription of MMPs, particularly MMP-9; this aberrant MMP expression can degrade extracellular matrix proteins *in vitro*, further breaking down the BBB (66) (**Figure 2**). Unfortunately, there is only limited *in vivo* evidence concerning the role of MMPs in BBB disruption (66). At a functional level however, MMP-9 gene deletion mice exposed to surgical trauma have been shown to exhibit better cognitive performance (in terms of fear conditioning) compared to wild-type mice (77).

Lastly, once the BBB is disrupted, circulating BMDMs in the periphery are able to enter the CNS and augment neuroinflammation *via* cytokine expression and microglial activation (**Figure 2**). While mast cells and microglia exist in the CNS, there are no normally occurring populations of dendritic cells or monocytes (78). In the setting of inflammation and BBB breakdown however, BMDMs are recruited to the CNS (79) *via* interactions between the chemokine monocyte chemo-attractant protein 1 [MCP-1, also called C-C motif ligand 2 (CCL2)] and the BMDM cell surface receptor chemokine receptor type 2 (CCR2) (**Figure 2**). Once the BMDMs are present in the CNS, they continue to secrete pro-inflammatory cytokines *via* upregulation of NF-κB transcription (34), and activate microglia in the CNS, further amplifying the neuroinflammation. In mice it has been shown that preoperative depletion of BMDMs reduced POCD (80), suggesting that BMDM migration plays a pivotal role in POCD. Taken together, once the BBB is disrupted, cytokines can freely enter the CNS, causing trafficking of BMDMs to neural tissues and initiating poorly regulated immune functions.

Microglial Activation

Microglia are known as the "resident macrophages" of the CNS (81) and have many important contributory functions in the CNS, including synaptic pruning during development (82) and synaptic scaling in neural plasticity (83). Derived from yolk-sac cells, microglia migrate to the CNS early in development, before the differentiation of many cell types in the CNS (81). As a part of the innate immune system, microglia surveil brain parenchyma (84) and are the first responders to pathogens in the CNS. Although a fully differentiated cell, microglia have the unique ability to self-replenish within the CNS (85).

Normally, microglia are in an inactive state maintained by binding of the CX3CR1 protein to the microglial CX3CR1 receptor (86). However, in the setting of inflammation and BBB breakdown, they can differentiate into one of two activated phenotypes, M1 and M2 (87). The M1 phenotype has high phagocytic properties and is pro-inflammatory (88, 89), while the M2 phenotype is involved in tissue repair and remodeling and is anti-inflammatory (90). Not surprisingly, pro-inflammatory mediators such as TNFα or lipopolysaccharide promote microglial differentiation into the M1 phenotype (91). Moreover, TNFα blockade can suppress microglial activation in mice (35). Conversely, anti-inflammatory cytokines such as IL-4 are known to play a role in promoting the alternative M2 phenotype (88). However, recent evidence is beginning to challenge the dichotomy of the M1/M2 phenotypes, suggesting that there are many overlapping phenotypes with various functions and activation pathways (92). One such new area is the role of mast-cell degeneration in activating microglia: In a recent rat study, Zhang et al. (93) showed that peripheral surgery induced CNS mast cell degranulation and subsequent microglial activation. Further, administration of cromolyn sodium (which inhibits mast cell degranulation) inhibits microglial activation in rats (93, 94), demonstrating a new microglial interaction and a possible new therapeutic target for POCD.

Once microglia are activated, they continue to upregulate expression of pro-inflammatory cytokines, thus amplifying neuroinflammation and contributing to the development of POCD (**Figure 2**). Activated microglia are known to release HMGB1, TNFα, and IL-1β in a variety of rodent models (95–97). Further, astrocytes and microglia both upregulate expression of MCP-1/CCL2 (98), and astrocyte CCL2 can induce further microglial activation *in vitro* (99, 100). These chemokines cause further influx of BMDMs into the CNS: Trafficked BMDMs in turn can activate microglia to the M1 phenotype *via* TNFα/IL-1 expression, and activated microglia recruit more BMDMs into the CNS *via* reciprocal TNFα expression (101). In aged mice, microglial activation is increased in POCD (37, 49, 102). Moreover, in mice, both perioperative microglial depletion (103) and promotion of an M2 phenotype *via* erythropoietin administration (99) improved memory dysfunction as measured by passive avoidance and novel object recognition tests.

The Role of Oxidative Stress

In addition to the inflammatory pathways described above, surgical trauma can also produce oxidative stress and deplete the body of antioxidants (57); these oxidative processes, when superimposed on the inflammatory pathway, can contribute to the development of POCD. Surgical stimulation in rodents can raise the levels of CNS nicotinamide adenine dinucleotide phosphate (NADPH) oxidase, an enzyme compound that

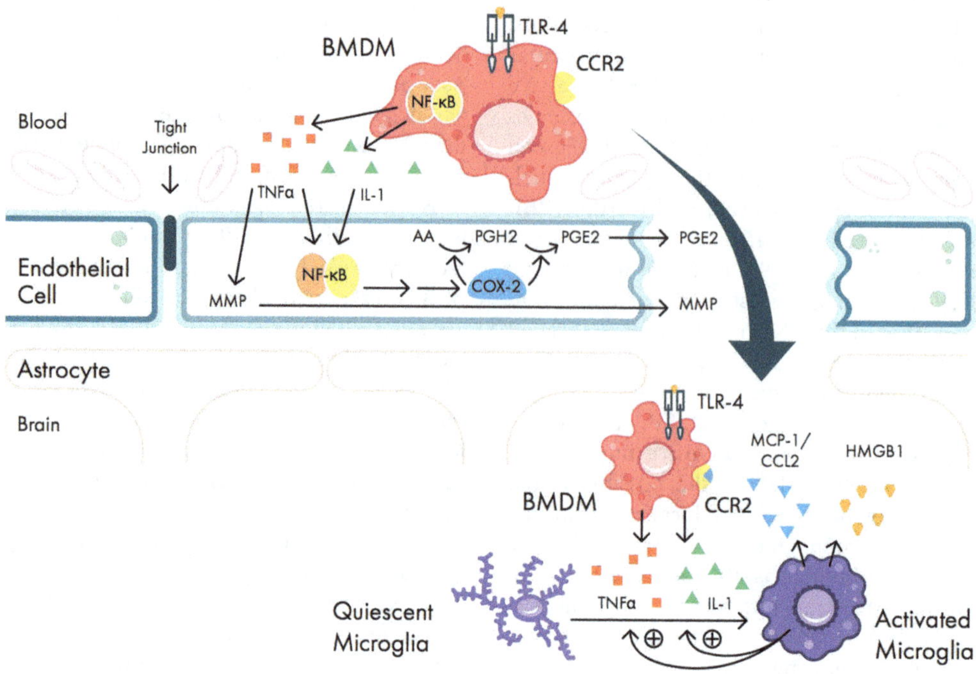

FIGURE 2 | Signaling pathways involved in blood-brain barrier (BBB) breakdown. Pro-inflammatory cytokines interleukin-1 (IL-1) and tumor necrosis factor alpha (TNFα) are secreted by bone marrow derived monocytes (BMDMs) and cause upregulation of nuclear factor-kappa B (NF-κB) and matrix metalloproteinase (MMP) expression in vascular endothelial cells. NF-κB activation causes downstream upregulation of cyclooxygenase 2 isozyme (COX-2) expression, which promotes prostaglandin synthesis and disrupts BBB permeability. Once the BBB is disrupted, BMDMs can enter the central nervous system (CNS); here, the pro-inflammatory cytokines IL-1 and TNFα promote the activation of quiescent microglia. These microglia promote further release of IL-1 and TNFα from BMDMs, as well as secrete high mobility group box-1 protein (HMGB1) and the chemokine monocyte chemo-attractant protein 1 (MCP-1, also called C-C motif ligand 2 (CCL2)). MCP-1/CCL2 binds to the BMDM cell surface receptor chemokine receptor type 2 (CCR2), further promoting BMDM migration into the CNS. AA, arachidonic acid; PGE2, prostaglandin E2; PGH2, prostaglandin H2; TLR-4, Toll-like receptor 4.

generates superoxide in response to stress (104). The superoxide radicals in turn generate other reactive oxygen species (ROS), potentially causing direct damage of neural tissues. Additionally, peripheral oxidative stress can also disrupt the BBB (105), representing a convergence of oxidative stress with the neuroinflammatory pathway. Within the CNS, microglia have been shown to release ROS (106) in response to both HMGB1 (107) and S100β (108). Of note, activated microglia are known to release HMGB1 (97), creating the opportunity for yet another neuroinflammatory positive feedback loop.

Recent evidence from animal and human studies suggests that oxidative stress alone can contribute to POCD. Hippocampal neurons are very metabolically active and are some of the most sensitive neurons to oxidative stress (109); it follows that hippocampal injury from oxidative stress can have profound effects on memory formation and spatial navigation. In aged rats, tibial fracture surgery was associated with memory impairments (measured by open field task and novel object recognition task) on postoperative day 1 with corresponding increases in oxidative damage in the hippocampus and prefrontal cortex (109). Oxidative injury from hypoglycemia has also been shown to induce cognitive impairment in rats, and inhibition of NADPH oxidase has been shown to mitigate such impairments (110). In humans, levels of the ROS nitric oxide are correlated with development of POCD (*via* neurocognitive battery) at 4 days and 3 months following cardiac surgery (111).

Functional Consequences of CNS Inflammation

Memory formation occurs in the hippocampus and is achieved by a process known as long-term potentiation (LTP). Although the mechanisms of induction and maintenance of LTP at various synapses in the CNS are very complex and somewhat controversial, LTP is thought to be achieved by high frequency glutamatergic activation of hippocampal neurons (112). At rest, presynaptic glutamatergic Schaffer cells signal to post-synaptic CA1 collateral neurons. The CA1 neurons themselves contain three types of glutamate receptors: the metabotropic Glu2 receptor and the ionotropic AMPA and NMDA receptors. During normal, low-frequency stimulation of CA1 neurons, glutamate acts on all receptors, but the NMDA channels are blocked by magnesium. With high frequency stimulation however, postsynaptic depolarization causes an activation of NMDA receptors, which causes an influx of calcium and activation of second messenger systems (112). Downstream, the number and sensitivity of AMPA receptors is increased through phosphorylation, and synaptic strength is increased, resulting in memory formation (113).

The presence of pro-inflammatory cytokines can have detrimental effects on the regulation of neurotransmitter signaling in the hippocampus, ultimately resulting in excitotoxic neuronal damage and resulting cognitive impairment. First, the hippocampus has a large number of cytokine receptors, rendering it susceptible to high concentrations of pro-inflammatory cytokines such as IL-1 and TNFα in neuroinflammatory processes (114, 115). Once these cytokine receptors are activated at high levels, there is a downregulation of metabotropic Glu2 receptors causing enhanced AMPA/NMDA signaling, disrupting the process of LTP (116). Meanwhile, HMGB1 can also potentiate glutamate signaling through NMDA, causing an increased influx of glutamate in hippocampal neurons, which ultimately results in glutamate toxicity (117). Further, TNFα can depress inhibitory neurotransmission *via* downregulation of GABA receptors, disrupting the delicate balance of excitatory and inhibitory neurotransmission and ultimately favoring glutamate toxicity (118). These detrimental effects are compounded by the T-cell mediated release of glutamate from activated microglia *via* a separate glutamate transporter subtype (119). Collectively, the aforementioned mechanisms contribute to glutamate toxicity in the hippocampus, resulting in neuronal death and cognitive impairment.

Cholinergic Anti-inflammatory Pathway

Although peripheral pro-inflammatory cytokines are the primary initiator of neuroinflammation, they are also involved in regulating the inflammatory response *via* a vagal reflex arc (34) (**Figure 3**). This serves to help limit the degree of inflammation and protect organ systems from further damage. In this arc, DAMPs released from surgical trauma are sensed by vagal afferents that terminate on the nucleus tractus solitarius (NTS) (120). The efferent arc of this reflex originates from fibers within the dorsal motor nucleus of the vagus, sending signals to the celiac ganglion. Within the celiac ganglion, vagal efferents regulate postganglionic catecholaminergic fibers *via* functional connections within the splenic nerve (121). The splenic nerve endings are in close anatomical position with T lymphocytes, which express β2 adrenergic receptors (122). When activated, T lymphocytes upregulate transcription of choline acetyltransferase, facilitating synthesis of acetylcholine (ACh) (120); this newly synthesized ACh can then activate circulating macrophages that express alpha-7 nicotinic ACh receptors (α7 nAChRs). Ultimately, activation of α7 nAChR-expressing macrophages causes inactivation of NF-kB, which decreases cytokine release (34). In addition, vagal stimulation is known to induce regulatory T-cells and secretion of anti-inflammatory cytokines IL-4 (which promotes microglial differentiation to the M2 phenotype) and IL-10 (123, 124). One experiment in rats treated with the cholinesterase inhibitor physostigmine following laparotomy showed a reduction in hippocampal IL-1β and TNF α expression and hippocampal damage (125). In humans, anticholinergic drugs are widely known to precipitate POCD (126), although it is unclear whether the cholinergic anti-inflammatory pathway is involved in this process. Thus, it has been proposed that vagal stimulation may mitigate the development of POCD (127), although this remains untested in human literature.

The vagus nerve also regulates pro-resolving lipid mediators known as resolvins, lipoxins, and macrophage mediators in resolving inflammation (maresins), all of which are derived from polyunsaturated fatty acids (4, 128). Resolvins act to block the migration of neutrophils and monocytes, and can reduce the oxidative burst of neutrophils (129). Similarly to α7 nAChR-expressing cells, maresins can inhibit NF-kB activity in macrophages and help promote microglial differentiation

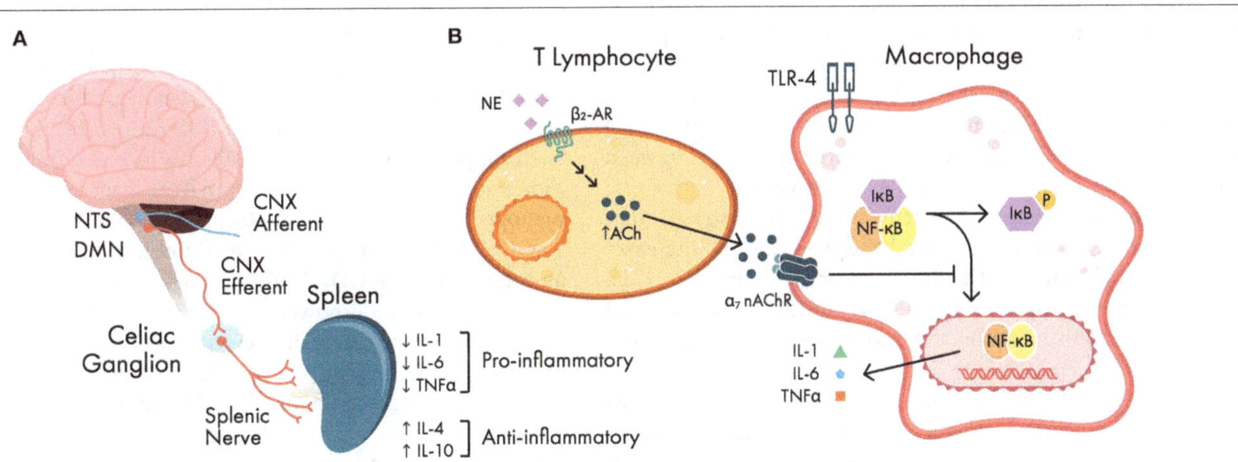

FIGURE 3 | Cholinergic anti-inflammatory pathway. **(A)** schema of vagal reflex arc. Damage-associated molecular patterns (DAMPs) are sensed by vagal afferents; the efferent vagal arc terminates in the celiac ganglion onto splenic nerve fibers, ultimately causing downregulation of pro-inflammatory cytokines and upregulation of anti-inflammatory cytokines. **(B)** cellular signaling within the cholinergic anti-inflammatory pathway. Splenic nerve endings terminate near T lymphocytes and increase acetylcholine (ACh) production *via* β_2 adrenergic receptors (β_2-ARs). The expressed ACh can activate circulating macrophages *via* alpha-7 nicotinic ACh receptors (α7 nAChRs). Activation of α7 nAChRs causes downstream inhibition of NF-kB activation, ultimately decreasing pro-inflammatory cytokine release. CNX, cranial nerve X (vagus nerve); DMN, dorsal motor nucleus of the vagus; IL, interleukin; NE, norepinephrine; NTS, nucleus tractus solitarius; P, phosphate group; TLR-4, Toll-like receptor 4; TNFα, tumor necrosis factor alpha.

to the M2 phenotype (130). Together, these lipid mediators represent possible new therapeutic targets for POCD. Lastly, the vagus nerve can also promote the restoration of BBB integrity *via* netrin-1, a protein involved in cell migration and axonal pathfinding during development (34), however netrin-1 has yet to be explored as a therapeutic target for POCD in human studies.

ETIOLOGY OF POCD

It is difficult to determine the etiology of POCD as surgery and anesthesia are virtually inseparable in modern society. As a result, surgery and anesthesia act as natural confounders of each other, hindering an understanding of a causal relationship and spurring controversy in the literature. Carefully designed animal and human studies have been developed to tease out the contributions of surgery or anesthesia to the development of POCD, however there is great variability in experimental design, limiting the interpretation of these results.

Evidence From Animal Models

Animal models can provide strong insight into the etiology of POCD by exposing a genetically identical group to different anesthetic or surgical regimens and comparing the rates of POCD across groups. Moreover, animal models have the advantage of assessing neuroinflammation at the level of brain parenchyma in terminal experiments, creating a vital link to the neuroinflammatory hypothesis. Much of the evidence supports the notion that surgery and not anesthesia causes both neuroinflammation and POCD: For example, studies in rodents have shown that hippocampal pro-inflammatory cytokines IL-1β, IL-6, and TNFα (70) and HMGB1 (56) are increased with surgery and isoflurane anesthesia, but not with isoflurane anesthesia alone. Moreover, the same studies have shown a higher incidence of POCD (measured using spatial learning paradigms) with surgery and isoflurane compared to isoflurane alone. Increases in hippocampal IL-1β, and TNFα and impaired spatial learning have also been observed in carotid exploration surgery with propofol anesthesia but not propofol anesthesia alone (63), and no differences have been observed in POCD (measured by fear conditioning and spatial learning) between total intravenous anesthesia (TIVA) and volatile anesthetic (131). More convincingly, a recent study demonstrated that open abdominal surgery under local anesthesia caused increases in hippocampal IL-6, TNFα, and memory impairments (71), suggesting that anesthesia *per se* is not necessary for the production of neuroinflammation and subsequent development of POCD.

However, studies looking solely at the effects of anesthesia yield mixed conclusions, with anesthesia being implicated as either a causal or protective agent. Administration of "balanced anesthesia" (consisting of both intravenous and volatile anesthetic agents) during early postnatal life has been shown to produce neurotoxic effects in rats (132), and repeated exposure to the volatile anesthetic sevoflurane has been shown to affect the cognitive function of young, but not adult, mice (133). Similarly, repeated exposure to 5 h of isoflurane (end-tidal isoflurane = 0.7–1.5 vol %) in infant Rhesus macaque monkeys exposed on postnatal day (P)6, P9, and P12 resulted in evidence of motor and socioemotional deficits when tested 12 months later; infants that were only exposed once on P5 had no such alterations (134). In older mice, isoflurane alone has been associated with hippocampal inflammation and impairment of spatial memory (135), however in rats, isoflurane alone did not have an effect on spatial memory processes, even with repeat anesthetics (136). In contrast, in the setting of myocardial ischemia-reperfusion injury in rats, sevoflurane seems to exert a protective effect, mitigating impairments in long-term potentiation (LTP) and improving memory function (137, 138). While the discrepancies between these studies may be partially explained by the different experimental paradigms and the different metrics used to evaluate POCD, it may also be possible that anesthesia induces more subtle changes in cognitive function compared to surgery. One study showed that the combination of isoflurane and intraperitoneal ketamine alone decreased spatial memory and learning, but to a lesser degree than with combined anesthesia and surgery (139). Moreover, hippocampal pro-inflammatory cytokines were only increased with the combination of surgery and anesthesia, suggesting that if anesthesia alone can cause POCD, it may do so *via* non-inflammatory mechanisms. A summary of the findings of relevant animal studies can be found in **Table 1**.

Evidence From Human Studies

Although human studies rely on heterogeneous populations and are limited in scope by ethical considerations, it is possible to tease out the relative contributions of surgery vs. anesthesia to the development of POCD by comparing outcomes in patients undergoing different anesthetic regimens, including general anesthesia, neuraxial anesthesia, and sedation. Indeed, a large ($n = 636$) prospective observational study comparing coronary artery bypass grafting (CABG) under general anesthesia, hip replacement under spinal anesthesia, and percutaneous coronary angiography under sedation showed no difference in POCD rates between groups (7). This result was especially interesting as rates of POCD were long thought to be higher in cardiac surgery due to the inflammation associated with CPB (2, 13). These results have been supported by prospective observational studies showing no difference in POCD between spinal vs. general anesthesia for orthopedic surgery (41, 42). Moreover, a large systematic review was unable to demonstrate a clear connection between general anesthesia and POCD (140), although the majority of studies examined were underpowered and used variable methodologies. As in animal studies, it has even been proposed that volatile anesthesia may be protective in the setting of ischemic organ damage, ultimately mitigating POCD from organ ischemia (141).

Results from randomized controlled trials, while rigorous, are inconsistent and merit further investigation into the causes of POCD. As seen in observational studies, a prospective randomized clinical trial comparing the use of general vs. spinal anesthesia in extracorporeal shock wave lithotripsy showed no significant difference in the incidence of POCD defined by a neurocognitive battery (142), suggesting that surgery and not anesthesia causes POCD. In a separate study of patients undergoing CABG using high-dose vs. low-dose fentanyl

TABLE 1 | Selected relevant pre-clinical studies on etiology of POCD.

Study	Animal model	Experimental model	Cognitive testing	Cellular/Molecular findings	Neurocognitive findings
Cao et al. (70)	Adult (3–6 month) and aged (20–24 month) old Sprague Dawley rats	Partial hepatectomy under sevoflurane anesthesia vs. sevoflurane alone	Morris water maze	Upregulated expression of IL-1β and IL-6 on postoperative day 1 in all rats, and in aged rats until postoperative day 3	Surgery and anesthesia, but not anesthesia alone, caused impairments in latency and distance in all rats on postoperative day 1, and in aged rats until postoperative day 3
He et al. (56)	22–23 month old Sprague-Dawley rats	Splenectomy under general anesthesia vs. 2 h isoflurane anesthesia vs. naïve control	Reversal learning version of Morris water maze	Upregulation of HMGB1 and RAGE levels in surgical group BBB disruption (by TEM) in surgical group	Surgery and anesthesia, but not anesthesia alone, caused cognitive impairments from surgery to postoperative day 3
Qian et al. (139)	20–22 month old BALB/c mice	Splenectomy with isoflurane vs. isoflurane alone vs. control	Y-maze testing	Splenectomy increased hippocampal expression of IL-1β and TNFα	Splenectomy with anesthesia and anesthesia alone both impaired cognitive testing on postoperative days 1 and 3
Tasbihgou et al. (138)	Adult male Wistar rats	Deep vs. light propofol anesthesia, with and without subsequent exposure to hypoxia	Novel object recognition test	Light anesthesia group with hypoxia had lower neurogenesis, but higher BDNF and microglia-ramification	No impairment in cognitive function in either deep or light anesthesia
Walters et al. (136)	Adult Sprague-Dawley rats	Four exposures to isoflurane anesthesia (2, 2, 4, and 6 h) over 7 weeks	Fixed consecutive number, incremental repeated acquisition, progressive ratio tasks†	none	No deficits in any cognitive tasks after single or repeat anesthetic exposure
Wang et al. (135)	6–8 month old male C57BL/6 mice; 14 month old male C57BL/6 mice	Isoflurane vs. no anesthetic exposure	Morris water maze	Older but not younger mice had increased hippocampal expression of NLRP3‡	Older but not younger mice had cognitive impairment after isoflurane anesthesia compared to no anesthetic exposure
Xu et al. (71)	9 and 18 month old female C57BL/6J mice	Laparotomy under local anesthesia (no sedation) vs. sham procedure (no incision)	Fear conditioning system	Surgery increased hippocampal levels of IL-6 and TNFα in all mice, with larger increases in older mice	Cognitive deficits with surgery alone in both young and older mice
Zhang et al. (63)	4 month old male Fischer 344 rats	Right carotid exploration with propofol and buprenorphine anesthesia vs. anesthesia alone	Barnes maze Fear conditioning system	Surgery decreased cytoplasmic hippocampal NF-κB, increased IL-1β, IL-6, MMP-9	Surgery and anesthesia, but not anesthesia alone caused impairments in cognitive metrics
Zhang et al. (131)	20 month old male Fischer 344 rats	Right carotid exploration with propofol-buprenorphine anesthesia vs. isoflurane-buprenorphine anesthesia	Barnes maze Fear conditioning system	No difference in hippocampal TNFα and IL-1β expression in propofol vs. isoflurane anesthesia	Surgery caused impairments in cognitive metrics independent of anesthetic type
Zhu et al. (137)	Adult male Wistar rats	Transient coronary artery occlusion with and without sevoflurane preconditioning vs. sham operation	N/A	Coronary occlusion increased hippocampal TNFα and IL-1β mRNA expression 1–3 days postoperatively; cytokine levels attenuated by sevoflurane	Coronary occlusion inhibited LTP compared to sham operation; sevoflurane preconditioning reversed this effect on postoperative days 1 and 3

BBB, blood-brain barrier; BDNF, brain-derived neurotrophic factor; HMGB1, high mobility group box-1 protein; IL-1β, interleukin-1 beta; IL-6, interleukin 6; LTP, long-term potentiation; MMP-9, matrix metalloproteinase 9; N/A, non-applicable; NF-κB, nuclear factor-kappa B; NLRP3, NOD-like receptor protein 3 inflammasome; RAGE, receptor for advanced glycosylation end products; TEM, transmission electron microscopy; TNFα, tumor necrosis factor alpha.

† Rats were trained to perform these tasks for at least 15 months prior to anesthetic exposure.

‡ NLRP3 causes maturation and secretion of cytokines IL-1β and IL-18.

anesthesia, the same group showed no difference in POCD at 3 and 12 months following surgery, although low-dose fentanyl did have higher rates of POCD at 1 week following surgery (143). However, randomized controlled trials comparing propofol and volatile anesthesia in laparoscopic cholecystectomy (144) and esophageal resection (145) have shown a higher incidence of POCD and pro-inflammatory markers with volatile anesthesia. It is important to note that these trials used different neurocognitive assessments to identify POCD, including the mini-mental status exam (MMSE) and the Montreal Cognitive Assessment (MoCA). Other randomized clinical trials attempting to show a dose-response effect with volatile anesthesia have shown that high-dose anesthetic is associated with an increased incidence of POCD (146, 147). However, these trials used the Bispectral Index™ (BIS™) as a proxy for anesthetic depth, which has been shown to be influenced by a variety of non-anesthetic factors (148–150) and is often discordant with brain activity observed under anesthesia (151); thus, BIS™ may not be an accurate representation of anesthetic depth and may limit the interpretation of these studies. A summary of the findings of relevant clinical studies can be found in **Table 2**.

PROPOSED TREATMENTS FOR POCD

The neuroinflammatory hypothesis provides many varied targets for candidate treatments for POCD. These treatments largely fall into one of three strategies: blocking inflammation by inhibiting inflammatory mediators (anti-inflammatory), preventing the oxidative component of inflammation (anti-oxidative), or protecting neurons during and promoting neuronal health before surgery (pro-neuronal). We present an overview of multiple candidate treatments, with a brief discussion of their hypothesized mechanisms of action and their plausibility established from pre-clinical models where appropriate. We will focus on the existing human data for each treatment, where available, including ongoing human trials from the United States National Library of Medicine (ClinicalTrials.gov), the European Union Clinical Trials Register (clinicaltrialsregister.eu), and the Australian New Zealand Clinical Trials Registry (anzctr.org.au). Please see **Table 3** for a summary of clinical studies for proposed treatments. For an in-depth review of the pre-clinical and human data supporting various treatments for POCD, please see Skvarc et al. (57).

Anti-inflammatory

COX-2 Inhibitors

The cyclooxygenase 2 (COX-2) enzyme is responsible for catalyzing the conversion of arachidonic acid to pro-inflammatory prostaglandins (68) and can increase BBB permeability (69). For these reasons, COX-2 is considered an important mediator of neuroinflammation and a potential target for treatment of POCD. Indeed, rodent models have shown that the COX-2 inhibitor parecoxib is capable of downregulating IL-1 β and TNFα expression (168); furthermore, meloxicam, a non-steroidal anti-inflammatory drug (NSAID) with relative selectivity for COX-2 has been shown to decrease short-term deficits in recognition memory following surgery (169). So far, two human trials have evaluated the efficacy of COX-2 inhibition on POCD, both in geriatric patients undergoing total knee arthroplasty (152, 153). In a trial of 134 elderly patients, parecoxib was shown to decrease pro-inflammatory markers and POCD incidence (as assessed using a neurocognitive battery) compared to placebo at 1 week, but not 3 months following surgery (152), although this negative result was largely due to improved cognitive performance in the placebo group. Similarly, a trial of 178 elderly patients showed that celecoxib reduced pro-inflammatory markers and POCD (determined by reduction in performance of $\geq$2 of 5 cognitive tests) at 1 week following surgery compared to placebo (153). There are no ongoing registered clinical trials testing the use of NSAIDs or selective COX-2 inhibitors in POCD.

Minocycline

Minocycline is a second-generation tetracycline antibiotic that has anti-inflammatory properties; it has shown to be useful in reducing cognitive deficits in animal models of cerebral ischemia, Alzheimer's disease, and Parkinson's disease (170). Minocycline readily crosses the BBB, and thus may also be useful in inhibiting neuroinflammation. In rats, minocycline has been shown to block IL-1β, with a concomitant reduction in surgery-induced hippocampal-dependent memory impairment (determined by fear conditioning test) (73). In mice undergoing appendectomy, preoperative administration of minocycline has been shown to downregulate production of IL-1β, IL-6, and TNFα, inhibit microglial activation, and impair learning (measured *via* Morris water maze and fear conditioning test) (171). However, it has been recently demonstrated in aged rats undergoing abdominal surgery that minocycline may simply delay microglial activation (172). Thus, while it has been proposed that minocycline may be useful for reducing POCD, it may not prevent development of delayed POCD. Currently, there is a multicenter randomized Phase 3 clinical trial recruiting patients to investigate the efficacy of preoperative minocycline in reducing POCD in patients with colon cancer undergoing colorectal surgery (ClinicalTrials.gov identifier NCT02928692).

Dexamethasone

Dexamethasone is a corticosteroid with glucocorticoid actions and powerful (>30 times more potent than cortisol) anti-inflammatory properties. As with other steroid hormones, dexamethasone inhibits the infiltration of leukocytes into the target inflammatory region (173); moreover, it can downregulate the transcription of cytokines and other cell adhesion molecules (174). Although dexamethasone has well-demonstrated anti-inflammatory actions, it is unclear whether it may have an effect on the development of POCD. In a study by Karaman et al. (175), male rats given sevoflurane were shown to develop memory deficits (measured *via* Morris water maze) at 7 and 30 days post anesthesia. Administration of 0.1 mg/kg dexamethasone before anesthetic administration reversed these deficits at both time points, suggesting its utility in

TABLE 2 | Relevant clinical studies on etiology of POCD.

Study	Study Type	Cohort	Sample size (*n*)	Surgical procedure(s)	Anesthetic exposure	Cognitive metrics	Key findings
Evered et al. (7)	Prospective observational	CABG, hip replacement: adults > 55 CA: adults > 50	636	Elective CABG, hip replacement, CA	CABG: general anesthesia Hip replacement: spinal anesthesia CA: sedation	Battery of seven neuropsychological tests	No difference in POCD rates between groups (CABG–16%; hip replacement–16%; CA–21%)
Geng et al. (144)	Prospective randomized	Adults > 60	150	Laparoscopic cholecystectomy	Propofol vs. sevoflurane vs. isoflurane anesthesia	Battery of eight neuropsychological tests	Lower POCD in propofol compared to sevoflurane or isoflurane on postoperative days 1 and 3
Hirsch et al. (42)	Prospective observational	Adults ≥ 55	10	Elective major knee surgery	Spinal anesthesia with propofol sedation and femoral nerve catheter	Word list test Verbal fluency test Digit symbol test	40% POCD on postoperative day 1; 20% POCD on postoperative day 2; 40% POCD on postoperative day 3
Hou et al. (147)	Prospective randomized	Adults ≥ 60; ASA 1-2	66	Elective total knee arthroplasty	Deep vs. light anesthesia† with sevoflurane and propofol, femoral and sciatic nerve blocks	MoCA Z-score < 1.96	Higher POCD in deep (20%) compared to light (3%) anesthesia
Ji et al. (41)	Prospective observational	Adults ≥ 65	83	Elective total hip replacement	Spinal anesthesia	Digit symbol substitution test Concentration endurance test Number connection test‡	POCD rate 24.6% on postoperative day 7
Qiao et al. (145)	Prospective randomized	Adults 65–75	90	Esophageal resection	Sevoflurane vs. methylprednisone and sevoflurane vs. propofol	MoCA MMSE	Higher POCD in sevoflurane group on postoperative days 1, 3, 7
Shu et al. (146)	Prospective randomized	Females 20–60	192	Gynecologic laparoscopic surgery	Sevoflurane with remifentanil, titrated to BIS††	MMSE Trail-making test	Lower POCD in 40 ≤ BIS ≤ 50 group on postoperative day 1
Silbert et al. (142)	Prospective randomized	Adults > 55 without previous neurologic deficit	100	Extracorporeal shock wave lithotripsy	General vs. spinal anesthesia	Battery of eight neuropsychological tests	No difference in POCD rates between groups
Silbert et al. (143)	Prospective randomized	Adults > 55 without previous neurologic deficit	350	Elective CABG	High-dose vs. low-dose fentanyl anesthesia	Battery of eight neuropsychological tests	Higher POCD in low-dose fentanyl group 1 week following surgery. No difference in POCD at 3 and 12 months following surgery

ASA, American Society of Anesthesiologists Classification Scale; BIS, Bispectral Index; CA, coronary angiography; CABG, coronary artery bypass graft; MMSE, Mini-mental Status Examination; MoCA, Montreal Cognitive Assessment.
†Deep vs. light anesthesia determined by BIS values 40–50 vs. 55–65, respectively. ††BIS values stratified to three groups: 30 ≤ BIS ≤ 40, 40 ≤ BIS ≤ 50, 50 ≤ BIS ≤ 50.
‡Neurocognitive tests in this study amended to a Chinese protocol.

mitigating POCD. However, a randomized clinical trial of patients given 1 mg/kg intraoperative dexamethasone during cardiac surgery failed to demonstrate a difference in cognitive performance both at 1 month and at 12 months following surgery (154). There is only one registered clinical trial on dexamethasone and POCD (ClinicalTrials.gov identifier NCT01332812); this Phase 4 study of 300 patients compared administration of 8 mg of dexamethasone following anesthesia induction vs. no injection and measured POCD *via* a cognitive battery up to 180 days post-surgery. Currently no results are reported.

Cholinergic Agents

The cholinergic anti-inflammatory pathway provides a variety of potential therapeutic targets for POCD. Both the α7 nAChR agonist PHA 586487 (176) and physostigmine (125) have been

TABLE 3 | Clinical studies for proposed treatments for POCD.

Treatment	Published clinical studies and relevant findings	Registered ongoing clinical trials (if applicable)
ANTI-INFLAMMATORY		
COX-2 inhibitors	Zhu et al. (152): intraoperative and postoperative parecoxib vs. placebo in total knee arthroplasty (reduction in POCD at 1 week but not 3 months postoperatively) Zhu et al. (153): 1 week of preoperative celecoxib vs. placebo in total knee arthroplasty (reduction in POCD at postoperative day 7)	none
Minocycline	none	NCT02928692: preoperative minocycline vs. no treatment in colorectal surgery
Dexamethasone	Ottens et al. (154): intraoperative dexamethasone bolus vs. no treatment during cardiac surgery (no difference in cognitive performance at 1 and 12 months postoperatively)	NCT01332812: intraoperative dexamethasone bolus vs. no treatment in general surgery
Cholinergic agents	Doraiswamy et al. (155): 12-week course of donepezil >6 months vs. no treatment after CABG (improved memory recall, no improved cognition)	NCT02419352: sugammadex vs. neostigmine/atropine at end of general anesthesia NCT02927522: donepezil vs. placebo for 7 days following general surgery
Targeted cytokine inhibition	None	None
ANTIOXIDATIVE		
Statins	Das et al. (156): postoperative statin vs. placebo in off-pump CABG (reduced POCD on postoperative day 6)	None
N-acetylcysteine	None	PANACEA trial ACTRN12614000411640: NAC vs. placebo twice daily for 4 days beginning on day of non-cardiac surgery
Edaravone	None	None
PRO-NEURONAL		
Dexmedetomidine	Li et al. (157): dexmedetomidine bolus and intraoperative infusion vs. saline in laparoscopic cholecystectomy (reduced POCD on postoperative day 1) Chen et al. (158): correlation between reduction of pro-inflammatory cytokines and reduced POCD on postoperative day 1 in general surgery	NCT02275182: intraoperative dexmetedomidine vs. placebo in general surgery NEUROPRODEX trial 2013-000823-15: intraoperative dexmetedomidine vs. placebo in cardiac and abdominal surgery NCT03480061: intraoperative dexmedetomidine bolus and postoperative infusion vs. standard sedation in cardiac surgery NCT02923128: postoperative dexmedetomidine vs. sufentanil infusion in elective non-cardiac surgery
Amantadine	None	NCT03527134: five-day postoperative amantadine vs. no treatment in general surgery
Enhancing cognitive reserve	None	NCT02747784: three-month postoperative cognitive training regimen vs. no treatment in breast/urogynecological surgery
VARIOUS TARGETS		
Local anesthetics	Wang et al. (159): lidocaine bolus and intraoperative infusion in CABG surgery (improved working memory, verbal associative learning compared to saline controls) Chen et al. (160): lidocaine bolus and intraoperative infusion in spinal surgery (slight improvement in cognitive function)	NCT00975910: lidocaine bolus and intraoperative infusion vs. placebo in supratentorial craniotomy NCT02848599: bupivacaine vs. morphine PCA for 72 h following general surgery
Ketamine	Hudetz et al. (161): ketamine bolus at anesthetic induction during cardiac surgery (improved memory/executive function) Nagels et al. (162): ketamine bolus and intraoperative infusion following anesthetic induction during cardiac surgery (no change in POCD compared to placebo)	NCT02892916: ketamine bolus following anesthetic induction vs. placebo in elective orthopedic surgery
Lipid mediators	none	None
Cannabinoid receptors	none	none
Melatonin	Hansen et al. (163): melatonin 6 mg/kg daily for 3 months improved sleep but had no effect on POCD in women having breast cancer surgery Fan et al. (164): melatonin 1 mg/kg daily for 6 days improved sleep and improves MMSE scores in patients undergoing hip arthroplasty	none
Turmeric	none	none
Acupuncture	Gao et al. (165): Electroacupuncture preserved MMSE scores 2 and 4 days following general surgery. Lin et al. (166): Electroacupuncture preserved MMSE scores on day 3 following intestinal surgery for cancer. (167): Electroacupuncture preserved MMSE scores in elderly patients on day 3 following colorectal surgery for cancer.	none

CABG, coronary artery bypass graft; MMSE, Mini-Mental State Exam; NAC, N-acetylcysteine; PCA, patient-controlled analgesia.

shown to reduce pro-inflammatory cytokines and neuronal damage in rat hippocampus following surgery. However, neither of these studies evaluated behavioral impairments, limiting their generalizability to POCD. In humans, during anesthetic emergence, patients are often given cholinesterase inhibitors such as neostigmine to reverse neuromuscular blocking agents (which are routinely administered to help provide optimal surgical conditions). However, the cyclic oligosaccharide sugammadex, which rapidly and profoundly reverses neuromuscular blockade by encapsulating nondepolarizing steroidal neuromuscular blocking agents such as rocuronium and vecuronium (177), has significantly reduced the use of cholinesterase inhibitors during surgery and provides a unique way to test the association of cholinesterase inhibitors on POCD. Indeed, one registered clinical trial (ClinicalTrials.gov identifier NCT02419352) has randomized 160 patients to receive either sugammadex or the combination of neostigmine and atropine at the end of surgery and anesthesia; results have not yet been published. Other human studies have focused on the anticholinesterase drug donepezil as a potential therapy. In a pilot randomized clinical trial of 44 patients, Doraiswamy et al. (155) showed that a 12-week course of donepezil given at least 6 months following CABG surgery improved memory recall but not cognition. A new Phase 3 clinical trial (ClinicalTrials.gov identifier NCT02927522) plans to randomize over 500 patients to receive donepezil or placebo for 7 days following surgery, and evaluate for POCD 1 week following surgery (although it is unclear what psychological tests are used to define POCD in this study). Again, although vagal stimulation has been proposed to mitigate the development of POCD (127), there are no current human trials designed to test this hypothesis.

Targeted Cytokine Inhibition

Although there are currently no human data and no registered clinical trials, drugs that block specific cytokines are already utilized as treatment for chronic inflammatory diseases such as rheumatoid arthritis (RA) and may be a potential target for POCD therapies. The IL-1 receptor antagonist anakinra represents one such target: It has been shown that IL-1 knockout mice have lower levels of IL-6 following peripheral surgery, and less memory impairment (73). Similarly, intracisternal administration of an IL-1 receptor antagonist immediately preceding abdominal surgery in aged rats prevented a decrease in memory consolidation on postoperative day 4 (178). The anti-TNFα antibody Etanercept (also used in RA) may be another target for POCD, as preoperative administration of anti-TNFα antibody inhibited IL-1β production in mice and mitigated memory impairments in mice (35). Further, the IL-6 receptor antibody toclizumab has been shown to reduce memory impairments in mice following surgery (179).

Antioxidative

Statins

Statins are reversible competitive inhibitors of the enzyme 3-hydroxy-3-methylglutaryl-CoA reductase (HMG-CoA reductase). This enzyme catalyzes the conversion of HMG-CoA to mevalonate, and is the rate-limiting step of cholesterol synthesis from fatty acids (180). As part of this enzymatic process, NADPH is produced; by inhibiting HMG-CoA reductase, NADPH production is lowered, which can reduce the levels of oxidative species (181). Statins have been widely proposed to be beneficial for neurological disorders including dementia (182) and postoperative delirium (183). In POCD, a small randomized controlled trial comparing postoperative statin vs. placebo administration in patients undergoing off-pump CABG showed a significant reduction in memory dysfunction (measured by postgraduate institute memory scale) on postoperative day 6 (156). Unfortunately, no other prospective clinical trials are currently underway to investigate the otherwise promising effects of a widely utilized drug.

N-Acetylcysteine

N-acetylcysteine (NAC) has antioxidant properties which are related to its role as a precursor for glutathione synthesis (184). Additionally, in pre-clinical studies, NAC has been shown to downregulate pro-inflammatory cytokine synthesis including HGMB-1 (185), upregulate anti-inflammatory cytokine synthesis (186), and reduce microglial activation (187). A systematic review of the human literature has suggested that NAC supplementation can have beneficial cognitive effects for patients with a wide variety of neurological and psychiatric disorders, including Alzheimer's disease, traumatic brain injury, Parkinson's disease, and addictive behavior (184), thus raising the possibility of NAC as a potential treatment for POCD. Only one randomized controlled trial, The Post-Anesthesia N-acetylcysteine Cognitive Evaluation (PANACEA) trial (Australian New Zealand Clinical Trials Registry identifier ACTRN12614000411640) is currently being conducted to investigate the utility of NAC in POCD. This single center trial has randomized patients recovering from non-cardiac surgery to receive 1,200 mg of NAC or placebo twice daily beginning on the day of surgery and continuing for four consecutive days. POCD will be assessed *via* a neurocognitive battery at 1 week, 3, and 12 months following surgery (188). The study is ongoing and no results have been reported at this time.

Edaravone

Edaravone is a free radical scavenger that is used as an adjunct therapy for acute ischemic stroke in Japan, and as therapy for amyotrophic lateral sclerosis (ALS) in Japan and the United States. These uses are based on small randomized clinical trials that have shown modest efficacy in stroke (189) and early-stage ALS (190). Edaravone readily crosses the BBB, and has been shown to mitigate or ameliorate impairments in spatial and working memory in rats at 3 and 7 days following left nephrectomy and lipopolysaccharide administration (38). Moreover, the same group showed an increase in hippocampal levels of the antioxidant superoxide dismutase and a decrease in microglial activation on postoperative day 3. Taken together, this evidence suggests that edaravone has antioxidative and anti-inflammatory properties and may be a potential treatment for POCD in humans, however there are no published human studies or registered clinical trials.

Pro-neuronal

Dexmedetomidine

Dexmedetomidine is a centrally-acting presynaptic α_2 adrenergic receptor antagonist used for sedation in the operating room and intensive care unit; its mechanism of action is inhibition of norepinephrine release from adrenergic neurons projecting from the locus coeruleus to the basal forebrain, anterior cortex, intralaminar nucleus of the thalamus, and the preoptic area of the hypothalamus (191). Dexmedetomidine's sedative properties are largely believed to be due to norepinephrine inhibition in the preoptic area of the hypothalamus, an important nucleus in regulating arousal and sleep pathways. Dexmedetomidine is also hypothesized to have actions in the spinal cord, and is used as an adjunct for intraoperative analgesia (192) and the prolongation of regional nerve blockade (193). Recently, dexmedetomidine has been shown to enhance HMGB1 resolution in mice, likely *via* a vagotonic mechanism (194), suggesting that it also has downstream effects on reducing inflammation. Human studies have shown that dexmedetomidine bolus followed by infusion throughout laparoscopic cholecystectomy reduces serum pro-inflammatory cytokines and POCD (as measured *via* MMSE scores) compared to saline on postoperative day 1 (157). Moreover, Chen et al. (158) showed a correlation between the level of reduction of pro-inflammatory cytokines and POCD on postoperative day 1 (measured *via* MMSE), providing a much-needed link between cytokine levels and the severity of cognitive dysfunction. There are several registered ongoing Phase 4 clinical trials examining the efficacy of dexmedetomidine on POCD, comparing intraoperative dexmedetomidine to placebo (ClinicalTrials.gov identifier NCT02275182, NEUROPRODEX trial–EudraCT number 2013-000823-15), looking at late (12 months following surgery) POCD (ClinicalTrials.gov identifier NCT03480061), and comparing postoperative dexmedetomidine vs. sufentanil infusion (ClinicalTrials.gov identifier NCT02923128). So far, no data have been reported from these clinical trials.

Amantadine

Amantadine was initially marketed as an antiviral agent but was found to have dopaminergic actions which led to its use in Parkinson's disease (74). *In vivo*, amantadine has also been demonstrated to promote the production of glial cell line-derived neurotrophic factor (GDNF), an important pro-neuronal agent that promotes glial growth, protects glia, and inhibits microglial activation (195). In a rat surgical model, animals treated with intraperitoneal amantadine or intracerebroventricular GDNF showed a reduction of memory impairment compared to controls 1 day following surgery (74). Further, amantadine inhibited surgery induced neuroinflammation on postoperative day 1. In humans, there is only one randomized clinical trial in the recruitment phase investigating the use of a 5-day course of amantadine (beginning with one dose preoperatively) on POCD (ClinicalTrials.gov identifier NCT03527134).

Enhancing Cognitive Reserve

Poor cognitive function preoperatively is a potential risk factor for development of POCD, and pro-cognitive activities such as sleep, exercise, and education level seem to have a protective effect on POCD (34). As a result, it has been proposed that preoperative cognitive training may have a beneficial effect on reducing the incidence and severity of POCD. In rats, a cognitively stimulating environment has shown to attenuate surgery induced cognitive memory impairments (measured *via* novel object recognition test) and hippocampal cytokine increases (196). There is one registered clinical trial (REACT trial, ClinicalTrials.gov identifier NCT02747784) currently recruiting female patients with breast or urogynecological surgery for a 3-month postoperative cognitive training regimen compared to no treatment. Patients will be measured for POCD *via* a neurocognitive battery at 3 months following surgery; data from this trial are not available at this time.

Candidate Treatments With Various Targets

Local Anesthetics

Local anesthetics such as lidocaine and bupivacaine work by stabilizing the open, inactive state of voltage-gated sodium channels; when injected peri-neuronally, the preferential local diffusion of local anesthetics to pain fibers produces its analgesic actions (197, 198). Because pain is a trigger for inflammatory pathways, it has been proposed that local anesthetics may reduce peripheral inflammation (and thus neuroinflammation and POCD). Despite the plausibility of this hypothesis, human data has not been convincing. Patients undergoing CABG surgery given lidocaine bolus 1.5 mg/kg and infusion of 4 mg/kg/h throughout surgery showed improvements in working memory and verbal associative learning compared to saline controls on postoperative day 9, however both groups had deficits in short-term memory, processing speed, and executive function (159). In spinal surgery, lidocaine bolus of 1 mg/kg followed by 1.5 mg/kg/h infusion showed a slight improvement in MMSE scores (160). Currently, there are two registered randomized controlled trials investigating the use of local anesthetics in preventing POCD. One Phase 2 trial of 100 patients with supratentorial craniotomy tested the efficacy of lidocaine bolus 1.5 mg/kg and infusion 2 mg/kg/h after induction of surgery until anesthetic emergence on POCD (ClinicalTrials.gov identifier NCT00975910), although no results have been published. Similarly, a small Phase 2 trial of 70 patients (currently under recruitment) is testing the use of postoperative bupivacaine vs. morphine patient-controlled analgesia for 72 h following surgery on POCD (ClinicalTrials.gov identifier NCT02848599), although the primary cognitive endpoint is MMSE scores at postoperative day 5.

Ketamine

Ketamine is an NMDA receptor antagonist with sedative, hypnotic, and analgesic properties; it is used as an anesthetic agent as well as an adjunct for neuropathic pain (191, 199). By virtue of its NMDA receptor antagonism, ketamine reduces glutamate transmission in the brain; coupled with its analgesic properties, ketamine has been proposed to reduce neuroinflammation (200). In pre-clinical models, ketamine seems to have differential effects on the levels of pro-inflammatory cytokines (201, 202), however ketamine has been shown to attenuate cognitive impairment in rodents (202, 203). Human data are equally unclear: one small clinical trial ($n = 60$) using a bolus of 0.5 mg/kg ketamine at the induction of cardiac surgery showed improved metrics of memory and executive function compared to control 1 week following surgery (161), however in a similar (but smaller) population, a 2.5 mg/kg ketamine bolus followed by 0.125 mg/kg infusion throughout the intraoperative period showed no change in POCD (measured by neurocognitive battery) compared to placebo at 1 or 10 weeks following surgery (162). It is unclear whether the discrepancies observed may be due to different dosing regimens, different cognitive assessments, or small sample size. There is currently a large ($n = 900$) randomized Phase 3 clinical trial (ClinicalTrials.gov identifier NCT02892916) recruiting patients undergoing elective orthopedic surgeries to receive a 0.5 mg/kg ketamine bolus following anesthetic induction with POCD assessment as a secondary outcome (determined by MoCA score) at 1 week and 3 months following surgery. Results are not available at this time.

Lipid Mediators (Resolvins, Lipoxins, Maresins)

As opposed to preventing the production of pro-inflammatory cytokines or oxidative species, lipid mediators such as resolvins, lipoxins, and maresins have begun to receive attention as possible resolvers of neuroinflammation (4, 129). In a rat model of CPB with deep hypothermic circulatory arrest, the resolution agonist annexin A1 was shown to (1) reduce systemic and neural pro-inflammatory cytokines due to inhibition of NF-κB, (2) inhibit microglial activation, and mitigate declines in Morris water maze performance at postoperative day 3 (204). Currently, no human trials exist on the role of these lipid mediators in POCD, although these agents may become more promising as more animal data become available.

Cannabinoid Receptors

Cannabinoids are a variety of substances that can modulate neurotransmitter release *via* cannabinoid receptors and regulate a variety of physiological processes including appetite, mood, and pain (205). The most widely known cannabinoid is tetrahydrocannabinol (THC), the psychoactive ingredient in plants of the genus Cannabis. Cannabinoids are known to suppress TLR-mediated inflammatory responses, and immune cells themselves can produce endogenous cannabinoids, possibly representing homeostatic mechanisms (206). In mice, the activation of cannabinoid receptor 2 (CR2) was shown to attenuate hippocampal memory impairment (*via* fear conditioning test) and decrease pro-inflammatory cytokines in the hippocampus and prefrontal cortex at 1, 3, and 7 days following tibial fracture surgery (207). Due to the controlled nature of exogenous and synthetic cannabinoids, there are no human data on the effects of cannabinoids on POCD, although this may represent a new area of study as cannabinoids are beginning to be used as therapy for a range of disorders including depression, anorexia, epilepsy, and multiple sclerosis (208, 209).

Melatonin

Melatonin is an endogenous hormone synthesized from L-tryptophan and secreted from the pineal gland. Its production is inhibited by 460–480 nm light in the blue portion of the electromagnetic spectrum and functions in maintaining circadian rhythms (210). Melatonin is also known to modulate production of pro- and anti-inflammatory cytokines and reduce cell adhesion molecules, and scavenge free radicals (211). In rodents, exogenous melatonin attenuates volatile (isoflurane)-induced memory impairment in adult and aged animals (212–214); this effect appears to result from improvements in the sleep-wake cycle (213, 214). Results from two published trials in human subjects offer no insight as to the efficacy of melatonin for the prevention of POCD. In the first instance, 54 women aged 30–75 years undergoing surgery for breast cancer were given 6 mg/day melatonin vs. placebo for 3 months beginning preoperatively again improved sleep-efficiency but without a discernable effect on POCD as measured using the ISPOCD test battery (163). In a more age-appropriate cohort of patients scheduled for hip arthroplasty (age > 65 years; $n = 139$), melatonin (1 mg/day taken orally beginning the day before surgery and continued for 5 days consecutively postoperatively) again improved sleep quality and appeared to preserve basic aspects of cognition as measured by the MMSE in the immediate (within 7 days) postoperative period (164); however, a lack of more appropriate neurocognitive assessments over a more extended time frame, preclude supporting melatonin as prophylaxis against POCD. There are no registered clinical trials currently investigating the use of melatonin in POCD.

Turmeric

Turmeric is a plant of the ginger family whose roots are boiled and ground for coloring and flavoring in many Eastern cultures. As such, it is comprised of many biological compounds with varying concentrations depending on the manufacturing method. One compound, curcumin, has been shown to have antioxidant and anti-inflammatory properties, possibly by inhibition of NF-κB (215). In "aged" male ICR mice (age 12 months) who underwent midline laparotomy, curcumin attenuated surgery-induced impairment in novel object recognition as well as spatial learning and memory (216); here, the anesthetic consisted solely of a neuroleptic anesthetic using fentanyl plus droperidol, so the relevance to current clinical practice is unclear. There are no published or open registered clinical trials currently investigating the use of turmeric or curcumin in POCD.

Acupuncture

Acupuncture is a well-known therapy in alternative medicine, having been developed more than 3,000 years ago in China. It is gaining popularity in the Western world and is being tested as a treatment for a variety of inflammatory disorders including asthma, carpal tunnel syndrome, and fibromyalgia (217). While little is known about acupuncture and POCD, recent evidence suggests that electroacupuncture increases hippocampal expression of α7 nAChRs, downregulates TNFα and IL-1β expression in hippocampal neurons, and can improve spatial memory at 1, 3, and 7 days following partial hepatectomy in rats (218). While there are no animal studies on acupuncture and POCD, three human studies (published in Chinese) were identified (165–167); sample sizes were 120, 124, and 83 subjects, respectively. Although subjects were randomized, the reported methods in each report raise enough concern as to render the validity of the data uncertain, thereby precluding a clear assessment as to the efficacy of the technique. There are no registered clinical trials currently investigating the use of acupuncture in POCD.

CONCLUSION

POCD is a widespread phenomenon following the surgical experience and can have detrimental effects on an individual's functional status and quality of life. People with preexisting neurocognitive impairments seem to be exceptionally prone to developing POCD, and POCD may unmask such impairments even in the absence of clinical detection. A large and growing body of evidence from pre-clinical and clinical studies has implicated the roles of neuroinflammation in the pathogenesis of POCD, from peripheral injury to neuronal death and functional manifestations. However, the data are not entirely conclusive because of heterogeneities in animal models and human populations studied, as well as variability in pre-clinical and clinical assessments of POCD. While both animal and human studies demonstrate a variety of neuroinflammatory mechanisms at play in the perioperative period, the root causes of that inflammation, whether surgery, anesthesia, or even prior inflammation from sources such as infection are unknown. Data from randomized clinical trials seem to more strongly favor surgery as the main inciting factor of POCD, but again these data are not wholly consistent across populations, surgeries, and time scales. An alternative hypothesis is that the combination of surgery and anesthesia contributes to the pathogenesis of POCD: anesthesia may weaken the BBB by modulating tight junction protein expression (219) in a dose-dependent manner (220), while surgery provides the peripheral nidus for inflammation that is ultimately amplified in the CNS. Whatever the cause, neuroinflammation has been shown to be a common feature underlying many chronic and neurodegenerative diseases; a better understanding of such mechanisms may aid in improved diagnosis and treatment of a family of neurocognitive disorders.

The neuroinflammatory hypothesis has already generated a variety of potential candidates for treatment of POCD. The utility of many of these proposed treatment options have shown promising results in animal studies, however when applied to human populations, the treatment options yield more modest results. At this time, the lack of a formal definition of POCD is a critical barrier to future research; without a formal definition, the results of any one study may not be applicable to any other population than the one tested. Moreover, without a formal definition our understanding of the pathogenesis of POCD lacks generalizability to other neurodegenerative disorders that share common cellular mechanisms and clinical features. Only by standardizing our metrics and timepoints of POCD assessment will we be able to better understand the true incidence of POCD, compare the contributions of potential risk factors, and evaluate treatments across a large patient cohort (49, 221). Nevertheless, the sheer number of proposed treatments is suggestive of a growing interest in understanding POCD, and will hopefully benefit patients *via* a diverse array of therapies.

AUTHOR CONTRIBUTIONS

SAS drafted the manuscript. SAS and PAG contributed to the literature review, manuscript revision, and read and approved the submitted manuscript.

FUNDING

This work was supported by the Department of Anesthesiology, Weill Cornell Medical College.

ACKNOWLEDGMENTS

We gratefully acknowledge Mo' Safavynia for all figure preparation associated with this manuscript.

REFERENCES

1. Edwards ML, Bause GS. From dental to mental institutions: an american dentist and a british psychiatrist highlight insanity following nitrous-oxide administration. *J Anesth Hist.* (2018) 4:133–4. doi: 10.1016/j.janh.2018.02.002
2. Bedford PD. Adverse cerebral effects of anaesthesia on old people. *Lancet* (1955) 269:259–63.
3. Evered L, Silbert B, Knopman D, Scott D, DeKosky S, Rasmussen L, et al. Recommendations for the nomenclature of cognitive change associated with anaesthesia and surgery. *Br J Anaesth.* (2018) 121:1005–12. doi: 10.1016/j.bja.2017.11.087
4. Vacas S, Degos V, Feng X, Maze M. The neuroinflammatory response of postoperative cognitive decline. *Br Med Bull.* (2013) 106:161–78. doi: 10.1093/bmb/ldt006
5. Berger M, Nadler JW, Browndyke J, Terrando N, Ponnusamy V, Cohen HJ, et al. Postoperative cognitive dysfunction: minding the gaps in our knowledge of a common postoperative complication in the elderly. *Anesthesiol Clin.* (2015) 33:517–50. doi: 10.1016/j.anclin.2015.05.008
6. Androsova G, Krause R, Winterer G, Schneider R. Biomarkers of postoperative delirium and cognitive dysfunction. *Front Aging Neurosci.* (2015) 7:1347–16. doi: 10.3389/fnagi.2015.00112
7. Evered L, Scott DA, Silbert B, Maruff P. Postoperative cognitive dysfunction is independent of type of surgery and anesthetic. *Anesth Analg.* (2011) 112:1179–85. doi: 10.1213/ANE.0b013e318215217e
8. Moller JT, Cluitmans P, Rasmussen LS, Houx P, Rasmussen H, Canet J, et al. Long-term postoperative cognitive dysfunction in the elderly: ISPOCD1 study. *Lancet* (1998) 351:857–61. doi: 10.1016/S0140-6736(97)07382-0
9. Silbert B, Evered L, Scott DA, McMahon S, Choong P, Ames D, et al. Preexisting cognitive impairment is associated with postoperative cognitive dysfunction after hip joint replacement surgery. *Anesthesiology* (2015) 122:1224–34. doi: 10.1097/ALN.0000000000000671
10. Newman MF, Kirchner JL, Phillips-Bute B, Gaver V, Grocott H, Jones RH, et al. Longitudinal assessment of neurocognitive function after

coronary-artery bypass surgery. *N Engl J Med.* (2001) 344:395–402. doi: 10.1056/NEJM200102083440601

11. Steinmetz J, Christensen KB, Lund T, Lohse N, Rasmussen LS, Group I. Long-term consequences of postoperative cognitive dysfunction. *Anesthesiology* (2009) 110:548–55. doi: 10.1097/ALN.0b013e318195b569
12. Sprung J, Roberts RO, Knopman DS, Olive DM, Gappa JL, Sifuentes VL, et al. Association of mild cognitive impairment with exposure to general anesthesia for surgical and nonsurgical procedures: a population-based study. *Mayo Clin Proc.* (2016) 91:208–17. doi: 10.1016/j.mayocp.2015.10.023
13. Nussmeier NA, Arlund C, Slogoff S. Neuropsychiatric complications after cardiopulmonary bypass: cerebral protection by a barbiturate. *Anesthesiology* (1986) 64:165–70.
14. Monk TG, Weldon BC, Garvan CW, Dede DE, van der Aa MT, Heilman KM, et al. Predictors of cognitive dysfunction after major noncardiac surgery. *Anesthesiology* (2008) 108:18–30. doi: 10.1097/01.anes.0000296071.19434.1e
15. Robinson TN, Walston JD, Brummel NE, Deiner S, Brown CH, Kennedy M, et al. Frailty for surgeons: review of a national institute on aging conference on frailty for specialists. *J Am Coll Surg.* (2015) 221:1083–92. doi: 10.1016/j.jamcollsurg.2015.08.428
16. Hall DE, Arya S, Schmid KK, Blaser C, Carlson MA, Bailey TL, et al. Development and initial validation of the risk analysis index for measuring frailty in surgical populations. *JAMA Surg.* (2017) 152:175–82. doi: 10.1001/jamasurg.2016.4202
17. Hall DE, Arya S, Schmid KK, Carlson MA, Lavedan P, Bailey TL, et al. Association of a frailty screening initiative with postoperative survival at 30:180, and 365 Days. *JAMA Surg.* (2017) 152:233–40. doi: 10.1001/jamasurg.2016.4219
18. Esses G, Andreopoulos E, Lin HM, Arya S, Deiner S. A comparison of three frailty indices in predicting morbidity and mortality after on-pump aortic valve replacement. *Anesth Analg.* (2018) 126:39–45. doi: 10.1213/ANE.0000000000002411
19. Moskven E, Bourassa-Moreau Md MFE, Charest-Morin R, Flexman A, and Street J. The impact of frailty and sarcopenia on postoperative outcomes in adult spine surgery. A systematic review of the literature. *Spine J.* (2018) 18:2354–69. doi: 10.1016/j.spinee.2018.07.008
20. Rothrock RJ, Steinberger JM, Badgery H, Hecht AC, Cho SK, Caridi JM, et al. Frailty status as a predictor of 3-month cognitive and functional recovery following spinal surgery: a prospective pilot study. *Spine J.* (2019) 19:104-112. doi: 10.1016/j.spinee.2018.05.026
21. Robinson TN, Wu DS, Pointer LF, Dunn CL, and Moss M. Preoperative cognitive dysfunction is related to adverse postoperative outcomes in the elderly. *J Am Coll Surg.* (2012) 215:12–7; discussion 17–18. doi: 10.1016/j.jamcollsurg.2012.02.007
22. Culley DJ, Flaherty D, Fahey MC, Rudolph JL, Javedan H, Huang CC, et al. Poor performance on a preoperative cognitive screening test predicts postoperative complications in older orthopedic surgical patients. *Anesthesiology* (2017) 127:765–74. doi: 10.1097/ALN.0000000000001859
23. Gasparini M, Vanacore N, Schiaffini C, Brusa L, Panella M, Talarico G, et al. A case-control study on Alzheimer's disease and exposure to anesthesia. *Neurol Sci.* (2002) 23:11–4. doi: 10.1007/s100720200017
24. Horsburgh K, McCarron MO, White F, Nicoll JA. The role of apolipoprotein E in Alzheimer's disease, acute brain injury and cerebrovascular disease: evidence of common mechanisms and utility of animal models. *Neurobiol Aging* (2000) 21:245–55. doi: 10.1016/S0197-4580(00)00097-X
25. Heyer EJ, Wilson DA, Sahlein DH, Mocco J, Williams SC, Sciacca R, et al. APOE-epsilon4 predisposes to cognitive dysfunction following uncomplicated carotid endarterectomy. *Neurology* (2005) 65:1759–63. doi: 10.1212/01.wnl.0000184579.23624.6b
26. Avidan MS, Searleman AC, Storandt M, Barnett K, Vannucci A, Saager L, et al. Long-term cognitive decline in older subjects was not attributable to noncardiac surgery or major illness. *Anesthesiology* (2009) 111:964–70. doi: 10.1097/ALN.0b013e3181bc9719
27. Berger M, Nadler JW, Friedman A, McDonagh DL, Bennett ER, Cooter M, et al. The effect of propofol versus isoflurane anesthesia on human cerebrospinal fluid markers of alzheimer's disease: results of a randomized trial. *J Alzheimers Dis.* (2016) 52:1299–310. doi: 10.3233/JAD-151190
28. Whittington RA, Bretteville A, Dickler MF, Planel E. Anesthesia and tau pathology. *Prog Neuropsychopharmacol Biol Psychiatry* (2013) 47:147–55. doi: 10.1016/j.pnpbp.2013.03.004
29. Whittington RA, Bretteville A, Virag L, Emala CW, Maurin TO, Marcouiller F, et al. Anesthesia-induced hypothermia mediates decreased ARC gene and protein expression through ERK/MAPK inactivation. *Sci Rep.* (2013) 3:1388. doi: 10.1038/srep01388
30. Whittington RA, Virag L, Gratuze M, Petry FR, Noel A, Poitras I, et al. Dexmedetomidine increases tau phosphorylation under normothermic conditions *in vivo* and *in vitro*. *Neurobiol Aging* (2015) 36:2414–28. doi: 10.1016/j.neurobiolaging.2015.05.002
31. Hudetz JA, Iqbal Z, Gandhi SD, Patterson KM, Byrne AJ, Pagel PS. Postoperative delirium and short-term cognitive dysfunction occur more frequently in patients undergoing valve surgery with or without coronary artery bypass graft surgery compared with coronary artery bypass graft surgery alone: results of a pilot study. *J Cardiothorac Vasc Anesth.* (2011) 25:811–6. doi: 10.1053/j.jvca.2010.05.003
32. Hudetz JA, Patterson KM, Iqbal Z, Gandhi SD, Pagel PS. Metabolic syndrome exacerbates short-term postoperative cognitive dysfunction in patients undergoing cardiac surgery: results of a pilot study. *J Cardiothorac Vasc Anesth.* (2011) 25:282–7. doi: 10.1053/j.jvca.2010.06.008
33. Dallmeier D, Larson MG, Vasan RS, Keaney JF, Fontes JD, Meigs JB, et al. Metabolic syndrome and inflammatory biomarkers: a community-based cross-sectional study at the Framingham Heart Study. *Diabetol Metabol Syndr.* (2012) 4:28. doi: 10.1186/1758-5996-4-28
34. Saxena S, Maze M. Impact on the brain of the inflammatory response to surgery. *La Presse Med.* (2018) 47:e73–e81. doi: 10.1016/j.lpm.2018.03.011
35. Terrando N, Monaco C, Ma D, Foxwell BMJ, Feldmann M, Maze M. Tumor necrosis factor-alpha triggers a cytokine cascade yielding postoperative cognitive decline. *Proc Natl Acad Sci USA.* (2010) 107:20518–22. doi: 10.1073/pnas.1014557107
36. Fidalgo AR, Cibelli M, White JPM, Nagy I, Maze M, Ma D. Systemic inflammation enhances surgery-induced cognitive dysfunction in mice. *Neurosci. Lett.* (2011) 498:63–6. doi: 10.1016/j.neulet.2011.04.063
37. Hovens IB, van Leeuwen BL, Nyakas C, Heineman E, van der Zee EA, Schoemaker RG. Prior infection exacerbates postoperative cognitive dysfunction in aged rats. *Am J Physiol. Regul Integr. Compar Physiol.* (2015) 309:R148–59. doi: 10.1152/ajpregu.00002.2015
38. Wang P, Cao J, Liu N, Ma L, Zhou X, Zhang H, et al. Protective effects of edaravone in adult rats with surgery and lipopolysaccharide administration-induced cognitive function impairment. *PLoS ONE* (2016) 11:e0153708. doi: 10.1371/journal.pone.0153708
39. Buvanendran A, Kroin JS, Berger RA, Hallab NJ, Saha C, Negrescu C, et al. Upregulation of prostaglandin E2 and interleukins in the central nervous system and peripheral tissue during and after surgery in humans. *Anesthesiology* (2006) 104:403–10.
40. van Harten AE, Scheeren TWL, Absalom AR. A review of postoperative cognitive dysfunction and neuroinflammation associated with cardiac surgery and anaesthesia. *Anaesthesia* (2012) 67:280–93. doi: 10.1111/j.1365-2044.2011.07008.x
41. Ji M-H, Yuan H-M, Zhang G-F, Li X-M, Dong L, Li W-Y, et al. Changes in plasma and cerebrospinal fluid biomarkers in aged patients with early postoperative cognitive dysfunction following total hip-replacement surgery. *J Anesth.* (2013) 27:236–42. doi: 10.1007/s00540-012-1506-3
42. Hirsch J, Vacas S, Terrando N, Yuan M, Sands LP, Kramer J, et al. Perioperative cerebrospinal fluid and plasma inflammatory markers after orthopedic surgery. *J Neuroinflammat.* (2016) 13:211. doi: 10.1186/s12974-016-0681-9
43. Peng L, Xu L, Ouyang W. Role of peripheral inflammatory markers in postoperative cognitive dysfunction (POCD): a meta-analysis. *PLoS ONE* (2013) 8:e79624–e79610. doi: 10.1371/journal.pone.0079624
44. Liu X, Yu Y, Zhu S. Inflammatory markers in postoperative delirium (POD) and cognitive dysfunction (POCD): a meta-analysis of observational studies. *PLoS One* (2018) 13:e0195659. doi: 10.1371/journal.pone.0195659
45. Goto T, Maekawa K. Cerebral dysfunction after coronary artery bypass surgery. *J Anesthes.* (2014) 28:242–8. doi: 10.1007/s00540-013-1699-0
46. Öztürk S, and Saçar M, Baltalarli A, and Öztürk I. (2016). Effect of the type of cardiopulmonary bypass pump flow on postoperative cognitive function

in patients undergoing isolated coronary artery surgery. *Anatol J Cardiol.* 16:875–80. doi: 10.14744/AnatolJCardiol.2015.6572

47. Rasmussen LS, Larsen K, Houx P, Skovgaard LT, Hanning CD, Moller JT, et al. The assessment of postoperative cognitive function. *Acta Anaesthesiol Scand.* (2001) 45:275–89. doi: 10.1034/j.1399-6576.2001.045003275.x
48. Evered L, Scott DA, Silbert B. Cognitive decline associated with anesthesia and surgery in the elderly. *Curr Opin Psychiatry* (2017) 30:220–6. doi: 10.1097/YCO.0000000000000321
49. Hovens IB, Schoemaker RG, van der Zee EA, Heineman E, Izaks GJ, van Leeuwen BL. Thinking through postoperative cognitive dysfunction: how to bridge the gap between clinical and pre-clinical perspectives. *Brain Behav Immunity* (2012) 26:1169–79. doi: 10.1016/j.bbi.2012.06.004
50. APA. *Diagnostic and Statistical Manual of Mental Disorders (DSM-5®), American Psychiatric Pub.* Arlington, VA: American Psychiatric Association, (2013).
51. Berger M, Terrando N, Smith SK, Browndyke JN, Newman MF, Mathew JP. Neurocognitive function after cardiac surgery: from phenotypes to mechanisms. *Anesthesiology* (2018) 129:829–51. doi: 10.1097/ALN.0000000000002194
52. Evered LA, Silbert BS. Postoperative cognitive dysfunction and noncardiac surgery. *Anesth Analg.* (2018) 127:496–505. doi: 10.1213/ANE.0000000000003514
53. Maldonado JR. Neuropathogenesis of delirium: review of current etiologic theories and common pathways. *Am J Geriatr Psychiatry* (2013) 21:1190–222. doi: 10.1016/j.jagp.2013.09.005
54. Zhang Q, Raoof M, Chen Y, Sumi Y, Sursal T, Junger W, et al. Circulating mitochondrial DAMPs cause inflammatory responses to injury. *Nature* (2010) 464:104–7. doi: 10.1038/nature08780
55. Lotze MT, Tracey KJ. High-mobility group box 1 protein (HMGB1): nuclear weapon in the immune arsenal. *Nat Rev Immunol.* (2005) 5:331–42. doi: 10.1038/nri1594
56. He H-J, Wang Y, Le Y, Duan K-M, Yan X-B, Liao Q, et al. Surgery upregulates high mobility group box-1 and disrupts the blood-brain barrier causing cognitive dysfunction in aged rats. *CNS Neurosci Therapeut.* (2012) 18:994–1002. doi: 10.1111/cns.12018
57. Skvarc DR, Berk M, Byrne LK, Dean OM, Dodd S, Lewis M, et al. Post-operative cognitive dysfunction_ an exploration of the inflammatory hypothesis and novel therapies. *Neurosci Biobehav Rev.* (2018) 84:116–33. doi: 10.1016/j.neubiorev.2017.11.011
58. Li R-L, Zhang Z-Z, Peng M, Wu Y, Zhang J-J, Wang C-Y, et al. Postoperative impairment of cognitive function in old mice: a possible role for neuroinflammation mediated by HMGB1, S100B, and RAGE. *J Surg Res.* (2013) 185:815–24. doi: 10.1016/j.jss.2013.06.043
59. Terrando N, Yang T, Wang X, Fang J, Cao M, Andersson U, et al. Systemic HMGB1 neutralization prevents postoperative neurocognitive dysfunction in aged rats. *Front Immunol.* (2016) 7:441. doi: 10.3389/fimmu.2016.00441
60. Lin G-X, Wang T, Chen M-H, Hu Z-H, Ouyang W. Serum high-mobility group box 1 protein correlates with cognitive decline after gastrointestinal surgery. *Acta Anaesthesiol. Scand.* (2014) 58:668–74. doi: 10.1111/aas.12320
61. Hem S, Albite R, Loresi M, Rasmussen J, Ajler P, Yampolsky C, et al. Pathological changes of the hippocampus and cognitive dysfunction following frontal lobe surgery in a rat model. *Acta Neurochirurg.* (2016) 158:2163–71. doi: 10.1007/s00701-016-2938-6
62. Li Z, Ni C, Xia C, Jaw J, Wang Y, Cao Y, et al. Calcineurin/nuclear factor-κB signaling mediates isoflurane-induced hippocampal neuroinflammation and subsequent cognitive impairment in aged rats. *Mol Med Rep.* (2017) 15:201–9. doi: 10.3892/mmr.2016.5967
63. Zhang J, Jiang W, Zuo Z. Pyrrolidine dithiocarbamate attenuates surgery-induced neuroinflammation and cognitive dysfunction possibly via inhibition of nuclear factor κB. *Neuroscience* (2014) 261:1–10. doi: 10.1016/j.neuroscience.2013.12.034
64. Ma Y, Cheng Q, Wang E, Li L, Zhang X. Inhibiting tumor necrosis factor-α signaling attenuates postoperative cognitive dysfunction in aged rats. *Mol Med Rep.* (2015) 12:3095–100. doi: 10.3892/mmr.2015.3744
65. Cheon SY, Kim JM, Kam EH, Ho C-C, Kim EJ, Chung S, et al. Cell-penetrating interactomic inhibition of nuclear factor-kappa B in a mouse model of postoperative cognitive dysfunction. *Sci Rep* (2017) 7:13482. doi: 10.1038/s41598-017-14027-2
66. Rempe RG, Hartz AM, Bauer B. Matrix metalloproteinases in the brain and blood–brain barrier: versatile breakers and makers. *J Cereb Blood Flow Metabol.* (2016) 36:1481–507. doi: 10.1177/0271678X16655551
67. Zlokovic BV. The blood-brain barrier in health and chronic neurodegenerative disorders. *Neuron* (2008) 57:178–201. doi: 10.1016/j.neuron.2008.01.003
68. Engblom D, Ek M, Saha S, Ericsson-Dahlstrand A, Jakobsson P-J, Blomqvist A. Prostaglandins as inflammatory messengers across the blood-brain barrier. *J Mol Med.* (2002) 80:5–15. doi: 10.1007/s00109-001-0289-z
69. Terrando N, Eriksson LI, Kyu Ryu J, Yang T, Monaco C, Feldmann M, et al. Resolving postoperative neuroinflammation and cognitive decline. *Ann Neurol.* (2011) 70:986–95. doi: 10.1002/ana.22664
70. Cao X-Z, Ma H, Wang J-K, Liu F, Wu B-Y, Tian A-Y, et al. Postoperative cognitive deficits and neuroinflammation in the hippocampus triggered by surgical trauma are exacerbated in aged rats. *Progr Neuropsychopharmacol Biol Psychiatry* (2010) 34:1426–32. doi: 10.1016/j.pnpbp.2010.07.027
71. Xu Z, Dong Y, Wang H, Culley DJ, Marcantonio ER, Crosby G, et al. Peripheral surgical wounding and age-dependent neuroinflammation in mice. *PLoS ONE* (2014) 9:e96752. doi: 10.1371/journal.pone.0096752
72. Reinsfelt B, Ricksten S-E, Zetterberg H, Blennow K, Fredén-Lindqvist J, Westerlind A. Cerebrospinal fluid markers of brain injury, inflammation, and blood-brain barrier dysfunction in cardiac surgery. *Ann Thorac Surg.* (2012) 94:549–55. doi: 10.1016/j.athoracsur.2012.04.044
73. Cibelli M, Fidalgo AR, Terrando N, Ma D, Monaco C, Feldmann M, et al. Role of interleukin-1beta in postoperative cognitive dysfunction. *Ann Neurol.* (2010) 68:360–8. doi: 10.1002/ana.22082
74. Zhang J, Tan H, Jiang W, Zuo Z. Amantadine alleviates postoperative cognitive dysfunction possibly by increasing glial cell line-derived neurotrophic factor in rats. *Anesthesiology* (2014) 121:773–85. doi: 10.1097/ALN.0000000000000352
75. Bayram H, Hidiroglu M, Cetin L, Kucuker A, Iriz E, Uguz E, et al. Comparing S-100 beta protein levels and neurocognitive functions between patients undergoing on-pump and off-pump coronary artery bypass grafting. *J Surg Res.* (2013) 182:198–202. doi: 10.1016/j.jss.2012.10.047
76. Silva FP, Schmidt AP, Valentin LS, Pinto KO, Zeferino SP, Oses JP, et al. S100B protein and neuron-specific enolase as predictors of cognitive dysfunction after coronary artery bypass graft surgery. *Eur J Anaesthesiol.* (2016) 33:681–9. doi: 10.1097/EJA.0000000000000450
77. Bi J, Shan W, Luo A, Zuo Z. Critical role of matrix metallopeptidase 9 in postoperative cognitive dysfunction and age-dependent cognitive decline. *Oncotarget* (2017) 8:51817–29. doi: 10.18632/oncotarget.15545
78. Dong H, Zhang X, Qian Y. Mast cells and neuroinflammation. *Med Sci Monit Basic Res.* (2014) 20:200–6. doi: 10.12659/MSMBR.893093
79. Wohleb ES, McKim DB, Sheridan JF, Godbout JP. Monocyte trafficking to the brain with stress and inflammation: a novel axis of immune-to-brain communication that influences mood and behavior. *Front Neurosci.* (2014) 8:447. doi: 10.3389/fnins.2014.00447
80. Degos V, Vacas S, Han Z, van Rooijen N, Gressens P, Su H, et al. Depletion of bone marrow-derived macrophages perturbs the innate immune response to surgery and reduces postoperative memory dysfunction. *Anesthesiology* (2013) 118:527–36. doi: 10.1097/ALN.0b013e3182834d94
81. Frost JL, Schafer DP. Microglia: architects of the developing nervous system. *Trends Cell Biol.* (2016) 26:587–97. doi: 10.1016/j.tcb.2016.02.006
82. Cunningham CL, Martínez-Cerdeño V, Noctor SC. Microglia regulate the number of neural precursor cells in the developing cerebral cortex. *J Neurosci.* (2013) 33:4216–33. doi: 10.1523/JNEUROSCI.3441-12.2013
83. Li Q, Barres BA. Microglia and macrophages in brain homeostasis and disease. *Nat Rev Immunol.* (2018) 18:225–42. doi: 10.1038/nri.2017.125
84. Nimmerjahn A, Kirchhoff F, Helmchen F. Resting microglial cells are highly dynamic surveillants of brain parenchyma *in vivo*. *Science* (2005) 308:1314–8. doi: 10.1126/science.1110647
85. Hashimoto D, Chow A, Noizat C, Teo P, Beasley MB, Leboeuf M, et al. Tissue-resident macrophages self-maintain locally throughout adult life with minimal contribution from circulating monocytes. *Immunity* (2013) 38:792–804. doi: 10.1016/j.immuni.2013.04.004
86. Biber K, Neumann H, Inoue K, Boddeke HWGM. Neuronal 'On' and 'Off' signals control microglia. *Trends Neurosci.* (2007) 30:596–602. doi: 10.1016/j.tins.2007.08.007

87. Szalay G, Martinecz B, Lénárt N, Környei Z, Orsolits B, Judák L, et al. Microglia protect against brain injury and their selective elimination dysregulates neuronal network activity after stroke. *Nat Commun.* (2016) 7:11499. doi: 10.1038/ncomms11499
88. Gordon S. Alternative activation of macrophages. *Nat Rev Immunol.* (2003) 3:23–35. doi: 10.1038/nri978
89. Thériault P, ElAli A, Rivest S. The dynamics of monocytes and microglia in Alzheimer's disease. *Alzheimer Res Ther.* (2015) 7:41. doi: 10.1186/s13195-015-0125-2
90. Martinez FO, Helming L, Gordon S. Alternative activation of macrophages: an immunologic functional perspective. *Ann Rev Immunol.* (2009) 27:451–83. doi: 10.1146/annurev.immunol.021908.132532
91. Machado-Pereira M, Santos T, Ferreira L, Bernardino L, Ferreira R. Anti-inflammatory strategy for M2 microglial polarization using retinoic acid-loaded nanoparticles. *Med Inflammat.* (2017) 2017:6742427–11. doi: 10.1155/2017/6742427
92. Tay TL, Savage JC, Hui CW, Bisht K, Tremblay M-È. Microglia across the lifespan: from origin to function in brain development, plasticity and cognition. *J Physiol.* (2017) 595:1929–45. doi: 10.1113/JP272134
93. Zhang X, Dong H, Li N, Zhang S, Sun J, Zhang S, et al. Activated brain mast cells contribute to postoperative cognitive dysfunction by evoking microglia activation and neuronal apoptosis. *J Neuroinflammat.* (2016) 13:127. doi: 10.1186/s12974-016-0592-9
94. Zhang S, Dong H, Zhang X, Li N, Sun J, and Qian Y. Cerebral mast cells contribute to postoperative cognitive dysfunction by promoting blood brain barrier disruption. *Behav Brain Res.* (2016) 298:158–66. doi: 10.1016/j.bbr.2015.11.003
95. Clausen BH, Lambertsen KL, Babcock AA, Holm TH, Dagnaes-Hansen F, Finsen B. Interleukin-1beta and tumor necrosis factor-alpha are expressed by different subsets of microglia and macrophages after ischemic stroke in mice. *J Neuroinflammat.* (2008) 5:46. doi: 10.1186/1742-2094-5-46
96. Henkel JS, Beers DR, Zhao W, Appel SH. Microglia in ALS: the good, the bad, and the resting. *J Neuroimmune Pharmacol.* (2009) 4:389–98. doi: 10.1007/s11481-009-9171-5
97. Terrando N, Rei Fidalgo A, Vizcaychipi M, Cibelli M, Ma D, Monaco C, et al. The impact of IL-1 modulation on the development of lipopolysaccharide-induced cognitive dysfunction. *Crit Care* (2010) 14:R88. doi: 10.1186/cc9019
98. Prinz M, Priller J. Tickets to the brain: role of CCR2 and CX3CR1 in myeloid cell entry in the CNS. *J Neuroimmunol.* (2010) 224:80–4. doi: 10.1016/j.jneuroim.2010.05.015
99. Lee JH, Kam EH, Kim SY, Cheon SY, Kim EJ, Chung S, et al. Erythropoietin attenuates postoperative cognitive dysfunction by shifting macrophage activation toward the M2 phenotype. *Front Pharmacol.* (2017) 8:839. doi: 10.3389/fphar.2017.00839
100. Xu J, Dong H, Qian Q, Zhang X, Wang Y, Jin W, et al. Astrocyte-derived CCL2 participates in surgery-induced cognitive dysfunction and neuroinflammation via evoking microglia activation. *Behav Brain Res.* (2017) 332:145–53. doi: 10.1016/j.bbr.2017.05.066
101. D'Mello C, Le T, Swain MG. Cerebral microglia recruit monocytes into the brain in response to tumor necrosis factoralpha signaling during peripheral organ inflammation. *J Neurosci.* (2009) 29:2089–102. doi: 10.1523/JNEUROSCI.3567-08.2009
102. Wang H-L, Ma R-H, Fang H, Xue Z-G, Liao Q-W. Impaired spatial learning memory after isoflurane anesthesia or appendectomy in aged mice is associated with microglia activation. *J Cell Death* (2015) 8:9–19. doi: 10.4137/JCD.S30596
103. Feng X, Valdearcos M, Uchida Y, Lutrin D, Maze M, Koliwad SK. Microglia mediate postoperative hippocampal inflammation and cognitive decline in mice. *JCI Insight* (2017) 2:e91229. doi: 10.1172/jci.insight.91229
104. Zhang T, Leng Z, Liu W, Wang X, Yan X, Yu L. Suppressed expression of mitogen-activated protein kinases in hyperthermia induced defective neural tube. *Neurosci Lett.* (2015) 594:6–11. doi: 10.1016/j.neulet.2015.03.046
105. Abdul-Muneer PM, Chandra N, Haorah J. Interactions of oxidative stress and neurovascular inflammation in the pathogenesis of traumatic brain injury. *Mol Neurobiol.* (2015) 51:966–79. doi: 10.1007/s12035-014-8752-3
106. Heneka MT, Kummer MP, Latz E. Innate immune activation in neurodegenerative disease. *Nat Rev Immunol.* (2014) 14:463–77. doi: 10.1038/nri3705
107. Gao H-M, Zhou H, Zhang F, Wilson BC, Kam W, Hong J-S. HMGB1 acts on microglia Mac1 to mediate chronic neuroinflammation that drives progressive neurodegeneration. *J Neurosci.* (2011) 31:1081–92. doi: 10.1523/JNEUROSCI.3732-10.2011
108. Adami C, Bianchi R, Pula G, Donato R. S100B-stimulated NO production by BV-2 microglia is independent of RAGE transducing activity but dependent on RAGE extracellular domain. *Biochim Biophys Acta* (2004) 1742:169–77. doi: 10.1016/j.bbamcr.2004.09.008
109. Netto MB, de Oliveira Junior AN, Goldim M, Mathias K, Fileti ME, da Rosa N, et al. Oxidative stress and mitochondrial dysfunction contributes to postoperative cognitive dysfunction in elderly rats. *Brain Behav Immunity* (2018) 73:661–9. doi: 10.1016/j.bbi.2018.07.016
110. Won SJ, Yoo BH, Kauppinen TM, Choi BY, Kim JH, Jang BG, et al. Recurrent/moderate hypoglycemia induces hippocampal dendritic injury, microglial activation, and cognitive impairment in diabetic rats. *J Neuroinflammat.* (2012) 9:182. doi: 10.1186/1742-2094-9-182
111. Harmon D, Eustace N, Ghori K, Butler M, O'Callaghan S, O'Donnell A, et al. Plasma concentrations of nitric oxide products and cognitive dysfunction following coronary artery bypass surgery. *Eur J Anaesthesiol.* (2005) 22:269–76.
112. Nicoll RA. A brief history of long-term potentiation. *Neuron* (2017) 93:281–90. doi: 10.1016/j.neuron.2016.12.015
113. Segal M. Dendritic spines and long-term plasticity. *Nat Rev Neurosci.* (2005) 6:277–84. doi: 10.1038/nrn1649
114. Rothwell NJ, Luheshi G, Toulmond S. Cytokines and their receptors in the central nervous system: physiology, pharmacology, and pathology. *Pharmacol Ther.* (1996) 69:85–95.
115. Rachal Pugh C, Fleshner M, Watkins LR, Maier SF, Rudy JW. The immune system and memory consolidation: a role for the cytokine IL-1beta. *Neurosci Biobehav Rev.* (2001) 25:29–41.
116. Riazi K, Galic MA, Kentner AC, Reid AY, Sharkey KA, Pittman QJ. Microglia-dependent alteration of glutamatergic synaptic transmission and plasticity in the hippocampus during peripheral inflammation. *J Neurosci.* (2015) 35:4942–52. doi: 10.1523/JNEUROSCI.4485-14.2015
117. Pedrazzi M, Averna M, Sparatore B, Patrone M, Salamino F, Marcoli M, et al. Potentiation of NMDA receptor-dependent cell responses by extracellular high mobility group box 1 protein. *PLoS ONE* (2012) 7:e44518. doi: 10.1371/journal.pone.0044518
118. Pribiag H, Stellwagen D. TNF-alpha downregulates inhibitory neurotransmission through protein phosphatase 1-dependent trafficking of GABA(A) receptors. *J Neurosci.* (2013) 33:15879–93. doi: 10.1523/JNEUROSCI.0530-13.2013
119. Evonuk KS, Baker BJ, Doyle RE, Moseley CE, Sestero CM, Johnston BP, et al. Inhibition of system Xc(-) transporter attenuates autoimmune inflammatory demyelination. *J Immunol.* (2015) 195:450–63. doi: 10.4049/jimmunol.1401108
120. Wu H, Li L, Su X. Vagus nerve through α7 nAChR modulates lung infection and inflammation: models, cells, and signals. *BioMed. Res. Int.* (2014) 2014:283525. doi: 10.1155/2014/283525
121. Rosas-Ballina M, Ochani M, Parrish WR, Ochani K, Harris YT, Huston JM, et al. Splenic nerve is required for cholinergic antiinflammatory pathway control of TNF in endotoxemia. *Proc Natl Acad Sci USA.* (2008) 105:11008–13. doi: 10.1073/pnas.0803237105
122. Sanders VM. The beta2-adrenergic receptor on T and B lymphocytes: do we understand it yet? *Brain Behav Immun.* (2012) 26:195–200. doi: 10.1016/j.bbi.2011.08.001
123. Ghia J-E, Blennerhassett P, El-Sharkawy RT, Collins SM. The protective effect of the vagus nerve in a murine model of chronic relapsing colitis. *Am J Physiol Gastrointest Liver Physiol.* (2007) 293:G711–718. doi: 10.1152/ajpgi.00240.2007
124. O'Mahony C, van der Kleij H, Bienenstock J, Shanahan F, O'Mahony L. Loss of vagal anti-inflammatory effect: *in vivo* visualization and adoptive transfer. *Am J Physiol Regul Integr Compar Physiol.* (2009) 297, R1118–26. doi: 10.1152/ajpregu.90904.2008
125. Kalb A, von Haefen C, Sifringer M, Tegethoff A, Paeschke N, Kostova M, et al. Acetylcholinesterase inhibitors reduce neuroinflammation and -degeneration in the cortex and hippocampus of a surgery stress rat model. *PLoS ONE* (2013) 8:e62679. doi: 10.1371/journal.pone.0062679

126. Kashyap M, Belleville S, Mulsant BH, Hilmer SN, Paquette A, Tu LM, et al. Methodological challenges in determining longitudinal associations between anticholinergic drug use and incident cognitive decline. *J Am Geriatr Soc.* (2014) 62:336–41. doi: 10.1111/jgs.12632
127. Xiong J, Xue FS, Liu JH, Xu YC, Liao X, Zhang YM, et al. Transcutaneous vagus nerve stimulation may attenuate postoperative cognitive dysfunction in elderly patients. *Med Hypotheses* (2009) 73:938–41. doi: 10.1016/j.mehy.2009.06.033
128. Serhan CN. Treating inflammation and infection in the 21st century: new hints from decoding resolution mediators and mechanisms. *FASEB J.* (2017) 31:1273–88. doi: 10.1096/fj.201601222R
129. Terrando N, Gómez-Galán M, Yang T, Carlström M, Gustavsson D, Harding RE, et al. Aspirin-triggered resolvin D1 prevents surgery-induced cognitive decline. *FASEB J.* (2013) 27:3564–71. doi: 10.1096/fj.13-230276
130. Serhan CN, Yang R, Martinod K, Kasuga K, Pillai PS, Porter TF, et al. Maresins: novel macrophage mediators with potent antiinflammatory and proresolving actions. *J Exp Med.* (2009) 206:15–23. doi: 10.1084/jem.20081880
131. Zhang J, Tan H, Jiang W, Zuo Z. The choice of general anesthetics may not affect neuroinflammation and impairment of learning and memory after surgery in elderly rats. *J Neuroimm Pharmacol.* (2015) 10:179–89. doi: 10.1007/s11481-014-9580-y
132. Jevtovic-Todorovic V, Hartman RE, Izumi Y, Benshoff ND, Dikranian K, Zorumski CF, et al. Early exposure to common anesthetic agents causes widespread neurodegeneration in the developing rat brain and persistent learning deficits. *J Neurosci.* (2003) 23:876–82. doi: 10.1523/JNEUROSCI.23-03-00876.2003
133. Shen X, Dong Y, Xu Z, Wang H, Miao C, Soriano SG, et al. Selective anesthesia-induced neuroinflammation in developing mouse brain and cognitive impairment. *Anesthesiology* (2013) 118:502–15. doi: 10.1097/ALN.0b013e3182834d77
134. Coleman K, Robertson ND, Dissen GA, Neuringer MD, Martin LD, Cuzon Carlson VC, et al. Isoflurane anesthesia has long-term consequences on motor and behavioral development in infant rhesus macaques. *Anesthesiology* (2017) 126:74–84. doi: 10.1097/ALN.0000000000001383
135. Wang Z, Meng S, Cao L, Chen Y, Zuo Z, Peng S. Critical role of NLRP3-caspase-1 pathway in age-dependent isoflurane-induced microglial inflammatory response and cognitive impairment. *J Neuroinflammat.* (2018) 15:109. doi: 10.1186/s12974-018-1137-1
136. Walters JL, Chelonis JJ, Fogle CM, Orser BA, Paule MG. Single and repeated exposures to the volatile anesthetic isoflurane do not impair operant performance in aged rats. *Neurotoxicology* (2016) 56:159–69. doi: 10.1016/j.neuro.2016.07.012
137. Zhu J, Jiang X, Shi E, Ma H, Wang J. Sevoflurane preconditioning reverses impairment of hippocampal long-term potentiation induced by myocardial ischaemia-reperfusion injury. *Eur J Anaesthesiol.* (2009) 26:961–8. doi: 10.1097/EJA.0b013e328330e968
138. Tasbihgou SR, Netkova M, Kalmar AF, Doorduin J, Struys MMRF, Schoemaker RG, et al. Brain changes due to hypoxia during light anaesthesia can be prevented by deepening anaesthesia; a study in rats. *PLoS ONE* (2018) 13:e0193062. doi: 10.1371/journal.pone.0193062
139. Qian X-L, Zhang W, Liu M-Z, Zhou Y-B, Zhang J-M, Han L, et al. Dexmedetomidine improves early postoperative cognitive dysfunction in aged mice. *Eur J Pharmacol.* (2015) 746:206–12. doi: 10.1016/j.ejphar.2014.11.017
140. Newman S, Stygall J, Hirani S, Shaefi S, Maze M. Postoperative cognitive dysfunction after noncardiac surgery: a systematic review. *Anesthesiology* (2007) 106:572–90.
141. Sanders RD, Maze M. Neuroinflammation and postoperative cognitive dysfunction: can anaesthesia be therapeutic? *Eur J Anaesthesiol.* (2010) 27:3–5. doi: 10.1097/EJA.0b013e3283318ef9
142. Silbert BS, Evered LA, Scott DA. Incidence of postoperative cognitive dysfunction after general or spinal anaesthesia for extracorporeal shock wave lithotripsy. *Br J Anaesth.* (2014) 113:784–91. doi: 10.1093/bja/aeu163
143. Silbert BS, Scott DA, Evered LA, Lewis MS, Kalpokas M, Maruff P, et al. A comparison of the effect of high- and low-dose fentanyl on the incidence of postoperative cognitive dysfunction after coronary artery bypass surgery in the elderly. *Anesthesiology* (2006) 104:1137–45.
144. Geng Y-J, Wu Q-H, Zhang R-Q. Effect of propofol, sevoflurane, and isoflurane on postoperative cognitive dysfunction following laparoscopic cholecystectomy in elderly patients: a randomized controlled trial. *J Clin Anesth.* (2017) 38:165–71. doi: 10.1016/j.jclinane.2017.02.007
145. Qiao Y, Feng H, Zhao T, Yan H, Zhang H, Zhao X. Postoperative cognitive dysfunction after inhalational anesthesia in elderly patients undergoing major surgery: the influence of anesthetic technique, cerebral injury and systemic inflammation. *BMC Anesthesiol.* (2015) 15:154. doi: 10.1186/s12871-015-0130-9
146. Shu A-H, Wang Q, Chen X-B. Effect of different depths of anesthesia on postoperative cognitive function in laparoscopic patients: a randomized clinical trial. *Curr Med Res Opin.* (2015) 31:1883–7. doi: 10.1185/03007995.2015.1075968
147. Hou R, Wang H, Chen L, Qiu Y, Li S. POCD in patients receiving total knee replacement under deep vs. light anesthesia: a randomized controlled trial. *Brain Behav.* (2018) 8:e00910. doi: 10.1002/brb3.910
148. Erdogan MA, Demirbilek S, Erdil F, Aydogan MS, Ozturk E, Togal T, et al. The effects of cognitive impairment on anaesthetic requirement in the elderly. *Eur J Anaesthesiol.* (2012) 29:326–31. doi: 10.1097/EJA.0b013e32835475c6
149. Babiloni C, Carducci F, Lizio R, Vecchio F, Baglieri A, Bernardini S, et al. Resting state cortical electroencephalographic rhythms are related to gray matter volume in subjects with mild cognitive impairment and Alzheimer's disease. *Hum Brain Mapp.* (2013) 34:1427–46. doi: 10.1002/hbm.22005
150. Schuller PJ, Newell S, Strickland PA, Barry JJ. Response of bispectral index to neuromuscular block in awake volunteers. *Br J Anaesth.* (2015) 115 Suppl 1:i95–103. doi: 10.1093/bja/aev072
151. Avidan MS, Graetz TJ. Monitoring the brain strikes a discordant note for anesthesiologists. *Can J Anaesth.* (2018) 65:501–6. doi: 10.1007/s12630-018-1086-2
152. Zhu Y-Z, Yao R, Zhang Z, Xu H, Wang L-W. Parecoxib prevents early postoperative cognitive dysfunction in elderly patients undergoing total knee arthroplasty: a double-blind, randomized clinical consort study. *Medicine* (2016) 95:e4082. doi: 10.1097/MD.0000000000004082
153. Zhu Y, Yao R, Li Y, Wu C, Heng L, Zhou M, et al. Protective effect of celecoxib on early postoperative cognitive dysfunction in geriatric patients. *Front Neurol.* (2018) 9:633. doi: 10.3389/fneur.2018.00633
154. Ottens TH, Dieleman JM, Sauer AM, Peelen LM, Nierich AP, de Groot WJ, et al. Effects of dexamethasone on cognitive decline after cardiac surgery: a randomized clinical trial. *Anesthesiology* (2014) 121:492–500. doi: 10.1097/ALN.0000000000000336
155. Doraiswamy PM, Babyak MA, Hennig T, Trivedi R, White WD, Mathew JP, et al. Donepezil for cognitive decline following coronary artery bypass surgery: a pilot randomized controlled trial. *Psychopharmacol Bull.* (2007) 40:54–62.
156. Das S, Nanda SK, Bisoi AK, Wadhawan AN. Effect of preoperative statin therapy on early postoperative memory impairment after off-pump coronary artery bypass surgery. *Ann Card Anaesth.* (2016) 19:38–44. doi: 10.4103/0971-9784.173018
157. Li Y, He R, Chen S, Qu Y. Effect of dexmedetomidine on early postoperative cognitive dysfunction and peri-operative inflammation in elderly patients undergoing laparoscopic cholecystectomy. *Exp Therapeut Med.* (2015) 10:1635–42. doi: 10.3892/etm.2015.2726
158. Chen W, Liu B, Zhang F, Xue P, Cui R, Lei W. The effects of dexmedetomidine on post-operative cognitive dysfunction and inflammatory factors in senile patients. *Int J Clin Exp Med.* (2015) 8:4601–5.
159. Wang HL, Yan HD, Liu YY, Sun BZ, Huang R, Wang XS, et al. Intraoperative intravenous lidocaine exerts a protective effect on cell-mediated immunity in patients undergoing radical hysterectomy. *Mol Med Rep.* (2015) 12:7039–44. doi: 10.3892/mmr.2015.4235
160. Chen K, Wei P, Zheng Q, Zhou J, Li J. Neuroprotective effects of intravenous lidocaine on early postoperative cognitive dysfunction in elderly patients following spine surgery. *Med Sci Monit.* (2015) 21:1402–7. doi: 10.12659/MSM.894384
161. Hudetz JA, Iqbal Z, Gandhi SD, Patterson KM, Byrne AJ, Hudetz AG, et al. Ketamine attenuates post-operative cognitive dysfunction

after cardiac surgery. *Acta Anaesthesiol Scand.* (2009) 53:864–72. doi: 10.1111/j.1399-6576.2009.01978.x

162. Nagels W, Demeyere R, Van Hemelrijck J, Vandenbussche E, Gijbels K, Vandermeersch E. Evaluation of the neuroprotective effects of S(+)-ketamine during open-heart surgery. *Anesth Analg.* (2004) 98:1595–603, table of contents. doi: 10.1213/01.ANE.0000117227.00820.0C
163. Hansen MV, Madsen MT, Andersen LT, Hageman I, Rasmussen LS, Bokmand S, et al. Effect of melatonin on cognitive function and sleep in relation to breast cancer surgery: a randomized, double-blind, placebo-controlled trial. *Int J Breast Cancer* (2014) 2014:416531. doi: 10.1155/2014/416531
164. Fan Y, Yuan L, Ji M, Yang J, Gao D. The effect of melatonin on early postoperative cognitive decline in elderly patients undergoing hip arthroplasty: a randomized controlled trial. *J Clin Anesth.* (2017) 39:77–81. doi: 10.1016/j.jclinane.2017.03.023
165. Gao XQ, Zhang ZY, Ma WH. Effects of electroacupuncture assistant general anesthesia on postoperative cognitive dysfunction of aged patients. *Zhongguo Zhong Xi Yi Jie He Za Zhi* (2012) 32:591–3.
166. Lin SY, Gao J, Yin ZL, Zhou LJ, Chen X. [Impacts of the different frequencies of electroacupunctrue on cognitive function in patients after abdominal operation under compound anesthesia of acupuncture and drugs]. *Zhongguo Zhen Jiu* (2013) 33:1109–12.
167. Lin SY, Yin ZL, Gao J, Zhou LJ, Chen X. [Effect of acupuncture-anesthetic composite anesthesia on the incidence of POCD and TNF-alpha, IL-1beta, IL-6 in elderly patients]. *Zhongguo Zhong Xi Yi Jie He Za Zhi* (2014) 34:795–9.
168. Peng M, Wang Y-L, Wang F-F, Chen C, Wang C-Y. The cyclooxygenase-2 inhibitor parecoxib inhibits surgery-induced proinflammatory cytokine expression in the hippocampus in aged rats. *J Surg Res.* (2012) 178:e1–8. doi: 10.1016/j.jss.2012.08.030
169. Kamer AR, Galoyan SM, Haile M, Kline R, Boutajangout A, Li Y-S, et al. Meloxicam improves object recognition memory and modulates glial activation after splenectomy in mice. *Eur J Anaesthesiol.* (2012) 29:332–7. doi: 10.1097/EJA.0b013e3283534f56
170. Fan L, Wang T-L, Xu YC, Ma YH, Ye WG. Minocycline may be useful to prevent/treat postoperative cognitive decline in elderly patients. *Med Hypotheses* (2011) 76:733–6. doi: 10.1016/j.mehy.2011.02.010
171. Wang H-L, Liu H, Xue Z-G, Liao Q-W, Fang H. Minocycline attenuates post-operative cognitive impairment in aged mice by inhibiting microglia activation. *J Cell Mol Med.* (2016) 20:1632–9. doi: 10.1111/jcmm.12854
172. Li W, Chai Q, Zhang H, Ma J, Xu C, Dong J, et al. High doses of minocycline may induce delayed activation of microglia in aged rats and thus cannot prevent postoperative cognitive dysfunction. *J Int Med Res.* (2018) 46:1404–13. doi: 10.1177/0300060517754032
173. Tsurufuji S, Kurihara A, Kiso S, Suzuki Y, Ohuchi K. Dexamethasone inhibits generation in inflammatory sites of the chemotactic activity attributable to leukotriene B4. *Biochem Biophys Res Commun.* (1984) 119:884–90.
174. Barnes PJ. Anti-inflammatory actions of glucocorticoids: molecular mechanisms. *Clin Sci.* (1998) 94:557–72.
175. Karaman T, Karaman S, Dogru S, Tapar H, Sahin A, Süren M. Short-term and long-term effects of dexamethasone on cognitive dysfunction induced by sevoflurane in adult rats. *Turk J Anaesthesiol Reanimat.* (2017) 45:158–63. doi: 10.5152/TJAR.2017.98624
176. Han Z, Li L, Wang L, Degos V, Maze M, Su H. Alpha-7 nicotinic acetylcholine receptor agonist treatment reduces neuroinflammation, oxidative stress, and brain injury in mice with ischemic stroke and bone fracture. *J Neurochem.* (2014) 131:498–508. doi: 10.1111/jnc.12817
177. Puhringer FK, Rex C, Sielenkamper AW, Claudius C, Larsen PB, Prins ME, et al. Reversal of profound, high-dose rocuronium-induced neuromuscular blockade by sugammadex at two different time points: an international, multicenter, randomized, dose-finding, safety assessor-blinded, phase II trial. *Anesthesiology* (2008) 109:188–97. doi: 10.1097/ALN.0b013e31817f5bc7
178. Barrientos RM, Hein AM, Frank MG, Watkins LR, Maier SF. Intracisternal interleukin-1 receptor antagonist prevents postoperative cognitive decline and neuroinflammatory response in aged rats. *J Neurosci.* (2012) 32:14641–8. doi: 10.1523/JNEUROSCI.2173-12.2012
179. Hu J, Feng X, Valdearcos M, Lutrin D, Uchida Y, Koliwad SK, et al. Interleukin-6 is both necessary and sufficient to produce perioperative neurocognitive disorder in mice. *Br J Anaesth.* (2018) 120:537–45. doi: 10.1016/j.bja.2017.11.096
180. Cerqueira NM, Oliveira EF, Gesto DS, Santos-Martins D, Moreira C, Moorthy HN, et al. Cholesterol biosynthesis: a mechanistic overview. *Biochemistry* (2016) 55:5483–506. doi: 10.1021/acs.biochem.6b00342
181. Margaritis M, Channon KM, Antoniades C. Statins as regulators of redox state in the vascular endothelium: beyond lipid lowering. *Antioxid Redox Signal.* (2014) 20:1198–215. doi: 10.1089/ars.2013.5430
182. Swiger KJ, Manalac RJ, Blumenthal RS, Blaha MJ, Martin SS. Statins and cognition: a systematic review and meta-analysis of short- and long-term cognitive effects. *Mayo Clin Proc.* (2013) 88:1213–21. doi: 10.1016/j.mayocp.2013.07.013
183. Katznelson R, Djaiani GN, Borger MA, Friedman Z, Abbey SE, Fedorko L, et al. Preoperative use of statins is associated with reduced early delirium rates after cardiac surgery. *Anesthesiology* (2009) 110:67–73. doi: 10.1097/ALN.0b013e318190b4d9
184. Skvarc DR, Dean OM, Byrne LK, Gray L, Lane S, Lewis M, et al. The effect of N-acetylcysteine (NAC) on human cognition-A systematic review. *Neurosci Biobehav Rev.* (2017) 78:44–56. doi: 10.1016/j.neubiorev.2017.04.013
185. Gabryel B, Bielecka A, Bernacki J, Labuzek K, Herman ZS. Immunosuppressant cytoprotection correlates with HMGB1 suppression in primary astrocyte cultures exposed to combined oxygen-glucose deprivation. *Pharmacol Rep.* (2011) 63:392–402. doi: 10.1016/S1734-1140(11)70505-9
186. Santiago FM, Bueno P, Olmedo C, Muffak-Granero K, Comino A, Serradilla M, et al. Effect of N-acetylcysteine administration on intraoperative plasma levels of interleukin-4 and interleukin-10 in liver transplant recipients. *Transplant Proc.* (2008) 40:2978–80. doi: 10.1016/j.transproceed.2008.08.103
187. Berman AE, Chan WY, Brennan AM, Reyes RC, Adler BL, Suh SW, et al. N-acetylcysteine prevents loss of dopaminergic neurons in the EAAC1-/- mouse. *Ann Neurol.* (2011) 69:509–20. doi: 10.1002/ana.22162
188. Skvarc DR, Dean OM, Byrne LK, Gray LJ, Ives K, Lane SE, et al. The Post-Anaesthesia N-acetylcysteine cognitive evaluation (PANACEA) trial: study protocol for a randomised controlled trial. *Trials* (2016) 17:395. doi: 10.1186/s13063-016-1529-4
189. Edaravone Acute Infarction Study G. Effect of a novel free radical scavenger, edaravone (MCI-186), on acute brain infarction. Randomized, placebo-controlled, double-blind study at multicenters. *Cerebrovasc Dis.* (2003) 15:222–9. doi: 10.1159/000069318
190. Abe K, Itoyama Y, Sobue G, Tsuji S, Aoki M, Doyu M, et al. Confirmatory double-blind, parallel-group, placebo-controlled study of efficacy and safety of edaravone (MCI-186) in amyotrophic lateral sclerosis patients. *Amyotroph Lateral Scler Frontotemporal Degener.* (2014) 15:610–7. doi: 10.3109/21678421.2014.959024
191. Purdon PL, Sampson A, Pavone KJ, Brown EN. Clinical Electroencephalography for Anesthesiologists: Part I: background and basic signatures. *Anesthesiology* (2015) 123:937–60. doi: 10.1097/ALN.0000000000000841
192. Wang X, Liu N, Chen J, Xu Z, Wang F, Ding C. Effect of intravenous dexmedetomidine during general anesthesia on acute postoperative pain in adults: a systematic review and meta-analysis of randomized controlled trials. *Clin J Pain* (2018). doi: 10.1097/AJP.0000000000000630
193. Schnabel A, Reichl SU, Weibel S, Kranke P, Zahn PK, Pogatzki-Zahn EM, et al. Efficacy and safety of dexmedetomidine in peripheral nerve blocks: a meta-analysis and trial sequential analysis. *Eur J Anaesthesiol.* (2018) 35:745–58. doi: 10.1097/EJA.0000000000000870
194. Hu J, Vacas S, Feng X, Lutrin D, Uchida Y, Lai IK, et al. Dexmedetomidine prevents cognitive decline by enhancing resolution of high mobility group box 1 protein-induced inflammation through a vagomimetic action in mice. *Anesthesiology* (2018) 128:921–31. doi: 10.1097/ALN.0000000000002038
195. Rocha SM, Cristovao AC, Campos FL, Fonseca CP, Baltazar G. Astrocyte-derived GDNF is a potent inhibitor of microglial activation. *Neurobiol Dis.* (2012) 47:407–15. doi: 10.1016/j.nbd.2012.04.014
196. Kawano T, Eguchi S, Iwata H, Tamura T, Kumagai N, Yokoyama M. Impact of preoperative environmental enrichment on prevention of development of cognitive impairment following abdominal surgery in a rat model. *Anesthesiology* (2015) 123:160–70. doi: 10.1097/ALN.00000000000 00697

197. Sheets MF, Hanck DA. Molecular action of lidocaine on the voltage sensors of sodium channels. *J Gen Physiol.* (2003) 121:163–75. doi: 10.1085/jgp.20028651
198. Amir R, Argoff CE, Bennett GJ, Cummins TR, Durieux ME, Gerner P, et al. The role of sodium channels in chronic inflammatory and neuropathic pain. *J Pain* (2006) 7(5 Suppl. 3):S1–29. doi: 10.1016/j.jpain.2006.01.444
199. Maher DP, Chen L, Mao J. Intravenous ketamine infusions for neuropathic pain management: a promising therapy in need of optimization. *Anesth Analg.* (2017) 124:661–74. doi: 10.1213/ANE.0000000000001787
200. Bell JD. In Vogue: ketamine for neuroprotection in acute neurologic injury. *Anesth Analg.* (2017) 124:1237–43. doi: 10.1213/ANE.0000000000001856
201. De Kock M, Loix S, and Lavand'homme P. (2013). Ketamine and peripheral inflammation. *CNS Neurosci Ther.* 19:403–410. doi: 10.1111/cns.12104
202. Li Y, Shen R, Wen G, Ding R, Du A, Zhou J, et al. Effects of ketamine on levels of inflammatory cytokines IL-6, IL-1beta, and TNF-alpha in the hippocampus of mice following acute or chronic administration. *Front Pharmacol.* (2017) 8:139. doi: 10.3389/fphar.2017.00139
203. Della Giustina A, Goldim MP, Danielski LG, Florentino D, Mathias K, Garbossa L, et al. Alpha-lipoic acid attenuates acute neuroinflammation and long-term cognitive impairment after polymicrobial sepsis. *Neurochem Int.* (2017) 108:436–47. doi: 10.1016/j.neuint.2017.06.003
204. Zhang Z, Ma Q, Shah B, Mackensen GB, Lo DC, Mathew JP, et al. Neuroprotective effects of annexin A1 tripeptide after deep hypothermic circulatory arrest in rats. *Front Immunol.* (2017) 8:1050. doi: 10.3389/fimmu.2017.01050
205. Aizpurua-Olaizola O, Elezgarai I, Rico-Barrio I, Zarandona I, Etxebarria N, Usobiaga A. Targeting the endocannabinoid system: future therapeutic strategies. *Drug Discov Today* (2017) 22:105–10. doi: 10.1016/j.drudis.2016.08.005
206. McCoy KL. Interaction between cannabinoid system and toll-like receptors controls inflammation. *Med Inflamm.* (2016) 2016:5831315. doi: 10.1155/2016/5831315
207. Sun L, Dong R, Xu X, Yang X, Peng M. Activation of cannabinoid receptor type 2 attenuates surgery-induced cognitive impairment in mice through anti-inflammatory activity. *J Neuroinflammat.* (2017) 14:138. doi: 10.1186/s12974-017-0913-7
208. Papaseit E, Perez-Mana C, Perez-Acevedo AP, Hladun O, Torres-Moreno MC, Muga R, et al. Cannabinoids: from pot to lab. *Int J Med Sci.* (2018) 15:1286–95. doi: 10.7150/ijms.27087
209. Poleszak E, Wosko S, Slawinska K, Szopa A, Wrobel A, Serefko A. Cannabinoids in depressive disorders. *Life Sci.* (2018) 213:18–24. doi: 10.1016/j.lfs.2018.09.058
210. Cipolla-Neto J, and do Amaral FG. (2018). Melatonin as a hormone: new physiological and clinical insights. *Endocr Rev.* 39:990–1028. doi: 10.1210/er.2018-00084
211. Esposito E, Cuzzocrea S. Antiinflammatory activity of melatonin in central nervous system. *Curr Neuropharmacol.* (2010) 8:228–42. doi: 10.2174/157015910792246155
212. Liu Y, Ni C, Tang Y, Tian X, Zhou Y, Qian M, et al. Melatonin attenuates isoflurane-induced acute memory impairments in aged rats. *Basic Clin Pharmacol Toxicol.* (2013) 113:215–20. doi: 10.1111/bcpt.12079
213. Xia T, Cui Y, Chu S, Song J, Qian Y, Ma Z, et al. Melatonin pretreatment prevents isoflurane-induced cognitive dysfunction by modulating sleep-wake rhythm in mice. *Brain Res.* (2016) 1634:12–20. doi: 10.1016/j.brainres.2015.10.036
214. Song J, Chu S, Cui Y, Qian Y, Li X, Xu F, et al. Circadian rhythm resynchronization improved isoflurane-induced cognitive dysfunction in aged mice. *Exp Neurol.* (2018) 306:45–54. doi: 10.1016/j.expneurol.2018.04.009
215. Kim JH, Gupta SC, Park B, Yadav VR, Aggarwal BB. Turmeric (Curcuma longa) inhibits inflammatory nuclear factor (NF)-kappaB and NF-kappaB-regulated gene products and induces death receptors leading to suppressed proliferation, induced chemosensitization, and suppressed osteoclastogenesis. *Mol Nutr Food Res.* (2012) 56:454–65. doi: 10.1002/mnfr.201100270
216. Wu X, Chen H, Huang C, Gu X, Wang J, Xu D, et al. Curcumin attenuates surgery-induced cognitive dysfunction in aged mice. *Metab Brain Dis.* (2017) 32:789–98. doi: 10.1007/s11011-017-9970-y
217. Sierpina VS, Frenkel MA. Acupuncture: a clinical review. *South Med J.* (2005) 98:330–7. doi: 10.1097/01.SMJ.0000140834.30654.0F
218. Liu P-R, Zhou Y, Zhang Y, Diao S. Electroacupuncture alleviates surgery-induced cognitive dysfunction by increasing α7-nAChR expression and inhibiting inflammatory pathway in aged rats. *Neurosci Lett.* (2017) 659:1–6. doi: 10.1016/j.neulet.2017.08.043
219. Thal SC, Luh C, Schaible E-V, Timaru-Kast R, Hedrich J, Luhmann HJ, et al. Volatile Anesthetics influence blood-brain barrier integrity by modulation of tight junction protein expression in traumatic brain injury. *PLoS ONE* (2012) 7:e50752–e50712. doi: 10.1371/journal.pone.0050752
220. Tetrault S, Chever O, Sik A, Amzica F. Opening of the blood-brain barrier during isoflurane anaesthesia. *Eur J Neurosci.* (2008) 28:1330–41. doi: 10.1111/j.1460-9568.2008.06443.x
221. Royall DR, Palmer R, Chiodo LK, Polk MJ. Declining executive control in normal aging predicts change in functional status: the Freedom House Study. *J Am Geriatr Soc.* (2004) 52:346–52. doi: 10.1111/j.1532-5415.2004.52104.x

10

Intellectual Disability Associated with Pyridoxine-Responsive Epilepsies: The Need to Protect Cognitive Development

Bjørnar Hassel[1,2]*, Ane Gretesdatter Rogne[1] and Sigrun Hope[1]

[1] *Department for Neurohabilitation, Oslo University Hospital and University of Oslo, Oslo, Norway,* [2] *Norwegian Defence Research Establishment (FFI), Kjeller, Norway*

Correspondence:
Bjørnar Hassel
bjornar.hassel@medisin.uio.no

Pyridoxine (vitamin B6)-responsive epilepsies are severe forms of epilepsy that manifest as seizures immediately after birth, sometimes *in utero*, sometimes months, or years after birth. Seizures may be treated efficiently by life-long supplementation with pyridoxine or its biologically active form, pyridoxal phosphate, but even so patients may become intellectually disabled, for which there currently is no effective treatment. The condition may be caused by mutations in several genes (*TNSALP*, *PIGV*, *PIGL*, *PIGO*, *PNPO*, *PROSC*, *ALDH7A1*, *MOCS2*, or *ALDH4A1*). Mutations in *ALDH7A1*, *MOCS2*, and *ALDH4A1* entail build-up of reactive aldehydes (α-aminoadipic semialdehyde, γ-glutamic semialdehyde) that may react non-enzymatically with macromolecules of brain cells. Such reactions may alter the function of macromolecules, and they may produce "advanced glycation end products" (AGEs). AGEs trigger inflammation in the brain. This understanding points to aldehyde-quenching, anti-AGE, or anti-inflammatory therapies as possible strategies to protect cognitive development and prevent intellectual disability in affected children. Studies on how aldehydes traverse cell membranes and how they affect brain function could further the development of therapies for patients with pyridoxine-responsive epilepsies.

Keywords: vitamin B6, pyridoxine-responsive epilepsy, intellectual disability, lysine metabolism, α-aminoadipic semialdehyde, γ-glutamic semialdehyde, aldehydes, hyperprolinemia type II

INTRODUCTION

Pyridoxine-Responsive Epilepsy: Clinical Manifestations and Underlying Molecular Causes

Pyridoxine-responsive epilepsy is a severe form of epilepsy that manifests as generalized seizures immediately after birth, sometimes *in utero*. In some patients seizures begin some months or years after birth (1, 2). Life-long treatment with high doses of pyridoxine (vitamin B6) or its derivative pyridoxal 5′-phosphate (PLP) is efficient with respect to the epileptic seizures; withdrawal of pyridoxine may precipitate life-threatening *status epilepticus*, which is only reversed when pyridoxine is reinstated. Conventional antiepileptic drugs probably have no place in the treatment of this disorder. Pyridoxine-responsive epilepsy may entail intellectual disability and other neurodevelopmental impairments, such as attention deficit/hyperactivity disorder and autism (3, 4), which are not prevented by pyridoxine treatment alone, pointing to separate mechanisms underlying the epilepsy and the cognitive impairment. Only in some cases is the metabolic disturbance accompanied by structural changes (white matter changes, hippocampal sclerosis) that may contribute to the epilepsy or the intellectual disability.

PYRIDOXINE: THE BIOLOGICALLY ACTIVE FORM AND ITS ENTRY INTO THE BRAIN

To be biologically active, pyridoxine must be converted to PLP. This two-step conversion involves phosphorylation of pyridoxine to pyridoxine 5′-phosphate, which is then oxidized to PLP. PLP is a co-enzyme in more than 100 biochemical reactions, many involving amino acid metabolism (5). With respect to brain function, PLP is essential for the formation of various neurotransmitters and neuromodulators that are amino acids or derived from amino acids: monoamines, GABA, glutamate, glycine, D-serine, and taurine (5, 6). Through its involvement in amino acid metabolism PLP is necessary for energy production in all brain cells.

Pyridoxine's route from food ingredient to active coenzyme in the brain is somewhat complex. Pyridoxine is taken up in the gut and converted into PLP in the liver (**Figures 1A,B**). PLP is given off to the circulation, but for PLP to enter the brain, it has to lose its phosphate group and become pyridoxal. This dephosphorylation (from PLP to pyridoxal) is performed by an extracellular enzyme: tissue non-specific alkaline phosphatase, which is attached to cell surfaces by glycosylphosphatidylinositol (GPI) anchors. Once inside brain cells, pyridoxal is reconverted to PLP by the enzyme pyridoxal kinase (7). Reduced expression of pyridoxal kinase in mice leads to low levels of PLP in the brain and severe seizures (8); a similar condition has not yet been reported in humans.

GENETIC CAUSES OF PYRIDOXINE-RESPONSIVE EPILEPSY: SOME AFFECT METABOLISM OF PYRIDOXINE, SOME LEAD TO BUILD-UP OF REACTIVE METABOLITES THAT INACTIVATE PLP

Pyridoxine-responsive epilepsy is caused by rare, mostly recessive loss-of-function mutations in various genes. Some mutations affect the metabolism of pyridoxine, whereas some lead to accumulation of reactive metabolites that inactivate PLP (**Table 1**). The *PNPO* gene encodes the enzyme pyridoxine 5′-phosphate oxidase, which is rate-limiting for the formation of PLP in the liver (9) (**Figure 1**). Mutations affect the enzymes' ability to bind its cofactor (flavin mononucleotide) and its interaction with PLP-dependent enzymes (10). The result is reduced formation of PLP, a low circulating level of PLP, and

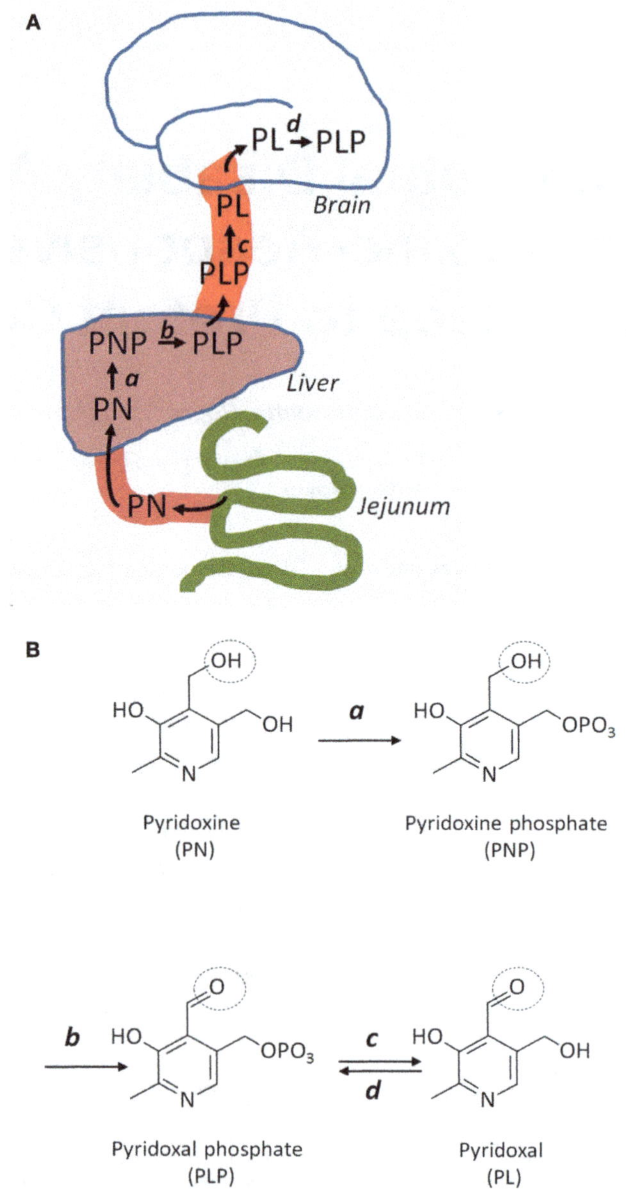

FIGURE 1 | Uptake, transport, and metabolism of pyridoxine and its derivatives. **(A)** Pyridoxine (PN) (or its closely related form pyridoxamine), is transported from the gut to the liver, where it is metabolized successively to pyridoxine phosphate (PNP) and pyridoxal phosphate (PLP). PLP is given off to the circulation, but cannot cross the blood-brain barrier and enter the brain unless it is converted to pyridoxal (PL). Once inside brain cells, PL is re-phosphorylated to PLP. **(B)** Molecular structures of pyridoxine and its metabolites. PN is phosphorylated to PNP by pyridoxine kinase (a) in the liver. PNP is oxidized to PLP by PNP oxidase (b). In brain capillaries, PLP is dephosphorylated to PL by tissue non-specific alkaline phosphatase (c). In brain cells, PL is re-phosphorylated to PLP by PL kinase (d). The circle shows the OH group that gives rise to the aldehyde function in PLP and PL.

Abbreviations: AGE, advanced glycation end product; CSF, cerebrospinal fluid; GABA, γ-amino butyric acid; GPI anchors, glycosylphosphatidylinositol anchors; MRI, magnetic resonance imaging; PLP, pyridoxal 5′-phosphate; P5C, Δ^1-pyrroline-5-carboxylate; P6C, L-Δ^1-piperidine-6-carboxylate; RAGE, receptor for advanced glycation end products.

TABLE 1 | Genes whose mutations cause defective PLP metabolism or inactivation of PLP through accumulation of reactive compounds.

	Gene	Protein	Protein function	Effect of mutation
Mutations related to PLP metabolism	*PNPO*	Pyridoxine phosphate oxidase	PLP synthesis from PNP	Lack of PLP in liver and hence in blood
	TNSALP	Tissue non-specific alkaline phosphatase	PL formation from PLP	Lack of PL formed at the blood-brain barrier
	PIGV, PIGL, PIGO	GPI-anchors	Anchoring tissue non-specific alkaline phosphatase at capillaries	Lack of PL formed at the blood-brain barrier
	PROSC	Proline synthase cotranscribed, aka "Pyridoxal phosphate homeostasis protein"	Cellular PLP homeostasis?	Increased cellular PLP consumption?
	PDXK	Pyridoxal kinase	PLP synthesis	Lack of PLP in cells (only in knock-out mouse model)
Mutations that cause PLP inactivation	*ALDH7A1*	α-Aminoadipic semialdehyde dehydrogenase	α-Aminoadipate	Accumulation of α-aminoadipic semialdehyde and P6C, which inactivates PLP
	MOCS2	Molybdenum cofactor synthesis 2	Involved in oxidation of sulphite to sulfate	Accumulation of sulphite, which inactivates α-aminoadipic semialdehyde dehydrogenase, causing accumulation of α-aminoadipic semialdehyde and P6C, which inactivates PLP
	ALDH4A1	P5C dehydrogenase	Metabolism of proline	Accumulation of γ-glutamic semialdehyde and P5C, which inactivates PLP

All mutations cause epilepsy, which (except in the case of experimental pyridoxal kinase deficiency) respond to pyridoxine therapy. GPI, glycosylphosphatidylinositol; PLP, pyridoxal phosphate; PL, pyridoxal; PNP, pyridoxine phosphate; P6C, L-Δ^1-piperidine-6-carboxylate; P5C, Δ^1-pyrroline-5-carboxylate.

a low availability of PLP (i.e., pyridoxal) to the brain. This deficiency may be amended with administration of PLP rather than pyridoxine.

The *TNSALP* gene encodes tissue non-specific alkaline phosphatase, which is present at the blood-brain barrier, among other tissues. This phosphatase dephosphorylates blood-borne PLP to pyridoxal, which may enter the brain. Loss-of-function *TNSALP* mutations lead to ineffective PLP dephosphorylation to pyridoxal, reduced pyridoxal transfer into the brain, and accumulation of PLP in blood (11). Pyridoxine treatment alleviates the ensuing epilepsy (12) probably by raising the serum level of PLP even further to achieve some increase in pyridoxal level. This approach may be effective, because the mechanism for transport of pyridoxal across the blood-brain barrier is not saturated, so that any increase in serum pyridoxal concentration will lead to increased uptake into the brain (13). The disorder, which is termed hypophosphatasia due to the low circulating level of alkaline phosphatase, may be treated with enzyme replacement therapy (14), which reduces the need for pyridoxine therapy (12).

Several proteins are involved in the formation of GPI anchors that tether extracellular tissue non-specific alkaline phosphatase to the cell membrane. Mutations in some genes (*PIGV, PIGL, PIGO*) (15, 16) that encode GPI-related proteins are known to cause pyridoxine-responsive epilepsy (17). Suboptimal GPI anchoring of tissue non-specific alkaline phosphatase at the blood-brain barrier probably explains the pyridoxine-responsiveness of the epilepsy of these patients (18). The dysfunctional anchoring of alkaline phosphatase is also the reason for the high circulating level of alkaline phosphatase in this disorder known as hyperphosphatasia or Mabry syndrome.

The *ALDH7A1* gene encodes the enzyme α-aminoadipic semialdehyde dehydrogenase (aka antiquitin), which is involved in lysine metabolism. The mutation, the incidence of which has recently been estimated at 1.6:100 000 (19), causes build-up of the lysine metabolite α-aminoadipic semialdehyde, its cyclic form L-Δ^1-piperidine-6-carboxylate (P6C), and their common precursor L-pipecolic acid. The level of these metabolites in plasma, urine, and cerebrospinal fluid (CSF) is typically elevated with *ALDH7A1* mutations (20, 21). P6C has been found to bind and inactivate PLP (22). This inactivation is thought to underlie the pyridoxine responsiveness of the seizures in this condition, which is often termed "pyridoxine-*dependent* epilepsy." A similar situation is caused by *MOCS2* mutations, which lead to molybdenum cofactor deficiency and sulphite accumulation. Sulphite has been shown to inhibit α-aminoadipic semialdehyde dehydrogenase (23), causing build-up of α-aminoadipic semialdehyde and hence of P6C, which inactivates PLP (24). In hyperprolinemia type II, mutations in *ALDH4A1* (Δ^1-pyrroline-5-carboxylate dehydrogenase) lead to accumulation of γ-glutamic semialdehyde and its cyclic form pyrroline-5-carboxylic acid (P5C). P5C reacts with PLP in a manner similar to P6C (25) to produces PLP deficiency in the brain (26).

The *PROSC* gene encodes a cytosolic protein that binds PLP. The function of the protein remains unknown, but it has been suggested to act as an intracellular PLP reservoir, preventing PLP, itself a reactive aldehyde, to react spontaneously with other cell constituents (27). *PROSC* mutations entail low CSF levels of PLP, possibly because PLP is consumed through spontaneous reactions with other cell constituents, and the epilepsy that accompanies the condition is therefore pyridoxine-responsive.

Thus, it seems that a lack of PLP in the brain is the cause of epilepsy in all the above-mentioned conditions: in *TNSALP* mutations and in mutations causing dysfunctional GPI anchoring of tissue non-specific alkaline phosphatase the transfer of PLP in the form of pyridoxal into the brain is suboptimal; in *PNPO* mutations, PLP is not produced normally in the liver; in *ALDH7A1*, *MOCS2*, and *ALDH4A1* mutations, PLP is inactivated by accumulating reactive metabolites. In *PROSC* mutations PLP may be consumed as it acts as a reactive metabolite toward other cell constituents (**Table 1**). In all cases treatment with pyridoxine or PLP itself alleviates the seizure tendency (2).

It has been hypothesized that a deficiency of PLP may cause seizures through suboptimal inhibitory GABAergic neurotransmission. However, in a study on one patient with pyridoxine-responsive epilepsy (reported before the genetic origin had been discovered) the CSF obtained by lumbar puncture had a level of glutamate that was 200 times higher than normal, indicative of dysfunctional glutamate metabolism, but the level of GABA was normal (28). With pyridoxine treatment the CSF level of glutamate was normalized, and that of GABA remained normal. Realizing that PLP is essential in more than 100 enzymatic reactions (5), ascribing pyridoxine-responsive seizures to one enzymatic dysfunction may seem reductionist. Intriguingly, in four patients with hyperprolinemia type II and pyridoxine-responsive epilepsy serum PLP was normal (29), and in two other cases of pyridoxine-responsive epilepsy, the level of PLP in CSF was normal (28, 30). The latter observation could suggest that CSF levels of PLP do not reliably reflect intracellular PLP levels in brain cells (which do not accumulate PLP, but pyridoxal) (13), or that the biochemistry of the mutations is more complex than one would expect from the (hitherto) known functions of the genes.

INTELLECTUAL DISABILITY IN PYRIDOXINE-RESPONSIVE EPILEPSY: THE NEED FOR NOVEL THERAPIES

Pyridoxine-responsive epilepsy is often associated with intellectual disability (2, 4, 10, 27, 29, 31). The intellectual disability is not prevented by pyridoxine treatment alone, and patients tend to be intellectually disabled although their epilepsy is well controlled. These observations point to unique mechanisms underlying the intellectual disability. Some effects of the metabolic derangement may be unspecific, such as lesions to periventricular white matter or to the hippocampus in the form of hippocampal sclerosis (27, 32), and such structural damage could play a role in the intellectual disability in addition to the biochemical alteration. In many cases, however, magnetic resonance imaging (MRI) of the brain is normal, and the cause of intellectual disability must be sought elsewhere.

Intellectual disability is diagnosed when a person has an IQ score below 70, when he/she has impaired adaptive skills, and when the disability was manifest before the person reached 18 years of age (33). Intellectual disability implies that development of complex brain functions, or cognitive functions, is slowed or arrested (34). Intellectual disability encompasses impairment in abstract thinking, language, numerical understanding, problem solving, and learning i.e., intellectual skills. It further implies impairment in executive functioning: the ability to initiate, prioritize, plan, and carry out actions, and the ability to regulate one's own emotions and impulses, and it affects the understanding of social cues and rules. Another area of disability is visuospatial understanding, or the comprehension of space and movement, manifesting as clumsiness in the execution of practical work and problem solving. Intellectual disability leaves the affected person with low psychomotor speed and limited attention span and working memory, which lead to slow information processing and vulnerability to distraction and fatigability. The degree of disability ranges from mild, through moderate and severe, to profound. Regardless of degree, the all-encompassing nature of intellectual disability renders the disabled person at an enormous disadvantage in managing his/her own adult life in an independent manner. Therefore, identification of ways to ameliorate or compensate for metabolic dysfunctions that entail intellectual disability is sorely needed. However, research into molecular mechanisms that may form the basis for therapy is scant. Below we therefore point to possibilities that arise from the understanding of the reactivity of the metabolites that accumulate in some of the pyridoxine-responsive epilepsies.

POSSIBLE TOXIC MECHANISMS OF α-AMINOADIPIC SEMIALDEHYDE, γ-GLUTAMIC SEMIALDEHYDE, P6C, AND P5C. THERAPEUTIC POSSIBILITIES

Several mutations that cause pyridoxine-responsive epilepsy lead to accumulation of reactive compounds: α-aminoadipic semialdehyde and P6C in *ALDH7A1* and *MOCS2* mutations (20, 23), γ-glutamyl semialdehyde and P5C in *ALDH4A1* mutations (25). These compounds must be assumed to accumulate in brain cells, and they emerge as likely pathogenic factors underlying the intellectual disability that accompanies pyridoxine-responsive epilepsy. Their levels would not be expected to decrease with pyridoxine therapy. An important mechanistic observation has come from intervention studies on patients with *ALDH7A1* mutations. These patients seem to improve cognitively on a diet that is poor in lysine, but enriched in arginine (32). The dose of dietary arginine was 150 mg arginine/kg bodyweight/day or higher in children that were from 288 days to 8 years of age (32). Arginine supplementation probably inhibits transfer of lysine across the blood-brain barrier, as the two amino acids travel competitively on the same transporter (35). The net result would be a reduction of the exposure of the brain to lysine, pointing to lysine metabolites (α-aminoadipic semialdehyde and its derivatives) as an important cause of intellectual disability in in *ALDH7A1* mutations. It cannot be ruled out, however, that such dietary measures may have biological effects in themselves that are not related to the effects of *ALDH7A1* mutations. Arginine supplementation has a number of biological effects in humans (36, 37), some of which may be related to arginine's role as a precursor for nitric oxide.

α-Aminoadipic semialdehyde and γ-glutamic semialdehyde may, because of their aldehyde groups, react non-enzymatically with proteins and probably other macromolecules, such as DNA, RNA and phospholipids, and with glutathione and other -SH-group-containing molecules (38–40). The reaction of proteins and other molecules with an aldehyde may change their function or turnover. Such reactions further lead to the formation of "advanced glycation end products" (AGEs). Other endogenous aldehydes, such as glucose in its open chain form (41), methylglyoxal (42), glyceraldehyde (43–45), and acetaldehyde (46), are known to participate in the formation of AGEs, a reactivity that is an important aspect of their pathogenicity. AGEs may trigger pathological inflammation reactions through their activation of AGE receptors [RAGEs; (47)]. This mechanism has been proposed to contribute to the cognitive derangement in Alzheimer disease and in the neuronal dysfunction observed in diabetes (44, 48). At present, a pathogenic role of spontaneous reactions between aldehydes and other cell constituents is only hypothetical. Even so, two possible therapeutic strategies emerge in the subset of pyridoxine-responsive epilepsies that are associated with aldehyde accumulation: prevention of AGE formation and inhibition of the downstream inflammatory reactions that AGEs may precipitate.

Prevention of AGE formation or inactivation of AGEs has proved possible with both metformin (49), a commonly used antidiabetic drug, and with trans-resveratrol, a polyphenol found in berries, and hesperetin, a flavonoid found in citrus fruit (50). Some studies suggest an anti-AGE effect of pyridoxine itself (51–53), while others do not confirm this (54–56). It may be possible to scavenge α-aminoadipic semialdehyde and γ-glutamic semialdehyde by other means as well, e.g., by increasing the availability of free SH groups in the form of glutathione or N-acetyl-cysteine. The reactivity of α-aminoadipic semialdehyde and γ-glutamic semialdehyde toward free -SH groups has not been determined, however. Treatments or diets that reduce the total exposure of the brain to AGE-forming compounds (e.g., from glucose, fructose, or their metabolites glyceraldehyde and methylglyoxal) may be beneficial when the level of α-aminoadipic semialdehyde or γ-glutamic semialdehyde is high. Such a diet may be one that keeps serum glucose low (57). The downstream inflammatory response to AGE formation may possibly be targeted by anti-inflammatory drugs, scavengers of reactive oxygen species, and RAGE antagonists (58–60).

The cyclic forms of α-aminoadipic semialdehyde, P6C, and γ-glutamic semialdehyde, P5C, are reactive toward PLP (22, 25), probably reflecting a general reactivity that could lead these compounds to modify other metabolites or cell constituents as well. However, this has not yet been studied in much detail.

It is not known where in the brain α-aminoadipic semialdehyde and γ-glutamic semialdehyde may exert their (supposed) toxic action, for instance, whether it occurs intra- or extracellularly. One missing factor that is necessary for the understanding of the toxicity of aldehydes is knowledge of how aldehydes cross cell membranes in the brain. From toxicological and metabolic studies (42, 61) it is clear that various aldehydes do cross cell membranes, but the transfer mechanism remains unknown and therefore escapes therapeutic manipulation.

A PATHOGENIC LACK OF DOWNSTREAM PRODUCTS DURING ENZYME DYSFUNCTION?

Although accumulation of toxic metabolites may be a primary mechanism of pathology in enzyme deficiencies, it cannot be ruled out that reduced formation of downstream metabolites contributes to the overall phenotype. In *ALDH7A1* mutation, α-aminoadipic semialdehyde is not converted into α-aminoadipate (and hence α-ketoadipate) at a normal rate. α-Aminoadipate may have important physiological functions as it may act as a ligand at the NMDA-type glutamate receptor, and it may modulate kynurenate metabolism (62). Further, α-aminoadipate is noted for its fairly selectively toxic effects on glial cells (63), which may be a reflection of a hitherto unexplored physiological effect of α-aminoadipate at lower concentrations. Therefore, a lack of α-aminoadipic semialdehyde dehydrogenase function may have biological consequences caused by downstream effect as well as by the accumulation of aldehyde substrate. A recently developed *aldh7a1* knock-out zebra fish (64) could be a suitable model for the testing of therapeutic effects of α-aminoadipate in loss of α-aminoadipic semialdehyde dehydrogenase function.

CAVEATS IN THE TREATMENT OF PYRIDOXINE-RESPONSIVE EPILEPSIES AND ASSOCIATED INTELLECTUAL DISABILITY

The use of pyridoxine at high doses must take into account that pyridoxine itself may be neurotoxic in the long run, causing polyneuropathy (65, 66), for which patients should be monitored. Further, the use of a diet that is rich in arginine to reduce transport of lysine across the blood-brain barrier (31) may lead to higher levels of γ-glutamic semialdehyde (and P5C), an arginine metabolite, that may lead to AGE formation. Lastly, the use of scavengers to reduce tissue concentration of α-aminoadipic semialdehyde in *ALDH7A1* mutations or γ-glutamic semialdehyde in *ALDH4A1* mutations must take into account that the scavenger might react with PLP itself, reducing the effectiveness of pyridoxine treatment.

The published reference values for PLP in CSF obtained through lumbar puncture cover a fairly narrow concentration range: 11–46 nmol/L in adults (67), 32–89 nmol/L (68), or 23–64 nmol/L (29) in children. In a recent study, we used HPLC and tandem mass spectrometry to measure PLP and other pyridoxine metabolites in CSF from the cerebral ventricles of 15 patients undergoing CSF drainage because of raised intracranial pressure (69); at the time of sampling the intracranial pressure was normal, and the CSF was clear and colorless. The range of PLP values in ventricular CSF was great: 3.65–132 nmol/L (median 11.3 nmol/L); pyridoxal range was 6.4–51 nmol/L (median 20 nmol/L); the range for pyridoxic acid, the metabolic product of pyridoxal, was 0.32–14.5 (median 1.77 nmol/L). Similar findings for PLP were reported by Footitt et al. (70). Thus, with a 36-fold difference between the lowest and the highest PLP value, it may be that the natural variation in CSF levels of PLP may explain differences in pyridoxine requirement among patients, and it may explain why some patients develop intellectual disability and others do not.

With respect to dietary treatment of patients suffering from *ALDH7A1* mutations with lysine restriction and arginine supplementation it should be realized that results on intellectual disability are preliminary, and that a better understanding of the variation in clinical response as well as possible side effects of the treatment is needed.

CONCLUSION

Pyridoxine-responsive epilepsies are often compounded by neurodevelopmental disorders, most importantly intellectual disability. The epilepsies may be treated efficiently with pyridoxine or PLP, but the intellectual disability does not respond to such treatment. In some forms of pyridoxine-responsive epilepsy the underlying mutation entails accumulation of certain aldehydes that may react non-enzymatically with brain cells constituents, altering their function. Alternatively, the aldehydes may, after binding to proteins and forming AGEs, produce inflammation upon activation of AGE receptors. Dietary measures to reduce the brain's exposure to lysine metabolite α-aminoadipic semialdehyde in *ALDH7A1* mutations has shown promise with respect to ameliorating intellectual disability; this was achieved by reducing dietary lysine and by dietary arginine supplementation upwards of 150 mg arginine/kg bodyweight/day in children that were from 288 days to 8 years of age (32).

Future therapies aimed at protecting cognitive development in affected children may exploit the possibility of inactivating the accumulating aldehydes, inhibiting AGE formation or AGE receptors, or dampening the inflammatory response that follows from AGE receptor activation.

AUTHOR CONTRIBUTIONS

All authors listed have made a substantial, direct and intellectual contribution to the work, and approved it for publication.

FUNDING

This work was supported by The Norwegian Health Association (Grant#1513).

REFERENCES

1. Stockler S, Plecko B, Gospe SM Jr, Coulter-Mackie M, Connolly M, van Karnebeek C, et al. Pyridoxine dependent epilepsy and antiquitin deficiency: clinical and molecular characteristics and recommendations for diagnosis, treatment and follow-up. *Mol Genet Metab.* (2011) 104:48–60. doi: 10.1016/j.ymgme.2011.05.014
2. Mills PB, Camuzeaux SS, Footitt EJ, Mills KA, Gissen P, Fisher L, et al. Epilepsy due to PNPO mutations: genotype, environment and treatment affect presentation and outcome. *Brain.* (2014) 137:1350–60. doi: 10.1093/brain/awu051
3. Burd L, Stenehjem A, Franceschini LA, Kerbeshian J. A 15-year follow-up of a boy with pyridoxine (vitamin B6)-dependent seizures with autism, breath holding, and severe mental retardation. *J Child Neurol.* (2000) 15:763–5. doi: 10.1177/088307380001501111
4. van Karnebeek CD, Tiebout SA, Niermeijer J, Poll-The BT, Ghani A, Coughlin CR II, et al. Pyridoxine-dependent epilepsy: an expanding clinical spectrum. *Pediatr Neurol.* (2016) 59:6–12. doi: 10.1016/j.pediatrneurol.2015.12.013
5. Clayton PT. B6-responsive disorders: a model of vitamin dependency. *J Inherit Metab Dis.* (2006) 29:317–26. doi: 10.1007/s10545-005-0243-2
6. Petroff OA. GABA and glutamate in the human brain. *Neuroscientist.* (2002) 8:562–73. doi: 10.1177/1073858402238515
7. Kwok F, Churchich JE. Brain pyridoxal kinase. Purification, substrate specificities, and sensitized photodestruction of an essential histidine. *J Biol Chem.* (1979) 254:6489–95.
8. Gachon F, Fonjallaz P, Damiola F, Gos P, Kodama T, Zakany J, et al. The loss of circadian PAR bZip transcription factors results in epilepsy. *Genes Dev.* (2004) 18:1397–412. doi: 10.1101/gad.301404
9. Choi JD, Bowers-Komro M, Davis MD, Edmondson DE, McCormick DB. Kinetic properties of pyridoxamine (pyridoxine)-5'-phosphate oxidase from rabbit liver. *J Biol Chem.* (1983) 258:840–5.
10. di Salvo ML, Mastrangelo M, Nogués I, Tolve M, Paiardini A, Carducci C, et al. Pyridoxine-5'-phosphate oxidase (Pnpo) deficiency: clinical and biochemical alterations associated with the C.347g> A (P.·Arg116gln) mutation. *Mol Genet Metab.* (2017) 122:135–42. doi: 10.1016/j.ymgme.2017.08.003
11. Whyte MP, Landt M, Ryan LM, Mulivor RA, Henthorn PS, Fedde KN, et al. Alkaline phosphatase: placental and tissue-non-specific isoenzymes hydrolyze phosphoethanolamine, inorganic pyrophosphate, and pyridoxal 5'-phosphate. Substrate accumulation in carriers of hypophosphatasia corrects during pregnancy. *J Clin Invest.* (1995) 95:1440–5. doi: 10.1172/JCI117814
12. Oyachi M, Harada D, Sakamoto N, Ueyama K, Kondo K, Kishimoto K, et al. A case of perinatal hypophosphatasia with a novel mutation in the ALPL gene: clinical course and review of the literature. *Clin Pediatr Endocrinol.* (2018) 27:179–86. doi: 10.1297/cpe.27.179
13. Spector R, Johanson CE. Vitamin transport and homeostasis in mammalian brain: focus on vitamins B and E. *J Neurochem.* (2007) 103:425–38. doi: 10.1111/j.1471-4159.2007.04773.x
14. Whyte MP, Greenberg CR, Salman NJ, Bober MB, McAlister WH, Wenkert D, et al. Enzyme-replacement therapy in life-threatening hypophosphatasia. *N Engl J Med.* (2012) 366:904–13. doi: 10.1056/NEJMoa1106173
15. Krawitz PM, Schweiger MR, Rödelsperger C, Marcelis C, Kölsch U, Meisel C, et al. Identity-by-descent filtering of exome sequence data identifies PIGV mutations in hyperphosphatasia mental retardation syndrome. *Nat Genet.* (2010) 42:827–9. doi: 10.1038/ng.653
16. Horn D, Krawitz P, Mannhardt A, Korenke GC, Meinecke P. Hyperphosphatasia-mental retardation syndrome due to PIGV mutations: expanded clinical spectrum. *Am J Med Genet.* (2011) 155A:1917–22. doi: 10.1002/ajmg.a.34102
17. Kuki I, Takahashi Y, Okazaki S, Kawawaki H, Ehara E, Inoue N, et al. Vitamin B6-responsive epilepsy due to inherited GPI deficiency. *Neurology.* (2013) 81:1467–9. doi: 10.1212/WNL.0b013e3182a8411a
18. Thompson MD, Killoran A, Percy ME, Nezarati M, Cole DE, Hwang PA. Hyperphosphatasia with neurologic deficit: a pyridoxine-responsive seizure disorder? *Pediatr Neurol.* (2006) 34:303–7. doi: 10.1016/j.pediatrneurol.2005.08.020
19. Coughlin CR II, Swanson MA, Spector E, Meeks NJL, Kronquist KE, Aslamy M, et al. The genotypic spectrum of ALDH7A1 mutations resulting in pyridoxine dependent epilepsy: a common epileptic encephalopathy. *J Inherit Metab Dis.* (2018). doi: 10.1007/s10545-018-0219-7. [Epub ahead of print].
20. Plecko B, Paul K, Paschke E, Stoeckler-Ipsiroglu S, Struys E, Jakobs C, et al. Biochemical and molecular characterization of 18 patients with pyridoxine-dependent epilepsy and mutations of the antiquitin (ALDH7A1) gene. *Hum Mutat.* (2007) 28:19–26. doi: 10.1002/humu.20433
21. Struys EA, Bok LA, Emal D, Houterman S, Willemsen MA, Jakobs C. The measurement of urinary Δ^1-piperideine-6-carboxylate, the alter ego of α-aminoadipic semialdehyde, in Antiquitin deficiency. *J Inherit Metab Dis.* (2012) 35:909–16. doi: 10.1007/s10545-011-9443-0
22. Mills PB, Struys E, Jakobs C. Mutations in antiquitin in individuals with pyridoxine-dependent seizures. *Nat Med.* (2006) 12:307–9. doi: 10.1038/nm1366

23. Mills PB, Footitt EJ, Ceyhan S, Waters PJ, Jakobs C, Clayton PT, et al. Urinary AASA excretion is elevated in patients with molybdenum cofactor deficiency and isolated sulphite oxidase deficiency. *J Inherit Metab Dis.* (2012) 35:1031–6. doi: 10.1007/s10545-012-9466-1
24. Struys EA, Nota B, Bakkali A, Al Shahwan S, Salomons GS, Tabarki B. Pyridoxine-dependent epilepsy with elevated urinary α-amino adipic semialdehyde in molybdenum cofactor deficiency. *Pediatrics.* (2012) 130:e1716–9. doi: 10.1542/peds.2012-1094
25. Farrant RD, Walker V, Mills GA, Mellor JM, Langley GJ. Pyridoxal phosphate de-activation by pyrroline-5-carboxylic acid. Increased risk of vitamin B6 deficiency and seizures in hyperprolinemia type II. *J Biol Chem.* (2001) 276:15107–16. doi: 10.1074/jbc.M010860200
26. Walker V, Mills GA, Peters SA, Merton WL. Fits, pyridoxine, and hyperprolinaemia type II. *Arch Dis Child.* (2000) 82:236–7. doi: 10.1136/adc.82.3.236
27. Darin N, Reid E, Prunetti L, Samuelsson L, Husain RA, Wilson M, et al. Mutations in PROSC disrupt cellular pyridoxal phosphate homeostasis and cause vitamin-B_6-dependent epilepsy. *Am J Hum Genet.* (2016) 99:1325–37. doi: 10.1016/j.ajhg.2016.10.011
28. Baumeister FA, Gsell W, Shin YS, Egger J. Glutamate in pyridoxine-dependent epilepsy: neurotoxic glutamate concentration in the cerebrospinal fluid and its normalization by pyridoxine. *Pediatrics.* (1994) 94:318–21.
29. van de Ven S, Gardeitchik T, Kouwenberg D, Kluijtmans L, Wevers R, Morava E. Long-term clinical outcome, therapy and mild mitochondrial dysfunction in hyperprolinemia. *J Inherit Metab Dis.* (2014) 37:383–90. doi: 10.1007/s10545-013-9660-9
30. Levtova A, Camuzeaux S, Laberge AM, Allard P, Brunel-Guitton C, Diadori P, et al. Normal cerebrospinal fluid pyridoxal 5'-phosphate level in a PNPO-deficient patient with neonatal-onset epileptic encephalopathy. *JIMD Rep.* (2015) 22:67–75. doi: 10.1007/8904_2015_413
31. Pena IA, MacKenzie A, Van Karnebeek CDM. Current knowledge for pyridoxine-dependent epilepsy: a 2016 update. *Expert Rev Endocrinol Metab.* (2017) 12:5–20. doi: 10.1080/17446651.2017.1273107
32. Coughlin CR II, van Karnebeek CD, Al-Hertani W, Shuen AY, Jaggumantri S, Jack RM, et al. Triple therapy with pyridoxine, arginine supplementation and dietary lysine restriction in pyridoxine-dependent epilepsy: neurodevelopmental outcome. *Mol Genet Metab.* (2015) 116:35–43. doi: 10.1016/j.ymgme.2015.05.011
33. World Health Organization. *WHO Methods and Data Sources for Global Burden of Disease Estimates 2000–2011.* Global Health Estimates Technical Paper. (2013) WHO/HIS/HSI/GHE/2013.4
34. Salvador-Carulla L, Reed GM, Vaez-Azizi LM, Cooper SA, Martinez-Leal R, Bertelli M, et al. Intellectual developmental disorders: towards a new name, definition and framework for "mental retardation/intellectual disability" in ICD-11. *World Psychiatry.* (2011) 10:175–80. doi: 10.1002/j.2051-5545.2011.tb00045.x
35. O'Kane RL, Viña JR, Simpson I, Zaragozá R, Mokashi A, Hawkins RA. Cationic amino acid transport across the blood-brain barrier is mediated exclusively by system y^+. *Am J Physiol Endocrinol Metab.* (2006) 291:E412–9. doi: 10.1152/ajpendo.00007.2006
36. McNeal CJ, Meininger CJ, Reddy D, Wilborn CD, Wu G. Safety and effectiveness of arginine in adults. *J Nutr.* (2016) 146:2587S–93S. doi: 10.3945/jn.116.234740
37. Shah PS, Shah VS, Kelly LE. Arginine supplementation for prevention of necrotising enterocolitis in preterm infants. *Cochrane Database Syst Rev.* (2017) 4:CD004339. doi: 10.1002/14651858.CD004339.pub4
38. Daneshvar B, Frandsen H, Autrupand H, Dragsted LO. γ-Glutamyl semialdehyde and 2-amino-adipic semialdehyde: biomarkers of oxidative damage to proteins. *Biomarkers.* (1997) 2:117–23. doi: 10.1080/135475097231841
39. Akagawa M, Sasaki D, Kurota Y, Suyama K. Formation of alpha-aminoadipic and gamma-glutamic semialdehydes in proteins by the maillard reaction. *Ann N Y Acad Sci.* (2005) 1043:129–34. doi: 10.1196/annals.1333.016
40. Estévez M, Ollilainen V, Heinonen M. Analysis of protein oxidation markers alpha-aminoadipic and gamma-glutamic semialdehydes in food proteins using liquid chromatography (LC)-electrospray ionization (ESI)-multistage tandem mass spectrometry (MS). *J Agric Food Chem.* (2009) 57:3901–10. doi: 10.1021/jf804017p
41. Giri B, Dey S, Das T, Sarkar M, Banerjee J, Dash SK. Chronic hyperglycemia mediated physiological alteration and metabolic distortion leads to organ dysfunction, infection, cancer progression and other pathophysiological consequences: an update on glucose toxicity. *Biomed Pharmacother.* (2018) 107:306–28. doi: 10.1016/j.biopha.2018.07.157
42. Allaman I, Bélanger M, Magistretti PJ. Methylglyoxal, the dark side of glycolysis. *Front Neurosci.* (2015) 9:23. doi: 10.3389/fnins.2015.00023
43. Takeuchi M, Yamagishi S. Involvement of toxic AGEs (TAGE) in the pathogenesis of diabetic vascular complications and Alzheimer's disease. *J Alzheimers Dis.* (2009) 16:845–58. doi: 10.3233/JAD-2009-0974
44. Fawver JN, Schall HE, Petrofes Chapa RD, Zhu X, Murray IV. Amyloid-β metabolite sensing: biochemical linking of glycation modification and misfolding. *J Alzheimers Dis.* (2012) 30:63–73. doi: 10.3233/JAD-2012-112114
45. Koriyama Y, Furukawa A, Muramatsu M, Takino J, Takeuchi M. Glyceraldehyde caused Alzheimer's disease-like alterations in diagnostic marker levels in SH-SY5Y human neuroblastoma cells. *Sci. Rep.* (2015) 5:13313. doi: 10.1038/srep13313
46. Garaycoechea JI, Crossan GP, Langevin F, Mulderrig L, Louzada S, Yang F, et al. Alcohol and endogenous aldehydes damage chromosomes and mutate stem cells. *Nature.* (2018) 553:171–7. doi: 10.1038/nature25154
47. Srikanth V, Maczurek A, Phan T, Steele M, Westcott B, Juskiw D, et al. Advanced glycation endproducts and their receptor RAGE in Alzheimer's disease. *Neurobiol Aging.* (2011) 32:763–77. doi: 10.1016/j.neurobiolaging.2009.04.016
48. Frimat M, Daroux M, Litke R, Nevière R, Tessier FJ, Boulanger E. Kidney, heart and brain: three organs targeted by ageing and glycation. *Clin Sci.* (2017) 131:1069–92. doi: 10.1042/CS20160823
49. Kinsky OR, Hargraves TL, Anumol T, Jacobsen NE, Dai J, Snyder SA, et al. Metformin scavenges methylglyoxal to form a novel imidazolinone metabolite in humans. *Chem Res Toxicol.* (2016) 29:227–34. doi: 10.1021/acs.chemrestox.5b00497
50. Rabbani N, Thornalley PJ. Advanced glycation end products in the pathogenesis of chronic kidney disease. *Kidney Int.* (2018) 93:803–13. doi: 10.1016/j.kint.2017.11.034
51. Noori N, Tabibi H, Hosseinpanah F, Hedayati M, Nafar M. Effects of combined lipoic acid and pyridoxine on albuminuria, advanced glycation end-products, and blood pressure in diabetic nephropathy. *Int J Vitam Nutr Res.* (2013) 83:77–85. doi: 10.1024/0300-9831/a000147
52. Miyashita M, Arai M, Kobori A, Ichikawa T, Toriumi K, Niizato K, et al. Clinical features of schizophrenia with enhanced carbonyl stress. *Schizophr Bull.* (2014) 40:1040–946. doi: 10.1093/schbul/sbt129
53. Sadowska-Bartosz I, Galiniak S, Bartosz G. Kinetics of glycoxidation of bovine serum albumin by glucose, fructose and ribose and its prevention by food components. *Molecules.* (2014) 19:18828–49. doi: 10.3390/molecules191118828
54. Cetin E, Civelek S, Andican G, Candan Polizzi F, Yumuk V, Burçak G. Plasma AGE-peptides and C-peptide in early-stage diabetic nephropathy patients on thiamine and pyridoxine therapy. *Minerva Med.* (2013) 104:93–101.
55. Nascimento MM, Suliman ME, Murayama Y, Nihi M, Hayashi SY, Stenvinkel P, et al. Effect of high-dose thiamine and pyridoxine on advanced glycation end products and other oxidative stress markers in hemodialysis patients: a randomized placebo-controlled study. *J Ren Nutr.* (2006) 16:119–24. doi: 10.1053/j.jrn.2006.01.002
56. Tarwadi KV, Agte VV. Effect of micronutrients on methylglyoxal-mediated *in vitro* glycation of albumin. *Biol Trace Elem Res.* (2011) 143:717–25. doi: 10.1007/s12011-010-8915-7
57. Vlassara H, Uribarri J. Advanced glycation end products (AGE) and diabetes: cause, effect, or both? *Curr Diab Rep.* (2014) 14:453. doi: 10.1007/s11892-013-0453-1
58. Walker D, Lue LF, Paul G, Patel A, Sabbagh MN. Receptor for advanced glycation endproduct modulators: a new therapeutic target in Alzheimer's disease. *Expert Opin Investig Drugs.* (2015) 24:393–9. doi: 10.1517/13543784.2015.1001490
59. Schmidt AM. 2016 ATVB plenary lecture: receptor for advanced glycation endproducts and implications for the pathogenesis a treatment of cardiometabolic disorders: spotlight on the macrophage. *Arterioscler*

Thromb Vasc Biol. (2017) 37:613–21. doi: 10.1161/ATVBAHA.117.307263

60. Sanajou D, Ghorbani Haghjo A, Argani H, Aslani S. AGE-RAGE axis blockade in diabetic nephropathy: current status and future directions. *Eur J Pharmacol.* (2018) 833:158–64. doi: 10.1016/j.ejphar.2018.06.001
61. Hassel B, Elsais A, Frøland AS, Taubøll E, Gjerstad L, Quan Y, et al. Uptake and metabolism of fructose by rat neocortical cells *in vivo* and by isolated nerve terminals *in vitro*. *J Neurochem.* (2015) 133:572–81. doi: 10.1111/jnc.13079
62. Wu HQ, Ungerstedt U, Schwarcz R. L-alpha-aminoadipic acid as a regulator of kynurenic acid production in the hippocampus: a microdialysis study in freely moving rats. *Eur J Pharmacol.* (1995) 281:55–61. doi: 10.1016/0014-2999(95)00224-9
63. Sherpa AD, van de Nes P, Xiao F, Weedon J, Hrabetova S. Gliotoxin-induced swelling of astrocytes hinders diffusion in brain extracellular space via formation of dead-space microdomains. *Glia.* (2014) 62:1053–65. doi: 10.1002/glia.22661
64. Zabinyakov N, Bullivant G, Cao F, Fernandez Ojeda M, Jia ZP, Wen XY, et al. Characterization of the first knock-out *aldh7a1* zebrafish model for pyridoxine-dependent epilepsy using CRISPR-Cas9 technology. *PLoS ONE.* (2017) 12:e0186645. doi: 10.1371/journal.pone.0186645
65. Scott K, Zeris S, Kothari MJ. Elevated B6 levels and peripheral neuropathies. *Electromyogr Clin Neurophysiol.* (2008) 48:219–23. doi: 10.1002/9780470378014.ch14
66. Kulkantrakorn K. Pyridoxine-induced sensory ataxic neuronopathy and neuropathy: revisited. *Neurol Sci.* (2014) 35:1827–30. doi: 10.1007/s10072-014-1902-6
67. Jaeger B, Abeling NG, Salomons GS, Struys EA, Simas-Mendes M, Geukers VG, et al. Pyridoxine responsive epilepsy caused by a novel homozygous PNPO mutation. *Mol Genet Metab Rep.* (2016) 6:60–3. doi: 10.1016/j.ymgmr.2016.01.004
68. Ormazabal A, Oppenheim M, Serrano M, García-Cazorla A, Campistol J, Ribes A, et al. Pyridoxal 5'-phosphate values in cerebrospinal fluid: reference values and diagnosis of PNPO deficiency in paediatric patients. *Mol Genet Metab.* (2008) 94:173–7. doi: 10.1016/j.ymgme.2008.01.004
69. Dahlberg D, Struys EA, Jansen EE, Mørkrid L, Midttun Ø, Hassel B. Cyst fluid from cystic, malignant brain tumors: a reservoir of nutrients, including growth factor-like nutrients, for tumor cells. *Neurosurgery.* (2017) 80:917–24. doi: 10.1093/neuros/nyw101
70. Footitt EJ, Heales SJ, Mills PB, Allen GF, Oppenheim M, Clayton PT. Pyridoxal 5'-phosphate in cerebrospinal fluid; factors affecting concentration. *J Inherit Metab Dis.* (2011) 34:529–38. doi: 10.1007/s10545-011-9279-7

11

Neurological, Psychiatric and Biochemical Aspects of Thiamine Deficiency in Children and Adults

Shibani Dhir[1†], Maya Tarasenko[1†], Eleonora Napoli[1] and Cecilia Giulivi[1,2]*

[1] Department of Molecular Biosciences, School of Veterinary Medicine, University of California, Davis, Davis, CA, United States,
[2] Medical Investigations of Neurodevelopmental Disorders (MIND) Institute, University of California, Davis, Davis, CA, United States

***Correspondence:**
Cecilia Giulivi
cgiulivi@ucdavis.edu

†These authors have contributed equally to this work.*

Thiamine (vitamin B1) is an essential nutrient that serves as a cofactor for a number of enzymes, mostly with mitochondrial localization. Some thiamine-dependent enzymes are involved in energy metabolism and biosynthesis of nucleic acids whereas others are part of the antioxidant machinery. The brain is highly vulnerable to thiamine deficiency due to its heavy reliance on mitochondrial ATP production. This is more evident during rapid growth (i.e., perinatal periods and children) in which thiamine deficiency is commonly associated with either malnutrition or genetic defects. Thiamine deficiency contributes to a number of conditions spanning from mild neurological and psychiatric symptoms (confusion, reduced memory, and sleep disturbances) to severe encephalopathy, ataxia, congestive heart failure, muscle atrophy, and even death. This review discusses the current knowledge on thiamine deficiency and associated morbidity of neurological and psychiatric disorders, with special emphasis on the pediatric population, as well as the putative beneficial effect of thiamine supplementation in autism spectrum disorder (ASD) and other neurological conditions.

Keywords: autism spectrum disorders, brain, depressive disorders, encephalomyopathies, Krebs cycle, pentose phosphate pathway, thiamine transporter

INTRODUCTION

The essential nutrient thiamine (vitamin B1) is a water-soluble, sulfur-containing vitamin belonging to the vitamin B complex family (**Figure 1A**). Not being endogenously synthesized, the only available source of thiamine is dietary (beef, poultry, cereals, nuts, and beans). The body does not store thiamine in levels >30 mg, and the half-life for thiamine is only 9–18 days. For an average of ~2,000 kcal consumed daily, the minimum thiamine requirement is calculated at 0.66 mg (1), although the recommended daily intake for adult men and women is 1.2 and 1.1 mg, respectively (1, 2). During pregnancy or breast-feeding, this requirement increases to 1.4 mg/day (1). In children, the recommended dietary allowance (RDA) is age-dependent and spanning from 0.2 mg (from birth up to 6 months old) to 0.6 mg (from 6 months old to 8 years old) (3). In the human body, thiamine-rich tissues are skeletal muscles, heart, liver, kidney, and brain (4).

Despite the availability of dietary thiamine in wealthy countries, thiamine deficiency represents an important and usually overlooked issue. In developed countries, the predominant use of industrial food processing often depletes thiamine content along with other vitamins and nutrients. An increased consumption of processed food in the form of simple carbohydrates, not supplemented with adequate levels of thiamine, has been named "high calorie malnutrition" (7, 8).

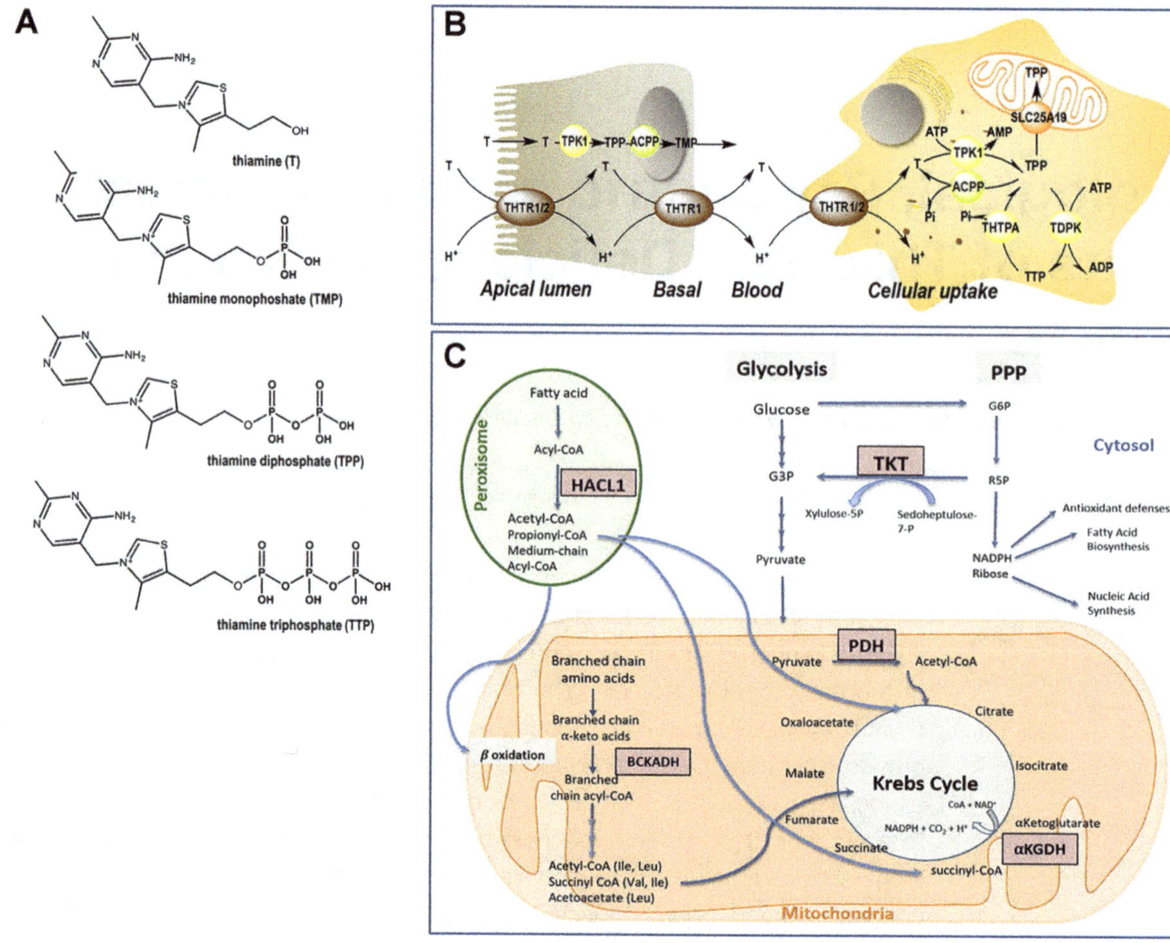

FIGURE 1 | Thiamine metabolism. **(A)** Chemical structure of thiamine and phosphorylated derivatives. **(B)** Absorption and cellular uptake of thiamine. Dietary thiamine is mainly in the form of phosphate derivatives and, before absorption, these are converted to free thiamine by intestinal phosphatases. Mammalians utilize THTR1 and THTR2 to transport thiamine. The THTR1 appears to function in the micromolar range, whereas the THTR-2 appears to function in the nanomolar range. Both transporters are expressed in the human small and large intestine, and the expression of THTR1 is higher than that of THTR2, with THTR1 found at both the apical and basolateral membranes of enterocytes (somewhat higher expression at the latter compared to the former domain). Expression of the THTR2 protein was found to be restricted to the apical membrane domain only [see (5) and references therein]. Free thiamine is converted to TPP by the action of TPK1 in the cytosol and dephosphorylation of TPP to TMP and thiamine by ACPP. At higher concentrations of thiamine, simple passive diffusion takes place [see (6) and references therein]. From blood, thiamine is taken up by either transporter (THTR1 or THTR2). Both carriers are widely distributed in the body, but the levels differ in different tissues. Once inside the target cells, thiamine is phosphorylated to TPP by TPK1 and to TTP by TDPK. Both TPP and TTP can be dephosphorylated by ACPP and THTPA, respectively. TPP in the cytosol is utilized as a cofactor for TKT, but it is also required as a cofactor in the mitochondrial compartment; hence, the mitochondrial SLC25A19 exists at the inner mitochondrial membrane. TPP must be bound to HACL1 and HACL2 for its transport to the peroxisomes. Abbreviations: ACPP, prostatic acid phosphatase; ADP, adenosine diphosphate; AMP, adenosine monophosphate; ATP, adenosine triphosphate; T, thiamine; TDPK, thiamine diphosphokinase; THTPA, thiamine triphosphatase; THTR, thiamine transporter; TMP, thiamine monophosphate; TPP, thiamine pyrophosphate. **(C)** Pathways involving TPP-dependent enzymes. In the cytosol, TPP is the cofactor of transketolase (TKT), an enzyme involved in the pentose phosphate pathway (PPP). The PPP produces nicotinamide adenine dinucleotide phosphate (NADPH) and ribose 5-phosphate (R5P), essential for antioxidant defense and fatty acid synthesis, and precursor in the biosynthesis of nucleotides, respectively. In mitochondria, TPP acts as a cofactor for branched-chain α-ketoacid dehydrogenase (BCKDH) complex, pyruvate dehydrogenase (PDH) complex, and α-ketoglutarate dehydrogenase. In peroxisomes, TPP is a cofactor for 2-hydroxyacyl-CoA lyase 1 (HACL1) as part of the fatty acid α-oxidation pathway.

Thus, despite the caloric density, the diet is often of poor nutrition quality and does not meet recommended dietary guidelines for micronutrient intake, making this an at-risk population for micronutrient malnutrition (8). For instance, at least 29% of obese subjects that will undergo bariatric surgery have been reported as thiamine deficient (9). This condition highlights the fine balance between adequate caloric intake and balanced nutritional diet. As thiamine is a key factor in the metabolism of glucose, an increased carbohydrate intake will proportionally increase thiamine's dietary demand (a minimum of 0.33 mg per

1,000 kcal) (1). Thus, rather than focusing on thiamine's RDA, it is critical to match its intake with carbohydrate consumption as well as total caloric intake.

In developing countries, thiamine deficiency remains a widespread concern due to high rates of white rice consumption (3). As home-pounding techniques are replaced with industrial rice milling and processing, essential nutrients (such as thiamine) within the bran are stripped away (10). Asian countries consume about 90% of the rice produced worldwide, fulfilling an estimated 60% of the population's daily dietary energy intake requirement, and consequently, thiamine deficiency has become prevalent in the 15% of the adolescent population (using the most conservative approximation) (11). Thiamine deficiency may develop by ingesting diets either contaminated with thiamine-metabolizing enzymes (e.g., thiaminase) (12) or that underwent thiamine inactivation by heat and/or sulfur dioxide (13). Heavy consumption of tannin-containing or food rich in caffeine, theobromine, and theophylline (such as those present in coffee, chocolate, and tea, respectively) can inactivate thiamine, thereby compromising the thiamine status (7, 14, 15).

Other risk factors that increase the likelihood of insufficient thiamine intake include aging, economic status, eating disorders, medical conditions affecting the gastrointestinal tract, subjects receiving parental nutrition, bariatric surgery, diabetes, and alcohol abuse (9, 16–23). Unmet needs for increasing the nutritional intake of thiamine are reported during lactation, pregnancy, and increased physical activity (11, 24). During lactation, infants have increased risks of developing beriberi from newly deficient but asymptomatic mothers (11). For instance, 27% of women of childbearing age are considered thiamine deficient in Cambodia, with 38% of infants being diagnosed as severely deficient in thiamine, a critical issue that contributes significantly to the mortality of 3-month-old babies (11).

However, even in the presence of an adequate thiamine intake, its deficiency can result from genetic factors, i.e., pathogenic gene mutations in key regulators of the thiamine pathway, including thiamine pyrophosphokinase 1 (TPK1), thiamine diphosphate kinase (TDPK), thiamine triphosphatase (THTPA), and thiamine transporters (SLC25A19, SLC19A2/THTR1, and SLC19A3/THTR2; **Figure 1B**). More recently, the organic cation transporter 1 (OCT1) has been claimed to act as a hepatic thiamine transporter (25).

Regardless of the underlying cause, thiamine deficits may have severe detrimental effects, with most of the symptoms manifesting at the neurological level (24, 26). Thiamine deficiency might cause brain tissue injury by inhibiting brain energy utilization given the critical role of thiamine-dependent enzymes associated within glucose utilization (27). This is supported by the significant rate of thiamine uptake by the blood–brain barrier emphasizing the high brain demand for thiamine and the need for its supply to sustain adequate brain functions (28, 29), especially in those brain areas with both high metabolic demands and high thiamine turnover (30–32).

This review will discuss the physiological and biochemical bases of thiamine metabolism and explore the pathophysiological implications of thiamine deficiency. In particular, we will highlight the effect of thiamine supplementation as a therapeutic strategy in the management of neurological disorders, with special emphasis on the pediatric population.

BIOCHEMICAL BASIS OF THIAMINE'S CELLULAR ROLE

Dietary Availability, Absorption, and Cellular Uptake

As with most hydrophilic micronutrients, thiamine absorption occurs mainly in the jejunum (33). Throughout the digestive tract, dietary proteins get hydrolyzed, releasing thiamine. In the intestinal lumen, alkaline phosphatases catalyze the hydrolysis of thiamine-phosphorylated derivatives into free thiamine (34). Unphosphorylated, free thiamine at concentrations higher than 1 μM enters the enterocyte by passive diffusion, whereas at lower levels, it is transported *via* the saturable thiamine/H^+ antiport system (thiamine transporter 1 or THTR1) through an energy-dependent process (33). Under conditions of thiamine deficiency, an upregulation of the expression of the thiamine transporter 2 (THTR2) was observed in Caco2 cells in culture, suggesting that diet can modulate the expression of this transporter (35). Within the enterocyte, thiamine is phosphorylated to thiamine pyrophosphate (TPP) by TPK1. Then, most TPP is dephosphorylated to thiamine monophosphate (TMP) to cross the basal membrane of the enterocyte. The TMP is released into the bloodstream through an ATPase-dependent transport system (36) (**Figure 1B**). Free thiamine can also reach the bloodstream *via* the thiamine transporter 2 (THTR2) located mainly at the basolateral membrane of the enterocyte. Once in blood, while very low levels of TMP and thiamine circulate free in plasma or serum, more than 90% of the phosphorylated thiamine (in the form of TPP) is present in erythrocytes and leukocytes (37). Notably, the isoform 3 of the carrier SLC44A4 has recently been described as a TPP carrier in the colon. Originally, SLC44A4 was described as a choline transporter linked to the non-neuronal synthesis of choline (38) and required to the efferent innervation of hair cells in the olivocochlear bundle for the maintenance of physiological function of outer hair cells and the protection of hair cells from acoustic injury (39). Recent evidence indicates that this carrier may mediate the absorption of microbiota-generated TPP (especially in infants) and contribute to host thiamine homeostasis (40).

The cellular uptake of thiamine from the bloodstream can be mediated by any of the two high-affinity carriers: THTR1 [encoded by *SLC19A2* (41)] and THTR2 [encoded by *SLC19A3* (42, 43)]. These transporters are ubiquitously expressed (42–44), but THTR1 is most abundant in the intestine, skeletal muscle, nervous system, and eye followed by the placenta, liver, and kidney, whereas THTR2 is located mostly in adipose tissue, breast tissue, liver, lymphocytes, spleen, gallbladder, placenta, pancreas, and brain (information collected from GeneCards). Once transported intracellularly, free thiamine is rapidly phosphorylated to TPP by thiamine pyrophosphokinase (TPK1). A second kinase, TDPK, adds a phosphate group to TPP to generate thiamine triphosphate (TTP). TPP and TTP can be dephosphorylated to, respectively, TMP and TPP by phosphatases [Prostatic Acid Phosphatase (ACPP) and THTPA, respectively; **Figure 1B**].

Biochemical Roles of Phosphorylated Forms of Thiamine

Up to 90% of the total thiamine in the body remains in its diphosphate, metabolically active form (TPP), whereas the rest is found as TMP and TTP (45). TPP is a cofactor of several thiamine-dependent enzymes involved in carbohydrate and fatty acid metabolism, namely, cytosolic transketolase (TKT), peroxisomal 2-hydroxyacyl-CoA lyase 1, and three mitochondrial enzymes (pyruvate dehydrogenase, α-ketoglutarate dehydrogenase, and branched-chain α-ketoacid dehydrogenase complexes; **Figure 1C**). As the biochemical role of TPP is well understood, the biological significance and contribution of TTP is not entirely clear. It was previously considered to be a specific neuroactive form of thiamine, but more recently, it has been reported that TTP (which is ~10% of the total brain thiamine pool) is involved in membrane excitability and nerve conduction by acting as a modulator of the permeability of sodium chloride channels (29, 32, 46).

Intracellular Location of TPP-Dependent Enzymes

Cytosol

In the cytosol, TPP acts as a cofactor for TKT, a key enzyme of the non-oxidative branch of the pentose phosphate pathway (PPP). This metabolic pathway generates nicotinamide adenine dinucleotide phosphate (NADPH) and ribose 5-phosphate (R5P) (47). NADPH is a key reducing agent in biosynthetic reactions and is a co-substrate of biosynthetic enzymes (fatty acid synthesis) and antioxidant enzymes such as the glutathione peroxidase–reductase system and thioredoxin peroxidases, among others. The crucial involvement of R5P in the biosynthesis of DNA and RNA highlights the critical role of thiamine in high-proliferating tissues.

Based on its role in the abovementioned biochemical pathways, it is expected that thiamine deficiency will result in increased oxidative stress and lower cell proliferation, as well as decreased fatty acid synthesis (including myelin) with severe consequences especially during brain development. Consistent with this premise, thiamine deficiency decreases TKT activity and leads to PPP impairment and reduced neurogenesis in murine cortex and hippocampus during neurodevelopment (48).

Peroxisomes

Peroxisomes play an important role in the catabolism of hydrogen peroxide, as well as in the shortening of very long fatty acids (which cannot undergo a direct mitochondrial β-oxidation catabolism) and α-oxidation (49). In the latter process, the TPP-dependent enzyme 2-hydroxyacyl-CoA lyase 1 (HACL1) catalyzes the cleavage of 3-methyl-branched and straight chain 2-hydroxy long-chain fatty acids (50). Phytanic acid (a 3-methyl-substituted, 20-carbon branched-chain fatty acid), unlike most fatty acids, is unable to undergo β-oxidation because of an existing methyl group in the 3-position (51). As such, it is broken down by HACL1 by an initial α-oxidation (52, 53). This branched-chain fatty acid is obtained through the diet, specifically from dairy products and red meat. The disruption of phytanic acid catabolism, due to inadequate levels of TPP, leads to triglyceride accumulation, which may cause deleterious effects such as cerebellar ataxia, peripheral polyneuropathy, vision and hearing loss, anosmia, and, in some instances, cardiac dysfunction and epiphyseal dysplasia (54). The symptoms caused by thiamine deficiency are shared by Refsum's disease, which is caused by pathogenic mutations in *HACL1* (55). Some of the symptoms are also observed in the autosomal recessive systemic disorder Zellweger syndrome and other peroxisomal-related diseases including the neonatal adrenoleukodystrophy. Zellweger syndrome is caused by pathogenic mutations in the pexin genes, which encode for proteins essential for the assembly of functional peroxisomes. It is characterized by deficits in the peroxisomal fatty acid oxidation pathway causing severe neurological and liver dysfunction as well as craniofacial abnormalities.

Mitochondria

Most (~90%) of the cytosolic TPP is transported into mitochondria *via* the mitochondrial thiamine pyrophosphate transporter [MTPPT, product of the *SLC25A19* gene (56)]. This transporter mediates the exchange of cytosolic TPP for the mitochondrial TMP; once in the cytosol, TMP is metabolized and converted back to TPP (56). In mitochondria, TPP is a critical cofactor for three enzymes, namely, pyruvate dehydrogenase, α-ketoglutarate dehydrogenase, and branched-chain α-ketoacid dehydrogenase (PDH, αKGDH, and BCKDH, respectively).

Studies in *SLC25A19* knockout mice and in carriers of the *SLC25A19* mutation, responsible for the Amish lethal microcephaly (MCPHA, see below) show, respectively, virtually undetectable and markedly reduced mitochondrial TPP levels in mouse embryonic fibroblasts and human lymphoblasts (56), which were completely restored upon addition of TPP to the PDH and KGDH complex assay mixtures (56).

Pyruvate dehydrogenase complex. This multisubunit complex catalyzes the TPP-dependent decarboxylation of pyruvate, generating acetyl-CoA, which then enters the Krebs cycle. The regulation of PDH activity constitutes a key metabolic switch influencing fuel choice, i.e., between fatty acid oxidation and glycolytic flux (57). The inability to adjust the choice of fuel for metabolic energy production has been proposed to underlie the "metabolic inflexibility" leading to the morbidity of metabolic disorders (58). Hence, thiamine-deficiency-mediated inhibition of the PDH complex will lock the system into the oxidation of glucose to pyruvate, leading to increases in lactate and decreases in cellular ATP production (59). As expected, in severe cases, the metabolic deficit presents as a fatal lactic acidosis in newborns, whereas in milder cases, neurological conditions may lead to structural abnormalities in the central nervous system (CNS), seizures, mental disability, and spasticity (60, 61).

α-Ketoglutarate dehydrogenase complex. This TPP-dependent enzyme catalyzes the formation of succinyl-CoA from α-ketoglutarate in the Krebs cycle and the consequent production of reduced nicotinamide adenine dinucleotide (NADH). Low TPP levels notably decrease αKGDH activity, thereby decreasing energy production and causing glutamate to accumulate (62), hampering oxidative metabolism and leading to neurodegeneration (63).

Branched-chain α-keto dehydrogenase complex. The TPP-dependent BCKDH enzyme, localized at the inner mitochondrial membrane, catalyzes one of the steps of the essential branched-chain amino acid (BCAAs; leucine, isoleucine, and valine) catabolic pathway. These amino acids are required for protein synthesis, and some of their catabolic products can be used for energy production *via* the citric acid cycle. In addition, their carbon skeletons (except Leu) can be used as precursors for gluconeogenesis (64). In a thiamine deficiency experimental model, medial thalamus was the brain region that shows the lowest levels of BCKDH with fivefold accumulation of Leu. This study suggested that the lower activity of this enzyme may be responsible for thalamic neuronal cell death observed in human cases of thiamine deficiency (65).

Similarly, a homozygous mutation in the BCKDH E1 α subunit results in the so-called maple syrup urine disease (MSUD, due to the distinct maple syrup smell to the urine as a result of keto acid buildup from unprocessed BCAA), characterized by physical and mental disabilities. A mild form of MSUD, called thiamine-responsive MSUD, is currently the only recognized variant that can be successfully treated with thiamine supplementation (OMIM 248600).

HIERARCHICAL ORDER OF THIAMINE-DEPENDENT ENZYMATIC DEFICIENCIES: EFFECT OF SPECIES, TISSUE, AND SUBCELLULAR COMPARTMENT

While it could be assumed that a deficiency in a given micronutrient affects its dependent enzymes equally, experimental evidence indicates otherwise. For instance, copper deficiency severely reduces cytochrome *c* oxidase activity affecting copper/zinc-superoxide dismutase to a lesser extent (66). Moreover, this hierarchical order is also tissue-specific as different brain areas (66). Similarly, in the case of thiamine deficiency, the most affected brain regions seem to be cerebellum, mammillary bodies, thalamus, hypothalamus, and brainstem in adults (1, 67). In children, MRI studies showed primary involvement of mammillary bodies as well as basal ganglia (68, 69) [preferentially the striatum and, to a lesser extent, the globus pallidus (68)], in addition to frontal lobes (69).

With regard to thiamine deficiency, Zhao et al. showed that, in mice, thiamine deprivation for 14 days led to different degrees of enzymatic deficiencies when testing for TKT, PDH, and αKGDH activities in the cortex and hippocampus (48). TKT activity was significantly more reduced in both brain regions compared to both mitochondrial enzymes PDH and αKGDH (48). Two studies reporting on a genetic mutation in SLC19A3.1 resulted in thiamine-deficient Alaskan huskies (26, 70). A greater reduction in TKT versus PDH activity was observed in the cortex. In the thalamus, however, PDH activity was affected twice as much as TKT activity (26). These studies support the concept of tissue-specific deficits of thiamine deficiency and also point to the species-specific differences that should be taken into account when making extrapolations to human studies.

In cases of severe thiamine deficiency, however, a broad enzymatic deficiency encompassing all three mitochondrial TPP-dependent enzymes would be expected to result in symptoms similar to those of the genetic disorder dihydrolipoamide dehydrogenase (DLDD) deficiency (OMIM 246900). This pathogenic mutation affects the E3 subunit, common to all three TPP-dependent dehydrogenases. Patients clinically present with lactic acidosis and neurodegeneration from inefficient oxidative metabolism, as well as increased BCAA concentrations and α-keto acids in the urine, with many of the same symptoms as MSUD, but with a more severe phenotype (71).

While BCKDH and HACL1 are (as indicated above) TPP-dependent enzymes, their activity is rarely reported in the context of thiamine deficiency, with the majority of studies focusing on TKT and PDH or αKGDH as indicators of oxidative stress (TKT) and mitochondrial dysfunction (PDH or αKGDH). However, a study by Navarro et al. noted significantly reduced BCKDH activity in the medial thalamus (compared to frontal cortex) accompanied by a fivefold increase in Leu levels following administration of a thiamine antagonist (65).

The consequences of thiamine deficiency on HACL1, however, remain mostly obscure. Recent work in HACL1-deficient mice revealed the presence of an additional TPP-dependent enzyme with lyase activity, localized in the endoplasmic reticulum, able to cleave 2-hydroxyphytanoyl-CoA (72). This process is not exactly like the one catalyzed by the peroxisomal HACL1 and involves a hydroxylation at position C2 carried out by the fatty acid 2-hydroxylase (FA2H), followed by the cleavage catalyzed by HACL1 (73). More recently, an orphan enzyme (HACL2) located in the endoplasmic reticulum known as bacterial acetolactate synthase-like was reported to cleave straight chain 2-hydroxyacyl-CoAs (74), and it is likely to be identical to the HACL1-like enzyme. A strong inverse association of C17:0 with diabetes and cardiovascular risk has been observed, suggesting a metabolic link between α-oxidation and these diseases (75, 76). More research is needed to elucidate the role of HADCL1 and HADCL2 in the context of thiamine deficiency.

DEFECTS IN GENES ASSOCIATED WITH THIAMINE METABOLISM

Pathogenic mutations in genes encoding for enzymes and transporters involved in thiamine metabolism result in symptoms similar to those found in nutrition-based thiamine deficiency and overlaps with disorders of mitochondrial dysfunction (**Table 1**). Those mutations affecting genes responsible for thiamine transporters 1 (*SLC19A2*; OMIM 249270) and 2 (*SLC19A3*; OMIM 607483) constitute the main cause of suboptimal intestinal thiamine absorption and, as a result, insufficient cellular distribution of thiamine through the body.

Carriers of homozygous or compound heterozygous loss-of-function or missense mutations in *SLC19A2* develop a rare condition known as thiamine-responsive megaloblastic anemia (TRMA) or Rogers syndrome (OMIM 249270). Most cases are currently found in isolated populations with consanguineous partners (85). This early-onset, autosomal recessive disorder is characterized by megaloblastic anemia, macrocytosis, diabetes mellitus, and sensorineural deafness. Other, more variable features include optic atrophy, congenital heart defects, short stature, and significant neurological deficits such as stroke and epilepsy during infancy (77, 86). The term "thiamine-responsive" refers to the observation of clinical, symptomatic improvement after administration of high doses of thiamine (86, 87).

The biotin–thiamine-responsive basal ganglia disease (BTBGD; OMIM: 607483) is a neurometabolic autosomal recessive disorder

TABLE 1 | Genetic mutations affecting thiamine metabolism.

Name of disease	Mutation	Protein	Age at onset	Clinical symptoms	Management (dose) (reference)
TRMA/Rogers syndrome	SLC19A2	THTR1	Birth to adolescence	Megaloblastic anemia, diabetes mellitus, sensorineural deafness, optic atrophy, congenital heart defects, short stature	Thiamine (50–100 mg/day) (77)
Biotin–thiamine-responsive basal ganglia disease	SLC19A3	THTR2	Birth to adolescence	Episodic encephalopathy associated with febrile illness, seizures, external ophthalmoplegia, dysphagia, gait ataxia, bilateral lesions of the basal ganglia	– Biotin (5–10 mg/kg/day), thiamine (300–900 mg) (78) – Biotin (5–10 mg/kg/day), thiamine (100–200 mg) (79)
Amish lethal microcephaly/THMD3	SLC25A19	Mitochondrial TPP carrier	Birth	Episodic encephalopathy associated with lactic acidosis and alpha-ketoglutaric aciduria, microcephaly, delayed psychomotor development, seizures, increased urinary lactate	– Phenobarbital (for seizures) and physical therapy (80) – High-fat diet (81)
Thiamine metabolism dysfunction syndrome 4/THMD4 (progressive polyneuropathy type)	SLC25A19	MTPC	Adolescence	Episodic encephalopathy associated with febrile illness, transient neurologic dysfunction, residual weakness, progressive axonal polyneuropathy, bilateral striatal degeneration	High-dose thiamine administered at the time of the study. Outcome not available (82)
Thiamine metabolism dysfunction syndrome 5 (episodic encephalopathy type) THMD5	TPK1	Thiamine phosphokinase 1	Early childhood	Episodic encephalopathy (Leigh-like) associated with high serum and CSF lactate with progressive neurologic and motor dysfunctions (gait disturbances, ataxia, dystonia, and spasticity, which, in some cases, may result in loss of ability to walk) triggered by infections. Cognitive function usually preserved; some developmental delay. Some patients may recover from some neurologic deficits; in others, the outcome is fatal.	Oral thiamine (100–200; 500 mg/day) (83, 84)

caused by a mutation in the *SLC19A3* gene, characterized by subacute encephalopathy with confusion, convulsions, muscle rigidity, ataxia, dysarthria, and dystonia, which can be fatal if left untreated. However, the disorder is completely reversible within by early treatment with biotin (5–10 mg/kg/day) in combination with thiamine [from 100–200 mg (79) to 300–900 mg (78); **Table 1**], underscoring the critical nature of a timely diagnosis. Signs and symptoms usually appear during childhood (between the ages of 3 and 10 years), although onset of the disease can vary between newborn period and adulthood (78, 88).

The Amish lethal microcephaly (MCPHA; OMIM 607196), also known as thiamine metabolism dysfunction syndrome-3 (THMD3; **Table 1**) (56), is caused by homozygous mutation in the *SLC25A19* gene. Amish type microcephaly is a severe autosomal recessive metabolic disorder characterized by severe microcephaly apparent at birth, profoundly delayed psychomotor development, brain malformations, and episodic encephalopathy associated with lactic acidosis and α-ketoglutaric aciduria (89). The clinical management is achieved by administering a high-fat diet (81), which sustains the production of ATP by mitochondria primarily through fatty acid β-oxidation, bypassing PDH to directly enter the Krebs cycle. Importantly, the metabolic similarity of MCPHA to PDH deficiency (OMIM 312070) indicates the relevance of administering a low-carbohydrate diet to patients with MCPHA to avoid a risk of exacerbating the lactic acidemia.

A less severe variant of the disease, thiamine metabolism dysfunction syndrome 4 (THMD4; OMIM 613710), is similarly caused by a homozygous mutation in the *SLC25A19* gene (**Table 1**). In THMD4, mitochondrial TPP uptake is reduced but not completely abolished. The disorder is characterized by childhood onset of episodic encephalopathy, causing transient neurologic dysfunction and a slight increase in cerebrospinal fluid (CSF) lactate levels during the acute phase of the disease. Most patients fully recover without therapeutic intervention; however, in some instances, mild residual weakness may persist (82).

Genetic defects in TPK1 (also known as THMD5) prevent the phosphorylation of thiamine to TPP, the active cofactor. It usually presents during childhood with acute encephalopathic episodes associated with increased serum and CSF lactate. These episodes result in progressive motor dysfunction (e.g., gait defects, ataxia, dystonia, and spasticity) associated with striatal, basal ganglial, and cerebellar regions of the brain, but cognition appeared to remain intact. Given that the phenotype is highly variable, it is likely that residual TPK1 activity and/or other cellular kinases (albeit at a lower extent and favored by the mass action of high thiamine doses) may also phosphorylate thiamine, thereby partly circumventing the metabolic block. This is based on the fact that i) some affected subjects improved with thiamine treatment [100–200 mg/day or 200 mg/twice daily (90, 91)] or with supplementation with thiamine and niacin, biotin, α-lipoic acid, and ketogenic diet (90), whereas others did not (83); and ii) deficiencies in other TPP-dependent enzymes, TKT and BCKADH, have not been observed in subjects with pathogenic mutations in TPK1 (83).

PATHOLOGY OF THIAMINE DEFICIENCY

As indicated above, the pathology of thiamine deficiency entails impaired energy-production from mitochondria in the form of ATP when using pyruvate-generating substrates (e.g., glucose) as well as increased oxidative stress (27). Under these conditions, glucose *via* glycolysis generates pyruvate, which cannot enter the Krebs cycle as acetyl-CoA due to the low activity of PDH. As such, pyruvate is transaminated to Ala or reduced to lactate *via* lactate dehydrogenase. This is consistent with the elevated lactate and organic acids observed in CSF, urine, and blood during thiamine deficiency (92–94).

Thiamine deficiency has been show to stabilize HIF-1α under normoxic conditions, thereby upregulating the expression of the glucose transporter GLUT1, VEGF, aldolase A, LDH, and THTR2 (95). This stabilization might be achieved by the inhibition of prolyl hydroxylase by increased oxidative stress conditions originated from the lower TKT activity within the PPP. These changes may be accompanied by increased glycolysis and fatty acid oxidation to sustain the cellular energy needs. The latter process may ensue with the ultimate formation of acetyl-CoA, skipping the PDH-catalyzed step. The increased flux of acetyl-CoA will then build up the levels of Krebs' intermediates including fumarate and succinate (also inhibitors of prolyl hydroxylase), especially if the biotin-dependent pyruvate carboxylase cannot sustain the production of oxaloacetate, the most limiting substrate of the cycle. This also provides a biochemical explanation for the efficacy of the biotin and thiamine supplementation in the treatment of the biotin–thiamine-responsive basal ganglia disease. Although lower thiamine deficiency also affects α-KGDH activity, which is essential to maintain the levels of Glu, Asp, and GABA, its activity seems to be less affected than PDC, thus providing an operational Krebs cycle albeit at a lower efficiency. The lower activity of BCKADH can explain the higher levels of BCAA (Leu, Ile, and Val) in human fluids.

The human central nervous system has a high-energy demand, with 2% of the body mass overseeing about 20% of the total metabolic expenditure, the majority of which is spent on firing action potentials, on neuron communication, through chemical synapses, axon growth, and myelination (96). With glucose being the primary fuel for energy production in the brain, it is not surprising that mitochondrial dysfunction and the consequent impaired glucose metabolism have been associated with several neurological and neurodevelopmental conditions (97) and major psychiatric illnesses, such as depression (98) and schizophrenia (99). The neurological symptoms in thiamine deficiency are similar to defects of PDH, which most frequently present as Leigh-like syndrome with basal ganglia involvement. Therefore, the nervous system, which is highly specialized in the use of glucose for energy generation, seems to be most vulnerable to PDHC deficiency due to TPP depletion. In the brain, the lower mitochondrial ATP production will limit the maintenance of membrane potential *via* the action of the Na^+,K^+-ATPase, thereby compromising nerve conduction and chemical synapses. Moreover, the increased oxidative stress due to the lower TKT activity will damage critical biomolecules, initiating lipid peroxidation and oxidative damage to proteins resulting in fragmentation, posttranslational modifications, and cross-linkings. The modification of epitopes on normal, endogenous molecules may result in the activation of the microglia and immune cells, compounding oxidative stress-mediated damage. The lower TKT has additional detrimental actions: by providing a suboptimal NADPH supply, biosynthetic reactions (nucleic acids and lipids) are undermined. This will limit not only cell proliferation but also the synthesis of fatty acids critical for the myelin sheath of axons. Thus, the combination of increased lipid peroxidation and the decreased fatty acid synthesis can result in demyelination, explaining some of the neurological issues caused by thiamine deficiency.

Altered thiamine metabolism has also been linked to growth of both neuronal soma and dendritic arbors in murine hippocampal neurons in culture. The individual silencing of TPK1 or each of the TPP carriers Slc25a19 and Slc19a3 in neurons significantly decreased dendrite arborization and soma size compared to controls (100). Conversely, overexpression of TPK1, Slc25a19, and Slc19a3 significantly reversed these changes, leading to increased dendritic branch length and number as well as soma size. Notably, these pathways are independent and nonredundant, as the overexpression of any of the proteins did not improve the dendritic damage caused by suppression of the other two. These findings are indicative of the crucial role that thiamine metabolism plays in soma and dendrite growth (100), and they are consistent with the microcephaly and neuronal damage reported in cases of thiamine deficiency.

In Adults

Symptoms and Consequences of Thiamine Deficiency

Thiamine deficiency can present with a broad range of neurological signs in children, such as anorexia, irritability, agitation, muscle pain, diminished or abolished deep tendon reflexes, ataxia, paralysis, and a progressively altered level of consciousness. Lactic acidosis may explain some of the generalized symptoms, including lethargy, irritability, anorexia, tachycardia, and tachypnea. These clinical manifestations are probably secondary to mitochondrial dysfunction in the heart and smooth muscle (particularly the gastrointestinal tract) and an autonomic nervous system insult (neurotransmitters). Others such as mood changes (agitation, confusion, and generalized malaise) may result from brain energy deficits as well as from a compromised synthesis of neurotransmitters (glutamate and GABA). Given the above-described varied clinical presentations, especially in children, any unexplained severe neurological signs or symptoms should raise the suspicion of thiamine deficiency [see Hiffler et al. (3) and references therein].

Generally, in blood from healthy adults, TPP levels <70 nmol/L are suggestive of thiamine deficiency [reference values: 70–180 nmol/L; https://www.mayocliniclabs.com (101, 102)]. Thiamine levels have also been assessed in CSF, in the context of Alzheimer's disease and in instances of *SLC19A3* mutations (103, 104). Although no universally accepted reference values exist for CSF, thiamine levels of 5–7 nM are considered normal in adults (105).

Blood and CSF thiamine levels provide limited information when assessing the thiamine status of a subject, as they not necessarily reflect thiamine metabolic function (102) or a direct association to its levels in the tissues. As such, assessments of erythrocytes' TKT and, if available, that of other tissue-specific TPP-dependent enzymes (PDH, αKGDH) are considered gold standards (24, 26). Basic TKT activity is usually expressed as units per gram of hemoglobin (g Hb), but more importantly, the percentage of activation of TKT to TPP supplementation are calculated (with 0–15% considered normal). One study reported that the HPLC detection of TPP in whole blood or red blood cells is equally effective to the TKT activation ratio at determining thiamine deficiency (37).

The TKT activation ratio (red blood cells) and/or the activities of TPP-dependent enzymes (leukocytes, skin fibroblasts, and muscle biopsies) are usually accompanied by testing the levels of serum lactate and pyruvate, BCAAs, organic acids, as well as brain imaging. The only cases in which the evaluation of free thiamine in plasma/serum and CSF seems to provide a valuable diagnostic tool is when dealing with pathogenic mutations in SLC19A3 (104). Similarly, urinary excretion of thiamine is also not a reliable method for the assessment of its bodily levels as it is dependent on its intake and absorption. Generally, it is expressed per unit of creatinine to account for renal function, and age should be taken into account as normal values differ in children [120 nmol/mmol creatinine in 1–13 years old (105)] and adults [220 nmol/mmol creatinine in >18 years old (105)].

Unfortunately, early symptoms of thiamine deficiency are not pronounced or distinctive enough to warrant a direct diagnosis. They include loss of appetite, nausea, weakness, apathy, fatigue, irritation, sleep disturbances, anorexia, and abdominal discomfort (106). Furthermore, the identification of specific clinical symptoms of thiamine deficiency is problematic because it is obscured by the contribution of other confounding conditions (comorbidities) such as infections and/or multiple nutritional deficiencies.

The clinical classification of thiamine deficiency falls usually into dry (or neuritic, characterized by polyneuropathy, reduced knee jerk and other tendon reflexes, and progressive severe weakness of muscles) and wet (or cardiac, characterized by edema of the legs, trunk, and face; high cardiac output; ventricular failure; and pulmonary congestion). This classification is based on the amount of fluid that accumulates in the body due to factors like cardiac function and kidney lesions, among others (107). However, many cases of thiamine deficiency are amply systemic and encompass the nervous and cardiovascular system, as well as the gastrointestinal tract (with symptoms spanning from anorexia, abdominal pain, and constipation) (108). Long-term consequences of severe thiamine deficiency are manifested by the appearance of hemorrhagic and/or necrotic lesions with neuronal and dendritic spine loss in the thalamus, hypothalamus, and cerebellum (109–111), as well as polyneuritis, peripheral edema, cardiac enlargement, and ophthalmoplegia (27).

When early, generalized thiamine deficiency is suspected, prompt administration of thiamine is advised and typically an effective treatment. A wide range of therapeutic approaches and thiamine doses are reported in the literature, spanning from 1.5 to 600 mg/day (112), with 10–20 mg/day as divided doses for several weeks for mild polyneuropathy and 20–30 mg/day for moderate to severe, usually until after disappearance of symptoms (106). Generally, thiamine deficiency is approached with doses of 5–30 mg/day intravenously (IV) or intramuscularly (IM), three times daily, followed by 5–30 mg/day orally until after disappearance of symptoms (112). However, this approach is notably less effective for individuals with chronic forms of thiamine deficiency-related disorders involving encephalopathies (see the section Wernicke Encephalopathy) (113) or TPK1 deficiencies. In the latter case, it would be worth to explore a treatment directly with TPP; however, it is not clear whether this phosphorylated thiamine form would cross the blood–brain barrier and/or reach subcellular targets such as PDH.

Wernicke Encephalopathy

Wernicke encephalopathy (WE) is a thiamine-deficiency-related acute neuropsychiatric condition, often associated with alcohol abuse (114). It is characterized by ataxia, loss of muscle coordination, memory loss, confusion, and ocular abnormalities (ophthalmoplegia). Failure to timely diagnose the disease and the lack of an appropriate therapy result in death in 17% of the cases, while 84% will undergo permanent brain damage involving severe short-term memory loss and hallucinations [or Korsakoff's syndrome (KS)], residual syndrome in patients previously affected with WE (115). Because of the close association between these two conditions, they often get referred to as Wernicke–Korsakoff syndrome (WKS). Recently, it has been suggested that WE may be underdiagnosed (116), with similar incidence in both adults and children (117), with ratification of the diagnosis in 0.4–2.8% of *postmortem* cases, but recognized only in 32% and 6% of patients with and without alcoholism, respectively. In particular, it would be critical to consider WE in any patient showing two of the following characteristics: nutritional deficiency, cerebellar or oculomotor abnormalities, or impaired mental state or memory (116). Only 16% of the WE cases are expected to fully recover after thiamine supplementation. As oral absorption is highly variable and patient-dependent (116), parenteral treatment is highly recommended with daily doses of 100–200 mg thiamine (IV) for non-alcoholics and 500 mg (up to three administrations daily) for alcoholics (114).

A substantial body of literature has been published in the past >50 years regarding WE. A detailed description of the clinical features, pathophysiology, and treatment of this syndrome is beyond the scope of this review.

Depression

A number of studies have shown an inverse association between thiamine levels and symptoms of depression in adults. A cross-sectional study on >1,500 elderly Chinese (age 50–70 years) showed that subjects with lower levels of erythrocyte thiamine (likely representing TPP bound to TKT) displayed more severe symptoms of depression (118). In this report, although no apparent differences were noted between individuals with and without depressive symptoms in dietary thiamine intake, the authors could not exclude errors in dietary assessment related to differences in food processing (118). In addition, other factors like diabetes, altered hormone profiles, and increased alcohol consumption observed in some individuals with depressive symptoms could play a critical role in the bioavailability of thiamine (118).

A direct correlation between thiamine deficiency and symptoms of major depressive disorder (MDD) had been previously found in a population of 74 individuals with history of malnutrition (119). These findings were confirmed by another study involving 118 geriatric patients (120), although in this particular instance, no information about dietary thiamine intake was provided.

Additionally, Ghaleiha and colleagues explored the interventional effect of thiamine supplementation in thiamine-deficient subjects with MDD in a 12-week, randomized, double-blind clinical trial (121). The study concluded that symptoms of depression improved significantly in subjects with MDD following 6 weeks of thiamine supplementation compared to placebo.

Finally, positive mood changes (clearheadedness, increased energy and appetite, improved sleep patterns, and decreased fatigue) have been observed following thiamine supplementation in healthy elderly (16) as well as younger (122) women, compared to the same population assigned to the placebo group. Interestingly, while in the elderly population, a marginal deficiency of thiamine was reportedly due to the lack of a national thiamine enrichment policy for grains and cereals at the time of the study, in the case of younger women, a normal thiamine intake was recorded for all participants at baseline.

In Children

In children, thiamine deficiency presents with acute symptoms and very rapid onset, and in the vast majority of cases, it affect infants who are breast-fed by thiamine-deficient mothers or with thiamine-deficient formulas.

A pivotal study that highlighted the crucial role of thiamine as an essential nutrient for infant development and discussed how TD phenotype may be confused or overlooked with other diseases was based on an epidemiological investigation on 24- to 39-month-old children presenting repeated vomiting, irritability, and lethargy, without major neurological abnormalities. All children who had consumed the same soy-based, thiamine-deficient formula (<0.5 mg/g formula) suffered from language and motor development deficits compared to sex- and age-matched children fed with other milk-based diets (123). Another study on the acute and long-term effects of thiamine-deficient formula-fed children who were not promptly diagnosed reported that a subset of patients (36%) died of cardiac and respiratory complications (124), and the remaining children developed intellectual disabilities, neurodevelopmental delay, and major motor dysfunction by the age of 9 (124). Recently, in another study by Harel et al. (125), more than 50% of a preschool children cohort, who were exposed to a thiamine-deficient diet for more than 1 month during the first 24 months of life, developed movement and motor skills difficulties compared to less than 10% among children with appropriate thiamine intake.

Infantile Thiamine Deficiency

Infantile thiamine deficiency (ITD) manifests after 2–3 weeks of thiamine deprivation with initially milder symptoms (refusal to eat, vomiting, and irritability), followed by rapid deterioration, with a high fatality rate (106). Newborns who are severely thiamine deprived may develop infantile beriberi. The disorder is rare in developed countries, as it can be readily treated with thiamine supplementation (126). However, it remains a concern in developing countries among infants breast-fed by thiamine-deficient mothers or fed with thiamine-deficient formula. Without proper thiamine supplementation, the deficiency is characterized by a rapid onset of symptoms involving vomiting, diarrhea, tachypnea, convulsions, ataxia, paralysis, cardiac dysfunction, and heart failure. In many cases, fatality occurs quickly (127). Those children who survive thiamine-deficiency-related WE [see the section Wernicke Encephalopathy and Vasconcelos et al. (128)] continue to live with developmental disabilities including severe epilepsy, language impairment, loss of motor function (to varying degrees), and mental retardation (mild to profound) (124).

In two separate case reports, one newborn (2 months old) with early infantile Leigh-like *SLC19A3* gene defect (129) and one (30 days old) with THTR2 deficiency (130) responded dramatically differently to thiamine supplementation. In the first case, the 2-month-old infant initially presenting with fever, feeding difficulties, and complex partial seizures (129) subsequently developed a severe encephalopathy. MRI showed abnormalities in both cerebral hemispheres as well as in brainstem and cerebellum, basal ganglia, and thalamus. A diffuse volume loss was also noted in both hemispheres. At the biochemical level, metabolic acidosis was diagnosed. Despite a prompt therapeutic regimen consisting of thiamine (37.5 mg/kg) and biotin (10 mg/kg) twice daily, the patient's conditions never improved and he died at 4 months of age. The lack of response to treatment in this instance seems to suggest that its effectiveness is completely halted in the presence of a null mutation leading to a complete loss of function of the thiamine transporter in the early-onset form [see Table 1 in Alfadhel (129)].

In the second case report, the infant showed acute mitochondrial encephalopathy, accompanied by increased level of lactate in the blood and cerebrospinal fluid as well as abnormal levels of α-ketoglutarate in the urine. Cortico-subcortical lesions were visualized by MRI, some of which seemed to have appeared in the perinatal period (130). Within 48 h after administration of thiamine (100 mg/day), biotin (10 mg/day), and carnitine (300 mg/day), a remarkable improvement was observed in both clinical and biochemical outcomes (130). After discontinuing biotin, the patient remained stable for 6 months on thiamine supplementation (20 mg/kg/day) (130).

It is now widely established that less severe cases of ITD can be treated (to varying degrees) with early thiamine supplementation. In general, therapeutic recommended doses are 10–25 mg/daily IV or IM for 2 weeks, or 10–50 mg/daily orally, followed by 5–10 mg/daily for 1 month (112).

Autism Spectrum Disorders

More recently, thiamine-based treatments have gained a great deal of attention as a therapeutic strategy for other developmental and neurological disorders linked to mitochondrial dysfunction. One such disorder is autism spectrum disorder (ASD), a group of complex neurological and developmental disabilities, with a prevalence of 1 in 54 and 1 in 252, respectively, for males and females age 8 years in the United States (131). "Spectrum" refers to the wide heterogeneity and range of symptoms within three characteristic patterns: atypical cognitive profile, executive dysfunction, and unusually restricted or repetitive behavior (131). Individuals with ASD show severe cognitive and verbal impairments and experience challenges in the development of critical social communication skills.

Limited findings are available on the link between thiamine bioavailability and the development of autism. However, studies show that the consumption of herbal supplements rich in thiaminase during pregnancy (132) or alcohol exposure *in utero* (133) may predispose a fetus to thiamine deficiency during pregnancy and increased risk for ASD. A study conducted on rat pups nursed by thiamine-deficient dams displayed comparable findings, in which the offspring exhibited behavioral abnormalities consistent with ASD symptoms (134).

A number of hypotheses have been put forward on the pathophysiological mechanisms linking thiamine deficiency and ASD (135), including i) increased apoptosis, due to the link of thiamine with p53 (136, 137), Bcl-2 (138, 139), and caspases (140); ii) deregulation of the serotoninergic system (141, 142); and iii) increased oxidative stress, due to the putative role of thiamine in prostaglandin expression, decreased lipid peroxidation as well as expression of nitric oxide synthase (143, 144), and its involvement as a cofactor for TKT in the PPP, master regulator of NADPH homeostasis.

More interestingly, a subset of children with ASD has been characterized by PDH deficiency and mitochondrial dysfunction (145, 146), suggesting that thiamine deficiency may also ensue in PDH deficits or that a borderline thiamine intake would compound the preexistent PDH deficit, precipitating energy metabolism and leading to ASD in genetically predisposed individuals. Furthermore, a more recent study has shown decreased TPP levels in plasma from ASD children compared to healthy controls (147), suggesting either lower consumption or an impaired absorption from the gastrointestinal tract, providing a link between thiamine metabolism and the gut microbiome, which has been considered in the context of ASD (148). While there is no evidence to suggest that a sole deficiency in thiamine may result in ASD, it could certainly be a contributing element in concert with other epigenetic factors in the presence of an already predisposed genetic background.

Based on the finding that children with ASD seem to have an impairment in the catabolism and excretion of thiol-containing heavy metals, Lonsdale et al. proposed that thiamine supplementation may be indicated for all children with ASD (149), with the idea that heavy metal toxicity can hamper TKT activity, increase oxidative stress, and, in turn, disrupt thiamine homeostasis. Hence, thiamine supplementation may, to some extent, improve carbohydrate metabolism, mitochondrial function, and brain energy production (150). In that study, children with ASD were administered a thiamine derivative, bi-daily for 2 months and noted improved communication skills, sociability, sensory/cognitive awareness, and behavior in 8 out of the 10 children studied as well as reduction in urine arsenic and mercury levels (149). In a separate, double-blind, placebo-controlled study, researchers noted decreased oxidative stress, increased ATP in plasma and NADH and NADPH production in red blood cells, and improved PGI-R (Parent Global Impressions—Revised) scores in hyperactivity, tantrum, and receptive language categories in autistic children administered vitamin/mineral supplementation, which included thiamine, over a 3-month period (151).

These pilot studies provide some support for a thiamine-based approach as a therapeutic intervention for ASD. However, further studies are warranted to clarify the role and specificity of thiamine supplementation for the management of the diverse and extensive range of ASD features.

Depression in Children and Child-Bearing Women

To our knowledge, to date, only one study has investigated the contribution of thiamine levels to pediatric depression (152). Surprisingly, and opposite to findings in adults, this study found a direct correlation between thiamine intake and depressive symptoms in Spanish schoolchildren (7–9 years old).

Although a fairly common condition among teenagers, little is known about depression and its treatment in children 12 years old and younger (153). Depression in children is often overlooked and oftentimes mistaken by teachers and parents and labeled as laziness, learning disabilities, or belligerence (154). Similarly, the "acting out" behavior observed in pediatric depression is often labeled as bullying, rebellion, or even psychotic behavior (154).

The effects of thiamine supplementation might be significant as palliative treatment in postpartum depression (PPD) and have a critical role on the infant's subsequent cognitive development. PPD has been associated with an increased risk of developing learning disabilities, Attention-Deficit/Hyperactivity Disorder (ADHD), and anxiety disorders in toddlers, which makes PPD a critical concern for both mother and infant (155). Nikseresht et al. investigated the therapeutic effects of Zn^{2+}, Mg^{2+}, and TPP supplementation in a PPD mouse model. Improvements in depressive symptoms and anxiety-like behaviors (tested by forced swimming test and elevated plus-maze), as well as total antioxidant capacity, were noted in the dams when the nutrients were administered on postpartum day 3 (156). Taken together, these findings indicate that thiamine supplementation may be a promising therapeutic strategy for PPD. However, future studies should address the role of thiamine in PPD independently and whether supplementation in instances of PPD positively impacts infant development.

CONCLUSIONS AND FUTURE PERSPECTIVES

Thiamine deficiency, regardless of the underlying mechanism (genetic or epigenetic), impairs critical TPP-dependent enzymes involved in intermediary metabolism and antioxidant defenses. The consequent decrease in ATP production and increased oxidative stress result in neurological deficits, which become especially detrimental during critical windows of neurodevelopment. In the recent years, thiamine supplementation has been contemplated, with some success, as a therapeutic approach for neurodevelopmental disorders, including ASD and major psychiatric disorders (i.e., depression). However, the vast heterogeneity of the pathogenic mechanisms underlying these conditions, along with the difficulty of diagnosis and the assumption that diets from developed countries supply enough thiamine to match the caloric intake (including perinatal periods), has not prompted enough research to address the role and effects of thiamine supplementation as a therapeutic strategy in the context of neurodevelopment/neurodegeneration. Of note, and an often overlooked issue, is the lack of incorporation of antioxidants into supplemental treatments that are deemed critical to minimize the thiamine-deficiency-dependent oxidative-stress-derived damage. This will also allow to shed light on the contribution of oxidative stress versus mitochondrial dysfunction to the morbidity of neurodegenerative disorders.

AUTHOR CONTRIBUTIONS

SD and MT equally contributed to the writing of the manuscript. EN contributed to writing and edited the text. CG conceptualized the paper, contributed to writing, and edited the text.

ACKNOWLEDGEMENTS

We would like to thank the technical assistance of Dr. E. Penna.

REFERENCES

1. Martin PR, Singleton CK, Hiller-Sturmhofel S. The role of thiamine deficiency in alcoholic brain disease. *Alcohol Res Health* (2003) 27:134–42.
2. Martel JL, Franklin DS. Vitamin B1 (thiamine). In: *StatPearls*. Treasure Island (FL), (2018).
3. Hiffler L, Rakotoambinina B, Lafferty N, Martinez Garcia D. Thiamine deficiency in tropical pediatrics: new insights into a neglected but vital metabolic challenge. *Front Nutr* (2016) 3:16. doi: 10.3389/fnut.2016.00016
4. Singleton CK, Martin PR. Molecular mechanisms of thiamine utilization. *Curr Mol Med* (2001) 1:197–207. doi: 10.2174/1566524013363870
5. Said HM, Nexo E. Chapter 64—Mechanisms and regulation of intestinal absorption of water-soluble vitamins: cellular and molecular aspects. In: Johnson LR, Ghishan FK, Kaunitz JD, Merchant JL, Said HM, Wood JD, editors. *Physiology of the gastrointestinal tract*, 5th ed. Boston: Academic Press (2012). p. 1711–56. doi: 10.1016/B978-0-12-382026-6.00064-6
6. Calhau C, Faria A, Keating E, Martel F. Chapter 39—Interaction of polyphenols with the intestinal and placental absorption of some nutrients and other compounds. In: Watson RR, Preedy VR, Zibadi S, editors. *Polyphenols in human health and disease*. San Diego: Academic Press (2014). p. 523–36. doi: 10.1016/B978-0-12-398456-2.00039-6
7. Lonsdale D. A review of the biochemistry, metabolism and clinical benefits of thiamin(e) and its derivatives. *Evid Based Complement Alternat Med* (2006) 3:49–59. doi: 10.1093/ecam/nek009
8. Lonsdale D, Marrs C. High-calorie malnutrition and its impact on health. In: Lonsdale D, Marrs C, editors. *Thiamine deficiency disease, dysautonomia, and high calorie malnutrition*. Cambridge, MA: Academic Press (2017). p. 213–61. doi: 10.1016/B978-0-12-810387-6.00006-X
9. Roust LR, DiBaise JK. Nutrient deficiencies prior to bariatric surgery. *Curr Opin Clin Nutr Metab Care* (2017) 20:138–44. doi: 10.1097/MCO.0000000000000352
10. Scrimshaw NS, Behar M. Malnutrition in underdeveloped countries. *N Engl J Med* (1965) 272:193–98 CONCL. doi: 10.1056/NEJM196501282720406
11. Whitfield KC, Smith G, Chamnan C, Karakochuk CD, Sophonneary P, Kuong K, et al. High prevalence of thiamine (vitamin B1) deficiency in early childhood among a nationally representative sample of Cambodian women of childbearing age and their children. *PLoS Negl Trop Dis* (2017) 11:e0005814. doi: 10.1371/journal.pntd.0005814
12. Fujita A. Thiaminase. *Adv Enzymol Relat Subj Biochem* (1954) 15:389–421.
13. Leichter J, Joslyn MA. Kinetics of thiamin cleavage by sulphite. *Biochem J* (1969) 113:611–15. doi: 10.1042/bj1130611
14. Hilker DM, Somogyi JC. Antithiamins of plant origin: their chemical nature and mode of action. *Ann N Y Acad Sci* (1982) 378:137–45. doi: 10.1111/j.1749-6632.1982.tb31192.x
15. Vimokesant S, Kunjara S, Rungruangsak K, Nakornchai S, Panijpan B. Beriberi caused by antithiamin factors in food and its prevention. *Ann N Y Acad Sci* (1982) 378:123–36. doi: 10.1111/j.1749-6632.1982.tb31191.x
16. Smidt LJ, Cremin FM, Grivetti LE, Clifford AJ. Influence of thiamin supplementation on the health and general well-being of an elderly Irish population with marginal thiamin deficiency. *J Gerontol* (1991) 46:M16–22. doi: 10.1093/geronj/46.1.M16
17. Thornalley PJ, Babaei-Jadidi R, Al Ali H, Rabbani N, Antonysunil A, Larkin J, et al. High prevalence of low plasma thiamine concentration in diabetes linked to a marker of vascular disease. *Diabetologia* (2007) 50:2164–70. doi: 10.1007/s00125-007-0771-4
18. Sequeira Lopes da Silva JT, Almaraz Velarde R, Olgado Ferrero F, Robles Marcos M, Perez Civantos D, Ramirez Moreno JM, et al. Wernicke's encephalopathy induced by total parental nutrition. *Nutr Hosp* (2010) 25:1034–36.
19. Junior EV, Cesar CL, Fisberg RM, Marchioni DM. Socio-economic variables influence the prevalence of inadequate nutrient intake in Brazilian adolescents: results from a population-based survey. *Public Health Nutr* (2011) 14:1533–8. doi: 10.1017/S1368980011000760
20. Renthal W, Marin-Valencia I, Evans PA. Thiamine deficiency secondary to anorexia nervosa: an uncommon cause of peripheral neuropathy and Wernicke encephalopathy in adolescence. *Pediatr Neurol* (2014) 51:100–3. doi: 10.1016/j.pediatrneurol.2014.03.025
21. Kerns JC, Arundel C, Chawla LS. Thiamin deficiency in people with obesity. *Adv Nutr* (2015) 6:147–53. doi: 10.3945/an.114.007526
22. Chandrakumar A, Bhardwaj A, t Jong GW. Review of thiamine deficiency disorders: Wernicke encephalopathy and Korsakoff psychosis. *J Basic Clin Physiol Pharmacol* (2018) 30:153–62. doi: 10.1515/jbcpp-2018-0075
23. Kamasak T, Kul S, Tusat M, Ozgun N, Cansu A. A case of Wernicke encephalopathy developing after ileal bypass surgery. *Pediatr Emerg Care* (2018) 34:e223–e225. doi: 10.1097/PEC.0000000000001472
24. Croft L, Napoli E, Hung CK, St Leger J, Gearhart S, Heym K, et al. Clinical evaluation and biochemical analyses of thiamine deficiency in Pacific harbor seals (*Phoca vitulina*) maintained at a zoological facility. *J Am Vet Med Assoc* (2013) 243:1179–89. doi: 10.2460/javma.243.8.1179
25. Chen L, Yee SW, Giacomini KM. OCT1 in hepatic steatosis and thiamine disposition. *Cell Cycle* (2015) 14:283–4. doi: 10.1080/15384101.2015.1006532
26. Vernau K, Napoli E, Wong S, Ross-Inta C, Cameron J, Bannasch D, et al. Thiamine deficiency-mediated brain mitochondrial pathology in Alaskan Huskies with mutation in SLC19A3.1. *Brain Pathol* (2015) 25:441–53. doi: 10.1111/bpa.12188
27. Butterworth RF. Thiamin deficiency and brain disorders. *Nutr Res Rev* (2003) 16:277–84. doi: 10.1079/NRR200367
28. Greenwood J, Love ER, Pratt OE. Kinetics of thiamine transport across the blood–brain barrier in the rat. *J Physiol* (1982) 327:95–103. doi: 10.1113/jphysiol.1982.sp014222
29. Rindi G, Comincioli V, Reggiani C, Patrini C. Nervous tissue thiamine metabolism *in vivo*. II. Thiamine and its phosphoesters dynamics in different brain regions and sciatic nerve of the rat. *Brain Res* (1984) 293:329–42. doi: 10.1016/0006-8993(84)91240-X

30. Butterworth RF, Giguere JF, Besnard AM. Activities of thiamine-dependent enzymes in two experimental models of thiamine-deficiency encephalopathy. 2. alpha-Ketoglutarate dehydrogenase. *Neurochem Res* (1986) 11:567–77. doi: 10.1007/BF00965326
31. Bettendorff L, Wins P, Lesourd M. Subcellular localization and compartmentation of thiamine derivatives in rat brain. *Biochim Biophys Acta* (1994) 1222:1–6. doi: 10.1016/0167-4889(94)90018-3
32. Bettendorff L, Mastrogiacomo F, Kish SJ, Grisar T. Thiamine, thiamine phosphates, and their metabolizing enzymes in human brain. *J Neurochem* (1996) 66:250–8. doi: 10.1046/j.1471-4159.1996.66010250.x
33. Rindi G, Laforenza U. Thiamine intestinal transport and related issues: recent aspects. *Proc Soc Exp Biol Med* (2000) 224:246–55. doi: 10.1046/j.1525-1373.2000.22428.x
34. Schaller K, Holler H. Thiamine absorption in the rat. II. Intestinal alkaline phosphatase activity and thiamine absorption from rat small intestine *in-vitro* and *in-vivo*. *Int J Vitam Nutr Res* (1975) 45:30–8.
35. Nabokina SM, Subramanian VS, Valle JE, Said HM. Adaptive regulation of human intestinal thiamine uptake by extracellular substrate level: a role for THTR-2 transcriptional regulation. *Am J Physiol Gastrointest Liver Physiol* (2013) 305:G593–599. doi: 10.1152/ajpgi.00237.2013
36. Laforenza U, Gastaldi G, Rindi G. Thiamine outflow from the enterocyte: a study using basolateral membrane vesicles from rat small intestine. *J Physiol* (1993) 468:401–12. doi: 10.1113/jphysiol.1993.sp019778
37. Talwar D, Davidson H, Cooney J, St JRD. Vitamin B(1) status assessed by direct measurement of thiamin pyrophosphate in erythrocytes or whole blood by HPLC: comparison with erythrocyte transketolase activation assay. *Clin Chem* (2000) 46:704–10.
38. Song P, Rekow SS, Singleton CA, Sekhon HS, Dissen GA, Zhou M, et al. Choline transporter-like protein 4 (CTL4) links to non-neuronal acetylcholine synthesis. *J Neurochem* (2013) 126:451–61. doi: 10.1111/jnc.12298
39. Ma Z, Xia W, Liu F, Ma J, Sun S, Zhang J, et al. SLC44A4 mutation causes autosomal dominant hereditary postlingual non-syndromic mid-frequency hearing loss. *Hum Mol Genet* (2017) 26:3234. doi: 10.1093/hmg/ddx232
40. Nabokina SM, Inoue K, Subramanian VS, Valle JE, Yuasa H, Said HM. Molecular identification and functional characterization of the human colonic thiamine pyrophosphate transporter. *J Biol Chem* (2017) 292:16526. doi: 10.1074/jbc.A113.528257
41. Fleming JC, Tartaglini E, Steinkamp MP, Schorderet DF, Cohen N, Neufeld EJ. The gene mutated in thiamine-responsive anaemia with diabetes and deafness (TRMA) encodes a functional thiamine transporter. *Nat Genet* (1999) 22:305–8. doi: 10.1038/10379
42. Subramanian VS, Marchant JS, Parker I, Said HM. Cell biology of the human thiamine transporter-1 (hTHTR1). Intracellular trafficking and membrane targeting mechanisms. *J Biol Chem* (2003) 278:3976–84. doi: 10.1074/jbc.M210717200
43. Subramanian VS, Marchant JS, Said HM. Targeting and trafficking of the human thiamine transporter-2 in epithelial cells. *J Biol Chem* (2006) 281:5233–45. doi: 10.1074/jbc.M512765200
44. Ganapathy V, Smith SB, Prasad PD. SLC19: the folate/thiamine transporter family. *Pflugers Arch* (2004) 447:641–6. doi: 10.1007/s00424-003-1068-1
45. Lu J, Frank EL. Rapid HPLC measurement of thiamine and its phosphate esters in whole blood. *Clin Chem* (2008) 54:901–6. doi: 10.1373/clinchem.2007.099077
46. Gangolf M, Czerniecki J, Radermecker M, Detry O, Nisolle M, Jouan C, et al. Thiamine status in humans and content of phosphorylated thiamine derivatives in biopsies and cultured cells. *PLoS One* (2010) 5:e13616. doi: 10.1371/journal.pone.0013616
47. Butterworth RF, Kril JJ, Harper CG. Thiamine-dependent enzyme changes in the brains of alcoholics: relationship to the Wernicke-Korsakoff syndrome. *Alcohol Clin Exp Res* (1993) 17:1084–88. doi: 10.1111/j.1530-0277.1993.tb05668.x
48. Zhao Y, Pan X, Zhao J, Wang Y, Peng Y, Zhong C. Decreased transketolase activity contributes to impaired hippocampal neurogenesis induced by thiamine deficiency. *J Neurochem* (2009) 111:537–46. doi: 10.1111/j.1471-4159.2009.06341.x
49. Fraccascia P, Casteels M, De Schryver E, Van Veldhoven PP. Role of thiamine pyrophosphate in oligomerisation, functioning and import of peroxisomal 2-hydroxyacyl-CoA lyase. *Biochim Biophys Acta* (2011) 1814:1226–33. doi: 10.1016/j.bbapap.2011.06.007
50. Fraccascia P, Sniekers M, Casteels M, Van Veldhoven PP. Presence of thiamine pyrophosphate in mammalian peroxisomes. *BMC Biochem* (2007) 8:10. doi: 10.1186/1471-2091-8-10
51. Foulon V, Antonenkov VD, Croes K, Waelkens E, Mannaerts GP, Van Veldhoven PP, et al. Purification, molecular cloning, and expression of 2-hydroxyphytanoyl-CoA lyase, a peroxisomal thiamine pyrophosphate-dependent enzyme that catalyzes the carbon-carbon bond cleavage during alpha-oxidation of 3-methyl-branched fatty acids. *Proc Natl Acad Sci U S A* (1999) 96:10039–44. doi: 10.1073/pnas.96.18.10039
52. Watkins PA, Howard AE, Mihalik SJ. Phytanic acid must be activated to phytanoyl-CoA prior to its alpha-oxidation in rat liver peroxisomes. *Biochim Biophys Acta* (1994) 1214:288–94. doi: 10.1016/0005-2760(94)90075-2
53. van den Brink DM, Wanders RJ. Phytanic acid: production from phytol, its breakdown and role in human disease. *Cell Mol Life Sci* (2006) 63:1752–65. doi: 10.1007/s00018-005-5463-y
54. Skjeldal OH, Stokke O, Refsum S, Norseth J, Petit H. Clinical and biochemical heterogeneity in conditions with phytanic acid accumulation. *J Neurol Sci* (1987) 77:87–96. doi: 10.1016/0022-510X(87)90209-7
55. Wierzbicki AS, Lloyd MD, Schofield CJ, Feher MD, Gibberd FB. Refsum's disease: a peroxisomal disorder affecting phytanic acid alpha-oxidation. *J Neurochem* (2002) 80:727–35. doi: 10.1046/j.0022-3042.2002.00766.x
56. Lindhurst MJ, Fiermonte G, Song S, Struys E, De Leonardis F, Schwartzberg PL, et al. Knockout of Slc25a19 causes mitochondrial thiamine pyrophosphate depletion, embryonic lethality, CNS malformations, and anemia. *Proc Natl Acad Sci U S A* (2006) 103:15927–32. doi: 10.1073/pnas.0607661103
57. Randle PJ, Garland PB, Hales CN, Newsholme EA. The glucose fatty-acid cycle. Its role in insulin sensitivity and the metabolic disturbances of diabetes mellitus. *Lancet* (1963) 1:785–89. doi: 10.1016/S0140-6736(63)91500-9
58. Muoio DM. Metabolic inflexibility: when mitochondrial indecision leads to metabolic gridlock. *Cell* (2014) 159:1253–62. doi: 10.1016/j.cell.2014.11.034
59. Jankowska-Kulawy A, Bielarczyk H, Pawelczyk T, Wroblewska M, Szutowicz A. Acetyl-CoA deficit in brain mitochondria in experimental thiamine deficiency encephalopathy. *Neurochem Int* (2010) 57:851–56. doi: 10.1016/j.neuint.2010.09.003
60. Brown GK, Brown RM, Scholem RD, Kirby DM, Dahl HH. The clinical and biochemical spectrum of human pyruvate dehydrogenase complex deficiency. *Ann N Y Acad Sci* (1989) 573:360–8. doi: 10.1111/j.1749-6632.1989.tb15011.x
61. De Meirleir L. Disorders of pyruvate metabolism. *Handb Clin Neurol* (2013) 113:1667–73. doi: 10.1016/B978-0-444-59565-2.00034-4
62. Gibson GE, Blass JP, Beal MF, Bunik V. The alpha-ketoglutarate-dehydrogenase complex: a mediator between mitochondria and oxidative stress in neurodegeneration. *Mol Neurobiol* (2005) 31:43–63. doi: 10.1385/MN:31:1-3:043
63. Shi Q, Karuppagounder SS, Xu H, Pechman D, Chen H, Gibson GE. Responses of the mitochondrial alpha-ketoglutarate dehydrogenase complex to thiamine deficiency may contribute to regional selective vulnerability. *Neurochem Int* (2007) 50:921–31. doi: 10.1016/j.neuint.2007.03.010
64. Sperringer JE, Addington A, Hutson SM. Branched-chain amino acids and brain metabolism. *Neurochem Res* (2017) 42:1697–709. doi: 10.1007/s11064-017-2261-5
65. Navarro D, Zwingmann C, Butterworth RF. Impaired oxidation of branched-chain amino acids in the medial thalamus of thiamine-deficient rats. *Metab Brain Dis* (2008) 23:445–55. doi: 10.1007/s11011-008-9105-6
66. Prohaska JR, Bailey WR. Persistent regional changes in brain copper, cuproenzymes and catecholamines following perinatal copper deficiency in mice. *J Nutr* (1993) 123:1226–34. doi: 10.1093/jn/123.7.1226
67. Kril JJ, Harper CG. Neuroanatomy and neuropathology associated with Korsakoff's syndrome. *Neuropsychol Rev* (2012) 22:72–80. doi: 10.1007/s11065-012-9195-0
68. Opdenakker G, Gelin G, De Surgeloose D, Palmers Y. Wernicke encephalopathy: MR findings in two patients. *Eur Radiol* (1999) 9:1620–4. doi: 10.1007/s003300050896

69. Kornreich L, Bron-Harlev E, Hoffmann C, Schwarz M, Konen O, Schoenfeld T, et al. Thiamine deficiency in infants: MR findings in the brain. *AJNR Am J Neuroradiol* (2005) 26:1668–74.
70. Vernau KM, Runstadler JA, Brown EA, Cameron JM, Huson HJ, Higgins RJ, et al. Genome-wide association analysis identifies a mutation in the thiamine transporter 2 (SLC19A3) gene associated with Alaskan Husky encephalopathy. *PLoS One* (2013) 8:e57195. doi: 10.1371/journal.pone.0057195
71. Robinson BH. Prenatal diagnosis of disorders of energy metabolism. *Semin Neurol* (2001) 21:269–73. doi: 10.1055/s-2001-17944
72. Mezzar S, De Schryver E, Asselberghs S, Meyhi E, Morvay PL, Baes M, et al. Phytol-induced pathology in 2-hydroxyacyl-CoA lyase (HACL1) deficient mice. Evidence for a second non-HACL1-related lyase. *Biochim Biophys Acta Mol Cell Biol Lipids* (2017) 1862:972–90. doi: 10.1016/j.bbalip.2017.06.004
73. Foulon V, Sniekers M, Huysmans E, Asselberghs S, Mahieu V, Mannaerts GP, et al. Breakdown of 2-hydroxylated straight chain fatty acids *via* peroxisomal 2-hydroxyphytanoyl-CoA lyase: a revised pathway for the alpha-oxidation of straight chain fatty acids. *J Biol Chem* (2005) 280:9802–12. doi: 10.1074/jbc.M413362200
74. Kitamura T, Seki N, Kihara A. Phytosphingosine degradation pathway includes fatty acid alpha-oxidation reactions in the endoplasmic reticulum. *Proc Natl Acad Sci U S A* (2017) 114:E2616–E2623. doi: 10.1073/pnas.1700138114
75. Khaw KT, Friesen MD, Riboli E, Luben R, Wareham N. Plasma phospholipid fatty acid concentration and incident coronary heart disease in men and women: the EPIC-Norfolk prospective study. *PLoS Med* (2012) 9. doi: 10.1371/journal.pmed.1001255
76. Forouhi NG, Koulman A, Sharp SJ, Imamura F, Kroger J, Schulze MB, et al. Differences in the prospective association between individual plasma phospholipid saturated fatty acids and incident type 2 diabetes: the EPIC-InterAct case-cohort study. *Lancet Diab Endocrin* (2014) 2:810–18. doi: 10.1016/S2213-8587(14)70146-9
77. Oishi K, Diaz GA. Thiamine-responsive megaloblastic anemia syndrome. In: Adam MP, Ardinger HH, Pagon RA, Wallace SE, Bean LJH, Stephens K, Amemiya A, editors. *GeneReviews((R))*. Seattle (WA): University of Washington, Seattle (1993).
78. Tabarki B, Al-Hashem A, Alfadhel M. Biotin-thiamine-responsive basal ganglia disease. In: Adam MP, Ardinger HH, Pagon RA, Wallace SE, Bean LJH, Stephens K, Amemiya A, editors. *GeneReviews((R))*. Seattle (WA): University of Washington, Seattle (1993). p. 1993–2019.
79. Alfadhel M, Almuntashri M, Jadah RH, Bashiri FA, Al Rifai MT, Al Shalaan H, et al. Biotin-responsive basal ganglia disease should be renamed biotin-thiamine-responsive basal ganglia disease: a retrospective review of the clinical, radiological and molecular findings of 18 new cases. *Orphanet J Rare Dis* (2013) 8:83. doi: 10.1186/1750-1172-8-83
80. Biesecker LG. Amish lethal microcephaly. In: Adam MP, Ardinger HH, Pagon RA, Wallace SE, Bean LJH, Stephens K, Amemiya A, editors. *GeneReviews((R))*. Seattle (WA): University of Washington, Seattle (1993).
81. Siu VM, Ratko S, Prasad AN, Prasad C, Rupar CA. Amish microcephaly: long-term survival and biochemical characterization. *Am J Med Genet A* (2010) 152A:1747–51. doi: 10.1002/ajmg.a.33373
82. Spiegel R, Shaag A, Edvardson S, Mandel H, Stepensky P, Shalev SA, et al. SLC25A19 mutation as a cause of neuropathy and bilateral striatal necrosis. *Ann Neurol* (2009) 66:419–24. doi: 10.1002/ana.21752
83. Mayr JA, Freisinger P, Schlachter K, Rolinski B, Zimmermann FA, Scheffner T, et al. Thiamine pyrophosphokinase deficiency in encephalopathic children with defects in the pyruvate oxidation pathway. *Am J Hum Genet* (2011) 89:806–12. doi: 10.1016/j.ajhg.2011.11.007
84. Banka S, de Goede C, Yue WW, Morris AA, von Bremen B, Chandler KE, et al. Expanding the clinical and molecular spectrum of thiamine pyrophosphokinase deficiency: a treatable neurological disorder caused by TPK1 mutations. *Mol Genet Metab* (2014) 113:301–6. doi: 10.1016/j.ymgme.2014.09.010
85. Alfadhel M, Babiker A. Inborn errors of metabolism associated with hyperglycaemic ketoacidosis and diabetes mellitus: narrative review. *Sudan J Paediatr* (2018) 18:10–23. doi: 10.24911/SJP.2018.1.3
86. Lorber A, Gazit AZ, Khoury A, Schwartz Y, Mandel H. Cardiac manifestations in thiamine-responsive megaloblastic anemia syndrome. *Pediatr Cardiol* (2003) 24:476–81. doi: 10.1007/s00246-002-0215-3
87. Ganie MA, Ali I, Ahangar AG, Wani MM, Ahmed S, Bhat MA, et al. Thiamine responsive megaloblastic anemia syndrome associated with patent ductus arteriosus: first case report from Kashmir Valley of the Indian subcontinent. *Indian J Endocrinol Metab* (2012) 16:646–50. doi: 10.4103/2230-8210.98033
88. Aljabri MF, Kamal NM, Arif M, AlQaedi AM, Santali EY. A case report of biotin-thiamine-responsive basal ganglia disease in a Saudi child: is extended genetic family study recommended? *Medicine (Baltimore)* (2016) 95:e4819. doi: 10.1097/MD.0000000000004819
89. Kelley RI, Robinson D, Puffenberger EG, Strauss KA, Morton DH. Amish lethal microcephaly: a new metabolic disorder with severe congenital microcephaly and 2-ketoglutaric aciduria. *Am J Med Genet* (2002) 112:318–26. doi: 10.1002/ajmg.10529
90. Fraser JL, Vanderver A, Yang S, Chang T, Cramp L, Vezina G, et al. Thiamine pyrophosphokinase deficiency causes a Leigh disease like phenotype in a sibling pair: identification through whole exome sequencing and management strategies. *Mol Genet Metab Rep* (2014) 1:66–70. doi: 10.1016/j.ymgmr.2013.12.007
91. Mahajan A, Sidiropoulos C. TPK1 mutation induced childhood onset idiopathic generalized dystonia: report of a rare mutation and effect of deep brain stimulation. *J Neurol Sci* (2017) 376:42–3. doi: 10.1016/j.jns.2017.02.063
92. Murata T. Influence of thiamine on the amount of lactic acid in urine. *J Vitaminol (Kyoto)* (1958) 4:109–13. doi: 10.5925/jnsv1954.4.109
93. Wendel OW. A study of urinary lactic acid levels in humans. I. Influence of thiamine and pyrithiamine. *J Vitaminol (Kyoto)* (1960) 6:16–23. doi: 10.5925/jnsv1954.6.16
94. Israels S, Haworth JC, Dunn HG, Applegarth DA. Lactic acidosis in childhood. *Adv Pediatr* (1976) 22:267–303.
95. Sweet RL, Zastre JA. HIF1-alpha-mediated gene expression induced by vitamin B1 deficiency. *Int J Vitam Nutr Res* (2013) 83:188–97. doi: 10.1024/0300-9831/a000159
96. Attwell D, Laughlin SB. An energy budget for signaling in the grey matter of the brain. *J Cereb Blood Flow Metab* (2001) 21:1133–45. doi: 10.1097/00004647-200110000-00001
97. Mergenthaler P, Lindauer U, Dienel GA, Meisel A. Sugar for the brain: the role of glucose in physiological and pathological brain function. *Trends Neurosci* (2013) 36:587–97. doi: 10.1016/j.tins.2013.07.001
98. Karabatsiakis A, Bock C, Salinas-Manrique J, Kolassa S, Calzia E, Dietrich DE, et al. Mitochondrial respiration in peripheral blood mononuclear cells correlates with depressive subsymptoms and severity of major depression. *Transl Psychiatry* (2014) 4:e397. doi: 10.1038/tp.2014.44
99. Prabakaran S, Swatton JE, Ryan MM, Huffaker SJ, Huang JT, Griffin JL, et al. Mitochondrial dysfunction in schizophrenia: evidence for compromised brain metabolism and oxidative stress. *Mol Psych* (2004) 9:684-97:643. doi: 10.1038/sj.mp.4001511
100. Liu H, Sang S, Lu Y, Wang Z, Yu X, Zhong C. Thiamine metabolism is critical for regulating correlated growth of dendrite arbors and neuronal somata. *Sci Rep* (2017) 7:5342. doi: 10.1038/s41598-017-05476-w
101. Gold M, Chen MF, Johnson K. Plasma and red blood cell thiamine deficiency in patients with dementia of the Alzheimer's type. *Arch Neurol* (1995) 52:1081–86. doi: 10.1001/archneur.1995.00540350075019
102. Whitfield KC, Bourassa MW, Adamolekun B, Bergeron G, Bettendorff L, Brown KH, et al. Thiamine deficiency disorders: diagnosis, prevalence, and a roadmap for global control programs. *Ann N Y Acad Sci* (2018) 1430:3–43. doi: 10.1111/nyas.13919
103. Molina JA, Jimenez-Jimenez FJ, Hernanz A, Fernandez-Vivancos E, Medina S, de Bustos F, et al. Cerebrospinal fluid levels of thiamine in patients with Alzheimer's disease. *J Neural Transm (Vienna)* (2002) 109:1035–44. doi: 10.1007/s007020200087
104. Ortigoza-Escobar JD, Molero-Luis M, Arias A, Oyarzabal A, Darin N, Serrano M, et al. Free-thiamine is a potential biomarker of thiamine transporter-2 deficiency: a treatable cause of Leigh syndrome. *Brain* (2016) 139:31–8. doi: 10.1093/brain/awv342
105. Magos L. Geigy scientific tables. In: Lentner C, editor. *Units of measurement. Body fluids. Composition of the body. Nutrition*, 8th ed. West Cadwell, N.J. (1987). p. 165–77.
106. Fattal-Valevski A. Thiamine (vitamin B1). *J Evidence-Based Compl Alt Med* (2011) 16:12–20. doi: 10.1177/1533210110392941

107. WHO. International nomenclature of diseases. In: *Metabolic, nutritional, and endocrine disorders*, (1991). p. 278.
108. Williams RR. The classical deficiency diseases. *Fed Proc* (1961) 20(Suppl 7):323–27.
109. Mulholland PJ. Susceptibility of the cerebellum to thiamine deficiency. *Cerebellum* (2006) 5:55–63. doi: 10.1080/14734220600551707
110. Nardone R, Holler Y, Storti M, Christova M, Tezzon F, Golaszewski S, et al. Thiamine deficiency induced neurochemical, neuroanatomical, and neuropsychological alterations: a reappraisal. *Sci World J* (2013) 2013:309143. doi: 10.1155/2013/309143
111. Inaba H, Kishimoto T, Oishi S, Nagata K, Hasegawa S, Watanabe T, et al. Vitamin B1-deficient mice show impairment of hippocampus-dependent memory formation and loss of hippocampal neurons and dendritic spines: potential microendophenotypes of Wernicke–Korsakoff syndrome. *Biosci Biotechnol Biochem* (2016) 80:2425–36. doi: 10.1080/09168451.2016.1224639
112. Stargrove MB, Treasure J, McKee DL. *Herb, nutrient, and drug interactions: clinical implications and therapeutic strategies*. St. Louis (MO): Mosby/Elsevier (2008). p. 255.
113. Thomson AD, Marshall EJ. The treatment of patients at risk of developing Wernicke's encephalopathy in the community. *Alcohol* (2006) 41:159–67. doi: 10.1093/alcalc/agh250
114. Galvin R, Brathen G, Ivashynka A, Hillbom M, Tanasescu R, Leone MA. EFNS guidelines for diagnosis, therapy and prevention of Wernicke encephalopathy. *Eur J Neurol* (2010) 17:1408–18. doi: 10.1111/j.1468-1331.2010.03153.x
115. Arts NJ, Walvoort SJ, Kessels RP. Korsakoff's syndrome: a critical review. *Neuropsychiatr Dis Treat* (2017) 13:2875–90. doi: 10.2147/NDT.S130078
116. Day GS, Del Campo CM. Wernicke encephalopathy: a medical emergency. *CMAJ* (2014) 186:E295. doi: 10.1503/cmaj.130091
117. Zuccoli G, Siddiqui N, Bailey A, Bartoletti SC. Neuroimaging findings in pediatric Wernicke encephalopathy: a review. *Neuroradiol* (2010) 52:523–29. doi: 10.1007/s00234-009-0604-x
118. Zhang G, Ding H, Chen H, Ye X, Li H, Lin X, et al. Thiamine nutritional status and depressive symptoms are inversely associated among older Chinese adults. *J Nutr* (2013) 143:53–8. doi: 10.3945/jn.112.167007
119. Carney MW, Williams DG, Sheffield BF. Thiamine and pyridoxine lack newly-admitted psychiatric patients. *Br J Psychiatry* (1979) 135:249–54. doi: 10.1192/bjp.135.3.249
120. Pepersack T, Garbusinski J, Robberecht J, Beyer I, Willems D, Fuss M. Clinical relevance of thiamine status amongst hospitalized elderly patients. *Gerontology* (1999) 45:96–101. doi: 10.1159/000022070
121. Ghaleiha A, Davari H, Jahangard L, Haghighi M, Ahmadpanah M, Seifrabie MA, et al. Adjuvant thiamine improved standard treatment in patients with major depressive disorder: results from a randomized, double-blind, and placebo-controlled clinical trial. *Eur Arch Psychiatry Clin Neurosci* (2016) 266:695–702. doi: 10.1007/s00406-016-0685-6
122. Benton D, Griffiths R, Haller J. Thiamine supplementation mood and cognitive functioning. *Psychopharmacology* (1997) 129:66–71. doi: 10.1007/s002130050163
123. Fattal-Valevski A, Azouri-Fattal I, Greenstein YJ, Guindy M, Blau A, Zelnik N. Delayed language development due to infantile thiamine deficiency. *Dev Med Child Neurol* (2009) 51:629–34. doi: 10.1111/j.1469-8749.2008.03161.x
124. Mimouni-Bloch A, Goldberg-Stern H, Strausberg R, Brezner A, Heyman E, Inbar D, et al. Thiamine deficiency in infancy: long-term follow-up. *Pediatr Neurol* (2014) 51:311–16. doi: 10.1016/j.pediatrneurol.2014.05.010
125. Harel Y, Zuk L, Guindy M, Nakar O, Lotan D, Fattal-Valevski A. The effect of subclinical infantile thiamine deficiency on motor function in preschool children. *Matern Child Nutr* (2017) 13. doi: 10.1111/mcn.12397
126. Luxemburger C, White NJ, ter Kuile F, Singh HM, Allier-Frachon I, Ohn M, et al. Beri-beri: the major cause of infant mortality in Karen refugees. *Trans R Soc Trop Med Hyg* (2003) 97:251–5. doi: 10.1016/S0035-9203(03)90134-9
127. Barennes H, Sengkhamyong K, Rene JP, Phimmasane M. Beriberi (thiamine deficiency) and high infant mortality in northern Laos. *PLoS Negl Trop Dis* (2015) 9:e0003581. doi: 10.1371/journal.pntd.0003581
128. Vasconcelos MM, Silva KP, Vidal G, Silva AF, Domingues RC, Berditchevsky CR. Early diagnosis of pediatric Wernicke's encephalopathy. *Pediatr Neurol* (1999) 20:289–94. doi: 10.1016/S0887-8994(98)00153-2
129. Alfadhel M. Early infantile Leigh-like SLC19A3 gene defects have a poor prognosis: report and review. *J Cent Nerv Syst Dis* (2017) 9:1179573517737521. doi: 10.1177/1179573517737521
130. Perez-Duenas B, Serrano M, Rebollo M, Muchart J, Gargallo E, Dupuits C, et al. Reversible lactic acidosis in a newborn with thiamine transporter-2 deficiency. *Pediatrics* (2013) 131:e1670–1675. doi: 10.1542/peds.2012-2988
131. Baio J, Wiggins L, Christensen DL, Maenner MJ, Daniels J, Warren Z, et al. Prevalence of autism spectrum disorder among children aged 8 years—autism and developmental disabilities monitoring network, 11 sites, United States, 2014. *MMWR Surveill Summ* (2018) 67:1–23. doi: 10.15585/mmwr.ss6706a1
132. Ortega Garcia JA, Angulo MG, Sobrino-Najul EJ, Soldin OP, Mira AP, Martinez-Salcedo E, et al. Prenatal exposure of a girl with autism spectrum disorder to 'horsetail' (*Equisetum arvense*) herbal remedy and alcohol: a case report. *J Med Case Rep* (2011) 5:129. doi: 10.1186/1752-1947-5-129
133. Aronson M, Hagberg B, Gillberg C. Attention deficits and autistic spectrum problems in children exposed to alcohol during gestation: a follow-up study. *Dev Med Child Neurol* (1997) 39:583–7. doi: 10.1111/j.1469-8749.1997.tb07493.x
134. Mahmood S, Dani HM, Mahmood A. Effect of dietary thiamin deficiency on intestinal functions in rats. *Am J Clin Nutr* (1984) 40:226–34. doi: 10.1093/ajcn/40.2.226
135. Lương KVQ, Nguyễn LTH. The role of thiamine in autism. *Am J Psych Neurosci* (2013) 1:22–37. doi: 10.11648/j.ajpn.20130102.11
136. McLure KG, Takagi M, Kastan MB. NAD+ modulates p53 DNA binding specificity and function. *Mol Cell Biol* (2004) 24:9958–67. doi: 10.1128/MCB.24.22.9958-9967.2004
137. Yang Z, Ge J, Yin W, Shen H, Liu H, Guo Y. The expression of p53, MDM2 and Ref1 gene in cultured retina neurons of SD rats treated with vitamin B1 and/or elevated pressure. *Yan Ke Xue Bao* (2004) 20:259–63.
138. Ishaque A, Al-Rubeai M. Role of vitamins in determining apoptosis and extent of suppression by bcl-2 during hybridoma cell culture. *Apoptosis* (2002) 7:231–9. doi: 10.1023/A:1015343616059
139. Rabie T, Muhlhofer W, Bruckner T, Schwab A, Bauer AT, Zimmermann M, et al. Transient protective effect of B-vitamins in experimental epilepsy in the mouse brain. *J Mol Neurosci* (2010) 41:74–9. doi: 10.1007/s12031-009-9286-4
140. Chornyy S, Parkhomenko J, Chorna N. Thiamine deficiency caused by thiamine antagonists triggers upregulation of apoptosis inducing factor gene expression and leads to caspase 3-mediated apoptosis in neuronally differentiated rat PC-12 cells. *Acta Biochim Pol* (2007) 54:315–22.
141. Plaitakis A, Nicklas WJ, Berl S. Thiamine deficiency: selective impairment of the cerebellar serotonergic system. *Neurology* (1978) 28:691–8. doi: 10.1212/WNL.28.7.691
142. Chugani DC, Muzik O, Rothermel R, Behen M, Chakraborty P, Mangner T, et al. Altered serotonin synthesis in the dentatothalamocortical pathway in autistic boys. *Ann Neurol* (1997) 42:666–9. doi: 10.1002/ana.410420420
143. Lukienko PI, Mel'nichenko NG, Zverinskii IV, Zabrodskaya SV. Antioxidant properties of thiamine. *Bull Exp Biol Med* (2000) 130:874–6. doi: 10.1007/BF02682257
144. Frustaci A, Neri M, Cesario A, Adams JB, Domenici E, Dalla Bernardina B, et al. Oxidative stress-related biomarkers in autism: systematic review and meta-analyses. *Free Radic Biol Med* (2012) 52:2128–41. doi: 10.1016/j.freeradbiomed.2012.03.011
145. Giulivi C, Zhang YF, Omanska-Klusek A, Ross-Inta C, Wong S, Hertz-Picciotto I, et al. Mitochondrial dysfunction in autism. *JAMA* (2010) 304:2389–96. doi: 10.1001/jama.2010.1706
146. Gu F, Chauhan V, Kaur K, Brown WT, LaFauci G, Wegiel J, et al. Alterations in mitochondrial DNA copy number and the activities of electron transport chain complexes and pyruvate dehydrogenase in the frontal cortex from subjects with autism. *Transl Psychiatry* (2013) 3:e299. doi: 10.1038/tp.2013.68
147. Anwar A, Marini M, Abruzzo PM, Bolotta A, Ghezzo A, Visconti P, et al. Quantitation of plasma thiamine, related metabolites and plasma protein oxidative damage markers in children with autism spectrum disorder and healthy controls. *Free Radic Res* (2016) 50:S85–S90. doi: 10.1080/10715762.2016.1239821

148. Mulle JG, Sharp WG, Cubells JF. The gut microbiome: a new frontier in autism research. *Curr Psychiatry Rep* (2013) 15:337. doi: 10.1007/s11920-012-0337-0
149. Lonsdale D, Shamberger RJ, Audhya T. Treatment of autism spectrum children with thiamine tetrahydrofurfuryl disulfide: a pilot study. *Neuro Endocrinol Lett* (2002) 23:303–8.
150. Obrenovich ME, Shamberger RJ, Lonsdale D. Altered heavy metals and transketolase found in autistic spectrum disorder. *Biol Trace Elem Res* (2011) 144:475–86. doi: 10.1007/s12011-011-9146-2
151. Adams JB, Audhya T, McDonough-Means S, Rubin RA, Quig D, Geis E, et al. Effect of a vitamin/mineral supplement on children and adults with autism. *BMC Pediatr* (2011) 11:111. doi: 10.1186/1471-2431-11-111
152. Rubio-Lopez N, Morales-Suarez-Varela M, Pico Y, Livianos-Aldana L, Llopis-Gonzalez A. Nutrient intake and depression symptoms in Spanish children: the ANIVA study. *Int J Environ Res Public Health* (2016) 13. doi: 10.3390/ijerph13030352
153. Cheung AH, Kozloff N, Sacks D. Pediatric depression: an evidence-based update on treatment interventions. *Curr Psychiatry Rep* (2013) 15:381. doi: 10.1007/s11920-013-0381-4
154. Colbert P, Newman B, Ney P, Young J. Learning disabilities as a symptom of depression in children. *J Learn Disabil* (1982) 15:333–6. doi: 10.1177/002221948201500605
155. Society CP. Maternal depression and child development. *Paediatr Child Health* (2004) 9:575–98. doi: 10.1093/pch/9.8.575
156. Nikseresht S, Etebary S, Karimian M, Nabavizadeh F, Zarrindast MR, Sadeghipour HR. Acute administration of Zn, Mg, and thiamine improves postpartum depression conditions in mice. *Arch Iran Med* (2012) 15:306–11. doi: 012155/AIM.0012

12

Review of Clinical Studies Targeting Inflammatory Pathways for Individuals with Autism

Sina Hafizi[1*†], *Dina Tabatabaei*[2†] *and Meng-Chuan Lai*[3,4,5]

[1] Department of Psychiatry, Rady Faculty of Health Sciences, Max Rady College of Medicine, University of Manitoba, Winnipeg, MB, Canada, [2] School of Medicine, Tehran University of Medical Sciences, Tehran, Iran, [3] Centre for Addiction and Mental Health and The Hospital for Sick Children, Department of Psychiatry, University of Toronto, Toronto, ON, Canada, [4] Autism Research Centre, Department of Psychiatry, University of Cambridge, Cambridge, United Kingdom, [5] Department of Psychiatry, National Taiwan University Hospital and College of Medicine, Taipei, Taiwan

***Correspondence:**
Sina Hafizi
sina.hafizi@gmail.com

†These authors have contributed equally to this work

Immune dysfunction and abnormal immune response may be associated with certain mechanisms underlying autism spectrum disorder (ASD). The early evidence for this link was based on the increased incidence of ASD in children with a history of maternal infection during pregnancy. Observational studies show increased prevalence of immune-related disorders—ranging from atopy, food allergy, viral infections, asthma, primary immunodeficiency, to autoimmune disorders—in individuals with ASD and their families. Evidence of neuroglial activation and focal brain inflammation in individuals with ASD implies that the central nervous system immunity may also be atypical in some individuals with ASD. Also, both peripheral and central inflammatory responses are suggested to be associated with ASD-related behavioral symptoms. Atypical immune responses may be evident in specific ASD subgroups, such as those with significant gastrointestinal symptoms. The present review aimed to evaluate current literature of potential interventions that target inflammatory pathways for individuals with ASD and to summarize whether these interventions were associated with improvement in autism symptoms and adaptation. We found that the current literature on the efficacy of anti-inflammatory interventions in ASD is still limited and large-scale randomized controlled trials are needed to provide robust evidence. We concluded that the role of immune-mediated mechanisms in the emergence of ASD or related challenges may be specific to subsets of individuals (e.g. those with concurrent immunological disorders, developmental regression, or high irritability). These subsets of individuals of ASD might be more likely to benefit from interventions that target immune-mediated mechanisms and with whom next-stage immune-mediated clinical trials could be conducted.

Keywords: autism, inflammation, neuroinflammation, autism spectrum disorder, immune system

INTRODUCTION

Autism spectrum disorder (ASD) is a neurodevelopmental condition characterized by early onset social-communication challenges, repetitive, stereotypical behaviors, and idiosyncratic sensory responsivity (1). Although several genetic and environmental factors have been linked to ASD, the underlying pathophysiology is still not well-understood (2). To date, although there have been great progress in developing behavioral and psychological support for individuals with ASD, no approved medication therapy exist for the core symptoms; established medication treatment aims at reducing concurrent challenges, such as increased irritability (3). Considering the heterogeneous nature of this condition and the paucity of biomarkers, development of a safe and effective "one-size-fits-all" medical therapy is challenging.

Several lines of evidence suggest a role of inflammation in the underlying developmental mechanisms of ASD (4–6). Epidemiological studies show an association between maternal infection [such as influenza (7) or cytomegalovirus (8)] during pregnancy and increased risk of offspring autism (9, 10). Also, family history of autoimmune diseases is associated with higher rate of ASD (11). In the animal models of ASD, offspring of animals with infection during pregnancy present physiological and behavioral alterations resemble ASD symptoms in human (12,13). People with ASD are suggested to have altered levels of inflammatory markers in which pro-inflammatory markers tend to increase while anti-inflammatory markers decrease (14, 15). Furthermore, postmortem studies of inflammation in the brain suggest alterations of brain immune response in ASD, including increased levels of proinflammatory markers (16) and increased microglial activation (17–19). Suzuki and colleagues showed increased microglial activation in the brain of individuals with ASD (20). Also, multiple studies on CSF and plasma/serum samples of individuals with ASD reported increased levels of proinflammatory markers (4, 21–23). Genetic studies reveal association between genomic variations in the immune-related genes and ASD (24). For example, human leucocyte antigen (HLA) DRB1 alleles are suggested to be associated with a higher risk of autism (25, 26). There is an emerging consensus that a better understanding of inflammation and its relation with the underlying pathophysiology of autism can provide new insight into the underlying mechanisms of the challenges faced by at least a subgroup of people with ASD (27), and help with developing new treatments. Given the current evidence, a growing body of literature has examined the role of medications with anti-inflammatory effects in the treatment of ASD-associated challenges, either alone or as an adjuvant therapy. In this narrative review, we aimed to summarize studies exploring the use of medications that target inflammatory pathways for people with ASD and evaluate the effectiveness and side effect profiles. Both medications with primary anti-inflammatory action (e.g. celecoxib) and those with additional anti-inflammatory properties beside their primary mechanisms of action (e.g. minocycline) have been included. These medications were selected based on the previous evidence indicating their anti-inflammatory properties in other psychiatric or medical disorders. Due to the availability of up-to-date meta-analysis on some of these agents, such as polyunsaturated fatty acids (28–31), they were not included in this review.

METHODS

This narrative review aimed to summarize the available evidence on the role of anti-inflammatory medications in the management of challenges associated with ASD. The literature search was performed using PubMed in July 2018. No publication date restriction was applied. We only included peer-reviewed studies on human subjects (with no age limitation) that were published in English language. The following search terms were used: (autism OR autistic OR autism spectrum disorder OR ASD OR pervasive OR pervasive developmental disorder OR pervasive developmental disorders OR Asperger OR Asperger's) AND (celecoxib OR minocycline OR NAC OR N-acetylcysteine OR ACTH OR prednisone OR prednisolone OR hydrocortisone OR methylprednisolone OR dexamethasone OR cortisone OR triamcinolone OR betamethasone OR flavonoid OR lenalidomide OR pentoxifylline OR pioglitazone OR IVIG OR spironolactone OR topiramate OR memantine OR amantadine OR galantamine OR riluzole OR palmitoylethanolamide). We also identified additional articles by reference list/hand searching.

STUDIES OF MEDICATIONS TARGETING INFLAMMATORY PATHWAYS IN PEOPLE WITH ASD (IN ALPHABETICAL ORDER)

Amantadine

Amantadine is an antiviral and anti-Parkinson medication that is widely used in the management of central nervous system disorders including multiple sclerosis (32) and traumatic brain injury (33). This medication is shown to be neuroprotective by the following mechanisms: (1) anti-inflammatory properties, mainly by inhibiting the release of proinflammatory factors (34, 35); (2) increasing the level of neurotrophic factors; and (3) inhibiting effect on N-methyl-D-aspartate (NMDA) receptors (34). In a placebo-controlled trial, King and colleagues studied the efficacy of amantadine in the management of ASD (36). They administered amantadine (n = 19) or placebo (n = 20) to individuals with ASD (age range of 5–19 years) over 4 weeks. The efficacy was measured using the Aberrant Behavior Checklist (ABC) and the Clinical Global Impression (CGI) scales. Amantadine group had slightly higher percentage of responders (equal or more than 25% reduction in irritability and/or hyperactivity according to parent-rated ABC). Based on the clinician-rated ABC, the amantadine group had significantly more improvement in absolute scores of hyperactivity and inappropriate speech. Also, amantadine group had higher improvement according to their CGI score. The side effects did not significantly differ between the amantadine and placebo groups.

Mohammadi and colleagues in a randomized controlled trial on children with severe behavioral issues (i.e. disruptive symptoms such as irritability) related to autism (age range of 4–12 years), compared risperidone plus amantadine (n = 20) with risperidone plus placebo (n = 19) over a 10-week period (37). They observed a significant improvement in hyperactivity and irritability as measured by ABC in the amantadine group as compared to placebo. Also, the amantadine group had significantly more improvement than the placebo group based on the CGI scores. Side effects were not significantly different between the groups.

Celecoxib

Celecoxib is a nonsteroidal anti-inflammatory drug that selectively inhibits cyclooxygenase-2 (COX-2) enzyme. It has been widely studied as an adjuvant therapy in several psychiatric disorders including schizophrenia and depression (38, 39). In a randomized and double-blind controlled trial, Asadabadi and colleagues investigated the effect of celecoxib as an adjuvant therapy to risperidone in the treatment of children (age range of 4–12 years) with ASD and severe behavioral issues over 10 weeks. They used ABC rating scale to assess the clinical symptoms (40) (**Table 1**). Autistic children under treatment with celecoxib as an adjuvant therapy (n = 20) had significantly improved scores in irritability, social withdrawal/lethargy, and stereotypic behavior compared to the placebo group (n = 20). The study groups did not differ in terms of inappropriate speech, hyperactivity/non-compliance, or medications side effects.

Corticosteroids and ACTH

Corticosteroids have been effectively used in the management of neurological disorders, such as Landau–Kleffner syndrome (LKS) (41). Due to similarities in the progression and development between LKS and *regressive* ASD, and considering the growing evidence on the link between inflammation and ASD, a number of studies have investigated the effects of corticosteroids or adrenocorticotrophic hormone (ACTH) in regressive ASD (42). In a series of trials, Buitelaar and colleagues studied the role of ORG 2766, an ACTH analog, in the management of children with ASD (43–45). In the first trial, they enrolled 14 children (age range of 5–13 years) with ASD in a double-blind crossover study (45). ORG 2766 was administered over a 4-week period. They reported significant improvement in clinical symptoms (i.e. irritability, stereotypic behaviors, hyperactivity, and excessive speech) as measured by the parent-reported ABC and playroom data. In the second crossover trial, they reported positive effects of ORG 2766 (administered over an 8-week period) on symptoms of 20 children (age range of 5–15 years) with ASD as measured by ABC and CGI (43). In their third study, they reported the effect of ORG 2766 on social interactions of autistic children enrolled in their first trial (44). They found that ORG 2766 therapy resulted in a significant increase in the quality and quantity of social interactions in the participants.

In a single-case study, Stefanatos and colleagues administered corticosteroid (i.e. prednisone) to a 6-year-old boy with regressive ASD over a 28-month period (46). The patient started losing his language abilities at age 22 months. The medical and neurological assessments were mostly unremarkable except for hypoperfusion of perisylvian cortical region in SPECT and abnormal steady-state auditory evoked potentials. Corticosteroid therapy resulted in significant improvement in language, social abilities, and stereotypic behaviors.

More recently, Shenoy and colleagues reported a case of regressive ASD that was diagnosed at the age of 18 months (47). He presented with progressive lymphadenopathy, microcytic anemia, mild thrombocytopenia, and low white blood cells count. He was started on corticosteroid at the age of 33 months. After about a month of steroid therapy, the patient started regaining his language and communication abilities. After 26 months of therapy, all the laboratory values returned back to normal.

Matarazzo described two cases of regressive ASD with histories of recurrent bacterial infections (48). Both individuals were initially started on corticosteroid therapy and later due to the side effects, were switched to ACTH. In both cases, corticosteroid therapy led to improvement in language and communication skills, as well as behavioral symptoms, such as stereotypic behaviors.

Mordekar and colleagues reported two cases of regressive ASD treated with corticosteroid (49). The first case was a 4.5-year-old boy with ASD and generalized tonic–clonic seizure that regained his personality and language abilities after treatment with corticosteroid. The second case was a 4-year-old girl with ASD who lost her language and communication abilities after experiencing neurological symptoms associated with ataxia and fluctuation of consciousness. Her symptoms started to improve after three weeks of treatment with prednisolone. Forty-eight months after treatment, she was back to her normal function and personality.

Most recently, a retrospective study (age range of participants, 3–5 years) compared 20 children with regressive ASD treated with corticosteroids (for a maximum period of 4 months) with 24 autistic children without corticosteroid treatment; the authors observed significant improvement in the frequency modulated auditory evoked response, language function, and ASD symptom score according to DSM-IV criteria after corticosteroid therapy (50).

Taken together, there is a lack of randomized controlled trials to inform the clinical utility of corticosteroid in individuals with ASD. Single case, case series, and observational studies indicate the potential of corticosteroid or ACTH as a treatment for *regressive* ASD, but this awaits rigorous controlled trials to validate and to investigate the potential underlying mechanisms of action.

Flavonoids

Flavonoids are a large group of nutrients found in vegetables and fruits. They are shown to have anti-inflammatory effects through inhibition of inflammatory pathways, including the synthesis/activity of c-reactive protein, proinflammatory cytokines, and microglia (51). Theoharides and colleagues studied the effects of a flavonoids mixture (luteolin, quercetin, and rutin) in an open-label case-series of 37 children (age range of 4–14 years) with ASD over a period of 4 months (52). They reported improvement in attention and eye contact (50%), allergy and gastrointestinal symptoms (75%), and social interaction (25%). No side effects due to the treatment were noted. More recently, using similar supplement, Taliou and colleagues in an open-label trial studied 40 children (age range of 4–10 years) with ASD over a 26-week period (53). They reported significant improvement in communication, daily living skills, and social skills as measured by the Vineland Adaptive Behavior Scales (VABS) and also in hyperactivity, irritability, lethargy, and stereotypical behavior as measured by the ABC. More recently, the same group using the same database reported that children with ASD that had the most

TABLE 1 | Summary of the studies on the role of anti-inflammatory medications in the management of ASD.

Drug	Participants	Type of study	Treatment	Outcomes	References	Benefit based on strength of evidence
Amantadine						
Amantadine	ASD (DSM-IV and ICD-10) N = 39 Age: 5–19 years	Double-Blind, Placebo-Controlled Trial Amantadine (n = 19), Placebo (n = 20)	Amantadine administered at 2.5 mg/kg/day for 1 week and then 5 mg/kg/day for 3 weeks.	Based on parent-rated ABC amantadine group had slightly higher (statistically non-significant) percentage of responders. However, based on the clinician-rated ABC, the amantadine group had significantly more improvement in absolute score of hyperactivity and inappropriate speech than placebo group. - Amantadine group had higher CGI score (not statistically significant) than placebo group.	King et al., 2001 (36)	Potential benefit
Amantadine plus risperidone	ASD (DSM-IV-R) and (6 or more DSM IV-TR symptoms) N = 39, Age: 4–12 years	Double-Blind, Placebo-Controlled Trial Risperidone plus Amantadine (n = 20) Risperidone plus placebo (n = 19)	Risperidone administered between 1 and 2.0 mg/day, Amantadine administered at 100 mg/d (if <30 kg) or 150 mg/d (if >30 kg), over 10 weeks	-Significant improvement in hyperactivity and irritability in the amantadine treated than the placebo group. - Significant improvement in the amantadine group on CGI	Mohammadi et al., 2013 (37)	
Celecoxib						
Celecoxib plus risperidone	Children with ASD ((DSM)-IV-TR) N = 40, Age: 4–12 years	Parallel-group, randomized, double-blind, placebo-controlled trial Risperidone plus Celecoxib (n = 20), Risperidone plus placebo (n = 20)	Celecoxib:100 mg/day to 200/300 mg/day Risperidone: 0.5 mg/day to 0.5 mg/week to 2–3 mg/day over 10 weeks	Significant improvement in: - Irritability -Lethargy/Social Withdrawal - Stereotypic Behavior as measured with ABC	Asadabadi et al., 2013 (40)	Potential benefit
Corticosteroids						
Chronic oral prednisolone treatment	A 6-year-old boy with autoimmune condition plus ASD	Case study	2 mg/kg/day for 10 weeks followed by 0.5 mg/kg every other day for 12 months 2 mg/kg of daily for 4 weeks, measured monthly by 0.5 mg/kg from weeks 4 through 12. Between weeks 12 to 28, alternate-day dosing was quantified in 0.25 mg/kg steps every 4 weeks.	Significantly improved: -Spontaneous speech, greater responsiveness to verbal communications (Token Test for Children), and improved social relatedness. -Receptive (Peabody Picture Vocabulary Test) and expressive Vocabulary -Visuomotor abilities and Performance IQ(WISC-R) -Decreased Stereotyped utterances (Diagnostic Checklist for Behavior-Disturbed Children)	Stefanatos et al., 1995 (46)	Unknown benefit
Low-dose steroid therapy	Autism with autoimmune lymphoproliferative syndrome (ALPS) Age: 18 months old	Case study	2 mg/kg/day for 10 weeks. the prednisolone dose was further reduced to 0.4 mg/kg every other day. Finally, the dose of 0.5 mg/kg every other day was the effective maintenance dose for treatment of the ASD and autoimmune condition	- Increased social interaction - Improvements in speech, gesturing, non-verbal communication, and language expression and comprehension subjective improvement, followed by objective improvement in speech and developmental milestones	Shenoy et al., 2000 (47)	

(Continued)

TABLE 1 | Continued

Drug	Participants	Type of study	Treatment	Outcomes	References	Benefit based on strength of evidence
Steroid	Children with regressive Autism Spectrum Disorder (R-ASD) based on (DSM-IV) Steroid-treated R-ASD (STAR) (N = 20) Not-treated ASD patients (NSA) (N = 25), Age: 3–5 years	Retrospective Study	Oral prednisolone administered at 2 mg/kg/day. Treatment group: 4 Hz frequency modulated evoked response (FMAER) derived from language cortex of the superior temporal gyrus (STG)	-Significant increase in the 4 Hz FMAER spectral response and a significant reduction in response distortion compared to STAR group relative to the NSA group. - Significant improvement in STAR group subjects' language ratings - Most STAR group children showed significant behavioral improvement after treatment. -STAR group language and behavior improvement were retained one year after treatment. - Groups did not differ in terms of minor EEG abnormalities. -Steroid treatment produced no lasting morbidity.	Duffy et al., 2014 (50)	
	Case 1: 4.5-year-old boy with Childhood disintegrative disorder (CDD) and generalized tonic clonic seizure Case 2: 4.5-year-old girl with CDD who was mildly encephalopathic	Case series	Case 1: Prednisolone (40 mg; 2 mg/kg/day for 2 weeks and then weaned by 5 mg a week over 8 weeks). Prednisolone (2 mg/kg for 2 weeks, tapered over 1 week	-Remained seizure free on Sodium Valproate (30 mg/kg/day) and at 2-year follow-up his behavior remained normal. -Normal academic school progress at 30 months follow-up. -Slow improvement with fewer periods of agitation in the next 3 weeks -Clear understanding of some verbal commands and developed a little speech. - No periods of agitation or ataxia,	Mordekar et al., 2009 (49)	
Adrenocorticotropic hormone (ACTH)						
ORG 2766	ASD (DSM-III) N = 14, Age: 5–13 years	Placebo-controlled double-blind cross-over trial	20 mg/day over 4 weeks period	Significant Improvement in irritability, stereotypic behaviors, hyperactivity, and excessive speech) as measured with ABC	Buitelaar et al., 1990 (45)	Potential benefit
ORG 2766	ASD N = 14 Age: 5–13 years	Double-blind, placebo-controlled cross-over trial	20 mg/day over 8 weeks period	- Significant Improvement in stereotypic behaviors - Social interaction-, play behavior, and stereotypy ($P < 0.05$ for each) compared with placebo (ABC and CGI); -Adverse effects were minimal	Buitelaar et al., 1992 (44)	
ORG 2766	ASD, N = 20 Age: 5–15 years	Controlled trial	40 mg/day for 8 weeks	-Significant improvement in the children's play behavior and a significant increase in the social interaction between child and experimenter. -Gaze coordination between child and experimenter —Parents' checklist ratings (ABC) as well as clinicians' ratings (CGI).	Buitelaar et al., 1992 (43)	

(Continued)

TABLE 1 | Continued

Drug	Participants	Type of study	Treatment	Outcomes	References	Benefit based on strength of evidence
ACTH	Case 1: 8-year-old boy with ASD Case 2: 2-year-old girl with ASD	Case studies	Case 1: prednisone l0 mg/day followed by ACTH 10 IU/day Case 2: 10 mg of prednisone plus ampicillin as prophylactic treatment daily for two months which was replaced by ACTH 10 IU i.m. daily	-He was attentive and had no more echolalia, or stereotypies, -He was able to communicate using simple phrases, and to perform simple tasks; to correctly use toys and was willing to play with other children -Improvement in pronouncing a few words, understanding demands, -Improved attentiveness, calmness, and less isolatedness.	Matarazzo et al., 2002 (48)	
Flavonoids						
	Children with ASD N = 37, Age: 4–14 years, 29 boys and 8 girls	Case studies	-luteolin (100 mg) + quercetin (70 mg) + Flavonoid (200 mg) –2 capsules/20 kg/weight, or at least 400 mg total flavonoid	-Significant improvement in bowel color, form and habits in 2–3 weeks (75%) -Significant reduction in Allergic-like symptoms in their skin -Significant improvement in eye contact, and attention to directions (50%) -Significant improvement in retained learned tasks and social interactions (30–50% of patients) -Significant improvement in speaking skills (10%)	Theoharides et al., 2012 (52)	Unknown benefit
	ASD children N = 40, Age: 4–10 years; 42 boys and 8 girls	Prospective, open-label trial Two age groups: 4–6 years (n = 25), 7–10 years (n = 25)	luteolin (100 mg/capsule, from chamomile) and quercetin (70 mg/ capsule), and the quercetin glycoside rutin (30 mg/capsule) for 26 weeks	-Significant improvement in adaptive functioning as measured by Vineland Adaptive Behavior Scale (VABS) age-equivalent scores in the communication domain, daily living skills, and the social domain -Significant improvement in overall behavior as demonstrated by the decline in ABC subscale scores. -Age had no significant effect on results	Taliou et al., 2013 (53)	
	10-year-old boy	Case study	Co-Ultramicronized Palmitoylethanolamide/ Luteolin: 700 mg + 70 mg for 1 year	-Significantly decrease both total and subgroup scores, in particular; sociability, demonstrating improved behavioral outcome, in particular sociability (as per ATEC) -Significantly reduced most indexes of hyperactivity, as shown by reduction in motor stereotypies -Improved cognition as reported by parents and teachers (e.g. understanding of simple commands and accomplishing them easily; -Improved eye contact and the child's behavior became more affectionate	Bertolino et al., 2017 (55)	

(Continued)

TABLE 1 | Continued

Drug	Participants	Type of study	Treatment	Outcomes	References	Benefit based on strength of evidence
Galantamine						
	Autism (DSM-IV-TR) Case 1: 21-year-old male Case 2: a 32-year-old male Case 3: 42-year-old male	Case series	Case 1: Initial dose of 4 mg each month to a maximum of 12 mg as an adjunct treatment to his asthma medications Case 2: 4 mg daily Galantamine followed by a trial of donepezil due to side effects Case 3: Initial does of 4 mg per day for a month to a maximum of 16 mg	Case 1: Improved speech and cognition: active speech sound production -Spontaneous articulation, proper to the context and complex verbalizations Case 2: -Improvements in verbalizations, which were restricted to one- or two appropriate word responses to the questions asked Case 3: -Slight improvement in spontaneous speech and drooling -Significant improvement in aggressive behavior within the first month of treatment.	Hertzman et al., 2003 (57)	Potential benefit
	Children with autism N = 13, Mean Age: 8.8 +/- 3.5 years	12- week Open-label trial		-Significant improvement in irritability and social withdrawal subscales of ABC -Significant progresses in inattention and emotional liability (Conners' Parent Rating Scale-R) -Improvement in the anger subscale of the Children's Psychiatric Rating Scale.	Nicolson et al., 2006 (58)	
	ASD (DSM IV-TR) N = 40, Age: 4–12 years	Parallel-group, placebo-controlled, and double-blind trial Risperidone plus galantamine (n = 20) Risperidone plus placebo (n = 20)	Galantamine administered up to 24 mg/day or placebo, plus Risperidone administered up to 2 mg/day, for 10 weeks	-Significant improvement in the Irritability and Lethargy/Social Withdrawal subscales in the galantamine treated patients than the placebo group as measured with ABC	Ghaleiha et al., 2014 (59)	
Intravenous immunoglobulin (IVIG)						
	ASD (DSM-III-R) and immunological abnormalities N = 10, Age: 3–12 years	Open-label Study	400 mg/kg/month for 6 months at 4 weeks intervals	-Improvements in speech (better articulation and improved vocabulary) -one child almost completely recovered speech -Improved social behavior, better eye contact, loss of echolalia, and response to commands. - Mild improvement on spontaneous meaningful speech	Gupta et al., 1996 (60)	Potential benefit in individual with concurrent immunological disorder
	ASD (DSM-IIIR) N = 10, -Age: 4–17 years	Open-label study	4 infusions of (154 to 375 mg/kg), every 6 weeks	Mild improvements in attention and hyperactivity (n = 4) -No improvements (n = 5) - Almost total amelioration of autistic symptoms (n = 1)	Piloplys et al., 1998 (61)	

(Continued)

TABLE 1 | Continued

Drug	Participants	Type of study	Treatment	Outcomes	References	Benefit based on strength of evidence
	ASD (DSM IV) N = 7 -Age: 3–6 years (6 male, 1 female),	Pilot Open Clinical Trial	400 mg/kg/month- for 6 months	Not beneficial for behaviors or severity	Delgiudice-Asch et al., 1999 (62)	
	Outpatient male children with autism (ICD-10), N = 12, Age: 4.2–14.9 years	Double-blind and placebo-controlled crossover study	0.4 g/kg at once	Significant improvement in Irritability, hyperactivity, Inadequate eye contact, and Inappropriate speech as measured with ABC	Niederhofer et al., 2003 (63)	
	ASD N = 26, Age: 3–17 years	Open retrospective study	400 mg/kg/month IVIG for 6 months	-Significant decrease in irritability, social withdrawal, stereotypy, hyper- activity, inappropriate speech as measured with ABC -Regressing to pre-IVIG level within 2 to 4 months of termination of IVIG (n = 22)	Boris et al., 2005 (64)	
	Children with ASD, N = 31	Open-label case series	Initiated with 2 g/kg monthly with 1 g/kg/day for 2 days monthly	Reports from parents: -Improvements in communication and/or language with fewer reporting -Improvements in aberrant behavior, repetitive behavior, and academics, social interactions, tics, motor function, and seizures -Significant Improvement in cognition and mannerisms on Social Responsiveness Scale, SRS) -Mild significant improvement in communication and motivation (SRS) -Significant improvement in irritability, lethargy/social withdrawal, hyperactivity, and inappropriate speech as measured with ABC	Connery et al., 2018 (65)	
Lenalidomide						
	ASD (DSM-IV-TR) N = 7, Age: 6–12 years	Open-label (Pilot Study)	2.5 mg/day for 12 weeks	-Significant improvement in socialization, expressive, and receptive language (CGI) -Significant decreased symptoms of autism based on the CARS scores in six children who completed the 6-week follow-up	Chez et al., 2007 (67)	Unknown benefit
Memantine						
	Children with ASD (DSM-IV-TR) N = 40, Age: 4–12 years	Double-blind, placebo-controlled study Risperidone plus Memantine (n = 20) Risperidone plus placebo (n = 20)	Risperidone was administered up to 3 mg/d and memantine was administered up to 20 mg/day Initiate Risperidone with dose of 0.5 mg with subsequent dose increase in 0.5 mg increments weekly Initiate Memantine with dose of 5 mg/day with subsequent dose increase in 5 mg increments weekly for 10 weeks	Significant improvement in irritability, stereotypic behavior, and hyperactivity as measured with ABC	Ghaleiha et al., 2013 (69)	Unknown benefit

(Continued)

TABLE 1 | Continued

Drug	Participants	Type of study	Treatment	Outcomes	References	Benefit based on strength of evidence
	Autistic disorder, or Asperger disorder ((DSM-IV-TR) plus Moderate to severe ASD based on Social Responsiveness Scale-Adult Research Version (SRS-A), and the clinician-rated CGI N = 18, Age: 18–50 years	12-week, open-label treatment trial	Initiated with a daily dose of 5 mg that was increased by 5 mg weekly up to a maximum daily dose of 20 mg twice daily. (average dose, 19.7 ± 1.2 mg/day; range, 15–20 mg)	-Significant improvement in the severity of core features of autism based on (SRS) and (CGI) -Significant improvement in impaired reading and nonverbal communication based on Diagnostic Analysis of Nonverbal Accuracy Scale test and in executive function per self-report (Behavior Rating Inventory of Executive Functioning–Adult Self-Report Global Executive) -Significant improvement in cognitive dysfunction in particular executive areas of emotional control, task initiation, cognitive flexibility, self-regulation, planning and organization, response inhibition, and working memory; -Significant improvement in global functioning -Significant improvement in anxiety and ADHD symptoms	Joshi et al., 2016 (70)	
	ASD ((DSM-IV-TR), Autism Diagnostic Observation Schedule (ADOS) and the Autism Diagnostic Interview-Revised (ADI-R) N = 121, Age: 6–12 years Study 2: ASD (DSM-IV-TR) N = 66 (completed the study) Age: 5–16 years	Study 1: 12- week, randomized, double-blind, placebo-controlled, parallel-group. Placebo (n = 61), Memantine (n = 60). Study 2: 48-week open-label extension trial (enrolled participants n = 102; n = 66, completed the study) Placebo/Memantine (n = 35), Memantine/Memantine (n = 31)	Memantine doses were administered based on bodyweight and ranged between 3 and 15 mg/day	Study 1: -No significant between-group difference on the efficacy outcome of caregiver/parent ratings based on the Social Responsiveness Scale (SRS), -A Significant improvement as compared to baseline at Week 12 in both groups Study 2: -A tendency for improvement at the end of the extension period (48 weeks). -No significant improvements in the active group - Significant worsening of one communication measure in memantine group relative to placebo after 12 weeks.	Aman et al., 2017 (71)	
Minocycline						
	ASD (Autism Diagnostic Interview - Revised (ADI-R)), DSM-IV, or the Autism Diagnostic Observation Schedule N = 10 Age: 3–12 years	Open-label trial	1.4 mg/kg over 6 months	No clinical improvement noticed	Pardo et al., 2013 (73)	Unknown benefit

(Continued)

TABLE 1 | Continued

Drug	Participants	Type of study	Treatment	Outcomes	References	Benefit based on strength of evidence
	ASD (DSM-IV-TR) N = 46	Randomized, double-blind placebo-controlled trial Risperidone plus minocycline (n = 23), Risperidone plus placebo (n = 23)	50 mg twice per day for 10 weeks plus Risperidone titrated up to 2 mg/day	-Significant improvement of irritability and hyperactivity/noncompliance	Ghaleiha et al., 2016 (74)	
N-acetylcysteine	Children with ASD (DSM-IV-TR), N = 29, Age: 3–12 years	Double-blind, randomized, placebo-controlled study NAC (n = 14) Placebo (n = 15)	Initiated with 900 mg/daily for 4 weeks, followed by 900 mg/twice daily for 4 weeks and then 900 mg/three times daily for 4 weeks	-Significant reduction in irritability in the treatment group as measured with ABC -Significant improvement on stereotypies as measured with RBS-R - Significant improvements in social cognition and autism mannerisms as measured with SRS	Hardan et al., 2012 (80)	Potential benefit
	8-year-old boy with ASD (DSM-IV)	Case study	800 mg per day over 6 weeks	- Significant reduction in his nail-biting behavior - Significant reduction in his autistic symptoms 1 month after the onset of treatment -Significant improvement in: social interaction (visual analog scale), verbal skills and communication (visual analog scale), aggressive behavior, hyperactivity and limited interests, and severity and frequency of his blinking tic (parents report)	Ghanizadeh et al., 2012 (78)	
	Children and adolescents with ASD (DSM-IV-TR), N = 40, Age: 3.5–16 years	Randomized double blind placebo controlled trial NAC plus Risperidone (n = 17) Placebo plus Risperidone (n = 14)	1200 mg/day NAC + Risperidone or placebo + Risperidone for 8 weeks	Significant improvement in irritability as measured with ABC	Ghanizadeh et al., 2013 (81)	
	4-year-old boy with self-injurious behavior	Case study	Initiated with 0.45 g/d and titrated up to 1.8 g/day over 3 weeks	Improvement in frequency and severity of self-injurious behavior	Marler et al., 2014 (77)	
	17 years old with ASD	Case study	Administered 20% acetylcysteine oral solution started at 600 mg twice daily as an add-on to Quetiapine therapy for six weeks. continued acetylcysteine with 900 mg twice a day plus Quetiapine 200 mg twice a day	Significantly improved tantrums, irritability, and aggressive behavior	Stutzman et al., 2015 (79)	
	Children with autism spectrum disorder (ASD) N = 40, Age: 4–12 years	A Randomized, Double-Blind, Placebo-Controlled Clinical Trial Risperidone plus NAC (n = 20) Risperidone plus placebo (n = 20)	Risperidone administered up to 1 and 2.0 mg/d, NAC dosage was 600 to 900 mg/day over 10 weeks	-Significant interaction of time and treatment on irritability, and hyperactivity/ Noncompliance subscales. -By the end of trial, the treatment group had more improvement in irritability and hyperactivity/ noncompliance subscales scores as measured with ABC	Nikoo et al., 2015 (82)	

(Continued)

TABLE 1 | Continued

Drug	Participants	Type of study	Treatment	Outcomes	References	Benefit based on strength of evidence
	Children with Asperger' s disorder, PDD NOS, ASD ((DSM-IV, (ADI-R))) N = 31, Age: 4–12 years	Randomized, double-blind, placebo-controlled trial NAC (n = 16), Placebo (n = 15)	Regular daily dose was 56.2 mg/kg over week 12, with dose varying between 33.6 - 64.3 mg/kg. Initiated with the dose of 300 mg/day for weights between 15 to 30 kg Initiated with the dose of 600 mg/day, > 30 kg	- No significant difference between the treatment and placebo groups on the CGI test	Wink et al., 2016 (83)	
	Children with ASD (DSM-IV-TR) N = 98, Age: 3–9 years	Placebo-controlled, randomized clinical trial NAC (n = 48) Placebo (n = 50)	500 mg/day orally administered over 6 months	-No significant differences between treatment and placebo-treated groups for, scores on the SRS, Children's Communication Checklist and the RBS -No significant difference found on the three global impression scales: DBC-P, CGI, and PGI-I	Dean et al., 2017 (84)	
Palmitoylethanolamide						
	Case 1: 13-year-old male with autism Case 2: 15-year-old male with autism	Case series	Case 1: Oral administration of 1/2 tablet (300 mg) twice daily, followed by (600 mg) tablet twice daily for a month Case 2: 600 mg tablet for 3 months	Case 1: -Improvement in his behavior and expressive language (parents and school teacher's reports) -Decrease in tantrums, outburst, self-talking, and stereotypies. -Improvement in skin eczema, nose-picking, asthmatic cough, and allergy stigmata Case 2: -Improvement in speech, sociability, sensory/cognitive, and overall behaviour -Improvement in aggression and cognitive and behavioral skills, and Language	Antonucci et al., 2015 (87)	Potential benefit
	Autistic children (DSM-V) N = 62, Age: 4–12 years	Randomized, parallel group, double-blind placebo-controlled trial Risperidone plus PEA (n = 31), Risperidone plus placebo group (n = 31)	Children in both groups received Risperidone equally with initial dose of 0.5 mg and stepwise 0.5-mg weekly increases for the first 3 weeks plus 600 mg PEA twice daily over 10 weeks	-Significant improvement on ABC irritability and hyperactivity/noncompliance, and inappropriate speech symptoms related to risperidone plus placebo group	Khalaj et al., 2018 (88)	
Pentoxifylline						
	Behavioral anomalies of biological basis or autism N = 36, Age: 3–15 years	Open-label study	150–600 mg/day over 1 month	-Remarkably effective in (N = 10) Fairly effective in (N = 8) Slightly effective in (N = 3) No effect (N = 2) -Improvement in sameness maintenance syndrome as well as in increasing the understanding of language and human relations and in their self-image to the extent (based on authors observations)	Sogame et al., 1978 (90)	Potential benefit
	ASD N = 30 Case reports: aged 12, 13, and 15 years	Open-label study	Not specified	-Marked improvement (n = 6) -Slight amelioration of symptoms (n = 14) -three out of six patients reported marked improvement	Nakane et al., 1980 (91)	
	Male autistics N = 20, Age: 3–22 years	Open-label study	200 mg/day for 3 months	–35% improvement in behavior and mental development	Shimoide et al., 1981 (92)	

(Continued)

TABLE 1 | Continued

Drug	Participants	Type of study	Treatment	Outcomes	References	Benefit based on strength of evidence
	Psychotic (N = 18) and autistic children (N = 2): a 5-year-old boy and a 7-year-old girl	Open-label study	Dose of 50 mg/day to 200 mg/day Over 4–10 months	-Significant improvement in pronunciation of syllables and words -Significant improvements in behavior and in language -Significant Increased in attention to others and speech -Improvement in pronunciation of syllables and words	Turek et al., 1981 (93)	
	ASD (based on DSM IV-TR) N = 40, Age: 4–12 years	Randomized double-blind, placebo-controlled Risperidone plus pentoxifylline (n = 20), risperidone plus placebo (n = 20)	Pentoxifylline: 200- 600 mg/day Risperidone: 0.5- 3 mg/day Over 10 weeks	Significant improvement in: -Irritability, social withdrawal, and stereotypic behavior -Hyperactivity and inappropriate speech As measured with ABC	Akhondzadeh et al., 2010 (94)	
Pioglitazone						
	ASD (DSM-IV) N = 25, Age: 3 –17 years	Open-label study	30 mg/day for individuals with age range of 3 to 5 years 60 mg/day for individuals with age range of 6–17 years -Over 4 months	-Significant decrease in hyperactivity, Irritability, lethargy, and stereotypy as measured with ABC	Boris et al., 2007 (98)	Potential benefit
	Outpatients with ASD N = 40, Age: 4–12 years	Randomized, double-blind, parallel-group, placebo-controlled trial Risperidone plus Pioglitazone (n = 20) Risperidone plus placebo (n = 20)	Risperidone: initial dose of 0.5 mg/day which was titrated in 0.5 mg increments every week over 10 weeks Pioglitazone: dose of 30 mg/day (15 mg two times daily) in one group	-Significant reduction in irritability, lethargy/social withdrawal and hyperactivity/non-compliance	Ghaleiha et al., 2015 (99)	
Riluzole						
	ASD (DSM-IV-TR), N = 40, Age: 5–12 years	Double-Blind, Placebo-Controlled, Randomized Trial Risperidone plus Riluzole (n = 20), Risperidone plus placebo (n = 20)	Riluzole administered up to 50 or 100 mg/day according to bodyweight. Risperidone administered up to 2 or 3 mg/day (according to bodyweight) for 10 weeks.	-Significant improvement in the irritability, lethargy/social withdrawal, stereotypic behavior, and hyperactivity/non-compliance subscale in Riluzole-treated patients - 11 individuals in Riluzole group and 5 individuals in the placebo group were categorized as responders according to their CGI scores	Ghaleiha et al., 2013 (110)	Potential benefit
Spironolactone						
	12-year-old boy with well-established autism, immune dysregulation, and food allergies	Case Report	2 mg/kg/day for 4 weeks	-Significant improvement in irritability, social withdrawal, stereotypy, hyperactivity, inappropriate speech as measured with ABC -Significant improvement in receptive language (as measured with Peabody Picture Vocabulary Test III)	Bradstreet et al., 2007 (103)	Unknown benefit
Topiramate						
	Autistic children (DSM IV), N = 40, Age: 3–12 years	Double-blind, placebo-controlled trial Risperidone plus Topiramate (n = 20) Risperidone plus placebo (n = 20)	Risperidone was administered up to 2 mg/d for children between 10 and 40 kg and 3 mg/day for >40 kg. Topiramate was administered up to 100 mg/day for individuals <30 kg and 200 mg/day for individuals >30 kg) over 8 weeks	Significant improvement on irritability, stereotypic behavior, and hyperactivity/non-compliance subscales as measured with ABC	Rezaei et al., 2010 (107)	Potential benefit

behavioral improvement were the ones that had reduction in the serum levels of IL-6 and TNF following treatment with luteolin (54). Most recently, Bertolino and colleagues reported a single case of a 10-year-old boy with regressive ASD and history of recurrent febrile seizure who underwent treatment with a flavonoid supplement (Palmitoylethanolamide/Luteolin) over a 12-month period (55). Treatment with the flavonoid supplement led to improvement in ASD symptoms as measured by ASD treatment evaluation checklist (ATEC) and a scale for stereotypic behavior and the frequency of enuresis. No side effects were reported.

Overall, there may be a potential for the use of flavonoid in the management of individuals with ASD that need to be further examined in robust clinical trials. Due to insufficient evidence, no clinical recommendations can be made so far with regard to the use of flavonoids.

Galantamine

Galantamine is an acetylcholinesterase inhibitor approved for the treatment of Alzheimer's disease. It also has anti-inflammatory properties by inhibiting the pro-inflammatory markers, such as TNF and cytokines (56). Hertzman studied the effect of galantamine on three adults with autism (57). The first patient was a 21-year-old male. Treatment with 4 mg of galantamine for a month led to improvement in verbal communication and the patient started making sound and responding. The second case was a 32-year-old male that after treatment with 4 mg of galantamine presented with improvement in verbalization; however, he experienced allergic reactions and the medication was discontinued. The third case was a 42-year-old male. He presented aggressive behaviors and never had verbal communication. Treatment with 4 mg of galantamine within a month led to reduction of aggressive behaviors. In a more recent study, Nicolson and colleagues studied galantamine effects in an open-label trial on 13 children (mean age, 8.8 ± 3.5 years) with autism over a 12-week period (58). Children presented significant improvement in irritability and social withdrawal as measured by ABC and emotional liability and attention as measured by Conners' parent-rating scale. Moreover, children presented improvement in aggression as measured by the children's psychiatric rating scale. Except for headache in one child, galantamine treatment was well tolerated. In the only randomized controlled trial available, Ghaleiha and colleagues compared risperidone plus galantamine (n = 20) with risperidone plus placebo (n = 20) over a 10-week period in children (age range of 4–12 years) with ASD (59). They observed a significant improvement in irritability and lethargy/social withdrawal subscales of ABC with galantamine as compared to placebo. The side effects were not significantly different between the groups. These initial findings indicate the potential to further evaluate the benefit and safety of galantamine for autistic individuals in robust clinical trials.

Intravenous Immunoglobulin

Several open-label trials have investigated intravenous immunoglobulin (IVIG) therapy in ASD, particularly those with concomitant immunological deficits. Gupta and colleagues administered IVIG to 10 children (age range of 3–6 years) with ASD and IgG deficiency and/or high levels of maternal rubella antibody at 4 weeks interval for a minimum period of 6 months (60). Behavior, cognition, and developmental characteristics of these children were evaluated using Peabody picture vocabulary test, the VBAS, skill evaluation, and preschool language test. Treatment with IVIG resulted in improvement in social behavior, eye contact, echolalia, response to commands, and speech.

Later, Plioplys and colleagues studied IVIG administration in 10 children (age range of 4–17 years) with ASD and immunologic abnormalities (61). The IVIG infusions were administered every 6 weeks. Six children received four infusions and one individual each received 1, 3, 5, and 6 infusions. While five individuals did not experience any changes in their symptoms, four children were reported by their parents to have mild improvement in attention and hyperactivity. One individual had a significant improvement in social behavior and language in a step-wise fashion after each infusion. However, the clinical improvement reversed 2 months after the last (6th) infusion, and he again presented with the same severe autistic symptoms as he presented before participating in the study.

DelGiudice-Asch and colleagues administered IVIG to seven children (age range of 3.5–6 years) with ASD without known immunological anomalies at monthly intervals over a 6-month period (62). Five children received the six infusions and finished the study. Overall there were no significant improvement in any of the clinical symptoms as measured by Ritvo-Freeman Real Life rating scale, the children Yale-Brown Obsessive-Compulsive Scale, CGI scale for autistic disorder, and the ASD modification of the NIMH global obsessive-compulsive scale.

In a double-blind, placebo-controlled crossover study, Niederhofer and colleagues studied the effects of a single dose of IVIG on clinical symptoms of 12 children (age range of 4.2–14.9 years) with ASD as measured by ABC (63). The participants were medication free and *had no immunological disorders*. They found a significant improvement in parent-reported irritability, hyperactivity, inadequate eye contact, and inappropriate speech as measured by ABC and drowsiness and decreased activity as measured by the symptom checklist. However, none of the clinician ratings showed significant differences between placebo and IVIG groups. No remarkable side effects were noted.

In an open-label study, Boris and colleagues administered IVIG to 26 children (age range of 3–17 years) with ASD (with history of developmental regression) at a monthly basis for 6 months (64). They observed a significant improvement in total aberrant score (37%), hyperactivity (39%), inappropriate speech (25%), irritability (42%), lethargy (35%), and stereotypic behavior (28%) on the ABC. Only a small number of the participants experienced side effects. However, most children's behavior returned to their pre-IVIG status within 2–4 months of discontinuing the IVIG.

In an open-label case-series study, Connery and colleagues administered IVIG to 31 children (mean age of 9 years and 9 months with standard deviation of 4 years and 5 months) with ASD and autoimmune encephalopathy on a monthly basis (65). Clinical outcomes were measured using ABC and the Social Responsiveness Scale (SRS) as completed by the caretakers. IVIG treatment resulted in significant improvement in cognition and mannerism sub-scales and the total score of SRS. Moreover, they reported a significant improvement in irritability, lethargy, hyperactivity, and speech sub-scores as well as the total score of ABC. The most common side effects were headache and vomiting, which were common but limited to the infusion period.

Taken together, current evidence suggests potential benefit of IVIG in children with ASD and concomitant immunological disorders, such as autoimmune encephalopathy; however, given the common side effects and the invasiveness of the intervention, IVIG treatment needs to be considered cautiously, weighing the risks and benefits. More robust clinical trials in large cohort are required to further establish the evidence. For children with ASD *without* known immunological deficits, current evidence is inconsistent and insufficient, and therefore, there is no clear rationale so far to recommend IVIG treatment for this subpopulation of ASD.

Lenalidomide

Lenalidomide, a derivative of thalidomide, is an immunomodulatory medication widely used in the treatment of hematologic disorders and malignancies (66). In an open-label study, Chez and colleagues administered lenalidomide to seven male children aged 6 to 12 years with ASD and history of developmental regression and elevated levels of TNF-alpha, for a 12-week period (67). They observed a significant improvement in ASD symptoms as measured by the Childhood Autism Rating Scale (CARS) and also in expressive language as measured by CGI. Moreover, although not significant, treatment with lenalidomide decreased the levels of TNF-alpha in both serum and CSF. However, it is important to note that among the seven children enrolled, two developed a rash and discontinued the study, and an additional one discontinued from the study after eight weeks due to transient drop of absolute neutrophil count to <1500.

Memantine

Memantine is an NMDA receptor blocker with suggested neuroprotective and anti-inflammatory effects (68). Ghaleiha and colleagues in a randomized controlled trial compared treatment with memantine plus risperidone (n = 20) with risperidone plus placebo (n = 20) in children (age range of 4–12 years) with ASD (69). They reported significant improvements in irritability, stereotypic behavior, and hyperactivity/non-compliance as measured by ABC in the memantine group compared to the placebo group. They did not find any significant difference in the side effects between groups. More recently, an open-label study evaluated the efficacy and tolerability of memantine on 18 adults (age range of 18–50 years) with autism over a 12-week period (70). Treatment with memantine was associated with significant improvement in autism severity as measured by the SRS, CGI, MGH ASD rating scale, and brief psychiatric rating scale as well as anxiety, ADHD symptoms, nonverbal communication (measured by Diagnostic Analysis of Nonverbal Accuracy Scale test) and in executive function (measured by the Behavioral Rating Inventory of Executive Functioning and Cambridge neuropsychological test automated battery). Treatment with memantine was not associated with any serious adverse event. Most recently, in the largest randomized controlled trials so far on the efficacy of memantine in children (age range of 6–12 years) with autism, Aman and colleagues compared treatment with memantine (n = 60) with placebo (n = 61) over a 12-week period (71). They did not observe any significant clinical improvement as measured by the SRS, although in the 48-week open-label follow up, a trend of improvement was observed. They reported two serious adverse events during the study that both were recognized to be unrelated to the treatment.

Taken together, the current evidence does not support a role for memantine in the treatment of core autism characteristics and associated challenges. It is notable that some large-scale randomized controlled trials are still ongoing (e.g. https://clinicaltrials.gov/ct2/show/NCT01972074).

Minocycline

Minocycline is a tetracycline-class antibiotic with anti-inflammatory effects (72). In an open-label trial, Pardo and colleagues investigated the effect of minocycline on clinical measures (as measured by CGI and VABS) and blood/cerebrospinal fluid (CSF) growth factors and markers of inflammation in autistic children (age range of 3–12 years) with history of regression (n = 10) over a 6-month period (73). While minocycline did not have a significant effect on core autism symptoms and adaptive functioning, it significantly reduced IL-8, an anti-inflammatory cytokine, and brain-derived neurotrophic factor (BDNF) in the CSF, and BDNF level (as normalized by alpha-2 macroglobulin level) in serum. In contrast to BDNF, hepatic growth factor (HGF) in the CSF significantly increased after treatment with minocycline.

In a randomized placebo-controlled trial, Ghaleiha and colleagues evaluated the effect of minocycline as an adjunctive therapy to risperidone in autistic children over a 10-week period (74). Minocycline significantly improved scores on irritability and hyperactivity/noncompliance on the ABC; however, it did not have any significant effect on lethargy/social withdrawal, stereotypic behavior, and inappropriate speech. The authors did not report any significant difference in side effects between groups. The observed difference in the effects of minocycline on clinical presentations of the participants in the above studies might be due to the difference in the administered dosage, 1.4 mg/kg/day in the Pardo et al. study (73) versus 100 mg/day in the Ghaleiha et al. study (74).

Taken together, there is still insufficient evidence to support the use of minocycline in the treatment of core autism symptoms or associated challenges.

N-Acetylcysteine

There is a growing interest in the potential use of N-acetylcysteine (NAC) in the treatment of psychiatric disorders (75). NAC acts as a precursor for glutathione, the most abundant antioxidant in the brain and is shown to have both anti-oxidant and anti-inflammatory properties in the body (76). Several case reports and trials have investigated the effect of NAC in individuals with ASD.

In a case study, Marler and colleagues administered NAC to a 4-year-old autistic child with self-injurious behavior over a 3-week period and observed improvement in frequency and severity of self-injurious behavior (77). In another case study, Ghanizadeh and Derakhshan examined NAC effects on clinical symptoms of an 8-year-old boy with ASD over a 6-week period (78). They observed significant improvement in social impairment, social interaction, nail-biting behavior, verbal skills and communication, tics, and aggression as measured with visual analog scale by the parents. Stutzman and Dophiede studied a 17-year-old boy with ASD and intellectual disability who was treated with NAC as an adjuvant therapy to quetiapine over 6 weeks (79). Treatment with NAC led to a reduction in irritability and aggressive behaviors.

Several small-scale clinical trials suggest a potentially positive role for NAC. Hardan and colleagues in a 12-week randomized controlled trial treated children (age range of 3.2–10.7 years) with ASD with NAC (n = 14) or placebo (n = 15) (80). They observed a significant improvement in irritability (as measured by the ABC) and a trend toward significance on stereotypic/repetitive behaviors (as measured by ABC and Repetitive Behavior Scale-Revised) in the NAC compared to the placebo group. Additionally, NAC significantly improved mannerism score (as measured by the SRS). Groups did not significantly differ in terms of medication side effects. In a more recent randomized controlled trial, Ghanizadeh and colleague observed a significant improvement in irritability score (as measured by ABC), but not the core autism symptoms, in children (age range of 3.5–16 years) with ASD treated with risperidone and NAC (n = 17) as compared to risperidone and placebo (n = 14) over an 8-week period (81). In this trial, the most commonly reported side effects were constipation, increased appetite, fatigue, nervousness, and daytime drowsiness. In a similar study, Nikoo and colleagues compared autistic children (age range of 4–12 years) under treatment with risperidone and NAC (n = 20) with those treated with risperidone and placebo (n = 20) over a 10-week period (82). They observed a significant improvement in irritability and hyperactivity/noncompliance as measured by the ABC. No significant differences in side effects were found between the groups. Wink and colleagues in a 12-week randomized controlled trial compared autistic children (age range of 4–12 years) on NAC (n = 16) versus placebo (n = 15) (6 patients were later excluded due to adverse effects or losing follow up) in terms of their social impairment as measured by CGI scale, and also oxidative stress markers in the blood (83). They did not find any significant difference between groups with regard to their CGI, ABC, SRS, or VABS-II scores. However, they observed a significant increase in the level of glutathione and a trend toward significance for increase in the level of oxidized glutathione (GSSG) in the NAC group.

Dean and colleagues in a randomized controlled trial compared treatment with NAC versus placebo in 98 children (age range of 3.1–9.9 years) with ASD (50 in the placebo group, 48 in the NAC group) (84) and observed no significant effect of NAC on their primary (i.e. SRS, RBS-R, and children's communication checklist (CCC-2)) or secondary (i.e. CGI or developmental behavior checklist) outcomes. There was no significant difference in the frequency or severity of adverse events between groups.

Overall, although initial small-scale clinical trials show the potential of NAC in reducing irritability in children with ASD (and possibly some aspects of autistic characteristics in the repetitiveness domain), follow-up larger-scale trials so far fail to show impact on ASD core characteristics. Considering the relatively safe side effect profile, NAC may have a positive role in the treatment of irritability in autistic children (85), but so far there is no evidence supporting its use in targeting ASD core symptoms.

Palmitoylethanolamide

Palmitoylethanolamide is a fatty acid amide with neuroprotective, anti-inflammatory, and anti-nociceptive properties that exert its effect through the peroxisome proliferator-activated receptors (PPAR)-dependent pathway (86). In a case report, Antonucci and colleagues studied efficacy of palmitoylethanolamide on two adolescents with autism. The first was a 13-year-old male with regressive autism and history of eczema and allergy. After treatment with palmitoylethanolamide (Normast®; initially 600 mg daily and then 1200 mg daily) for 1 month, they observed a significant improvement in the CARS-2 score, behavior (i.e. tantrums, stereotyped behaviors, self-talking, outbursts), language abilities, and allergic symptoms (87). The second child was a 15-year-old male with a history of epilepsy. Treatment with Normast for three months led to significant improvement in ATEC score, aggression, cognition, and behavioral skills as well as blood IgE levels. In a randomized controlled trial, Khalaj and colleagues compared risperidone plus palmitoylethanolamide versus risperidone plus placebo over a 10-week period in children (age range of 4–12 years) with ASD (88). Treatment with palmitoylethanolamide resulted in significant improvement in ABC irritability and hyperactivity/noncompliance compared to placebo. The groups did not differ with regard to the side effects.

Taken together, more randomized controlled trials are needed to evaluate the use of palmitoylethanolamide in the treatment of core autism characteristics or associated challenges, as current evidence is still too limited to support its clinical use.

Pentoxifylline

Pentoxifylline is a xanthine derivative which has an inhibitory effect on inflammatory responses in the body (e.g. by interfering with TNF-alpha effect) (89). In an early open-label trial, Sogame administered pentoxifylline to 36 children (age range of 3–15 years) with ASD or behavioral disorders with organic etiology (90). He observed improvement in maintenance of sameness, language, and relation with others in the majority of the participants. He observed side effects, such as nausea, vomiting, headache, and low blood pressure in a small number of the participants. Nakane reported results of an open-label study of pentoxifylline on 30 children with ASD (91). Children were also on haloperidol. The assessment was based on the parents' observation. While six children had significant improvement of symptoms, 14 children presented minor improvements. Shimoide administered pentoxifylline to 20 male individuals (age range of 3–22 years) with ASD over a 3-month period and observed improvement in at least two of their three assessments (i.e. patients' behavior in specific situations, mental developmental scale for young children, Seiken's critical list for autistic children) (92). Side effects were related to gastrointestinal symptoms. Turek studied the effects of pentoxifylline on 2 children (a 5-year-old boy and a 7-year-old girl) with ASD and 18 with psychosis (93). He observed significant improvement in syllables and words pronunciation of the autistic children. Observed side effects were limited to excitement and sleep disturbances. In the only randomized controlled trial, Akhondzadeh and colleagues compared treatment with risperidone plus pentoxifylline (n = 20) versus risperidone plus placebo (n = 20) (94). Treatment with pentoxifylline led to a significant improvement on ABC in irritability, lethargy/social withdrawal, stereotypic behavior, hyperactivity/noncompliance, and inappropriate speech. Side effects were not significantly different between groups.

Taken together, pentoxifylline may be a beneficial adjuvant therapy for ASD when combined with risperidone, but the evidence is still insufficient, and robust clinical trials are needed.

Pioglitazone

Pioglitazone is an antidiabetic medication of the thiazolidinedione class that is commonly used for reducing blood glucose in patients with type 2 diabetes mellitus. It exerts its effect mainly through the peroxisome proliferator-activated receptors (PPAR) pathway. Due to the anti-inflammatory properties of this medication, it is suggested to be potentially beneficial in the management of psychiatric disorders (95–97). In an open-label trial, Boris and colleagues administered pioglitazone to 25 children (age range of 3–17 years) with ASD over a 3- to 4-month period and observed a significant improvement in irritability, lethargy, stereotypy behaviors, and hyperactivity as measured by the ABC (98). Improvements in irritability, lethargy, and hyperactivity were significantly associated with age, suggesting younger participants may benefit more from pioglitazone than older children. No significant side effects were observed among the participants.

Most recently, a 10-week randomized controlled trial compared the efficacy of risperidone plus pioglitazone (n = 20) versus risperidone plus placebo (n = 20) (99). This study found a significant improvement in ABC irritability, lethargy/social withdrawal, and hyperactivity/non-compliance after treatment with pioglitazone as compared to placebo. There was no significant difference in the side effects (mostly vomiting and headache) between pioglitazone and placebo groups.

Collectively, initial findings suggest a potential beneficial role for pioglitazone in the management of ASD in children, yet robust clinical trials are needed to provide adequate evidence.

Riluzole

Riluzole is known as the only beneficial medication for increasing survival in patients with amyotrophic lateral sclerosis (ALS). It mainly exerts its effect by inhibiting presynaptic release of glutamate. It is also shown to have anti-inflammatory effects (100). In a randomized controlled trial, Ghaleiha and colleagues (110) compared risperidone plus riluzole (n = 20) versus risperidone plus placebo (n = 20) over a 10-week period in children (age range of 5–12 years) with ASD. They observed significant improvement in ABC irritability, lethargy/social withdrawal, stereotypic behavior, and hyperactivity/noncompliance. Regarding the side effects, the riluzole group had significantly higher increase in appetite and weight gain. It is noteworthy that a large phase 2 trial studying riluzole effects on 58 participants has been conducted recently (https://clinicaltrials.gov/ct2/show/NCT01661855).

Spironolactone

Spironolactone as an antagonist for aldosterone receptor has a primary use in the management of condition associated with elevated levels of aldosterone. It is shown to have anti-inflammatory properties, potentially due to its affinity for other steroid receptors (101, 102). In a single case report and hypothesis paper, Bradstreet and colleagues administered spironolactone to a 12-year-old child with ASD and elevated testosterone level, over a 4-week period and observed improvement in irritability (79%), lethargy (83%), stereotypic behavior (60%), hyperactivity (72%), and inappropriate speech (67%) as measured by the ABC (103). They also noted improvement in receptive language.

Topiramate

Topiramate is an anti-epilepsy medication which is known to have neuroprotective effects (104), exerting through anti-inflammatory and antioxidant effects (105, 106). In the only study in autistic individuals, Rezaei and colleagues compared risperidone plus topiramate (n = 20) with risperidone plus placebo (n = 20) over an 8-week period in children (age range of 3–12 years) with ASD and observed a significant improvement in ABC irritability, stereotypic behavior, and hyperactivity/noncompliance (107). The topiramate group had significantly higher number of somnolence and decreased appetite than the placebo group.

Although initial evidence implies a potentially positive adjuvant role for topiramate, more robust clinical trials are required to determine whether the benefits are consistent and outweigh the side effects.

CONCLUSIONS AND FUTURE DIRECTION

While pharmacological interventions are frequently used in the management of concomitant psychiatric and behavior challenges in individuals with ASD, they have limited effect on the core symptoms of ASD. Current evidence on the role of inflammation in the underlying mechanisms leading to autism, or more importantly, to specific subgroups/subtypes of autism (e.g. those with concurrent immunological disorders) (27), has fueled the research on the potential use of agents with anti-inflammatory effects in the management of this condition (108) [as in a recent example of the treatment for a subgroup of individuals with depression (109)]. The literature on anti-inflammatory medications in the management of ASD is still in its infancy, dominated by case reports and open-label studies, with only a small portion of double-blind randomized controlled trials (in which many acted as adjuvant agents combined with risperidone) for which the findings are often not replicated yet. Nevertheless, certain findings imply potential for future investigation with more robustly conducted trials, especially in ASD subgroups such as those with concurrent immunological disorders, developmental regression, or high irritability/behavioral challenges.

This literature implies potential benefits of the following medications for ASD children with severe behavioral challenges (alone or especially when acting as an adjuvant agent with risperidone): amantadine, celecoxib, galantamine, N-acetylcysteine, palmitoylethanolamide, pentoxifylline, pioglitazone, riluzole, and topiramate. A small number of case report and case-series studies suggests a potential role for corticosteroids and ACTH in the management of regressive autism. Flavonoids are suggested by a few open-label studies to be a safe medication to potentially improve behavioral symptoms such as irritability. IVIG might be beneficial in ASD individuals with concurrent immunological disorders. Lenalidomide appeared to be beneficial to ASD individuals with developmental regression and with elevated TNF-alpha. However, it is important to note that the current evidence for efficacy and safety of all these medications in individuals with ASD is still very preliminary and inconclusive. For clinical decision making, safety should be the primary concern. These medications should be considered only when 1) the medication is indicated for the co-occurring medical disorder (e.g. immunological disorders); or 2) standard treatments have been depleted or are insufficient, and the potential benefits are judged to outweigh potential harms [note: N-acetylcysteine has been recommended in the latest clinical care pathway for reducing irritability in autistic individuals (85)]. Current evidence on the role of anti-inflammatory agents in ASD should be interpreted considering the following limitations. First, across all medications reviewed here, there is a lack of rigorous randomized double-blind placebo-controlled trials and very few successful replications so far. The available literature is enriched with case reports and open-label studies. There are a few randomized controlled trials, but they are often of small sample sizes and are being tested in the context of an adjuvant agent (i.e., with risperidone). Therefore, based on the studies that evaluate anti-inflammatory medications as adjuvant therapy, it is unclear whether the effect of an anti-inflammatory medication comes from the medication (or the anti-inflammatory action) itself. Secondly, most clinical trials have focused on short-term effects (about 12 weeks) of the medications. It can be difficult to detect significant changes in a short period of time, and the evidence for long-term efficacy or safety is still lacking. Finally, for most of the medications reviewed here, the exact mechanisms of action (including the biological link between their anti-inflammatory mechanisms and behavior changes of the individual) are not clear, so the interpretation of the findings is challenging, especially when there are other potentially non-immune-mediated mechanisms of action that may contribute to the neurobiological basis of ASD (e.g. the glutamatergic system).

In conclusion, current evidence supporting the efficacy and safety of anti-inflammatory interventions in ASD is still limited. Robust large-scale clinical trials are much needed. Nevertheless, some findings imply that the role for immune-mediated mechanisms in the emergence of autism or autism-related challenges may be specific to a subset of people with autism (27, 111). It may be the case that the greatest potential of anti-inflammatory agents lies in this aspect, in the light of stratified psychiatry and precision medicine.

AUTHOR CONTRIBUTIONS

SH, DT, and MC-L designed the study, ran the literature review, prepared the manuscript, and approved the final manuscript.

REFERENCES

1. Takumi T, Tamada K, Hatanaka F, Nakai N, Bolton PF. Behavioral neuroscience of autism. *Neurosci Biobehav Rev* (2019). doi: 10.1016/j.neubiorev.2019.04.012
2. Zecavati N, Spence SJ. Neurometabolic disorders and dysfunction in autism spectrum disorders. *Curr Neurol Neurosci Rep* (2009) 9(2):129–36. doi: 10.1007/s11910-009-0021-x
3. Anagnostou E. Clinical trials in autism spectrum disorder: evidence, challenges and future directions. *Curr Opin Neurol* (2018) 31(2):119–25. doi: 10.1097/WCO.0000000000000542
4. Zimmerman AW. et al. Cerebrospinal fluid and serum markers of inflammation in autism. *Pediatr Neurol* (2005) 33(3):195–201. doi: 10.1016/j.pediatrneurol.2005.03.014
5. Rossignol DA, Frye RE. A review of research trends in physiological abnormalities in autism spectrum disorders: immune dysregulation, inflammation, oxidative stress, mitochondrial dysfunction and environmental toxicant exposures. *Mol Psychiatry* (2012) 17(4):389–401. doi: 10.1038/mp.2011.165
6. Estes ML, McAllister AK. Maternal immune activation: implications for neuropsychiatric disorders. *Science* (2016) 353(6301):772–7. doi: 10.1126/science.aag3194
7. Atladóttir HÓ, Henriksen TB, Schendel DE, Parner ET. Autism after infection, febrile episodes, and antibiotic use during pregnancy: an exploratory study. *Pediatrics* (2012) 130: (6):e1447. doi: 10.1542/peds.2012-1107
8. Slawinski BL, Talge N, Ingersoll B, Smith A, Glazier A, Kerver J, et al. Maternal cytomegalovirus sero-positivity and autism symptoms in children. *Am J Reprod Immunol* (2018) 79(5):e12840. doi: 10.1111/aji.12840
9. Jiang HY, Xu LL, Shao L, Xia RM, Yu ZH, Ling ZX, et al. Maternal infection during pregnancy and risk of autism spectrum disorders: a systematic review and meta-analysis. *Brain Behav Immun* (2016) 58:165–72. doi: 10.1016/j.bbi.2016.06.005
10. Lombardo MV, Moon HM, Su J, Palmer TD, Courchesne E, Pramparo T. Maternal immune activation dysregulation of the fetal brain transcriptome and relevance to the pathophysiology of autism spectrum disorder. *Mol Psychiatry* (2018) 23(4):1001–13. doi: 10.1038/mp.2017.15
11. Atladóttir HO, Pedersen MG, Thorsen P, Mortensen PB, Deleuran B, Eaton WW, et al. Association of family history of autoimmune diseases and autism spectrum disorders. *Pediatr* (2009) 124(2):687–94. doi: 10.1542/peds.2008-2445
12. Meyer U. Prenatal poly(i:C) exposure and other developmental immune activation models in rodent systems. *Biol Psychiatry* (2014) 75(4):307–15. doi: 10.1016/j.biopsych.2013.07.011
13. Jones KL, Pride MC, Edmiston E, Yang M, Silverman JL, Crawley JN, et al. Autism-specific maternal autoantibodies produce behavioral abnormalities in an endogenous antigen-driven mouse model of autism. *Mol Psychiatry* (2018) 1. doi: 10.1038/s41380-018-0126-1
14. Patterson PH. Maternal infection and immune involvement in autism. *Trends Mol Med* (2011) 17(7):389–94. doi: 10.1016/j.molmed.2011.03.001

15. Masi A, Quintana DS, Glozier N, Lloyd AR, Hickie IB, Guastella AJ. Cytokine aberrations in autism spectrum disorder: a systematic review and meta-analysis. *Mol Psychiatry* (2015) 20(4):440–6. doi: 10.1038/mp.2014.59
16. Li X, Chauhan A, Sheikh AM, Patil S, Chauhan V, Li XM, et al. Elevated immune response in the brain of autistic patients. *J Neuroimmunol* (2009) 207(1-2):111–6. doi: 10.1016/j.jneuroim.2008.12.002
17. Morgan JT, Chana G, Pardo CA, Achim C, Semendeferi K, Buckwalter J, et al. Microglial activation and increased microglial density observed in the dorsolateral prefrontal cortex in autism. *Biol Psychiatry* (2010) 68(4):368–76. doi: 10.1016/j.biopsych.2010.05.024
18. Edmonson C, Ziats MN, Rennert OM. Altered glial marker expression in autistic post-mortem prefrontal cortex and cerebellum. *Mol Autism* (2014) 5(1):3. doi: 10.1186/2040-2392-5-3
19. Young AM, Chakrabarti B, Roberts D, Lai MC, Suckling J, Baron-Cohen S. From molecules to neural morphology: understanding neuroinflammation in autism spectrum condition. *Mol Autism* (2016) 7(1):9. doi: 10.1186/s13229-016-0068-x
20. Suzuki K, Sugihara G, Ouchi Y, Nakamura K, Futatsubashi M, Takebayashi K, et al. Microglial activation in young adults with autism spectrum disorder. *JAMA Psychiatry* (2013)70(1):49–58. doi: 10.1001/jamapsychiatry.2013.272
21. Chez MG, Dowling T, Patel PB, Khanna P, Kominsky M. Elevation of tumor necrosis factor-alpha in cerebrospinal fluid of autistic children. *Pediatr Neurol* (2007) 36(6):361–5. doi: 10.1016/j.pediatrneurol.2007.01.012
22. Suzuki K, Matsuzaki H, Iwata K, Kameno Y, Shimmura C, Kawai S, et al. Plasma cytokine profiles in subjects with high-functioning autism spectrum disorders. *PloS One* (2011) 6(5):e20470. doi: 10.1371/journal.pone.0020470
23. Ashwood P, Krakowiak P, Hertz-Picciotto I, Hansen R, Pessah I, Van de Water J. Elevated plasma cytokines in autism spectrum disorders provide evidence of immune dysfunction and are associated with impaired behavioral outcome. *Brain Behav Immun* (2011) 25(1):40–5. doi: 10.1016/j.bbi.2010.08.003
24. Michel M, Schmidt MJ, Mirnics K. Immune system gene dysregulation in autism and schizophrenia. *Dev Neurobiol* (2012) 72(10):1277–87. doi: 10.1002/dneu.22044
25. Chien YL, Wu YY, Chen CH, Gau SS, Huang YS, Chien WH, et al. Association of HLA-DRB1 alleles and neuropsychological function in autism. *Psychiatr Genet* (2012) 22(1):46–9. doi: 10.1097/YPG.0b013e32834915ae
26. Mostafa GA, Shehab AA, Al-Ayadhi LY. The link between some alleles on human leukocyte antigen system and autism in children. *J Neuroimmunol* (2013) 255: (1-2):70–4. doi: 10.1016/j.jneuroim.2012.10.002
27. Thom RP, Keary CJ, Palumbo ML, Ravichandran CT, Mullett JE, Hazen EP, et al. Beyond the brain: a multi-system inflammatory subtype of autism spectrum disorder. *Psychopharmacol (Berl)* (2019) 236:1–17. doi: 10.1007/s00213-019-05280-6
28. Cheng Y-S, Tseng P-T, Chen Y-W, Stubbs B, Yang W-C, Chen T-Y, et al. Supplementation of omega 3 fatty acids may improve hyperactivity, lethargy, and stereotypy in children with autism spectrum disorders: a meta-analysis of randomized controlled trials. *Neuropsychiatr Dis Treat* (2017)13:2531. doi: 10.2147/NDT.S147305
29. Rahimloua M, Rayyanib E, Hosseinia SA, Husaina D. An updated systematic review of the effects of n-3 long-chain polyunsaturated fatty acids on Autistic Spectrum Disorder. *J Nutr Sci Diet*(2018) 4(1):15–19.
30. Agostoni C, Nobile M, Ciappolino V, Delvecchio G, Tesei A, Turolo S, et al. The Role of Omega-3 Fatty Acids in Developmental Psychopathology: a Systematic Review on Early Psychosis, Autism, and ADHD. *Int J Mol Sci* (2017) 18(12):2608. doi: 10.3390/ijms18122608
31. Horvath A, Łukasik J, Szajewska H. ω-3 fatty acid supplementation does not affect autism spectrum disorder in children: a systematic review and meta-analysis-3. *J Nutr* (2017) 147(3):367–76. doi: 10.3945/jn.116.242354
32. Krupp LB, Coyle PK, Doscher C, Miller A, Cross AH, Jandorf L, et al. Fatigue therapy in multiple sclerosis: results of a double-blind, randomized, parallel trial of amantadine, pemoline, and placebo. *Neurology* (1995) 45(11):1956–61. doi: 10.1212/WNL.45.11.1956
33. Giacino JT, Whyte J, Bagiella E, Kalmar K, Childs N, Khademi A, et al. Placebo-controlled trial of amantadine for severe traumatic brain injury. *N Engl J Med* (2012) 366(9):819–26. doi: 10.1056/NEJMoa1102609
34. Ossola B, Schendzielorz N, Chen S-H, Bird GS, Tuominen RK, Männistö PT, et al. Amantadine protects dopamine neurons by a dual action: reducing activation of microglia and inducing expression of GNDF in astroglia. *Neuropharmacol* (2011)61(4):574–82. doi: 10.1016/j.neuropharm.2011.04.030
35. Kubera M, Maes M, Budziszewska B, Basta-Kaim A, Leskiewicz M, Grygier B, et al. Inhibitory effects of amantadine on the production of pro-inflammatory cytokines by stimulated in vitro human blood. *Pharmacol Rep* (2009) 61(6):1105–12. doi: 10.1016/S1734-1140(09)70173-2
36. King BH, Wright DM, Handen BL, Sikich L, Zimmerman AW, McMahon W, et al. Double-blind, placebo-controlled study of amantadine hydrochloride in the treatment of children with autistic disorder. *J Am Acad Child Adolesc Psychiatry* (2001) 40(6):658–65. doi: 10.1097/00004583-200106000-00010
37. Mohammadi MR, Yadegari N, Hassanzadeh E, Farokhnia M, Yekehtaz H, Mirshafiee O, et al. Double-blind, placebo-controlled trial of risperidone plus amantadine in children with autism: a 10-week randomized study. *Clin Neuropharmacol* (2013) 36(6):179–84. doi: 10.1097/WNF.0b013e3182a9339d
38. Müller N, Schwarz MJ, Dehning S, Douhe A, Cerovecki A, Goldstein-Müller B, et al. The cyclooxygenase-2 inhibitor celecoxib has therapeutic effects in major depression: results of a double-blind, randomized, placebo controlled, add-on pilot study to reboxetine. *Mol Psychiatry* (2006) 11:(7):680. doi: 10.1038/sj.mp.4001805
39. Muller N, Riedel M, Scheppach C, Brandstatter B, Sokullu S, Krampe K, et al. Beneficial antipsychotic effects of celecoxib add-on therapy compared to risperidone alone in schizophrenia. *Am J Psychiatry* (2002)159(6):1029–34. doi: 10.1176/appi.ajp.159.6.1029
40. Asadabadi M, Mohammadi M-R, Ghanizadeh A, Modabbernia A, Ashrafi M, Hassanzadeh E, et al. Celecoxib as adjunctive treatment to risperidone in children with autistic disorder: a randomized, double-blind, placebo-controlled trial. *Psychopharmacol* (2013) 225 (1):51–9. doi: 10.1007/s00213-012-2796-8
41. Sinclair DB, Snyder TJ. Corticosteroids for the treatment of Landau-Kleffner syndrome and continuous spike-wave discharge during sleep. *Pediatr Neurol* (2005) 32(5):300–6. doi: 10.1016/j.pediatrneurol.2004.12.006
42. Golla S, Sweeney JA. Corticosteroid therapy in regressive autism: Preliminary findings from a retrospective study. *BMC Med* (2014) 12(1):79. doi: 10.1186/1741-7015-12-79
43. Buitelaar JK, van Engeland H, de Kogel K, de Vries H, van Hooff J, van Ree J. The adrenocorticotrophic hormone (4–9) analog ORG 2766 benefits autistic children: report on a second controlled clinical trial. *J Am Acad Child Adolesc Psychiatry* (1992) 31(6):1149–56. doi: 10.1097/00004583-199211000-00026
44. Buitelaar JK, van Engeland H, de Kogel KH, de Vries H, van Hooff JA, van Ree JM. The use of adrenocorticotrophic hormone (4–9) analog ORG 2766 in autistic children: effects on the organization of behavior. *Biol Psychiatry* (1992) 31(11):1119–29. doi: 10.1016/0006-3223(92)90156-T
45. Buitelaar JK, van Engeland H, van Ree JM, de Wied D. Behavioral effects of Org 2766, a synthetic analog of the adrenocorticotrophic hormone (4–9), in 14 outpatient autistic children. *J Autism Dev Disord* (1990) 20(4):467–78. doi: 10.1007/BF02216053
46. Stefanatos GA, Grover W, Geller E. Case study: corticosteroid treatment of language regression in pervasive developmental disorder. *J Am Acad Child Adolesc Psychiatry* (1995) 34(8):1107–11. doi: 10.1097/00004583-199508000-00022
47. Shenoy S, Arnold S, Chatila T. Response to steroid therapy in autism secondary to autoimmune lymphoproliferative syndrome. *J Pediatr* (2000) 136(5):682–7. doi: 10.1067/mpd.2000.105355
48. Matarazzo EB. Treatment of late onset autism as a consequence of probable autommune processes related to chronic bacterial infection. *World J Biol Psychiatry* (2002) 3(3):162–6. doi: 10.3109/15622970209150618
49. Mordekar SR, Prendergast M, Chattopadhyay AK, Baxter PS. Corticosteroid treatment of behaviour, language and motor regression in childhood disintegrative disorder. *Eur J Paediatr Neurol* (2009) 13(4):367–9. doi: 10.1016/j.ejpn.2008.06.001
50. Duffy FH, Shankardass A, McAnulty GB, Eksioglu YZ, Coulter D, Rotenberg A, et al. Corticosteroid therapy in regressive autism: a retrospective study of effects on the Frequency Modulated Auditory Evoked Response (FMAER), language, and behavior. *BMC Neurol* (2014) 14(1):70. doi: 10.1186/1471-2377-14-70
51. Serafini M, Peluso I, Raguzzini A. Flavonoids as anti-inflammatory agents. *Proc Nutr Soc* (2010) 69(3):273–8. doi: 10.1017/S002966511000162X

52. Theoharides T, Asadi S, Panagiotidou S. *A case series of a luteolin formulation (NeuroProtek®) in children with autism spectrum disorders*. London, England: SAGE Publications Sage UK (2012). doi: 10.1177/039463201202500201
53. Taliou A, Zintzaras E, Lykouras L, Francis K. An open-label pilot study of a formulation containing the anti-inflammatory flavonoid luteolin and its effects on behavior in children with autism spectrum disorders. *Clin Ther* (2013) 35(5):592–602. doi: 10.1016/j.clinthera.2013.04.006
54. Tsilioni I, Taliou A, Francis K, Theoharides TC. Children with autism spectrum disorders, who improved with a luteolin-containing dietary formulation, show reduced serum levels of TNF and IL-6. *Trans Psychiatry* (2015) 5(9):e647. doi: 10.1038/tp.2015.142
55. Bertolino B, Crupi R, Impellizzeri D, Bruschetta G, Cordaro M, Siracusa R, et al. Beneficial effects of co-ultramicronized Palmitoylethanolamide/Luteolin in a mouse model of autism and in a Case Report of Autism. *CNS Neurosci Ther* (2017) 23(1):87–98. doi: 10.1111/cns.12648
56. Pavlov VA, Parrish WR, Rosas-Ballina M, Ochani M, Puerta M, Ochani K, et al. Brain acetylcholinesterase activity controls systemic cytokine levels through the cholinergic anti-inflammatory pathway. *Brain Behav Immun* (2009) 23(1):41–5. doi: 10.1016/j.bbi.2008.06.011
57. Hertzman M.Galantamine in the treatment of adult autism: a report of three clinical cases. *Int J Psychiatry Med* (2003) 33(4):395–8. doi: 10.2190/JE5Q-1NFT-FL40-7PMW
58. Nicolson R, Craven-Thuss B, Smith J. A prospective, open-label trial of galantamine in autistic disorder. *J Child Adolesc Psychopharmacol* (2006) 16(5):621–9. doi: 10.1089/cap.2006.16.621
59. Ghaleiha A, Ghyasvand M, Mohammadi M-R, Farokhnia M, Yadegari N, Tabrizi M, et al. Galantamine efficacy and tolerability as an augmentative therapy in autistic children: a randomized, double-blind, placebo-controlled trial. *J Psychopharmacol* (2014) 28(7):677–85. doi: 10.1177/0269881113508830
60. Gupta S, Aggarwal S, Heads C. Brief report: dysregulated immune system in children with autism: beneficial effects of intravenous immune globulin on autistic characteristics. *J Autism Dev Disord* (1996) 26(4):439–52. doi: 10.1007/BF02172828
61. Plioplys AV. Intravenous immunoglobulin treatment of children with autism. *J Child Neurol* (1998) 13(2):79–82. doi: 10.1177/088307389801300207
62. DelGiudice-Asch G, Simon L, Schmeidler J, Cunningham-Rundles C, Hollander E. Brief report: a pilot open clinical trial of intravenous immunoglobulin in childhood autism.*J Autism Dev Disord* (1999) 29(2):157–60. doi: 10.1023/A:1023096728131
63. Niederhofer H, Staffen W, Mair AJN. Immunoglobulins as an alternative strategy of psychopharmacological treatment of children with autistic disorder. *Neuropsychopharmacol* (2003) 28(5):1014. doi: 10.1038/sj.npp.1300130
64. Boris M, Goldblatt A, Edelson SM. Improvement in children with autism treated with intravenous gamma globulin. *J Nutr Environ Med* (2005) 15(4):169–76. doi: 10.1080/13590840600681827
65. Connery K, Tippett M, Delhey LM, Rose S, Slattery JC, Kahler SG, et al. Intravenous immunoglobulin for the treatment of autoimmune encephalopathy in children with autism. *Transl Psychiatry* (2018) 8(1):148. doi: 10.1038/s41398-018-0214-7
66. List A, Kurtin S, Roe DJ, Buresh A, Mahadevan D, Fuchs D, et al. Efficacy of lenalidomide in myelodysplastic syndromes. *N Engl J Med* (2005) 352(6):549–57. doi: 10.1056/NEJMoa041668
67. Chez M, Low R, Parise C, Donnel T. Safety and observations in a pilot study of lenalidomide for treatment in autism. *Autism Res Treat* (2012) 2012:291601. doi: 10.1155/2012/291601
68. Wu HM, Tzeng NS, Qian L, Wei SJ, Hu X, Chen SH, et al. Novel neuroprotective mechanisms of memantine: increase in neurotrophic factor release from astroglia and anti-inflammation by preventing microglial activation. *Neuropsychopharmacol* (2009) 34(10):2344–57. doi: 10.1038/npp.2009.64
69. Ghaleiha A, Asadabadi M, Mohammadi M-R, Shahei M, Tabrizi M, Hajiaghaee R, et al. Memantine as adjunctive treatment to risperidone in children with autistic disorder: a randomized, double-blind, placebo-controlled trial. *Int J Neuropsychopharmacol* (2013) 16(4):783–9. doi: 10.1017/S1461145712000880
70. Joshi G, Wozniak J, Faraone SV, Fried R, Chan J, Furtak S, et al. A Prospective open-label trial of memantine hydrochloride for the treatment of social deficits in intellectually capable adults with autism spectrum disorder. *J Clin Psychopharmacol* (2016) 36(3):262–71. doi: 10.1097/JCP.0000000000000499
71. Aman MG, Findling RL, Hardan AY, Hendren RL, Melmed RD, Kehinde-Nelson O, et al. Safety and efficacy of memantine in children with autism: randomized, placebo-controlled study and open-label extension. *J Child Adolesc Psychopharmacol* (2017) 27(5):403–12. doi: 10.1089/cap.2015.0146
72. Garrido-Mesa N, Zarzuelo A, Galvez J. Minocycline: far beyond an antibiotic. *Br J Pharmacol* (2013) 169(2):337–52. doi: 10.1111/bph.12139
73. Pardo CA, Buckley A, Thurm A, Lee LC, Azhagiri A, Neville DM, et al. A pilot open-label trial of minocycline in patients with autism and regressive features. *J Neurodev Disord* (2013) 5(1):9. doi: 10.1186/1866-1955-5-9
74. Ghaleiha A, Alikhani R, Kazemi M-R, Mohammadi M-R, Mohammadinejad P, Zeinoddini A, et al. Minocycline as adjunctive treatment to risperidone in children with autistic disorder: A randomized, double-blind placebo-controlled trial. *J Child Adolesc Psychopharmacol* (2016) 26(9):784–91. doi: 10.1089/cap.2015.0175
75. Minarini A, Ferrari S, Galletti M, Giambalvo N, Perrone D, Rioli G, et al. N-acetylcysteine in the treatment of psychiatric disorders: current status and future prospects. *Expert Opin Drug Metab Toxicol* (2017) 13(3):279–92. doi: 10.1080/17425255.2017.1251580
76. Sommer IE, van Westrhenen R, Begemann MJ, de Witte LD, Leucht S, Kahn RS. Efficacy of anti-inflammatory agents to improve symptoms in patients with schizophrenia: an update. *Schizophr Bull* (2014) 40(1):181–91. doi: 10.1093/schbul/sbt139
77. Marler S, Sanders KB, Veenstra-VanderWeele J.N-acetylcysteine as treatment for self-injurious behavior in a child with autism. *J Child Adolesc Psychopharmacol* (2014) 24(4):231–4. doi: 10.1089/cap.2013.0137
78. Ghanizadeh A, Derakhshan N. N-acetylcysteine for treatment of autism, a case report. *J Res Med Sci* (2012) 17(10):985–7.
79. Stutzman D, Dopheide J.Acetylcysteine for treatment of autism spectrum disorder symptoms. *Am J Health Syst Pharm* (2015) 72(22):1956–9. doi: 10.2146/ajhp150072
80. Hardan AY, Fung LK, Libove RA, Obukhanych TV, Nair S, Herzenberg LA, et al. A randomized controlled pilot trial of oral N-acetylcysteine in children with autism. *Biol Psychiatry* (2012) 71(11):956–61. doi: 10.1016/j.biopsych.2012.01.014
81. Ghanizadeh A, Moghimi-Sarani E. A randomized double blind placebo controlled clinical trial of N-Acetylcysteine added to risperidone for treating autistic disorders. *BMC Psychiatry* (2013) 13:196. doi: 10.1186/1471-244X-13-196
82. Nikoo M, Radnia H, Farokhnia M, Mohammadi M-R, Akhondzadeh S. N-Acetylcysteine as an adjunctive therapy to risperidone for treatment of irritability in autism: a randomized, double-blind, placebo-controlled clinical trial of efficacy and safety. *Clin Neuropharmacol* (2015) 38(1):11–7. doi: 10.1097/WNF.0000000000000063
83. Wink LK, Adams R, Wang Z, Klaunig JE, Plawecki MH, Posey DJ, et al. A randomized placebo-controlled pilot study of N-acetylcysteine in youth with autism spectrum disorder. *Mol Autism* (2016) 7(1):26. doi: 10.1186/s13229-016-0088-6
84. Dean OM, Gray KM, Villagonzalo KA, Dodd S, Mohebbi M, Vick T, et al. A randomised, double blind, placebo-controlled trial of a fixed dose of N-acetyl cysteine in children with autistic disorder. *Aust N Z J Psychiatry* (2017) 51(3):241–9. doi: 10.1177/0004867416652735
85. McGuire K, Fung LK, Hagopian L, Vasa RA, Mahajan R, Bernal P, et al. Irritability and problem behavior in autism spectrum disorder: a practice pathway for pediatric primary care. *Pediatr* (2016)137 Suppl 2(Supplement 2):S136–48. doi: 10.1542/peds.2015-2851L
86. Petrosino S, Di Marzo V. The pharmacology of palmitoylethanolamide and first data on the therapeutic efficacy of some of its new formulations. *Br J Pharmacol* (2017) 174(11):1349–65. doi: 10.1111/bph.13580
87. Antonucci N, Cirillo A, Siniscalco D. Beneficial Effects of Palmitoylethanolamide on expressive language, cognition, and behaviors in autism: a report of two cases. *Case Rep Psychiatry* (2015) 2015:325061. doi: 10.1155/2015/325061
88. Khalaj M, Saghazadeh A, Shirazi E, Shalbafan MR, Alavi K, Shooshtari MH, et al. Palmitoylethanolamide as adjunctive therapy for autism: Efficacy and

safety results from a randomized controlled trial. *J Psychiatr Res* (2018) 103:104–11. doi: 10.1016/j.jpsychires.2018.04.022

89. Sullivan GW, Carper HT, Novick WJ Jr., Mandell GL. Inhibition of the inflammatory action of interleukin-1 and tumor necrosis factor (alpha) on neutrophil function by pentoxifylline. *Infect Immun* (1988) 56(7):1722–9.
90. Sogame S. Clinical experiences with administration of pentoxifylline against autism and behaviour abnormalities. *Jpn J Child Psych* (1978) 19:137–44.
91. Nakane A. Effect of pentoxifylline in autistic children. *Tokyoto Eisei Gakkashi* (1980)65:104–5.
92. Shimoide M. Effect of pentoxifylline (Trental) on infantile autism. *Clin Exp Med* (1981) 58:285–8.
93. Turek S. Treatment of psychotic and autistic children with pentoxifylline. *ASANA* (1981) 1:51–60.
94. Akhondzadeh S, Fallah J, Mohammadi MR, Imani R, Mohammadi M, Salehi B, et al. Double-blind placebo-controlled trial of pentoxifylline added to risperidone: effects on aberrant behavior in children with autism.*Prog Neuropsychopharmacol Biol Psychiatry* (2010) 34(1):32–6. doi: 10.1016/j.pnpbp.2009.09.012
95. Orasanu G, Ziouzenkova O, Devchand PR, Nehra V, Hamdy O, Horton ES, et al. The peroxisome proliferator-activated receptor-gamma agonist pioglitazone represses inflammation in a peroxisome proliferator-activated receptor-alpha-dependent manner in vitro and in vivo in mice. *J Am Coll Cardiol* (2008) 52(10):869–81. doi: 10.1016/j.jacc.2008.04.055
96. Sato T, Hanyu H, Hirao K, Kanetaka H, Sakurai H, Iwamoto T. Efficacy of PPAR-gamma agonist pioglitazone in mild Alzheimer disease. *Neurobiol Aging* (2011) 32(9):1626–33. doi: 10.1016/j.neurobiolaging.2009.10.009
97. Zeinoddini A, Sorayani M, Hassanzadeh E, Arbabi M, Farokhnia M, Salimi S, et al. Pioglitazone adjunctive therapy for depressive episode of bipolar disorder: a randomized, double-blind, placebo-controlled trial. *Depress Anxiety* (2015) 32(3):167–73. doi: 10.1002/da.22340
98. Boris M, Kaiser CC, Goldblatt A, Elice MW, Edelson SM, Adams JB, et al. Effect of pioglitazone treatment on behavioral symptoms in autistic children.*J Neuroinflammation* (2007) 4(1):3. doi: 10.1186/1742-2094-4-3
99. Ghaleiha A, Rasa SM, Nikoo M, Farokhnia M, Mohammadi M-R, Akhondzadeh S. A pilot double-blind placebo-controlled trial of pioglitazone as adjunctive treatment to risperidone: Effects on aberrant behavior in children with autism. *J Psychiatry Res* (2015) 229(1-2):181–7. doi: 10.1016/j.psychres.2015.07.043
100. Liu BS, Ferreira R, Lively S, Schlichter LC, Spironolactone/Arthritis Study, Group. Microglial SK3 and SK4 currents and activation state are modulated by the neuroprotective drug, riluzole. *J Neuroimmune Pharmacol* (2013) 8(1):227–37. doi: 10.1007/s11481-012-9365-0
101. Bendtzen K, Hansen PR, Rieneck K, Spironolactone/Arthritis Study, Group. Spironolactone inhibits production of proinflammatory cytokines, including tumour necrosis factor-alpha and interferon-gamma, and has potential in the treatment of arthritis. *Clin Exp Immunol* (2003) 134(1):151–8. doi: 10.1046/j.1365-2249.2003.02249.x
102. Young MJ. Mechanisms of mineralocorticoid receptor-mediated cardiac fibrosis and vascular inflammation. *Curr Opin Nephrol Hypertens* (2008) 17(2):174–80. doi: 10.1097/MNH.0b013e3282f56854
103. Bradstreet JJ, Smith S, Granpeesheh D, El-Dahr JM, Rossignol D. Spironolactone might be a desirable immunologic and hormonal intervention in autism spectrum disorders. *Med Hypotheses* (2007) 68(5):979–87. doi: 10.1016/j.mehy.2006.10.015
104. Motaghinejad M, Motevalian M. Neuroprotective effects of various doses of topiramate against methylphenidate-induced oxidative stress and inflammation in isolated rat amygdala: the possible role of CREB/BDNF signaling pathway.*J Neural Transm* (2016) 123(12):1463–77. doi: 10.1007/s00702-016-1619-1
105. Motaghinejad M, Motevalian M. Involvement of AMPA/kainate and GABAA receptors in topiramate neuroprotective effects against methylphenidate abuse sequels involving oxidative stress and inflammation in rat isolated hippocampus.*Eur J Pharmacol* (2016) 784:181–91. doi: 10.1016/j.ejphar.2016.04.036
106. Tian Y, Guo SX, Li JR, Du HG, Wang CH, Zhang JM, et al. Topiramate attenuates early brain injury following subarachnoid haemorrhage in rats via duplex protection against inflammation and neuronal cell death. *Brain Res* (2015) 1622:174–85. doi: 10.1016/j.brainres.2015.06.007
107. Rezaei V, Mohammadi MR, Ghanizadeh A, Sahraian A, Tabrizi M, Rezazadeh SA, et al. Double-blind, placebo-controlled trial of risperidone plus topiramate in children with autistic disorder. *Prog Neuropsychopharmacol Biol Psychiatry* (2010) 34(7):1269–72. doi: 10.1016/j.pnpbp.2010.07.005
108. Kapur S, Phillips AG, Insel TR. Why has it taken so long for biological psychiatry to develop clinical tests and what to do about it? *Mol Psychiatry* (2012) 17: (12):1174. doi: 10.1038/mp.2012.105
109. Chamberlain SR, Cavanagh J, de Boer P, Mondelli V, Jones DNC, Drevets WC, et al. Treatment-resistant depression and peripheral C-reactive protein. *Br J Psychiatry* (2019) 214(1):11–9. doi: 10.1192/bjp.2018.66
110. Ghaleiha A, Mohammadi E, Mohammadi M-R, Farokhnia M, Modabbernia A, Yekehtaz H, et al. Riluzole as an adjunctive therapy to risperidone for the treatment of irritability in children with autistic disorder: a double-blind, placebo-controlled, randomized trial.*Pediatr Drugs* (2013) 15(6):505–14. doi: 10.1007/s40272-013-0036-2
111. Russo FB, Freitas BC, Pignatari GC, Fernandes IR, Sebat J, Muotri AR, et al. Modeling the interplay between neurons and astrocytes in autism using human induced pluripotent stem cells. *Biol Psychiatry* (2018) 83(7):569–78. doi: 10.1016/j.biopsych.2017.09.021

13

Inheritance of HLA-Cw7 Associated with Autism Spectrum Disorder (ASD)

*Terry Harville[1,2], Bobbie Rhodes-Clark[1], Sirish C. Bennuri[3,5], Leanna Delhey[4,5], John Slattery[6], Marie Tippett[3,5], Rebecca Wynne[7], Shannon Rose[3,5], Stephen Kahler[3,5] and Richard E. Frye[8,9]**

[1] Department of Pathology, University of Arkansas for Medical Sciences, Little Rock, AR, United States, [2] Department of Internal Medicine, University of Arkansas for Medical Sciences, Little Rock, AR, United States, [3] Department of Pediatrics, College of Medicine, University of Arkansas for Medical Sciences, Little Rock, AR, United States, [4] School of Public Health, University of Arkansas for Medical Sciences, Little Rock, AR, United States, [5] Arkansas Children's Research Institute, Little Rock, AR, United States, [6] BioRosa Technologies Inc, San Francisco, CA, United States, [7] National Center for Toxicological Research, Jefferson, AR, United States, [8] Barrow Neurological Institute at Phoenix Children's Hospital, Phoenix, AZ, United States, [9] Department of Child Health, University of Arizona College of Medicine, Phoenix, AZ, United States

Correspondence:
Richard E. Frye
rfrye@phoenixchildrens.com

Autism spectrum disorder (ASD) is a behaviorally defined disorder that is now thought to affect approximately 1 in 69 children in the United States. In most cases, the etiology is unknown, but several studies point to the interaction of genetic predisposition with environmental factors. The immune system is thought to have a causative role in ASD, and specific studies have implicated T lymphocytes, monocytes, natural killer (NK) cells, and certain cytokines. The human leukocyte antigen (HLA) system is involved in the underlying process for shaping an individual's immune system, and specific HLA alleles are associated with specific diseases as risk factors. In this study, we determine whether a specific HLA allele was associated with ASD in a large cohort of patients with ASD. Identifying such an association could help in the identification of immune system components which may have a causative role in specific cohorts of patients with ASD who share similar specific clinical features. Specimens from 143 patients with ASD were analyzed with respect to race and ethnicity. Overall, HLA-Cw7 was present in a much greater frequency than expected in individuals with ASD as compared to the general population. Further, the cohort of patients who express HLA-Cw7 shares specific immune system/inflammatory clinical features including being more likely to have allergies, food intolerances, and chronic sinusitis as compared to those with ASD who did not express HLA-Cw7. HLA-Cw7 has a role in stimulating NK cells. Thus, this finding may indicate that chronic over-activation of NK cells may have a role in the manifestation of ASD in a cohort of patients with increased immune system/inflammatory features.

Keywords: autism (ASD), HLA, immune system, natural killer cells, innate immnuity

INTRODUCTION

Autism spectrum disorder (ASD) is a behaviorally defined disorder that affects approximately 1 in 69 children in the United States (1). The definition of ASD is outlined in the Diagnostic and Statistical Manual of Mental Disorders (DSM)-5 which requires that those diagnosed exhibit deficits in social communication along with the presence of restricted interests and/or repetitive behaviors and/or sensory disorders. In addition, the symptoms must significantly interfere with the individual's ability to function properly in school, work, and other areas of life (2). Despite decades of research, the etiology(ies) of ASD is(are) still unknown (3), but epidemiological studies suggest that genetic predisposition interacts with environmental influences to trigger the biological events that results in ASD (4). Several physiological systems that are known to be influenced by environmental factors have been implicated in ASD, including redox and mitochondrial metabolism, as well as, immune dysregulation (3, 4).

ASD is described as a "spectrum" due to the variability in the extent and severity of behavioral and medical symptoms. The diagnostic criteria for ASD is wide enough to capture an overall phenotype, but the variability in symptoms and severity, as well as, specific laboratory results indicates that multiple etiologies may be responsible, including one that involves immune dysfunction (5). One of the challenges is to define potential subtypes using behavioral and physiological biomarkers in order to better define the disorder and identify treatment targets.

Many studies have indicated involvement of the immune system in ASD. Early studies identified family histories of autoimmune disease, specific HLA associations, and autoantibodies to a wide range of brain and non-brain tissues in children with ASD (6–13). Other studies have demonstrated a reduction in immunoglobulin production (14) and a positive therapeutic response to intravenous immunoglobulin treatment (15). Perhaps the most pivotal study from the Kennedy Krieger Institute found that autopsy revealed inflammatory changes in the cerebellum with cytokine elevations in cortical areas and similar abnormal cytokine profiles in the cerebrospinal fluid of patients with ASD (16). However, the reason for this immune dysregulation remains unknown.

Most notably, T lymphocytes and monocytes have been implicated as immune system components involved with ASD. Another immune cell type, natural killer (NK) cells are also implicated (11, 13, 17–19). The human leukocyte antigen (HLA) system is the core of the development and maintenance of the immune system in humans. It is the most polymorphic of all human proteins, and specific polymorphisms have been demonstrated to have specific roles in the development of autoimmune disorders. For example, it is well known that the risk for developing ankylosing spondylitis is increased in individuals who have inherited HLA-B27. Thus, involvement of specific HLA components in the etiology of immune-associated ASD is plausible.

NK cells are thought to be most critical as part of the immune system's first-line defense and immunosurveillance. Essentially, all the cells of the body (except for RBC) express HLA class I proteins. The expressed HLA-C locus components interact with NK cell killer immunoglobulin-like receptor (KIR) ligands. The HLA-C locus proteins are divided into two groups, group I or group II, based on the expression of 77 Ser and 80 Asn, in the sequence of the former, and expression 77 Asn and 80 Lys in the sequence of the latter. Further, HLA-C group I and group II reciprocally act as inhibitors and activators with specific KIR ligands expressed on the NK cells.

During normal immunosurveillance, an NK cell interrogating a human cell. If it finds the correct level of expression of HLA-C group I and group II components that "balance" activation and inhibition signaling *via* its KIR ligands, it leaves the cell unaffected. The normal ratio of expression of HLA-C group I to group II is 0.86. The presumption is that this was decided *via* evolution to provide the optimal NK cell immunosurveillance. Significant deviations from this may result in delayed immune system activation or perhaps over activation of immunity. For example, if the cell was infected by a virus, or was transformed and becoming cancerous, then the "normal" levels of HLA-C expression on the cell's surface may be altered, and the NK cell may become activated *via* the KIR ligand interaction. This activation could generate inflammatory signals, and the NK cell may actively begin to kill the cell.

We hypothesized that a significant involvement of the immune system in ASD would be exhibited as bias in the distribution of specific HLA types. Further, we hypothesized that this would be occurring in a cohort of patients with similar clinical and laboratory features, rather than the entire population of ASD. To this end, we performed HLA typing on 126 patients with ASD and 17 lymphoblastoid cell lines (LCLs) derived from patients with ASD (143 total). We analyzed the typing results based on the normal expected frequencies for total and subpopulations of African-American, Asian, Caucasian, and Hispanic racial and ethnic distributions. We found that HLA-Cw7 was over-represented in patients with ASD, primarily in the Caucasian cohort. Further analyses for clinical and laboratory features indicate that those who express HLA-Cw7 have a higher rate of immune system–associated issues in comparison with those with ASD who do not express HLA-Cw7. Our data support the notion that the increased expression of HLA-Cw7 in a cohort of patients with ASD and immune system–associated issues may support chronic over-stimulation of NK cells, resulting in the phenotypic features of ASD.

METHODS

The study contains data derived from cell lines obtained from 126 participants diagnosed with ASD seen in at Arkansas Children's Research Institute (Little Rock, AR) as part of two clinical studies (NCT02000284, NCT01602016) as well as 17 LCLs from the Autism Genetic Resource Exchange (AGRE) and the National Institutes of Mental Health biorepository. The primary purpose of the clinical studies from which these samples were derived was to investigate the relationship between mitochondrial dysfunction and ASD (NCT02000284) and abnormalities in folate metabolism and ASD (NCT01602016). Results on the primary studies from which these samples were derived has been published previously

(20–28), but investigation of HLA types in relation to ASD has not been previously reported in these samples. Likewise, the LCLs used in this study have been used in previous laboratory studies examining mitochondrial dysfunction in relation to ASD (29–32), and the effect of environmental agents on mitochondrial (33–36) and immune (37) functions of the LCLs but investigation of the HLA types of these LCLs in relation to ASD has not been published previously. The Institutional Review Board (IRB) at the University of Arkansas for Medical Sciences (Little Rock, AR) approved the clinical studies and use of cell lines for the primary investigation and additional investigations such as HLA typing and other secondary genomic, metabolomic, and proteomic investigations. For clinical studies, parents of participants provided written informed consent. All experiments were performed in accordance with relevant guidelines and regulations.

ASD Participants

One hundred twenty-six individuals with ASD met inclusion and exclusion criteria. **Table 1** outlines the clinical characteristics of these participants. Comorbid conditions were both derived from a parent reported medical questionnaire and from review of conditions diagnosed in the medical records. Regression (defined as loss of already obtained skills) was defined in detail in our questionnaire. Questions regarding regression included the timing, specific skills lost, duration of the regression, trigger, and whether multiple regressions were identified. Since this paper is not specifically on regression, we have not summarized these details in the table, only whether regression(s) were present or not present. This method for assessing medical comorbidities has been used in several of our previous studies (20, 21, 24, 25). We then selected the medical conditions that affected 10% or more of the individuals in the sample. Conditions with sample prevalence of less than 10% were considered unlikely to differentiate any immune subgroups defined by the HLA-typing analysis. Data for all the comorbid conditions were not available for all participants, as some families did not complete the questionnaire or did not provide medical records for review, or the review of the medical records could not determine if the participant suffered from the comorbid condition or not. This information was missing at random and affected less than 10% of the participants. The total number of participants with the required information is outlined in the table below.

TABLE 1 | ASD participant characteristics (N = 126).

Variable	
Age, mean (SD), years and months	7 years and 8 months (3 years and 6 months)
Males, N (%)	82% (22/126)
Caucasian	83% (104/126)
African American	7% (9/126)
Hispanic	3% (4/126)
Asian	7% (9/126)
Comorbid conditions (parent report), % (N)	
Abdominal pain	19% (23/118)
Allergies	43% (51/118)
Anxiety	26% (30/117)
ADHD	32% (37/117)
Sinusitis	13% (15/118)
Immune problems	14% (17/118)
Headaches	21% (25/118)
Regression	62% (72/116)
Comorbid conditions (medical records), N (%)	
Food allergies/intolerances	49% (56/115)
Chronic constipation	43% (49/113)
Chronic persistent infections	34% (41/119)
Immune disorder	10% (12/118)
Epilepsy	25% (29/118)

Inclusion criteria were (i) age 3 to 14 years of age and (ii) ASD diagnosis. Exclusion criteria were (i) chronic treatment with medications that would detrimentally affect mitochondrial function for the mitochondrial study from which these samples were derived, such as, antipsychotic medications, (ii) vitamin or mineral supplementation exceeding the recommended daily allowance, and (iii) prematurity.

The ASD diagnosis was defined by one of the following: (i) a gold-standard diagnostic instrument such as the Autism Diagnostic Observation Schedule (ADOS) and/or Autism Diagnostic Interview-Revised (ADI-R); (ii) the state of Arkansas diagnostic standard, defined as agreement of a physician, psychologist, and speech therapist; and/or (iii) DSM diagnosis by a physician along with standardized validated questionnaires and diagnosis confirmation by the Principal Investigator at the time (REF). We have validated that this criteria captures an accurate diagnosis of ASD in our previous studies by re-evaluating a portion of the participants with the ADI-R and determining that they all were well within the diagnostic criteria for ASD (20, 21, 24, 25).

Cell Lines

As outlined in **Supplemental Table 1**, 17 LCLs were derived from white males diagnosed with autistic disorder with a pedigree having at least one other affected male sibling (i.e., multiplex family) (mean [SD] age 12.5 [3.0] years). These LCLs were obtained from the Autism Genetic Resource Exchange (AGRE; Los Angeles, CA, USA) and the National Institutes of Mental Health (NIMH; Bethesda, MD, USA) center for collaborative genomic studies on mental disorders. All relevant guidelines and regulations were followed. These de-identified human samples were determined to be exempt from IRB review. Boys from which these autistic disorder LCLs were derived were diagnosed with a gold-standard examination, either the ADOS or the ADI-R.

DNA Isolation

DNA was isolated from buffy coats of blood collected in EDTA tubes using the Purgene DNA Purification Kit (Gentra Systems, Inc., Minneapolis, MN). For cell lines, DNA was isolated from $5x10^6$ pelleted cells using the same kit.

HLA Typing

HLA typing was performed as previously reported using reagents and supplies from One Lambda®, in an American Society of Histocompatibility and Immunogenetics (ASHI) certified, and College of American Pathology (CAP) certified, laboratory using the LabType® rSSO technique (38).

Statistical Analyses

HLA-typing results for the patients and LCLs with ASD were compared with the distributions of HLA components reported by the United Network for Organ Sharing (UNOs) (https://unos.org/wp-content/uploads/unos/CPRA_frequencies.xls). These data are felt to reflect accurately the distributions of HLA types by race/ethnicity in the US. The racial/ethnic distribution in the specimens with ASD differs from those of the general population (**Supplemental Table 2**). Therefore, the expected frequency calculations were adjusted to accommodate the deviations by race/ethnicity from the general population. From 143 study subjects, 286 HLA alleles are present. The expected allele frequencies of the general population were determined by taking the fraction of each individual allele present and multiplying by 286, the total expected allele number. Thus, potential fractions of expected alleles are generated, and these are rounded to the nearest integer. Not all HLA types are found in the patients with ASD in our study. Thus, these cannot be analyzed, but the lack of these HLA types has potential to affect the expected values, since all HLA alleles at the serologic equivalence level were included in making the expected calculations. Therefore, the total numbers of expected alleles for each HLA-locus are projected not to completely add up to 286. Some HLA alleles are null alleles, and therefore not expressed. There were 2 HLA-C locus null alleles and 45 HLA-DR51/52/53 null alleles in the patients with ASD. Therefore, the total number of alleles in patients with ASD for HLA-C and HLA-DR51/52/53 were 284 and 241, respectively. HLA-DR51/52/53 were not analyzed separately by race ethnicity.

Chi-square analyses were performed for samples with larger numbers, and Fisher Exact Test analyses were performed with sample size approximately 20 or fewer. The p values were calculated using Microsoft Excel®, with $p < 0.001$ selected to represent the most stringent condition for determining an association with specific HLA types. Results were analyzed similar to previous studies searching for associations of HLA-typing results with disease (6–12, 13, 39).

To determine if the specific HLA subgroup identified was defined by specific medical symptoms, partial least squares discriminant analysis (PLSDA) using R version 3.5.0 mixOmics Omics Data Integration Project (version 6.3.2) was used to explore symptoms depicted in **Table 1** to determine if there were any specific symptoms that differentiated subgroups identified by the HLA-typing results.

RESULTS

HLA Typing

HLA typing was performed on 143 total subjects (patients with ASD and LCLs from those diagnosed with ASD). The results were compared with the frequencies of individual HLA components from a very large national database (https://unos.org/wp-content/uploads/unos/CPRA_frequencies.xls), adjusted for the race/ethnic distributions of the subjects with ASD. The total group of patients was analyzed (see **Supplementary Tables 3–8**), and the HLA types were separately analyzed based on the individual race/ethnicity of the patients (see **Supplementary Tables 9–13**). Overall, HLA-Cw7 was found to be greatly over-represented from the expected in the total group and in the Caucasian cohort ($p < 0.001$) with significant positive association (**Table 2** and **Supplemental Tables 5** and **11**). HLA-DQ5 and HLA-DQ6 (**Supplementary Tables 8** and **13**) were nominally statistically significant but did not achieve statistical significance at the increased level we set at $p < 0.001$. HLA-A, HLA-B, HLA-DR, and HLA-DQ loci were not found to be represented with a significantly different frequency in ASD as compared to the general population (see **Supplementary Tables 3, 4, 6, 7, 9, 10, 12**). Likewise, loci on HLA-C and HLA-DQ other than those mentioned above were not found to be represented with a significantly different frequency in ASD as compared to the general population (see **Supplementary Tables 5, 8, 11, 13**).

The HLA types from specimens from 143 subjects with ASD were analyzed and compared with the expected distributions of HLA types in the normal population. Only HLA-Cw7 was found to be increased with respect to the expected distributions. Further, this was primarily due to more Caucasians with ASD expressing HLA-Cw7. Two hundred eighty-six alleles are present in 143 subjects. The expected allele frequency was calculated from the known distributions in the United States population and then adjusted for the frequencies of the race/ethnic frequencies in the ASD cohort. Samples with large numbers were analyzed by *chi square, and those with small sample numbers were analyzed by **Fischer Exact Test. P <0.001 was considered for statistical significance (**Supplemental Tables 2–13**).

In patients with ASD, HLA-C locus group II activating alleles are found more frequently than expected in the general population (**Table 3** and **Supplementary Table 5**). This increase in HLA-C locus activating alleles is primarily due to the increased frequency of expression of HLA-Cw7 (**Table 3**). The increase is due to the greater expression in Caucasians (**Table 4; Supplementary Table 11**).

The HLA-C locus components from subjects with ASD compared with the expected frequencies indicate an increase in group II Activating HLA-Cw7. All others are not statistically significantly different from the expected frequencies.

The total numbers of group I and group II activating alleles are compared by race/ethnicity in subjects with ASD. The total

TABLE 2 | HLA-Cw7 is found more than expected in patients with ASD.

	ASD expected	ASD observed	p =
Total ASD alleles = 286	42	91	*0.000001
Caucasian alleles = 242	35	84	*0.0000002
African American alleles = 18	1	2	**0.3857
Hispanic alleles = 8	0	0	**1.0000
Asian alleles = 18	9	5	**0.1097

**p value by Chi Square, **p value by Fisher Exact Test.*

TABLE 3 | Increase in patients with ASD expressing HLA-Cw7 explains the increase in HLA-C group II activating alleles detected.

HLA-C	Total expected ASD	Group I activating	Group II activating	Total observed ASD	Group I activating	Group II activating	p =	HLA-C
1	10		10	10		10	*1.00	1
2	10	10		10	10		*1.00	2
4	32	32		32	32		**1.00	4
5	24	24		18	18		**0.86	5
6	24	24		25	25		**1.00	6
7	42		42	91		91	**0.0007	7
8	12		12	11		11	**1.00	8
9	19		19	19		19	**1.00	9
10	26		26	28		28	**1.00	10
12	16		16	17		17	**1.00	12
14	7		7	2		2	*0.44	14
15	8	8		5	5		*0.88	15
16	9	9		11	11		**0.98	16
17	5	5		3	3		*0.92	17
18	1	1		2	2		*0.95	18

*p value by Chi Square, **p value by Fisher Exact Test.*

number of group II activating alleles is greater than expected in the total ASD cohort and the effect appears to be driven by Caucasians.

HLA-DQ5 and HLA-DQ6 were also found to trend toward being found in greater proportions in the subjects with ASD but did not achieve $p < 0.001$ statistical significance in this study (see **Supplementary Tables 8** and **13**). Inheritance of HLA-DQ6 has been previously associated with risk for scleroderma and narcolepsy. More subjects in a larger study may help to clarify the meaningfulness of this observation with regard to ASD.

Clinical Characteristics of HLA Subgroups

One hundred eight participants had information on all clinical measures in order to enter into the PLSDA. Given the significant effect of the HLA-Cw7 allele, we divided the ASD participants in those that were negative for the HLA-Cw7 allele (N = 50) and those with at least one HLA-Cw7 allele (N = 58). The PLSDA found two components with the first and second components explaining 9 and 12% of the variance, respectively. The discriminant function demonstrated a 65% accuracy in discriminating the groups. The individual participant's values on the two components are depicted in **Supplemental Figure 1**, and the correspondence of each clinical characteristic loading on the two components is given in **Supplemental Figure 2**.

TABLE 4 | Over-representation of HLA-C group II activating alleles observed in ASD.

	Total group I activating alleles	Total group II activating alleles	p =
Total ASD	95	189	*0.000002
Caucasian	73	167	*0.0000002
African American	9	9	**0.26
Hispanic	6	2	**0.06
Asian	7	11	**0.11

*p value from Chi Square, **p value from Fisher Exact Test.*

Supplemental Table 15 outlines the loading for the two individual components of the discriminant function as well as the total loading for both components. This is sorted by the loading value for each clinical characteristic and presented graphically in **Figure 1**. Positive loadings represent characteristics that are more representative of HLA-Cw7-positive participants whereas negative loading represent characteristics more representative of the HLA-Cw7-negative participants. Considering the top loadings for those who are HLA-Cw7-positive, we find that two of the three characteristics of HLA-Cw7-positive participants in our sample are related to immune system activation, including allergies, food intolerances, and chronic sinusitis, whereas none of the characteristics of the HLA-Cw7-negative patients involve immune system activation.

To better depict the characteristics of individual participants, we created an index to describe the number of clinical symptoms attributed to HLA-Cw7-negative and HLA-Cw7-positive participants in the analysis. A value of −1 was assigned for each of the top four clinical characteristics of HLA-Cw7-negative participants (regression, chronic constipation, headaches, abdominal pain), and a value of +1 was assigned for each of the top four clinical characteristics of HLA-Cw7-positive participants (allergies, food intolerances sinusitis, ADHD). As seen in **Figure 2**, HLA-Cw7-positive participants demonstrated a more positive score, on average, but also were more variable in their characteristics.

DISCUSSION

The specific etiologies responsible for causing ASD remain to be fully determined. Patients with ASD, while having an overall similar neuropsychiatric phenotype resulting in the diagnosis, have quite a variability in other clinical features and laboratory studies. It is expected that the individual's genetics influenced by environmental exposures results in the disease.

Many factors have implicated the immune system involvement in ASD. Notably, inflammatory effects on the central nervous system incriminate some alteration in immune function or dysregulation of immunity (14). Identification of specific cell

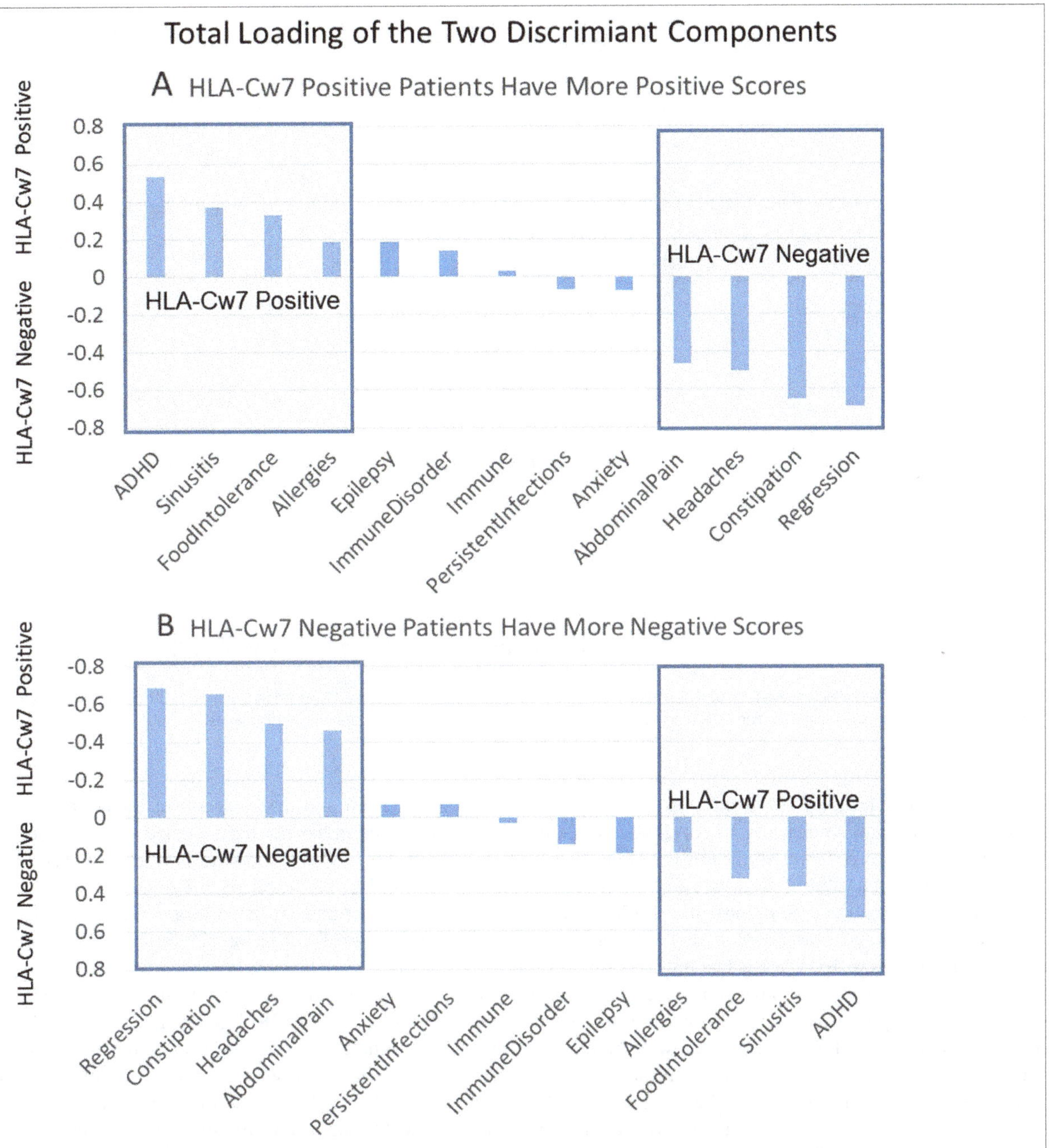

FIGURE 1 | Total components of the discriminant function. **(A)** Positive numbers represent components that are related to HLA-Cw7-positive participants. **(B)** Negative numbers represent components more representative of the HLA-Cw7-negative participants.

types and targets, as can be found in specific autoimmune disorders, has not been rewarding at this point in time. Further, it is doubtful that one specific immune dysfunctional cell type and target are responsible for all ASD. It is reasonable and plausible that specific cohorts of individuals with ASD united by similar clinical and laboratory features may have similar underlying forms of immune dysfunction resulting in some form of chronic inflammation, which results in the neurologic features of disease. Since ASD tends to occur early in life, the genetic features and environmental exposures would have to be part of this early presentation. Further, since HLA components are frequently found associated with specific autoimmune disorders, are expressed on the body's cells from the onset, and shape the immune system maturation and function, it is reasonable that specific HLA components could result in the immune system's response in such an adverse manner.

Previous studies have implicated specific HLA types to be associated with ASD (6–13). Perhaps, HLA-DR4 has been most commonly found in association (7, 8, 10, 11). HLA-A2 has also been commonly reported (6, 9, 10). Specific HLA haplotypes

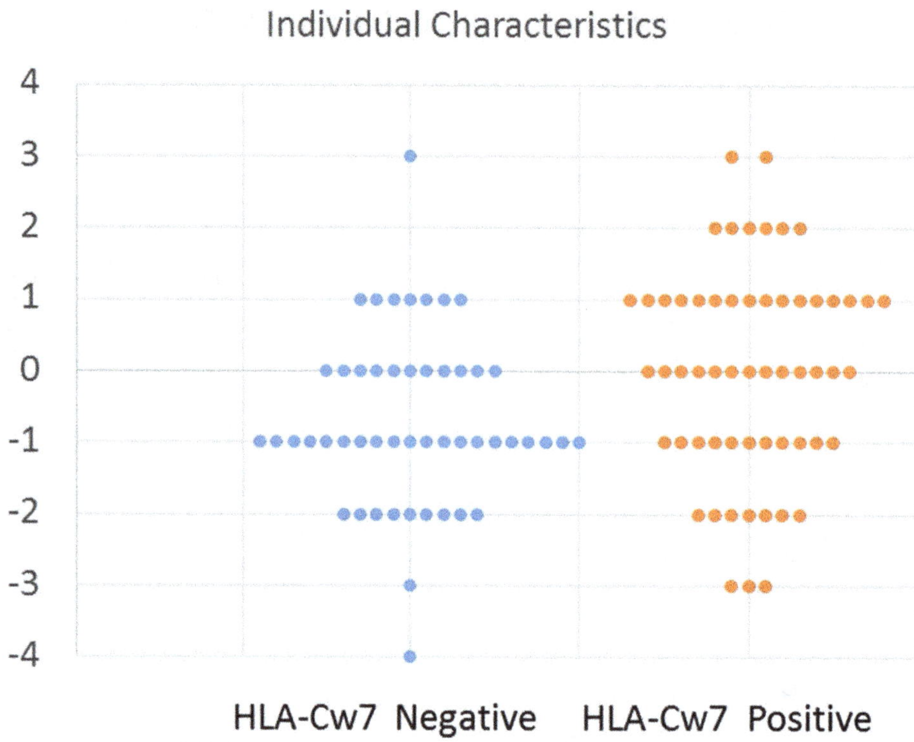

FIGURE 2 | Number of characteristics for HLA-Cw7-negative and HLA-Cw7-positive participants. Clinical characteristics that are more representative of absence of HLA-Cw7 indicate weighted negative, and clinical characteristics of presence of HLA-Cw7 indicate weighted positive.

have been reported (HLA- A*01-B*07-DRB1*0701-DQB1*0602) in patients from Saudi Arabia, and HLA-A2-B44-DR4 and HLA-B44-C30-DR4, from different studies in the United States (10–12). At the stringent p value of $p < 0.001$, we were unable to detect any of these associations (**Supplemental Tables 3–13**). From these reports, it may be ascertained that different geographic locations of patients with ASD may had predilection for different HLA type preferences. Although not specifically studied or stated in these reports, post-streptococcal immunoreactivity is correlated with HLA-DR4, and it is unknown whether PANDAS could be having a role in the bias toward finding an association with HLA-DR4 in some of the studies. Further, studies have not specifically sought for HLA-C locus associations, until the present study. Additionally, other studies have not specifically adjusted the expected control group HLA frequencies to the race/ethnic frequencies found in the ASD subjects. We believe that the careful adjustment for the race/ethnic distributions of the HLA types between the control/expected HLA distributions and the observed HLA types in our subjects with ASD has resulted in the difference found in our study *versus* those previously reported.

We found that a cohort of patients with ASD (primarily Caucasian) expresses HLA-Cw7 at more than twice the extent expected in the normal population. These patients share immune-associated clinical features, not found in patients who do not express HLA-Cw7. Interestingly, others have associated a subset of individuals with ASD and non-IgE-mediated food allergy (40) and chronic sinusitis (41) who have dysregulation in cytokine production and microRNA expression and dysregulation of innate immunity, although HLA distribution has not been studied in this subset. While HLA-DQ5 and HLA-DQ6 trended toward greater presence in subjects with ASD, since statistical significance was not achieved, we await further analyses with a larger number of subjects with ASD to pursue further the potential meaningfulness of these findings.

The HLA-C locus is expressed on all cell types (except RBC) and has a major role in immunosurveillance. HLA-C interacts with NK cell KIR ligands in an activating and inhibiting fashion. Thus, when an NK cell interrogates a cell in the body, the correct expression of HLA-C on the body cell prevents the NK cell from becoming activated. When a cell becomes infected with a virus, one of the viral strategies to prevent recognition is to decrease the expression of HLA on the cell surface. In doing so, the alteration in HLA-C expression can alert NK cells to attack. Cancerous cells are thought to be targeted by NK cells in a similar fashion, i.e., alteration in the normal levels of HLA-C expression.

The increased frequency of subjects with HLA-Cw7 expression also results in these subjects having an overall greater expression of the HLA-C group II activating alleles. While it remains to be proven, we suspect this cohort of patients may have a continuous and ongoing level of inflammation generated by NK cells in response to this increase in group II activating alleles. This could result in the overall increase in immune-associated clinical features in this cohort. Warren et al. (17) first investigated NK cell cytotoxic activity in ASD in 1987 and found reduced *ex vivo*

NK cell cytotoxic activity in 12/31 ASD subjects examined. This finding was supported by Vojdani et al. (18) who demonstrated reduced *ex vivo* NK cell cytotoxic activity in 45% of ASD children in a much larger cohort (1,027 ASD subjects). Shortly thereafter, Enstrom et al. (19) demonstrated increased numbers of NK cells as well as upregulation of NK cell receptors and cytolytic effector molecules in 52 children with ASD as compared to 27 controls. Importantly, while *ex vivo* NK cell cytotoxic activity was reduced in the ASD cohort, interferon-gamma-producing NK cells were increased under resting conditions in children with ASD suggesting that NK cells in the ASD cohort are maximally activated *in vivo* and, thus, chronically activated NK cells are down-regulated when stimulated *ex vivo*. Unfortunately, HLA typing was not performed in these three studies. Taken together, these data support the notion that a subset of ASD subjects with greater expression of HLA-C group II activating alleles may have chronically activated NK cells. Torres et al. have previously reported the association of activating KIR ligands and ASD (11, 13). Indeed, the KIR-activating gene 2DS1 was shown to be increased in frequency in patients with ASD, and this supports our findings as HLA-Cw7 is a cognate ligand for KIR 2DS1 (13). Thus, this could result in a greater level of NK cell activation in patients with ASD who express HLA-Cw7.

Further studies in patients with ASD who express HLA-Cw7 are needed with specific evaluation of NK cell activation *in vivo*. This could potentially lead to therapeutic intervention by specifically targeting over-active NK cells in patients with ASD who express HLA-Cw7. The overall decrease in chronic inflammation could then decrease the burden on the central nervous system in a cohort of patients with ASD.

AUTHOR CONTRIBUTIONS

All authors were involved in the design and conceptualization of the experiments. Laboratory experiments were conducted by TH, BR-C, SB, RW and SR. LD, JS, MT and RF were involved in subject recruitment and assessment. Data was analyzed by TH, LD, SR, SK and RF. All authors were involved in drafting, editing and finalizing the manuscript. All authors approved of the final manuscript.

FUNDING

We would like to thank the supporters of our research studies, including the Arkansas Biosciences Institute (Little Rock, AR, USA), the Jonty Foundation (St. Paul, MN), the Autism Research Institute (San Diego, CA), the Gupta Family Foundation (Atherton, CA), the Jane Bostford Johnson Foundation (New York, NY), the Jager Family Foundation (Chicago, IL) and the Phoenix Children's Hospital Foundation (Phoenix, AZ). HLA typing was in part funded by Department of Pathology, UAMS, Research Funds.

ACKNOWLEDGMENTS

We thank the families and individuals with ASD that participated in the Autism Genetic Research Exchange and the studies at the National Institutes of Mental Health for providing cell lines for research as well as families and individuals that were involved in clinical research at the Arkansas Children's Research Institute (Little Rock, AR).

REFERENCES

1. Christensen DL, Braun KVN, Baio J, Bilder D, Charles J, Constantino JN, et al. Prevalence and characteristics of autism spectrum disorder among children aged 8 years—autism and developmental disabilities monitoring network, 11 sites, United States, 2012. *MMWR Surveill Summ* (2018) 65(13):1–23. doi: 10.15585/mmwr.ss6513a1
2. Wiggins L, Christensen D, Van Naarden Braun K, Martin L, Baio J. Comparison of autism spectrum disorder surveillance status based on two different diagnostic schemes: findings from the metropolitan atlanta developmental disabilities surveillance program, 2012. *PLoS One* (2018) 13(11):e0208079. doi: 10.1371/journal.pone.0208079
3. Rossignol DA, Frye RE. A review of research trends in physiological abnormalities in autism spectrum disorders: immune dysregulation, inflammation, oxidative stress, mitochondrial dysfunction and environmental toxicant exposures. *Mol Psychiatry* (2012) 17(4):389–401. doi: 10.1038/mp.2011.165
4. Rossignol DA, Genuis SJ, Frye RE. Environmental toxicants and autism spectrum disorders: a systematic review. *Transl Psychiatry* (2014) 4:e360. doi: 10.1038/tp.2014.4
5. McDougle CJ, Landino SM, Vahabzadeh A, O'Rourke J, Zurcher NR, Finger BC, et al. Toward an immune-mediated subtype of autism spectrum disorder. *Brain Res* (2015) 1617:72–92. doi: 10.1016/j.brainres.2014.09.048
6. Stubbs EG, Magenis RE. HLA and autism. *J Autism Dev Disord* (1980) 10(1):15–9.
7. Torres AR, Maciulis A, Stubbs EG, Cutler A, Odell D. The transmission disequilibrium test suggests that HLA-DR4 and DR13 are linked to autism spectrum disorder. *Hum Immunol* (2002) 63(4):311–6.
8. Lee LC, Zachary AA, Leffell MS, Newschaffer CJ, Matteson KJ, Tyler JD, et al. HLA-DR4 in families with autism. *Pediatr Neurol* (2006) 35(5):303–7. doi: 10.1016/j.pediatrneurol.2006.06.006
9. Torres AR, Sweeten TL, Cutler A, Bedke BJ, Fillmore M, Stubbs EG, et al. The association and linkage of the HLA-A2 class I allele with autism. *Hum Immunol* (2006) 67(4-5):346–51. doi: 10.1016/j.humimm.2006.01.001
10. Chien YL, Wu YY, Chen CH, Gau SS, Huang YS, Chien WH, et al. Association of HLA-DRB1 alleles and neuropsychological function in autism. *Psychiatr Genet* (2012) 22(1):46–9. doi: 10.1097/YPG.0b013e32834915ae
11. Torres AR, Westover JB, Gibbons C, Johnson RC, Ward DC. Activating killer-cell immunoglobulin-like receptors (KIR) and their cognate HLA ligands are significantly increased in autism. *Brain Behav Immun* (2012) 26(7):1122–7. doi: 10.1016/j.bbi.2012.07.014
12. Al-Hakbany M, Awadallah S, Al-Ayadhi L. The relationship of HLA class I and II alleles and haplotypes with autism: a case control study. *Autism Res Treat* (2014) 2014:242048. doi: 10.1155/2014/242048
13. Torres AR, Sweeten TL, Johnson RC, Odell D, Westover JB, Bray-Ward P, et al. Common genetic variants found in HLA and KIR immune genes in autism spectrum disorder. *Front Neurosci* (2016) 10:463. doi: 10.3389/fnins.2016.00463
14. Edmiston E, Ashwood P, Van de Water J. Autoimmunity, autoantibodies, and autism spectrum disorder. *Biol Psychiatry* (2017) 81(5):383–90. doi: 10.1016/j.biopsych.2016.08.031
15. Connery K, Tippett M, Delhey LM, Rose S, Slattery JC, Kahler SG, et al. Intravenous immunoglobulin for the treatment of autoimmune encephalopathy in children with autism. *Transl Psychiatry* (2018) 8(1):148. doi: 10.1038/s41398-018-0214-7
16. Vargas DL, Nascimbene C, Krishnan C, Zimmerman AW, Pardo CA. Neuroglial activation and neuroinflammation in the brain of patients with autism. *Ann Neurol* (2005) 57(1):67–81. doi: 10.1002/ana.20315
17. Warren RP, Foster A, Margaretten NC. Reduced natural killer cell activity in autism. *J Am Acad Child Adolesc Psychiatry* (1987) 26(3):333–5. doi: 10.1097/00004583-198705000-00008

18. Vojdani A, Mumper E, Granpeesheh D, Mielke L, Traver D, Bock K, et al. Low natural killer cell cytotoxic activity in autism: the role of glutathione, IL-2 and IL-15. *J Neuroimmunol* (2008) 205(1–2):148–54. doi: 10.1016/j.jneuroim.2008.09.005
19. Enstrom AM, Lit L, Onore CE, Gregg JP, Hansen RL, Pessah IN, et al. Altered gene expression and function of peripheral blood natural killer cells in children with autism. *Brain Behav Immun* (2009) 23(1):124–33. doi: 10.1016/j.bbi.2008.08.001
20. Frye RE, Delhey L, Slattery J, Tippett M, Wynne R, Rose S, et al. Blocking and binding folate receptor alpha autoantibodies identify novel autism spectrum disorder subgroups. *Front Neurosci* (2016) 10:80. doi: 10.3389/fnins.2016.00080
21. Frye RE, Slattery J, Delhey L, Furgerson B, Strickland T, Tippett M, et al. Folinic acid improves verbal communication in children with autism and language impairment: a randomized double-blind placebo-controlled trial. *Mol Psychiatry* (2018) 23(2):247–56. doi: 10.1038/mp.2016.168
22. Burger BJ, Rose S, Bennuri SC, Gill PS, Tippett ML, Delhey L, et al. Autistic siblings with novel mutations in two different genes: insight for genetic workups of autistic siblings and connection to mitochondrial dysfunction. *Front Pediatr* (2017) 5:219. doi: 10.3389/fped.2017.00219
23. Delhey L, Kilinc EN, Yin L, Slattery J, Tippett M, Wynne R, et al. Bioenergetic variation is related to autism symptomatology. *Metab Brain Dis* (2017) 32(6):2021–31. doi: 10.1007/s11011-017-0087-0
24. Delhey LM, Nur Kilinc E, Yin L, Slattery JC, Tippett ML, Rose S, et al. The effect of mitochondrial supplements on mitochondrial activity in children with autism spectrum disorder. *J Clin Med* (2017) 6(2):pii:E18. doi: 10.3390/jcm6020018
25. Frye RE, Wynne R, Rose S, Slattery J, Delhey L, Tippett M, et al. Thyroid dysfunction in children with autism spectrum disorder is associated with folate receptor alpha autoimmune disorder. *J Neuroendocrinol* (2017) 29(3) :1-12. doi: 10.1111/jne.12461
26. Delhey LM, Tippett M, Rose S, Bennuri SC, Slattery JC, Melnyk S, et al. Comparison of treatment for metabolic disorders associated with autism:reanalysis of three clinical trials. *Front Neurosci* (2018) 12:19. doi: 10.3389/fnins.2018.00019
27. Howsmon DP, Vargason T, Rubin RA, Delhey L, Tippett M, Rose S, et al. Multivariate techniques enable a biochemical classification of children with autism spectrum disorder versus typically-developing peers: a comparison and validation study. *Bioeng Transl Med* (2018) 3(2):156–65. doi: 10.1002/btm2.10095
28. Vargason T, Kruger U, Roth E, Delhey LM, Tippett M, Rose S, et al. Comparison of three clinical trial treatments for autism spectrum disorder through multivariate analysis of changes in metabolic profiles and adaptive behavior. *Front Cell Neurosci* (2018) 12:503. doi: 10.3389/fncel.2018.00503
29. Rose S, Frye RE, Slattery J, Wynne R, Tippett M, Melnyk S, et al. Oxidative stress induces mitochondrial dysfunction in a subset of autistic lymphoblastoid cell lines. *Transl Psychiatry* (2014) 4:e377. doi: 10.1038/tp.2014.15
30. Rose S, Frye RE, Slattery J, Wynne R, Tippett M, Pavliv O, et al. Oxidative stress induces mitochondrial dysfunction in a subset of autism lymphoblastoid cell lines in a well-matched case control cohort. *PLoS One* (2014) 9(1):e85436. doi: 10.1371/journal.pone.0085436
31. Rose S, Bennuri SC, Wynne R, Melnyk S, James SJ, Frye RE. Mitochondrial and redox abnormalities in autism lymphoblastoid cells: a sibling control study. *FASEB J* (2017) 31(3):904–9. doi: 10.1096/fj.201601004R
32. Bennuri SC, Rose S, Frye RE. Mitochondrial dysfunction is inducible in lymphoblastoid cell lines from children with autism and may involve the TORC1 pathway. *Front Psychiatry* (2019) 10:269. doi: 10.3389/fpsyt.2019.00269
33. Rose S, Wynne R, Frye RE, Melnyk S, James SJ. Increased susceptibility to ethylmercury-induced mitochondrial dysfunction in a subset of autism lymphoblastoid cell lines. *J Toxicol* (2015) 2015:573701. doi: 10.1155/2015/573701
34. Frye RE, Rose S, Chacko J, Wynne R, Bennuri SC, Slattery JC, et al. Modulation of mitochondrial function by the microbiome metabolite propionic acid in autism and control cell lines. *Transl Psychiatry* (2016) 6(10):e927. doi: 10.1038/tp.2016.189
35. Frye RE, Rose S, Wynne R, Bennuri SC, Blossom S, Gilbert KM, et al. Oxidative stress challenge uncovers trichloroacetaldehyde hydrate-induced mitoplasticity in autistic and control lymphoblastoid cell lines. *Sci Rep* (2017) 7(1):4478. doi: 10.1038/s41598-017-04821-3
36. Rose S, Bennuri SC, Davis JE, Wynne R, Slattery JC, Tippett M, et al. Butyrate enhances mitochondrial function during oxidative stress in cell lines from boys with autism. *Transl Psychiatry* (2018) 8(1):42. doi: 10.1038/s41398-017-0089-z
37. Frye RE, Nankova B, Bhattacharyya S, Rose S, Bennuri SC, MacFabe DF. Modulation of immunological pathways in autistic and neurotypical lymphoblastoid cell lines by the enteric microbiome metabolite propionic acid. *Front Immunol* (2017) 8:1670. doi: 10.3389/fimmu.2017.01670
38. Harville TO. "HLA typing for cellular product characterization and identity testing,". In: EllenAreman MM, Loper K, editors. *Cellular Therapy: Principles, Methods, and Regulations*. AABB (2016).
39. Batra A, Cottler-Fox M, Harville T, Rhodes-Clark BS, Makhoul I, Nakagawa M. Autologous graft versus host disease: an emerging complication in patients with multiple myeloma. *Bone Marrow Res* (2014) 2014:891427. doi: 10.1155/2014/891427
40. Jyonouchi H, Geng L, Streck DL, Dermody JJ, Toruner GA. MicroRNA expression changes in association with changes in interleukin-1ss/interleukin10 ratios produced by monocytes in autism spectrum disorders: their association with neuropsychiatric symptoms and comorbid conditions (observational study). *J Neuroinflammation* (2017) 14(1):229. doi: 10.1186/s12974-017-1003-6
41. Jyonouchi H, Geng L, Streck DL, Toruner GA. Immunological characterization and transcription profiling of peripheral blood (PB) monocytes in children with autism spectrum disorders (ASD) and specific polysaccharide antibody deficiency (SPAD): case study. *J Neuroinflammation* (2012) 9:4. doi: 10.1186/1742-2094-9-4

14

Therapeutic Potential of Exogenous Ketone Supplement Induced Ketosis in the Treatment of Psychiatric Disorders

*Zsolt Kovács[1], Dominic P. D'Agostino[2,3], David Diamond[2,4], Mark S. Kindy[5,6,7], Christopher Rogers[2] and Csilla Ari[4]**

[1] Savaria Department of Biology, ELTE Eötvös Loránd University, Savaria University Centre, Szombathely, Hungary, [2] Department of Molecular Pharmacology and Physiology, Laboratory of Metabolic Medicine, Morsani College of Medicine, University of South Florida, Tampa, FL, United States, [3] Institute for Human and Machine Cognition, Ocala, FL, United States, [4] Department of Psychology, Hyperbaric Neuroscience Research Laboratory, University of South Florida, Tampa, FL, United States, [5] Department of Pharmaceutical Sciences, College of Pharmacy, University of South Florida, Tampa, FL, United States, [6] James A. Haley VA Medical Center, Tampa, FL, United States, [7] Shriners Hospital for Children, Tampa, FL, United States

***Correspondence:**
Csilla Ari
csari2000@yahoo.com

Globally, psychiatric disorders, such as anxiety disorder, bipolar disorder, schizophrenia, depression, autism spectrum disorder, and attention-deficit/hyperactivity disorder (ADHD) are becoming more prevalent. Although the exact pathological alterations are not yet clear, recent studies have demonstrated that widespread changes of very complex metabolic pathways may partially underlie the pathophysiology of many psychiatric diseases. Thus, more attention should be directed to metabolic-based therapeutic interventions in the treatment of psychiatric disorders. Emerging evidence from numerous studies suggests that administration of exogenous ketone supplements, such as ketone salts or ketone esters, generates rapid and sustained nutritional ketosis and metabolic changes, which may evoke potential therapeutic effects in cases of central nervous system (CNS) disorders, including psychiatric diseases. Therefore, the aim of this review is to summarize the current information on ketone supplementation as a potential therapeutic tool for psychiatric disorders. Ketone supplementation elevates blood levels of the ketone bodies: D-β-hydroxybutyrate (βHB), acetoacetate (AcAc), and acetone. These compounds, either directly or indirectly, beneficially affect the mitochondria, glycolysis, neurotransmitter levels, activity of free fatty acid receptor 3 (FFAR3), hydroxycarboxylic acid receptor 2 (HCAR2), and histone deacetylase, as well as functioning of NOD-like receptor pyrin domain 3 (NLRP3) inflammasome and mitochondrial uncoupling protein (UCP) expression. The result of downstream cellular and molecular changes is a reduction in the pathophysiology associated with various psychiatric disorders.

Abbreviations: A_1R and $A_{2A}R$, different types of adenosine receptors; AcAc, acetoacetate; ADHD, attention-deficit/hyperactivity disorder; BBB, blood–brain barrier; βHB, D-beta-hydroxybutyrate (R-3-hydroxybutyrate); β-OHBD, βHB dehydrogenase; CNS, central nervous system; COX-2, cyclooxygenase-2; FFAR3, free fatty acid receptor 3; HCAR2, hydroxycarboxylic acid receptor 2; HPA, hypothalamic-pituitary-adrenal; HMG-CoA, hydroxymethylglutaryl-CoA; HMGL, hydroxymethylglutaryl-CoA-lyase; HMGS, hydroxymethylglutaryl-CoA-synthase; KE, ketone ester; KS, ketone salt; IL-1β, interleukin-1β; MCT, medium chain triglyceride; NLRP3, NOD-like receptor pyrin domain 3; ROS, reactive oxygen species; SCOT: succinyl-CoA:3-ketoacid CoA transferase; SSRI, selective serotonin reuptake inhibitor; UCP, uncoupling proteins; WAG/Rij, Wistar Albino Glaxo/Rijswijk.

We conclude that supplement-induced nutritional ketosis leads to metabolic changes and improvements, for example, in mitochondrial function and inflammatory processes, and suggest that development of specific adjunctive ketogenic protocols for psychiatric diseases should be actively pursued.

Keywords: psychiatric diseases, exogenous ketone supplements, ketosis, mitochondrial dysfunction, inflammation

INTRODUCTION

With an increasing global prevalence, psychiatric disorders can present as serious medical conditions composed of emotional, cognitive, social, behavioral, and functional impairments (1). Lifetime onset of major depressive disorders in the general population is up to 11–16% (2, 3), with bipolar disorder present in 1% (4, 5), schizophrenia in 1% (6, 7), and anxiety disorder in 5–31% (1). In relation to attention-deficit/hyperactivity disorder (ADHD), worldwide prevalence of this disease in children/adolescence and adults is about 5.3% and 2.5%, respectively (8, 9), while about 1 in 68 children were diagnosed with autism in the United States in 2012 (10). It has been demonstrated that not only genetic factors but also environmental factors (e.g., infections, early traumas, and drugs), age, sociodemographic factors (e.g., ethnicity and socioeconomic status), and a complex interplay between these factors have a role in the pathophysiology of different psychiatric diseases, such as anxiety disorder (1, 11), bipolar disorder (5), schizophrenia (6, 12), major depressive disorder (2, 13, 14), autism spectrum disorder (15), and ADHD (16). Close association between different psychiatric disorders, such as anxiety disorder and major depressive disorder, has been demonstrated (5, 17–21).

However, while symptoms, characteristics, and classification of different psychiatric disorders are adequately described (1, 5, 7, 15, 16, 22), the pathophysiology of psychiatric diseases is not yet fully understood. Nevertheless, recent studies have demonstrated that the disturbance in the monoaminergic (23–26) and other neurotransmitter systems (e.g., glutamatergic, purinergic, and GABAergic) (27–34), in addition to widespread changes of very complex and connected metabolic pathways, may partially explain the general condition. For example, it has been suggested that mitochondrial dysfunction could play a major role (35). Mitochondrial dysfunction may decrease energy/ATP production, impair calcium homeostasis, increase levels of reactive oxygen species (ROS), and alter apoptotic pathways, inflammatory processes, neurotransmission, synaptic plasticity, and neuronal activity and connectivity (35, 36). Moreover, changes in hypothalamic–pituitary–adrenal (HPA) axis activity were also demonstrated in patients with psychiatric diseases, in which alterations may influence mitochondrial functions: a chronic increase in glucocorticoid levels may decrease mitochondrial energy production (35, 37). Membrane lipid dysregulation may affect the levels of pro-inflammatory cytokines, as well as the function of mitochondria, ion channels, and neurotransmitter systems implicated in the pathophysiology of psychiatric diseases (38, 39). In addition, changes in membrane fatty acid composition may alter the function of different cell-surface receptors, ion pumps, and special enzymes, such as 5'-nucleotidase, adenylate cyclase, and Na^+/K^+-ATPase (38, 40). Increased activity of the inflammatory system and redox pathways may enhance oxidative and nitrosative stress, mitochondrial dysfunction, neurodegeneration and neuronal death, production of pro-inflammatory cytokines, and activity of the HPA axis, whereas it may decrease neurogenesis and serotonin levels (35, 37). In addition, functional brain imaging studies demonstrated abnormalities in regional cerebral glucose metabolism in the prefrontal cortex in patients with mood disorders, providing evidence of persistent hypometabolism, particularly in the frontal gyrus, in depressed patients (41). Recent transcriptomic, proteomic, and metabolomics studies have also highlighted an abnormal cerebral glucose and energy metabolism as one of the potential pathophysiological mechanisms of schizophrenia, raising the possibility that a metabolically based intervention might have therapeutic value in the management of the disease (42).

Consequently, different metabolic changes and their downstream effects may generate complex, interlinked molecular and cellular processes, which may lead to different psychiatric diseases. It can be concluded that alterations in multiple interactive metabolic pathways and their effects on different physiological processes may largely underlie the pathophysiology in patients with psychiatric diseases. Indeed, if defective metabolism is the cause of such pathologies, then utilization of therapies designed to address deficiencies of metabolism (known as metabolic therapies) would be a rational approach for the treatment of these diseases.

In a process known as ketogenesis, the ketone bodies [D-β-hydroxybutyrate (βHB), acetoacetate (AcAc), and acetone] are catabolized under normal physiological conditions by the liver from fatty acids as a source of fuel (43–45). Higher levels of ketones are produced during starvation, fasting, and neonatal development (46, 47). Moreover, although most of βHB, which is used as an energy source in the brain, is synthesized by the liver, ketone body synthesis and release by astrocytes have also been demonstrated (48, 49). Ketone bodies can transport to the bloodstream from the liver, cross the blood–brain barrier (BBB), enter brain cells through monocarboxylic transporters, convert to acetyl CoA in the mitochondria, and enter the Krebs cycle (43–44, 45, 50). Through this process, ketosis (increased ketone body levels in the blood) provides energy by metabolism of ketone bodies to acetyl-CoA and synthesis of ATP for cells in the central nervous system (CNS) (43, 51, 52). It has been demonstrated in animal—and/or human studies—that ketogenic diets and supplements may have metabolism-based therapeutic potential in the treatment of several diseases, such as Alzheimer's disease (53–57), Parkinson's disease (54, 58–60), glucose transporter type 1-deficiency syndrome (61–63), amyotrophic lateral sclerosis (60, 64), cancer (44, 58, 65, 66), epilepsy (54, 67, 68), schizophrenia (42, 69–74), anxiety (55, 75–77), autism spectrum disorder (78–81), and depression (69, 77, 82).

Ketogenic diets are high-fat, adequate protein and very low carbohydrate diets that may have an alleviating role on psychiatric diseases (69, 73), likely through bioenergetics, ketone metabolism, and signaling, as well as their effects on, for example, neuronal activity, neurotransmitter balance, and inflammatory processes (43, 52, 83–91). Strict patient compliance to the KD is the primary factor in achieving therapeutic ketosis, and this is often difficult or impossible in the psychiatric population (69). Therefore, the administration of exogenous ketone supplements including medium chain triglycerides (MCTs), ketone salt (KS), ketone ester (KE), and their combination with MCT oil (e.g., KSMCT) presents a strategy to circumvent dietary restriction to rapidly induce and sustain nutritional ketosis (65, 75, 84, 92). Ketone bodies not only enhance cell energy metabolism through anaplerotic effects but also suppress oxidative stress, decrease inflammatory processes, and regulate functions of ion channels and neurotransmitter systems (45, 93, 94)—all processes implicated in the pathophysiology of psychiatric diseases (1, 5, 6, 15, 16, 22). Therefore, the rationale exists for the use of exogenous ketone supplementation, which induces a nutritional ketotic state similar to that derived from the ketogenic diet and may mimic the effects of ketogenic diet on several CNS diseases through ketone body-evoked metabolic and signaling alterations (54, 55, 67, 75, 95–99) and epigenetic effects (100).

In contrast to diabetic ketosis, which can induce pathological levels of blood βHB (ranging >25 mM) and potentially lead to life-threatening acidosis, nutritional ketosis elevates blood βHB from the normal range (0.1–0.2 mM) to a safe and—in many cases—therapeutic range (1–7 mM: therapeutic ketosis) (44, 54, 101). While rigorous adherence to ketogenic diets is typically difficult to follow and requires clear medical guidance and strong motivation, consumption of exogenous ketogenic agents effectively induces ketosis with little difficulty (65, 75, 84, 92, 102). Moreover, prolonged consumption of ketogenic diets may generate side effects, such as weight loss, alteration of mentation, growth retardation, nephrolithiasis, nausea, constipation, gastritis, hyperlipidemia, hypoglycemia, hyperuricemia, and ulcerative colitis (44, 69, 103, 104). Consequently, developing a safer alternative method using ketone body precursors and exogenous ketone supplements, such as KSs or KEs, to circumvent dietary restriction is appealing.

Recent research has demonstrated that it is possible to rapidly increase and maintain blood levels of ketone bodies in a dose-dependent manner in both animals and humans (54, 84, 99) for the treatment of several CNS diseases (55, 64, 67, 75). Thus, it is possible that exogenous ketone supplementation-induced ketosis may be an effective therapeutic tool against psychiatric diseases. Indeed, exogenous ketone supplements have a modulatory influence on behavior and anxiolytic effect in animal studies (55, 75, 83). Moreover, in contrast to ketogenic diets, exogenous ketone supplements are relatively well-tolerated and can be formulated and titrated to minimize or avoid side effects (56, 65, 75, 84, 99, 105, 106).

There is limited evidence to support the beneficial effects of exogenous ketone supplements in psychiatric diseases at the moment [e.g., Refs. (55, 75, 76)], but the use of exogenous ketone supplements may be a viable alternative or adjuvant to pharmacotherapy in the treatment of these disorders. Consequently, in the following major section, we provide a short overview of the metabolism of exogenous ketone supplements, which results in rapid and safe mild therapeutic ketosis and, as a consequence, may be an alternative method to ketogenic diets for the treatment of psychiatric disorders. In the next major sections, therapeutic potential of exogenous ketone supplements in the treatment of each psychiatric disease is summarized. This is followed by a brief conclusions section with perspective and future outlook.

METABOLISM OF EXOGENOUS KETONE SUPPLEMENTS: GENERATION OF THERAPEUTIC KETOSIS

Under typical (high carbohydrate) diet conditions, glycogen-derived glucose is the main energy source of brain cells (43, 107). However, ketogenic diets, starvation, and fasting result in an increased reliance of the brain on fat-derived ketones for fuel (43, 44, 108). Free fatty acids are converted into acyl-CoA in the liver cells, and subsequently, acyl-CoA is metabolized to acetyl-CoA by mitochondrial β-oxidation (**Figure 1A**). Acetyl-CoA may generate energy (*via* Krebs cycle: tricarboxylic acid cycle/TCA cycle) or it gets converted into ketone bodies (43–44, 45, 50). As hepatocytes are not able to utilize the high levels of acetyl-CoA derived from ketogenic diet-, starvation-, and fasting-evoked increase in fatty acids, under these conditions, a large portion of acetyl-CoA can be converted to ketone bodies (44, 45, 107). Two acetyl-CoA molecules fuse into one acetoacetyl-CoA molecule by acetoacetyl-CoA-thiolase. Subsequently, hydroxymethylglutaryl-CoA-synthase (HMGS) condenses the third acetyl-CoA molecule with acetoacetyl-CoA to form hydroxymethylglutaryl-CoA (HMG-CoA) (this process, catalyzed by HMGS, is the rate-limiting step of ketogenesis) (43–44, 45, 50). AcAc is liberated from HMG-CoA by hydroxymethylglutaryl-CoA-lyase (HMGL). AcAc may reduce to βHB by a NADH molecule in a βHB dehydrogenase (β-OHBD) catalyzed reaction, or, in lesser amounts, a part of AcAc may metabolize to acetone by the spontaneous, non-enzymatic decarboxylation of AcAc (43–44, 45, 50). The major circulating water-soluble ketone body is βHB (44, 50). AcAc is a chemically unstable molecule, and acetone is a very volatile compound (eliminated mainly *via* respiration from the lungs) (44, 50). As the metabolic enzyme succinyl-CoA:3-ketoacid CoA transferase (SCOT) is not expressed in the liver, hepatocytes are not able to consume ketone bodies as an energy substrate (45, 50, 52); thus, AcAc and βHB can exit the liver, enter the bloodstream, and be distributed to various tissues, including the brain, after transport through monocarboxylate transporters (43–44, 45, 50). In the mitochondria of brain cells, ketone bodies are converted back to acetyl-CoA (**Figure 1A**) (43–44, 45, 50). As the first step of this metabolic pathway, βHB oxidizes to AcAc by NAD^+ and β-OHBD. AcAc is then metabolized to acetoacetyl-CoA, which converts to two acetyl-CoA molecules (by SCOT and acetoacetyl-CoA-thiolase, respectively). Finally, acetyl-CoA molecules enter the Krebs cycle as an energy source for ATP synthesis (43–44, 45, 50).

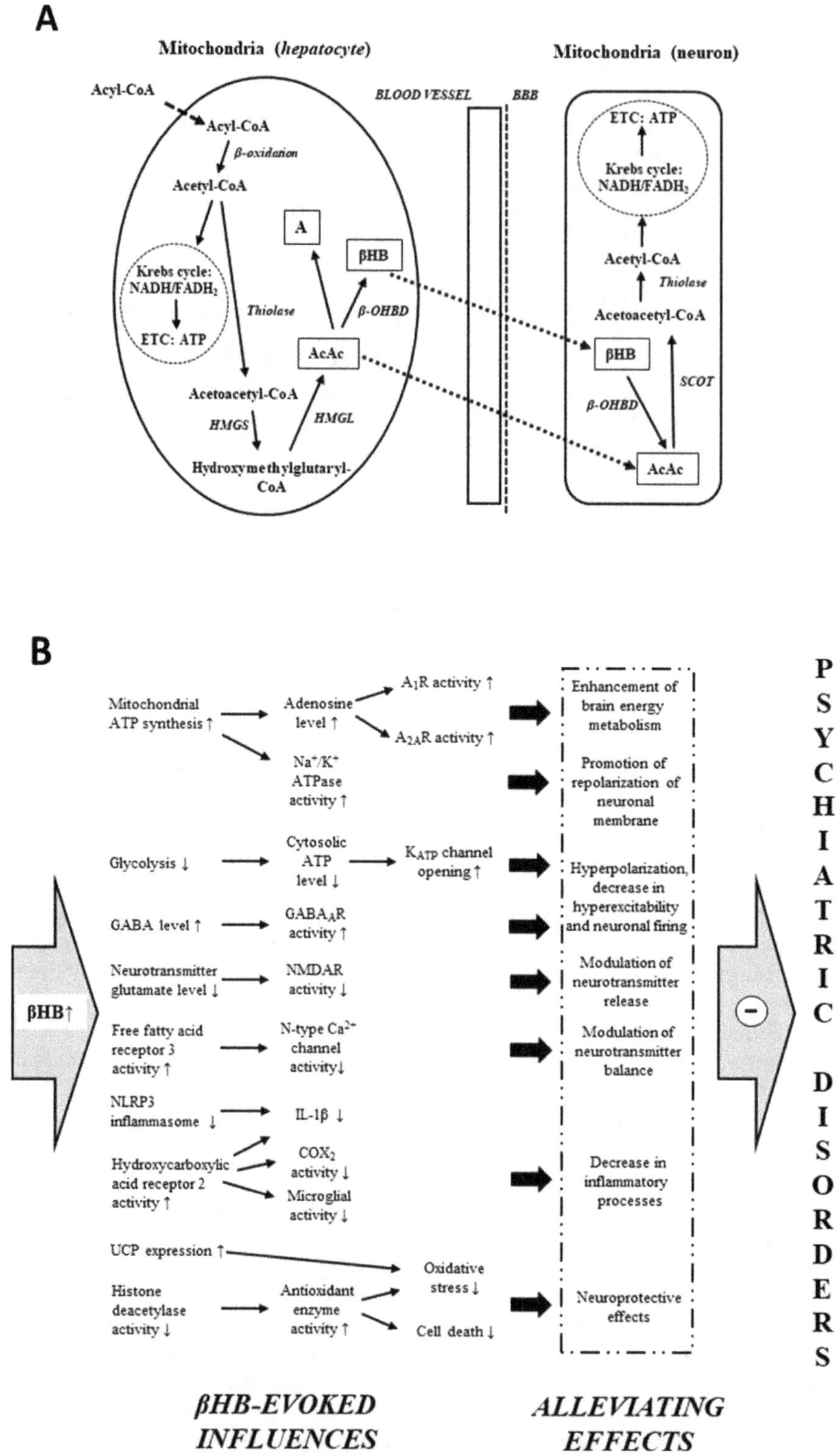

FIGURE 1 | Mitochondrial ketone body metabolism: ketogenesis in liver cells (*hepatocytes*) and ketolysis in brain cells (neuron) **(A)**. Main βHB-evoked metabolic effects and their consequences, which may evoke alleviating effects on different psychiatric diseases **(B)** (see text for more detailed putative mechanisms by which βHB may evoke alleviating effects on psychiatric diseases). Abbreviations: A, acetone; A_1R and $A_{2A}R$, different types of adenosine receptors; AcAc, acetoacetate; ATP, adenosine triphosphate; BBB, blood–brain barrier; βHB, D-beta-hydroxybutyrate (R-3-hydroxybutyrate); β-OHBD, βHB dehydrogenase; COX-2, cyclooxygenase-2; ETC, electron transport chain; GABA, gamma-aminobutyric acid; HMGL, hydroxymethylglutaryl-CoA-lyase; HMGS, hydroxymethylglutaryl-CoA-synthase; IL-1β, interleukin-1β; NADH/$FADH_2$, nicotinamide adenine dinucleotide/flavin adenine dinucleotide; NLRP3, NOD-like receptor pyrin domain 3; NMDAR, N-methyl-D-aspartate receptor; SCOT, succinyl-CoA:3-ketoacid CoA transferase; thiolase, acetoacetyl-CoA-thiolase; UCP, uncoupling proteins.

While a ketogenic diet could potentially confer numerous benefits to patients suffering from psychiatric disorders, compliance to the diet would likely be low. Reasons include the lack of knowledge, support, palatability, and different adverse effects such as gastrointestinal side effects (69, 103, 104). Most importantly, ketogenic diets must continuously restrict carbohydrates (typically 20 g/day) to sustain ketogenesis through elevated long-chain fatty acid oxidation (109). Nevertheless, the production of ketone bodies from KSs or KEs (e.g., by liver alcohol dehydrogenase and/or hydrolysis in the small intestine) is not inhibited by carbohydrates; thus, ketone supplements may be usable while maintaining a normal diet (105) to generate therapeutic ketosis.

After consumption or gavage administration, KEs are fully hydrolyzed in the small intestine by esterases, which can be transported to the systemic bloodstream, and converted to 1,3-butanediol. Following this, 1,3-butanediol is metabolized to AcAc and βHB in the liver by alcohol and aldehyde dehydrogenase (106, 110, 111). Moreover, MCTs/MCT oils are hydrolyzed to medium chain fatty acids (e.g., decanoic and octanoic acid) by lipases in the gastrointestinal tract, which are metabolized to ketone bodies in the liver (112). Thus, similar to ketogenic diets, metabolism of exogenous ketone supplements may result in increased levels of blood ketone bodies, which may serve the energy needs of brain cells (**Figure 1A**). For example, KS supplementation significantly increased the mitochondrial activity of both β-OHBD and acetoacetyl-CoA-thiolase in the brain of rats (83), and oral administration of exogenous ketone supplements is able to evoke and maintain rapid and safe mild ketosis in both animals and human (54, 64, 65, 75, 84, 92, 99, 101, 106, 108).

Unfortunately, MCTs are often not well tolerated because of their gastrointestinal side effects (e.g., diarrhea, dyspepsia, and flatulence) and supplementation of MCTs generates relatively low levels of ketone bodies in the blood (113). Oral administration of KEs fully metabolizes to βHB and AcAc and, as a consequence, more effectively increases ketone body levels compared to MCTs (56). KEs, such as (R)-3-hydroxybutyl-(R)-3-hydroxybutyrate and R,S-1,3-butanediol AcAc diester, are well-tolerated, safe, and efficient ketogenic agents in both animals and humans (56, 99, 105, 106). Moreover, it was demonstrated that a proper dose of KS alone (99) or in combination with other exogenous ketone supplements, such as KE and MCT (KEKS and KSMCT, respectively), may be a safe and efficacious way to achieve ketosis (65, 75, 84, 99). Thus, exogenous ketone supplements may be an effective alternative to ketogenic diets for therapeutic ketosis.

THERAPEUTIC POTENTIAL OF EXOGENOUS KETONE SUPPLEMENTS IN THE TREATMENT OF PSYCHIATRIC DISEASES

Although there has been remarkable progress in our knowledge on the biological effects and mechanisms of action of exogenous ketone supplements, their exact mechanisms on CNS diseases are largely unknown. It has been demonstrated that an increase in ketone body/βHB concentration may modulate neurotransmitter balance and release (43, 52, 85), decrease hyperexcitability, reduce firing rates of neurons (43, 84, 86), decrease neuroinflammation (43, 91), enhance brain energy metabolism (43, 50, 83, 84, 87), and provide neuroprotective effects (43, 45, 84, 88, 90), which together may protect different physiological processes under pathological conditions resulting in CNS diseases, such as psychiatric disorders (35–36, 37, 58, 69). Thus, it is possible that exogenous ketone supplement-evoked ketosis (65, 75, 84) and its significant metabolic effects, as well as their consequences, may have both preventive and therapeutic potential as a metabolic-based therapy in patients with psychiatric diseases (**Figure 1B**). In spite of the several metabolic alterations, the mechanism of action of exogenous ketone supplement-evoked ketosis on different psychiatric diseases was not investigated comprehensively. As a result, we have only limited results in relation to exact links between alleviating effects of ketone supplement-generated ketosis and pathological changes in psychiatric diseases. Nevertheless, both recent literature results on basic pathomechanisms of psychiatric diseases and mechanisms of therapeutic effects of exogenous ketone supplement-evoked ketosis strongly support the hypothesis that exogenous ketone supplement-evoked ketosis may modulate the background pathophysiological processes of psychiatric diseases. Indeed, an MCT diet caused anxiolytic effects (76) and βHB decreased anxiety-related and depressive behaviors in rats and mice (114, 115). It has also been demonstrated that sub-chronic (7 days) oral administration of exogenous ketone supplements, such as KE, KS, and KSMCT, evoked an anxiolytic effect in normal rats (Sprague–Dawley/SPD rats) and diseased rats (Wistar Albino Glaxo/Rijswijk rats: WAG/Rij rats; a rat model of human absence epilepsy) on elevated plus maze (EPM) test in correlation with increased levels of βHB (75, 95). Elevated ketone body levels were demonstrated in schizophrenic patients, suggesting that the energy supply of brain shifts from glucose towards ketone bodies in this disease (116). Based on correlation between βHB plasma levels and symptoms it was suggested that βHB may have a protective effect on executive functions in patients treated with schizophrenia (117). Other studies presented cases of patients with chronic schizoaffective disorders where the KD begin helping with mood and psychotic symptoms within 1 month or lead to remission of psychotic symptoms (73, 74). It has also been suggested that plasma level of βHB is associated with severity of depression in human and that βHB-evoked antidepressant-like effects may be in relation to its inhibitory effect on NOD-like receptor pyrin domain 3 (NLRP3)-induced neuro-inflammatory processes. The authors also suggested that modification of βHB levels by diet may be a novel therapeutic target for the treatment of mood disorders, such as depression (115, 118). In addition, ketosis (induction of βHB) may be the primary mediator of the therapeutic effect of the ketogenic diet and exogenous ketone supplements on different CNS diseases. From this viewpoint, the effect of exogenous ketone supplements mimics the ketogenic diet (43, 44, 51, 52, 54, 58, 72, 94, 96, 101, 119). Thus, ketogenic diet-evoked effects on psychiatric diseases may result (at least partly) from beneficial metabolic effects of βHB, for example, on mitochondrial functions, neuronal activity, neurotransmitter release, and inflammatory processes (43, 50, 52, 86, 91). Indeed, administration of a ketogenic diet not only increased the ketone body level but also was associated with improvements in anxiety disorder (75, 77), bipolar disorder (120), schizophrenia (42, 70, 73, 74, 121), depression (77, 122), autism spectrum disorder (78, 80, 123), and ADHD (124, 125) in animal models and/or humans, suggesting the beneficial effects of exogenous ketone supplement-induced ketosis on psychiatric diseases (**Figure 1B**).

However, thorough investigation of signaling pathways by which exogenous ketone supplement-evoked ketosis exerts beneficial effects on psychiatric diseases is needed. In the following subsection, we provide an overview of the main putative basic mechanisms, by which ketone supplement-evoked ketosis may alleviate different pathophysiological processes involved in psychiatric disorders.

Ketosis-Generated Effects on Mitochondrial Functions, Neurotransmitter Systems, Inflammatory Processes, and Their Consequences: Putative Alleviating Influences on Psychiatric Diseases

It has been demonstrated that ketone bodies serve as alternative fuel for brain cells when the glucose supply is insufficient: ketone bodies improve mitochondrial respiration and enhance mitochondrial ATP synthesis (**Figure 1B**) (47, 126). Increased mitochondrial ATP production may promote the repolarization of neuronal membrane after stimulation by means of Na^+/K^+ ATPase and may modulate the neurotransmitter levels (119). In addition, βHB may inhibit vesicular glutamate transporters (127). This effect, together with increased ATP production, decreases glutamate loading to vesicles and glutamate release and, as a consequence, suppresses neuronal excitability (68, 119, 127).

It was recently demonstrated that βHB inhibits the activity of N-type Ca^{2+} channels in sympathetic nerve terminals and may decrease the release of noradrenaline *via* activation of its G-protein-coupled receptor free fatty acid receptor 3 (FFAR3) (128). Increased levels of ketone bodies, such as βHB, may evoke other changes in metabolic pathways, such as inhibition of glycolysis (43). An inhibition of glycolysis may result in decreased levels of cytosolic ATP and, as a consequence, increased activity of ATP-sensitive potassium (K_{ATP}) channels generating hyperpolarization of neuronal membrane and decrease in neuronal activity (43, 129). As it was demonstrated, ketosis not only decreases glutamate release and extracellular glutamate levels and enhances the GABAergic effects by means of increased GABA levels and $GABA_A$ receptor activity (43, 68) but also increases adenosine levels (130) and may modulate metabolism of monoamines (**Figure 1B**). For example, increased levels of noradrenaline in mice brain (131) and decreased levels of metabolites of monoamine dopamine and serotonin (homovanillic acid/HVA and 5-hydroxyindole acetic acid/5-HIAA, respectively) in the human cerebrospinal fluid (132) were demonstrated under a ketotic state. Increased levels of extracellular adenosine lead to increased activity of adenosine receptors and may decrease hyperexcitability *via* A_1Rs, increase hyperpolarization of neuronal membrane, and decrease neuronal activity (133, 134). In addition, adenosine decreases the energy demand of brain tissue (e.g., *via* A_1R and A_{2A}R) (135), modulates immune system functions (e.g., activation of A_{2A}R decreases the inflammation-induced cytokine production from microglial cells) (136), and has a neuroprotective effect (e.g., evokes a decrease in oxidative stress and attenuates the harmful influence of ROS on brain cells *via* A_1R) (137, 138).

β-Hydroxybutyrate may exert its effects on numerous targets, including oxidative stress mediators (e.g., by inhibition of histone deacetylases and increased activity of antioxidant enzymes) and metabolic rate (e.g., increased NAD^+–NAD^+/NADH ratio) directly and/or indirectly *via* its G-protein-coupled receptors, such as hydroxycarboxylic acid receptor 2 (HCAR2, also known as PUMA-G or GPR109 receptor) (45, 90, 139, 140). As an endogenous ligand, βHB activates the HCAR2 receptor expressed on, for example, microglial cells (141). HCAR2 mediates the inhibitory effects of βHB on neurodegeneration, microglial activation, and inflammatory processes [e.g., decreases the expression/level of interleukins, such as interleukin-1β (IL-1β), and lipopolysaccharide/LPS-induced increase in cyclooxygenase-2/COX-2 activity and interleukin levels] (141–143) (**Figure 1B**). NOD-like receptor pyrin domain 3 inflammasome is a multiprotein complex, which may evoke cleavage of pro-IL-1β to its active form (IL-1β) for secretion by caspase-1 (144, 145). It was demonstrated that βHB decreases inflammatory processes likely through inhibition of NLRP3: βHB decreased not only the expression of NLRP3 and caspase-1 but also the level/release of proinflammatory cytokines, such as IL-1β (91, 146).

In general, oxidative stress damages proteins, lipids, and nucleic acids. One putative downstream effect of this damage is the opening of the mitochondrial permeability transition (mPT) pore and, as a consequence, activation of the apoptotic cascade processes pursuant to release of cytochrome c to the cytoplasm (147). It was demonstrated that increased production of ROS may activate mPT pore (97, 147). Ketone bodies decreased oxidative stress and ROS formation by enhancing complex I (NADH dehydrogenase)-driven mitochondrial respiration (140). It has also been demonstrated that KE increased both ketone body levels and expression of mitochondrial uncoupling proteins (UCPs; e.g., UCP 4 and UCP 5 in rat brain), which can decrease the production of ROS (50, 148) (**Figure 1B**). In addition, it was suggested that βHB not only prevents neuronal loss but also preserves synaptic function: βHB mitigates effects, which may evoke cell death/apoptosis (e.g., glutamate excitotoxicity, enhanced ROS production, impaired mitochondrial energetic functions, pathogenic mutations on mitochondrial DNA, and activation of mPT pore) (44, 97, 119, 149), and βHB may restore impairment of hippocampal long-term potentiation (150).

The changes induced by ketosis may lead to enhanced brain energy metabolism, promotion of repolarization of neuronal membrane, neuronal hyperpolarization, decreased hyperexcitability and neuronal firing, modulation of neurotransmitter release/balance, neuroprotective effects, and decreased inflammatory processes (**Figure 1B**). Downstream effects may include increased

GABA and ATP/adenosine levels, decreased levels of glutamate and IL-1β, and reductions in neuronal excitability and ROS formation. Based on these putative alleviating effects, which may have therapeutic potential in the treatment of different psychiatric diseases, this subsection is followed by a brief overview of the main pathological changes in different psychiatric diseases, which may be modulated or improved by ketosis-evoked beneficial effects and their consequences. Currently, we lack detailed information for understanding the exact mechanisms by which ketosis evokes beneficial effects on psychiatric disorders. However, we can be reasonably confident that the alleviating effects of exogenous ketone supplements on these disorders affect several interacting factors, including mitochondrial function, neurotransmitter levels, and inflammatory processes.

Anxiety Disorders

An increasing body of evidence suggests that dysregulation of the glutamatergic, serotonergic, purinergic, and GABAergic systems plays a role in the pathophysiology of anxiety disorders (33, 34, 151–153). For example, inhibition of NMDA and AMPA receptors by their antagonists (e.g., DL-2-amino-5-phosphonovaleric acid/APV and 6-cyano-7-nitroquinoxaline-2,3-dione/CNQX, respectively) fully or partially blocked the expression and/or acquisition of fear conditioning (30, 154). Activation of the serotonergic system (e.g., *via* increased levels of serotonin by selective serotonin reuptake inhibitors/SSRIs and activation of serotonin 5-HT1A receptors by buspirone or tandospirone) and increased activity of adenosinergic system (e.g., *via* activation of A_1 type of adenosine receptors/A_1R) have an anxiolytic effect (34, 155). Moreover, enhanced GABAergic neurotransmission evoked an anxiolytic effect, whereas decreased GABAergic transmission generated anxiogenic responses in animals (151, 153, 156). Altered functions are present in many regions, including the extended amygdala, ventromedial prefrontal cortex, hippocampus, hypothalamus, and the midbrain, and changed connections between these areas are implicated in the pathophysiology of anxiety disorders (157–159). Specific changes, such as underactivation (e.g., in ventromedial prefrontal cortex), overactivaton (e.g., in amygdala), and deficient functional connectivity (e.g., between hippocampus and amygdala), have also been demonstrated (157, 158, 160, 161). Changes in gray matter volume (e.g., in the right orbitofrontal cortex, amygdala, and hippocampus) (160, 162, 163), as well as dysfunction or hyperactivation of HPA axis and inflammatory system (e.g., increased level of proinflammatory cytokines) (14, 164), may have a role in pathophysiology of anxiety disorders. It was also demonstrated that mitochondrial dysfunctions and oxidative stress may be key factors in the emergence of anxiety disorders (165, 166).

Schizophrenia

It has been demonstrated that alterations in the neurotransmitter systems governed by GABA, glutamate, and the monoamines are involved in the development of schizophrenia (7, 23, 27, 32, 167–169). For example, in the prefrontal cortex, which partially mediates the negative symptoms of schizophrenia, low serotonin and dopamine levels were detected (7, 23). Cognitive symptoms may be linked with decreased level of GABA and serotonin (e.g., in the dorsolateral prefrontal cortex) (7, 170). Moreover, decrease in serotonin level was demonstrated in amygdala, which may lead to aggressive symptoms (7). It was concluded that, among others, hypofunction of the inhibitory GABAergic interneurons and changes in activity of implicated brain areas (e.g., because of decreased activity of inhibitory effects and imbalance between inhibitory/excitatory processes) have a role in the pathophysiology of schizophrenia (7, 167). Another recent study using an acute NMDA receptor hypofunction model of schizophrenia showed that feeding C57BL/6 mice a low carbohydrate/high-fat KD for 7 weeks prevented a variety of behavioral abnormalities induced by pharmacological inhibition of NMDA glutamate receptors (42). In the study, they found a lack of correlation between the measured prepulse inhibition of startle and body weight changes, providing evidence against the role of calorie restriction in its mechanism of action (42). Case studies on human patients with schizophrenia also supported the efficacy of using KD to improve symptoms (73, 74). Reduction in the volume of brain areas encompassing cortical gray and white matter (e.g., in amygdala and hippocampus/sensorimotor and dorsolateral prefrontal cortices) (171–173), gliosis (174), and increased neuronal apoptosis (7, 175) were also demonstrated in patients with schizophrenia. A great deal of evidence suggests that microglial activation, oxidative stress (e.g., increase in ROS activity), and mitochondrial dysfunction (e.g., changes in activity of complex I and cytochrome-c-oxidase/IV of electron transport chain) may also be involved in the pathophysiology of schizophrenia (167, 176–178). Increased activation of HPA axis by psychological stress, inflammatory processes, and increased level of cytokines (e.g., tumor necrosis factor alpha/TNF-α and IL-1β), as well as enhanced levels of glutamate and dopamine auto-oxidation, could lead to enhanced production of ROS and subsequently neurodegeneration and apoptosis (7, 167, 178–180).

Major Depressive Disorder

Structural brain alterations, such as decreased volume and cell number of brain areas (e.g., in hippocampus and several cortical areas) (3, 181–183) and abnormalities in activation or connectivity of brain structures and networks (e.g., chronic hyperactivity of limbic centers and brainstem) (13, 22, 184–186), may underlie the functional and behavioral changes observed in depressed patients. It has been demonstrated that changes in several components, including the glutamatergic system (e.g., increased glutamate level) (29), monoaminergic system (e.g., decrease in the level of serotonin, noradrenaline, and dopamine) (3, 13, 24, 187, 188), GABAergic system (e.g., reduced plasma and cerebrospinal fluid GABA levels) (189, 190), and purinergic system (e.g., overexpression of A_{2A} type of adenosine receptors/$A_{2A}R$) (28) have a role in the pathophysiology of major depressive disorder. Activation of microglia and astrocytes and inflammatory pathways (14, 164, 191, 192) may be associated with major depressive disorder. For example, increased activation and expression of NLRP3 inflammasome and interleukins (e.g., IL-1β) were revealed in both animal models and patients with depression (13, 193, 194). Hyperactivity of HPA system was also demonstrated (195). Neurodegeneration and neuronal death (e.g., through increased oxidative/nitrosative stress) and alterations in mitochondrial functions (e.g., decreased ATP production as well as enhanced apoptosis and oxidative stress) (35, 177, 196) also play a role in the emergence of major depressive disorder. It has been demonstrated that enhancement of inflammatory processes is associated with depression by modulation of different neurotransmitter systems: for example, inflammatory cytokines (e.g., IL-1β) reduce synaptic availability of monoamines and increase excitotoxicity (*via* extrasynaptic NMDA receptors) by increasing levels of extracellular glutamate (164, 197, 198). Moreover, cytokines may evoke decreased motivation and anhedonia *via* different pathways (e.g., by decreased release of dopamine in the basal ganglia) (164, 199).

Bipolar Disorder

It has been demonstrated that imbalance in monoaminergic neurotransmitter system (e.g., serotonergic, dopaminergic, and noradrenergic) (200–202), GABAergic system (e.g., decreased GABAergic transmission) (190), purinergic system (e.g., increased level of uric acid and reduced adenosinergic activity at A_1Rs) (31), and glutamatergic system (e.g., increased glutamate levels and NMDA receptor activity) (29) are associated with bipolar disorder. These alterations may be associated with mitochondrial dysfunction (e.g., deficit in activity of complexes I and IV), apoptosis, increase in ROS, oxidative damage, hyperexcitability (5, 177, 203, 204), and, as a consequence, decrease in glial cell or neuron number and gray matter, as well as changes in connectivity between implicated brain areas (e.g., hippocampus, prefrontal cortex, and amygdala) (205–207). Changes in endocrine functions (e.g., dysregulation of HPA axis) and inflammatory processes (e.g., increased proinflammatory cytokine levels, such as IL-1β) were demonstrated in association with bipolar disorder (203, 208).

Autism Spectrum Disorder

It has been demonstrated that agenesis of corpus callosum, changes in brain volume, thinning of several brain cortical areas (e.g., in the frontal parietal lobe), and decreased functional connectivity between brain areas (e.g., within frontal cortex) contribute to pathophysiology of autism spectrum disorder (209–212). It was also demonstrated that dysfunction in glutamatergic system (e.g., exaggerated signaling) (213–215) and GABAergic system (e.g., decreased GABA receptor expression and GABA-evoked inhibitory effects) (215, 216) may have a role in the pathophysiology of autism spectrum disorder by alterations in the excitation/inhibition balance. In addition, decreased level of serotonin/adenosine in implicated brain areas (e.g., medial frontal cortex) have also been demonstrated/suggested in this disease (25, 217–220). Impaired immune response, inflammation, and oxidative stress may be causative factors of autism spectrum disorder (15, 221). In fact, recent studies suggest that autism spectrum disorder is associated with inflammation (e.g., activation of glial cells and increased levels of cytokines) (222–224), mitochondrial dysfunction, and oxidative stress (e.g., increased ROS activity) (79, 225–227).

Attention Deficit/Hyperactivity Disorder

Reduction of brain volume and gray matter (e.g., in putamen and caudate nucleus) and underactivation or hyperactivation of different brain networks (e.g., in the frontoparietal and ventral attention network and the somatomotor system) were demonstrated in patients with ADHD (228, 229). Numerous studies have shown that increased glutamatergic tone/glutamate level (230), dopamine hypofunction (e.g., decreased stimulation-evoked release of dopamine) (26), and changes in GABAergic (e.g., decrease in GABA level) (230, 231), noradrenergic, and serotonergic system (16, 232–235) in the implicated brain areas may be causative factors of ADHD. Furthermore, increased oxidative stress (e.g., enhanced production of ROS) was demonstrated in a rat model of ADHD (236).

CONCLUSION

The effects of nutritional ketosis on CNS diseases, whether through diet or supplementation, have not been fully investigated. Consequently, only limited results have demonstrated the existence of alleviating effects of exogenous ketone supplement administration on animal models of psychiatric diseases and patients with psychiatric disorders. Nevertheless, there are several common pathophysiological metabolic alterations, such as changes in neurotransmitter release, increased inflammatory processes, abnormal cerebral glucose metabolism, and decreased mitochondrial-associated brain energy metabolism, which may have a role in the emergence of psychiatric diseases. Consequently, ketogenic interventions that can modulate a broad array of metabolic and signaling changes underlying the pathophysiology of psychiatric diseases may alleviate the onset of symptoms.

Based on our review of the literature, we hypothesize that utilizing exogenous ketone supplements alone or with ketogenic diet, either as a primary or an adjunctive therapy for selected psychiatric disorders, may potentially be an effective treatment. Thus, adding ketone supplements as an additional agent to the therapeutic regimen may alleviate symptoms of psychiatric diseases *via* modulation of different metabolic routes implicated in psychiatric disorders. Therefore, detailed investigation of exogenous ketone supplement-evoked direct and/or indirect alterations in molecular pathways and signaling processes associated with psychiatric diseases is needed.

The use of exogenous ketone supplements in psychiatric diseases is only in its infancy. Nevertheless, our increasing understanding of how exogenous ketone supplement-evoked ketosis/βHB exerts its effects on CNS diseases, combining with new results on pathophysiology of psychiatric diseases and their complex interplay with each other, suggests that exogenous ketone supplements may be ideal and effective adjuvants to drugs used in the treatment of psychiatric diseases. Thus, because exogenous ketone supplements modulate endogenous processes, their administration is a safe method to promote disease-alleviating effects without considerable risk, as well as minimal or no side effects compared to pharmacological treatments. Consequently, exogenous ketone supplements may help to both manage the side effects and increase the efficacy of drugs used in psychiatric diseases, especially in cases of treatment resistance.

Future research should explore the effects of exogenous ketones on the metabolic processes that underlie the diseases leading to psychiatric disorders in order to restore abnormal cerebral glucose and energy metabolism. Moreover, new studies are needed to investigate the effects, therapeutic efficacy, and exact mechanism(s) of action of exogenous ketone supplements alone or in combination with a ketogenic diet not only on animal models of psychiatric diseases, but also on patients with different psychiatric disorders. Future studies are needed to reveal which factors (e.g., age, sex, lifestyle, drugs, other diseases, and so on) can modify the effects of exogenous ketone supplements on psychiatric diseases; to develop new, more effective, and safe ketone supplements, which can be used in special ketogenic foods for treatment of CNS disorders, including psychiatric diseases. There is urgent need to develop therapeutic strategies and broadly accepted protocols guiding the administration of different types and combinations of exogenous ketone supplements. As a result of new studies in the near future, a better understanding of the pathophysiology of different psychiatric diseases and the connections between the underlying metabolic/signaling pathways may promote the development of novel metabolism-based adjuvant therapies, such as the administration of exogenous ketone supplements against psychiatric diseases.

AUTHOR CONTRIBUTIONS

ZK contributed to the conception of the manuscript, comprehensive search of the electronic databases, and writing of the manuscript. DPD contributed to the writing of the manuscript. DD, MK, and CR were in charge of revising the manuscript. CA was in charge of writing and revising the manuscript.

ACKNOWLEDGMENTS

This work was supported by OTKA K124558 Research Grant (to Zsolt Kovács) and ONR Grant N000141310062 and GLUT1D Foundation Grant #6143113500 (to Dominic D`Agostino). We thank Quest Nutrition LLC for supporting ongoing studies on this topic (to Csilla Ari).

REFERENCES

1. Craske MG, Stein MB, Eley TC, Milad MR, Holmes A, Rapee RM, et al. Anxiety disorders. *Nat Rev Dis Primers* (2017) 3:17024. doi: 10.1038/nrdp.2017.24
2. Bromet E, Andrade LH, Hwang I, Sampson NA, Alonso J, de Girolamo G, et al. Cross-national epidemiology of DSM-IV major depressive episode. *BMC Med* (2011) 9:90. doi: 10.1186/1741-7015-9-90
3. Kupfer DJ, Frank E, Phillips ML. Major depressive disorder: new clinical, neurobiological, and treatment perspectives. *Lancet* (2012) 379(9820):1045–55. doi: 10.1016/S0140-6736(11)60602-8
4. Merikangas KR, Jin R, He JP, Kessler RC, Lee S, Sampson NA, et al. Prevalence and correlates of bipolar spectrum disorder in the world mental health survey initiative. *Arch Gen Psychiatry* (2011) 68(3):241–51. doi: 10.1001/archgenpsychiatry.2011.12
5. Vieta E, Berk M, Schulze TG, Carvalho AF, Suppes T, Calabrese JR, et al. Bipolar disorders. *Nat Rev Dis Primers* (2018) 4:18008. doi: 10.1038/nrdp.2018.8
6. Kahn RS, Sommer IE, Murray RM, Meyer-Lindenberg A, Weinberger DR, Cannon TD, et al. Schizophrenia. *Nat Rev Dis Primers* (2015) 1:15067. doi: 10.1038/nrdp.2015.67
7. Patel S, Sharma D, Kalia K, Tiwari V. Crosstalk between endoplasmic reticulum stress and oxidative stress in schizophrenia: the dawn of new therapeutic approaches. *Neurosci Biobehav Rev* (2017b) 83:589–603. doi: 10.1016/j.neubiorev.2017.08.025
8. Polanczyk G, de Lima MS, Horta BL, Biederman J, Rohde LA. The worldwide prevalence of ADHD: a systematic review and metaregression analysis. *Am J Psychiatry* (2007) 164(6):942–8. doi: 10.1176/appi.ajp.164.6.942
9. Simon V, Czobor P, Bálint S, Mészáros A, Bitter I. Prevalence and correlates of adult attention-deficit hyperactivity disorder: meta-analysis. *Br J Psychiatry* (2009) (3):204–11. doi: 10.1192/bjp.bp.107.048827
10. Christensen DL, Baio J, Van Naarden Braun K, Bilder D, Charles J, Constantino JN, et al. Prevalence and characteristics of autism spectrum disorder among children aged 8 years—autism and developmental disabilities monitoring network, 11 sites, United States, 2012. *MMWR Surveill Summ* (2016) 65(3):1–23. doi: 10.15585/mmwr.ss6503a1
11. Craske MG, Stein MB. Anxiety. *Lancet* (2016) 388(10063):3048–59. doi: 10.1016/S0140-6736(16)30381-6
12. Lichtenstein P, Yip BH, Björk C, Pawitan Y, Cannon TD, Sullivan PF, et al. Common genetic determinants of schizophrenia and bipolar disorder in Swedish families: a population-based study. *Lancet* (2009) 373(9659):234–9. doi: 10.1016/S0140-6736(09)60072-6
13. Dean J, Keshavan M. The neurobiology of depression: an integrated view. *Asian J Psychiatr* (2017) 27:101–11. doi: 10.1016/j.ajp.2017.01.025
14. Hodes GE, Kana V, Menard C, Merad M, Russo SJ. Neuroimmune mechanisms of depression. *Nat Neurosci* (2015) 18(10):1386–93. doi: 10.1038/nn.4113
15. Bhat S, Acharya UR, Adeli H, Bairy GM, Adeli A. Autism: cause factors, early diagnosis and therapies. *Rev Neurosci* (2014) 25(6):841–50. doi: 10.1515/revneuro-2014-0056
16. Faraone SV, Asherson P, Banaschewski T, Biederman J, Buitelaar JK, Ramos-Quiroga JA, et al. Attention-deficit/hyperactivity disorder. *Nat Rev Dis Primers* (2015) 1:15020. doi: 10.1038/nrdp.2015.20
17. Brown KA, Samuel S, Patel DR. Pharmacologic management of attention deficit hyperactivity disorder in children and adolescents: a review for practitioners. *Transl Pediatr* (2018a) 7(1):36–47. doi: 10.21037/tp.2017.08.02
18. Moffitt TE, Harrington H, Caspi A, Kim-Cohen J, Goldberg D, Gregory AM, et al. Depression and generalized anxiety disorder: cumulative and sequential comorbidity in a birth cohort followed prospectively to age 32 years. *Arch Gen Psychiatry* (2007) 64(6):651–60. doi: 10.1001/archpsyc.64.6.651
19. Patel DR, Feucht C, Brown K, Ramsay J. Pharmacological treatment of anxiety disorders in children and adolescents: a review for practitioners. *Transl Pediatr* (2018) 7(1):23–35. doi: 10.21037/tp.2017.08.05
20. Whitehead C, Moss S, Cardno A, Lewis G. Antidepressants for the treatment of depression in people with schizophrenia: a systematic review. *Psychol Med* (2003) 33(4):589–99. doi: 10.1017/S0033291703007645
21. Wilczynski SM, Menousek K, Hunter M, Mudgal D. Individualized education programs for youth with autism spectrum disorders. *Psychol Schools* (2007) 44(7):653. doi: 10.1002/pits.20255
22. Otte C, Gold SM, Penninx BW, Pariante CM, Etkin A, Fava M, et al. Major depressive disorder. *Nat Rev Dis Primers* (2016) 2:16065. doi: 10.1038/nrdp.2016.65
23. Brisch R, Saniotis A, Wolf R, Bielau H, Bernstein HG, Steiner J, et al. The role of dopamine in schizophrenia from a neurobiological and evolutionary perspective: old fashioned, but still in vogue. *Front Psychiatry* (2014) 5:47. doi: 10.3389/fpsyt.2014.00047

24. Delgado PL. Depression: the case for a monoamine deficiency. *J Clin Psychiatry* (2000) 61 (Suppl 6):7–11. doi: 10.4088/JCP.v61n0103
25. Nakamura K, Sekine Y, Ouchi Y, Tsujii M, Yoshikawa E, Futatsubashi M, et al. Brain serotonin and dopamine transporter bindings in adults with high-functioning autism. *Arch Gen Psychiatry* (2010) 67(1):59–68. doi: 10.1001/archgenpsychiatry.2009.137
26. Russell VA. Dopamine hypofunction possibly results from a defect in glutamate-stimulated release of dopamine in the nucleus accumbens shell of a rat model for attention deficit hyperactivity disorder–the spontaneously hypertensive rat. *Neurosci Biobehav Rev* (2003) 27(7):671–82. doi: 10.1016/j.neubiorev.2003.08.010
27. Chiapponi C, Piras F, Piras F, Caltagirone C, Spalletta G. GABA system in schizophrenia and mood disorders: a mini review on third-generation imaging studies. *Front Psychiatry* (2016) 7:61. doi: 10.3389/fpsyt.2016.00061
28. Coelho JE, Alves P, Canas PM, Valadas JS, Shmidt T, Batalha VL, et al. Overexpression of adenosine A2A receptors in rats: effects on depression, locomotion, and anxiety. *Front Psychiatry* (2014) 5:67. doi: 10.3389/fpsyt.2014.00067
29. Hashimoto K, Sawa A, Iyo M. Increased levels of glutamate in brains from patients with mood disorders. *Biol Psychiatry* (2007) 62(11):1310–6. doi: 10.1016/j.biopsych.2007.03.017
30. Kim M, Campeau S, Falls WA, Davis M. Infusion of the non-NMDA receptor antagonist CNQX into the amygdala blocks the expression of fear-potentiated startle. *Behav Neural Biol* (1993) 59(1):5–8. doi: 10.1016/0163-1047(93)91075-X
31. Machado-Vieira R, Lara DR, Souza DO, Kapczinski F. Purinergic dysfunction in mania: an integrative model. *Med Hypotheses* (2002) 58(4):297–304. doi: 10.1054/mehy.2001.1543
32. Moghaddam B, Javitt D. From revolution to evolution: the glutamate hypothesis of schizophrenia and its implication for treatment. *Neuropsychopharmacology* (2012) 37(1):4–15. doi: 10.1038/npp.2011.181
33. Möhler H. The GABA system in anxiety and depression and its therapeutic potential. *Neuropharmacology* (2012) 62(1):42–53. doi: 10.1016/j.neuropharm.2011.08.040
34. Vincenzi F, Ravani A, Pasquini S, Merighi S, Gessi S, Romagnoli R, et al. Positive allosteric modulation of A1 adenosine receptors as a novel and promising therapeutic strategy for anxiety. *Neuropharmacology* (2016) 111:283–92. doi: 10.1016/j.neuropharm.2016.09.015
35. Adzic M, Brkic Z, Bulajic S, Mitic M, Radojcic MB. Antidepressant action on mitochondrial dysfunction in psychiatric disorders. *Drug Dev Res* (2016) 77(7):400–6. doi: 10.1002/ddr.21332
36. Zuccoli GS, Saia-Cereda VM, Nascimento JM, Martins-de-Souza D. The energy metabolism dysfunction in psychiatric disorders postmortem brains: focus on proteomic evidence. *Front Neurosci* (2017) 11:493. doi: 10.3389/fnins.2017.00493
37. Maes M, Yirmyia R, Noraberg J, Brene S, Hibbeln J, Perini G, et al. The inflammatory & neurodegenerative (I&ND) hypothesis of depression: leads for future research and new drug developments in depression. *Metab Brain Dis* (2009) 24(1):27–53. doi: 10.1007/s11011-008-9118-1
38. Murphy MG. Dietary fatty acids and membrane protein function. *J Nutr Biochem* (1990) 1(2):68–79. doi: 10.1016/0955-2863(90)90052-M
39. Müller CP, Reichel M, Mühle C, Rhein C, Gulbins E, Kornhuber J. Brain membrane lipids in major depression and anxiety disorders. *Biochim Biophys Acta* (2015) (8):1052–65. doi: 10.1016/j.bbalip.2014.12.014
40. Mocking RJT, Assies J, Ruhé HG, Schene AH. Focus on fatty acids in the neurometabolic pathophysiology of psychiatric disorders. *J Inherit Metab Dis* (2018) (4):597–611. doi: 10.1007/s10545-018-0158-3
41. Hosokawa T, Momose T, Kasai K. Brain glucose metabolism difference between bipolar and unipolar mood disorders in depressed and euthymic states. *Prog Neuropsychopharmacol Biol Psychiatry* (2009) 33(2):243–50. doi: 10.1016/j.pnpbp.2008.11.014
42. Kraeuter AK, van den Buuse M, Sarnyai Z. Ketogenic diet prevents impaired prepulse inhibition of startle in an acute NMDA receptor hypofunction model of schizophrenia. *Schizophr Res* (2018) 206:244–500. doi: 10.1016/j.schres.2018.11.011
43. Achanta LB, Rae CD. β-Hydroxybutyrate in the brain: one molecule, multiple mechanisms. *Neurochem Res* (2017) 42:35–49. doi: 10.1007/s11064-016-2099-2
44. Branco AF, Ferreira A, Simões RF, Magalhães-Novais S, Zehowski C, Cope E, et al. Ketogenic diets: from cancer to mitochondrial diseases and beyond. *Eur J Clin Invest* (2016) 46(3):285–98. doi: 10.1111/eci.12591
45. Newman JC, Verdin E. Ketone bodies as signaling metabolites. *Trends Endocrinol Metab* (2014) 25:42–52. doi: 10.1016/j.tem.2013.09.002
46. Augustin K, Khabbush A, Williams S, Eaton S, Orford M, Cross JH, et al. Mechanisms of action for the medium-chain triglyceride ketogenic diet in neurological and metabolic disorders. *Lancet Neurol* (2018) 17(1):84–93. doi: 10.1016/S1474-4422(17)30408-8
47. VanItallie TB, Nufert TH. Ketones: metabolism's ugly duckling. *Nutr Rev* (2003) (10):327–41. doi: 10.1301/nr.2003.oct.327-341
48. Guzmán M, Blázquez C. Ketone body synthesis in the brain: possible neuroprotective effects. *Prostaglandins Leukot Essent Fatty Acids* (2004) 70(3):287–92. doi: 10.1016/j.plefa.2003.05.001
49. Le Foll C, Levin BE. Fatty acid-induced astrocyte ketone production and the control of food intake. *Am J Physiol Regul Integr Comp Physiol* (2016) 310(11):R1186–92. doi: 10.1152/ajpregu.00113.2016
50. Koppel SJ, Swerdlow RH. Neuroketotherapeutics: a modern review of a century-old therapy. *Neurochem Int* (2018) 117:114–125. doi: 10.1016/j.neuint.2017.05.019
51. Veech RL. The therapeutic implications of ketone bodies: the effects of ketone bodies in pathological conditions: ketosis, ketogenic diet, redox states, insulin resistance, and mitochondrial metabolism. *Prostaglandins Leukot Essent Fatty Acids* (2004) 70:309–19. doi: 10.1016/j.plefa.2003.09.007
52. Yudkoff M, Daikhin Y, Melø TM, Nissim I, Sonnewald U, Nissim I. The ketogenic diet and brain metabolism of amino acids: relationship to the anticonvulsant effect. *Annu Rev Nutr* (2007) 27:415–30. doi: 10.1146/annurev.nutr.27.061406.093722
53. Broom GM, Shaw IC, Rucklidge JJ. The ketogenic diet as a potential treatment and prevention strategy for Alzheimer's disease. *Nutrition* (2019) 60:118–21. doi: 10.1016/j.nut.2018.10.003
54. Hashim SA, VanItallie TB. Ketone body therapy: from the ketogenic diet to the oral administration of ketone ester. *J Lipid Res* (2014) 55:1818–26. doi: 10.1194/jlr.R046599
55. Kashiwaya Y, Bergman C, Lee JH, Wan R, King MT, Mughal MR, et al. A ketone ester diet exhibits anxiolytic and cognition-sparing properties, and lessens amyloid and tau pathologies in a mouse model of Alzheimer's disease. *Neurobiol Aging* (2013) 34(6):1530–9. doi: 10.1016/j.neurobiolaging.2012.11.023
56. Newport MT, VanItallie TB, Kashiwaya Y, King MT, Veech RL. A new way to produce hyperketonemia: use of ketone ester in a case of Alzheimer's disease. *Alzheimers Dement* (2015) 11:99–103. doi: 10.1016/j.jalz.2014.01.006
57. Penke B, Paragi G, Gera J, Berkecz R, Kovács Z, Crul T, et al. The role of lipids and membranes in the pathogenesis of Alzheimer's disease: a comprehensive view. *Curr Alzheimer Res* (2018) 15(13):1191–212. doi: 10.2174/1567205015666180911151716
58. Stafstrom CE, Rho JM. The ketogenic diet as a treatment paradigm for diverse neurological disorders. *Front Pharmacol* (2012) 3:59. doi: 10.3389/fphar.2012.00059
59. Vanitallie TB, Nonas C, Di Rocco A, Boyar K, Hyams K, Heymsfield SB. Treatment of Parkinson disease with diet-induced hyperketonemia: a feasibility study. *Neurology* (2005) 64(4):728–30. doi: 10.1212/01.WNL.0000152046.11390.45
60. Veyrat-Durebex C, Reynier P, Procaccio V, Hergesheimer R, Corcia P, Andres CR, et al. How can a ketogenic diet improve motor function? *Front Mol Neurosci* (2018) 11:15. doi: 10.3389/fnmol.2018.00015
61. Bekker YAC, Lambrechts DA, Verhoeven JS, van Boxtel J, Troost C, Kamsteeg EJ, et al. Failure of ketogenic diet therapy in GLUT1 deficiency syndrome. *Eur J Paediatr Neurol* (2019) (in press). doi: 10.1016/j.ejpn.2019.02.012
62. Klepper J, Leiendecker B. Glut1 deficiency syndrome and novel ketogenic diets. *J Child Neurol* (2013) 28(8):1045–8. doi: 10.1177/0883073813487600
63. Veggiotti P, De Giorgis V. Dietary treatments and new therapeutic perspective in GLUT1 deficiency syndrome. *Curr Treat Options Neurol* (2014) 16(5):291. doi: 10.1007/s11940-014-0291-8
64. Ari C, Pilla R, D'Agostino D. Nutritional/metabolic therapies in animal models of amyotrophic lateral sclerosis, Alzheimer's disease, and seizures. In: *Bioactive Nutraceuticals and Dietary Supplements in Neurological*

and Brain Disease. Elsevier, Chapter 47 (2015). p. 449–59. doi: 10.1016/B978-0-12-411462-3.00047-3

65. Poff AM, Ward N, Seyfried TN, Arnold P, D'Agostino DP. Non-toxic metabolic management of metastatic cancer in VM mice: novel combination of ketogenic diet, ketone supplementation, and hyperbaric oxygen therapy. *PLoS One* (2015) 10:e0127407. doi: 10.1371/journal.pone.0127407
66. Sremanakova J, Sowerbutts AM, Burden S. A systematic review of the use of ketogenic diets in adult patients with cancer. *J Hum Nutr Diet* (2018) 31(6):793–802. doi: 10.1111/jhn.12587
67. Kovács Z, D'Agostino DP, Dobolyi A, Ari C. Adenosine A1 receptor antagonism abolished the anti-seizure effects of exogenous ketone supplementation in Wistar Albino Glaxo Rijswijk rats. *Front Mol Neurosci* (2017) 10:235. doi: 10.3389/fnmol.2017.00235
68. McNally MA, Hartman AL. Ketone bodies in epilepsy. *J Neurochem* (2012) 121:28–35. doi: 10.1111/j.1471-4159.2012.07670.x
69. Bostock EC, Kirkby KC, Taylor. BV. The current status of the ketogenic diet in psychiatry. *Front Psychiatry* (2017) 8:43. doi: 10.3389/fpsyt.2017.00043
70. Kraft BD, Westman EC. Schizophrenia, gluten, and low-carbohydrate, ketogenic diets: a case report and review of the literature. *Nutr Metab (Lond)* (2009) 6:10. doi: 10.1186/1743-7075-6-10
71. Pacheco A, Easterling WS, Pryer MW. A pilot study of the ketogenic diet in schizophrenia. *Am J Psychiatry* (1965) 121:1110–1. doi: 10.1176/ajp.121.11.1110
72. Włodarczyk A, Wiglusz MS, Cubała WJ. Ketogenic diet for schizophrenia: nutritional approach to antipsychotic treatment. *Med Hypotheses* (2018) 118:74–7. doi: 10.1016/j.mehy.2018.06.022
73. Palmer CM. Ketogenic diet in the treatment of schizoafective disorder: two case studies. *Schizophr Res* (2017) 189:208–9. doi: 10.1016/j.schres.2017.01.053
74. Palmer CM, Gilbert-Jaramillo J, Westman EC. The ketogenic diet and remission of psychotic symptoms in schizophrenia: two case studies. *Schizophr Res* (2019) (in press). doi: 10.1016/j.schres.2019.03.019
75. Ari C, Kovács Z, Juhasz G, Murdun C, Goldhagen CR, Koutnik AP, et al. Exogenous ketone supplements reduce anxiety-related behavior in Sprague-Dawley and Wistar Albino Glaxo/Rijswijk rats. *Front Mol Neurosci* (2016) 9:137. doi: 10.3389/fnmol.2016.00137
76. Hollis F, Mitchell ES, Canto C, Wang D, Sandi C. Medium chain triglyceride diet reduces anxiety-like behaviors and enhances social competitiveness in rats. *Neuropharmacology* (2018) 138:245–56. doi: 10.1016/j.neuropharm.2018.06.017
77. Sussman D, Germann J, Henkelman M. Gestational ketogenic diet programs brain structure and susceptibility to depression & anxiety in the adult mouse offspring. *Brain Behav* (2015) 5(2):e00300. doi: 10.1002/brb3.300
78. Ahn Y, Narous M, Tobias R, Rho JM, Mychasiuk R. The ketogenic diet modifies social and metabolic alterations identified in the prenatal valproic acid model of autism spectrum disorder. *Dev Neurosci* (2014) 36(5):371–80. doi: 10.1159/000362645
79. Cheng N, Rho JM, Masino SA. Metabolic dysfunction underlying autism spectrum disorder and potential treatment approaches. *Front Mol Neurosci* (2017) 10:34. doi: 10.3389/fnmol.2017.00034
80. Evangeliou A, Vlachonikolis I, Mihailidou H, Spilioti M, Skarpalezou A, Makaronas N, et al. Application of a ketogenic diet in children with autistic behavior: pilot study. *J Child Neurol* (2003) 18(2):113–8. doi: 10.1177/08830738030180020501
81. Ruskin DN, Murphy MI, Slade SL, Masino SA. Ketogenic diet improves behaviors in a maternal immune activation model of autism spectrum disorder. *PLoS One* (2017b) 12(2):e0171643. doi: 10.1371/journal.pone.0171643
82. Brietzke E, Mansur RB, Subramaniapillai M, Balanzá-Martínez V, Vinberg M, González-Pinto A, et al. Ketogenic diet as a metabolic therapy for mood disorders: evidence and developments. *Neurosci Biobehav Rev* (2018) 94:11–6. doi: 10.1016/j.neubiorev.2018.07.020
83. Brownlow ML, Jung SH, Moore RJ, Bechmann N, Jankord R. Nutritional ketosis affects metabolism and behavior in Sprague-Dawley rats in both control and chronic stress environments. *Front Mol Neurosci* (2017) 10:129. doi: 10.3389/fnmol.2017.00129
84. D'Agostino D, Pilla R, Held H, Landon C, Puchowicz M, Brunengraber H, et al. Therapeutic ketosis with ketone ester delays central nervous system oxygen toxicity seizures in rats. *Am J Phys Reg Integr Comp Phys* (2013) 304:829–36. doi: 10.1152/ajpregu.00506.2012
85. Erecińska M, Nelson D, Daikhin Y, Yudkoff M. Regulation of GABA level in rat brain synaptosomes: fluxes through enzymes of the GABA shunt and effects of glutamate, calcium, and ketone bodies. *J Neurochem* (1996) 67(6):2325–34. doi: 10.1046/j.1471-4159.1996.67062325.x
86. Ma W, Berg J, Yellen G. Ketogenic diet metabolites reduce firing in central neurons by opening K(ATP) channels. *J Neurosci* (2007) 27:3618–25. doi: 10.1523/JNEUROSCI.0132-07.2007
87. Marosi K, Kim SW, Moehl K, Scheibye-Knudsen M, Cheng A, Cutler R, et al. 3-Hydroxybutyrate regulates energy metabolism and induces BDNF expression in cerebral cortical neurons. *J Neurochem* (2016) 139(5):769–81. doi: 10.1111/jnc.13868
88. Puchalska P, Crawford PA. Multi-dimensional roles of ketone bodies in fuel metabolism, signaling, and therapeutics. *Cell Metab* (2017) 25(2):262–84. doi: 10.1016/j.cmet.2016.12.022
89. Samoilova M, Weisspapir M, Abdelmalik P, Velumian AA, Carlen PL. Chronic *in vitro* ketosis is neuroprotective but not anti-convulsant. *J Neurochem* (2010) (4):826–35. doi: 10.1111/j.1471-4159.2010.06645.x
90. Shimazu T, Hirschey MD, Newman J, He W, Shirakawa K, Le Moan N, et al. Suppression of oxidative stress by β-hydroxybutyrate, an endogenous histone deacetylase inhibitor. *Science* (2013) 339(6116):211–4. doi: 10.1126/science.1227166
91. Youm YH, Nguyen KY, Grant RW, Goldberg EL, Bodogai M, Kim D, et al. The ketone metabolite β-hydroxybutyrate blocks NLRP3 inflammasome-mediated inflammatory disease. *Nat Med* (2015) 21(3):263–9. doi: 10.1038/nm.3804
92. Kesl SL, Poff AM, Ward NP, Fiorelli TN, Ari C, Van Putten AJ, et al. Effects of exogenous ketone supplementation on blood ketone, glucose, triglyceride, and lipoprotein levels in Sprague-Dawley rats. *Nutr Metab (Lond)* (2016) 13:9. doi: 10.1186/s12986-016-0069-y
93. Bough KJ, Rho JM. Anticonvulsant mechanisms of the ketogenic diet. *Epilepsia* (2007) 48:43–58. doi: 10.1111/j.1528-1167.2007.00915.x
94. Rogawski MA, Löscher W, Rho JM. Mechanisms of action of antiseizure drugs and the ketogenic diet. *Cold Spring Harb Perspect Med* (2016) 6:1–28. doi: 10.1101/cshperspect.a022780
95. Kovács Z, D'Agostino DP, Ari C. Anxiolytic effect of exogenous ketone supplementation is abolished by adenosine A1 receptor inhibition in Wistar Albino Glaxo/Rijswijk rats. *Front Behav Neurosci* (2018) 12:29. doi: 10.3389/fnbeh.2018.00029
96. Lutas A, Yellen G. The ketogenic diet: metabolic influences on brain excitability and epilepsy. *Trends Neurosci* (2013) 36(1):32–40. doi: 10.1016/j.tins.2012.11.005
97. Maalouf M, Rho JM, Mattson MP. The neuroprotective properties of calorie restriction, the ketogenic diet, and ketone bodies. *Brain Res Rev* (2009) 59(2):293–315. doi: 10.1016/j.brainresrev.2008.09.002
98. Simeone TA, Simeone KA, Stafstrom CE, Rho JM. Do ketone bodies mediate the anti-seizure effects of the ketogenic diet? *Neuropharmacology* (2018) 133:233–41. doi: 10.1016/j.neuropharm.2018.01.011
99. Stubbs BJ, Cox PJ, Evans RD, Santer P, Miller JJ, Faull OK, et al. On the metabolism of exogenous ketones in humans. *Front Physiol* (2017) 8:848. doi: 10.3389/fphys.2017.00848
100. Benjamin JS, Pilarowski GO, Carosso GA, Zhang L, Huso DL, Goff LA, et al. A ketogenic diet rescues hippocampal memory defects in a mouse model of Kabuki syndrome. *Proc Natl Acad Sci U S A* (2017) 114(1):125–30. doi: 10.1073/pnas.1611431114
101. Veech RL, Chance B, Kashiwaya Y, Lardy HA, Cahill GF, Jr. Ketone bodies, potential therapeutic uses. *IUBMB Life* (2001) 51(4):241–7. doi: 10.1080/152165401753311780
102. Kovács Z, D'Agostino DP, Diamond DM, Ari C. Exogenous ketone supplementation decreased the lipopolysaccharide-induced increase in absence epileptic activity in Wistar Albino Glaxo Rijswijk rats. *Front Mol Neurosci* (2019) 12:45. doi: 10.3389/fnmol.2019.00045
103. Hartman AL, Vining EP. Clinical aspects of the ketogenic diet. *Epilepsia* (2007) 48(1):31–42. doi: 10.1111/j.1528-1167.2007.00914.x
104. Nordli DR Jr, Kuroda MM, Carroll J, Koenigsberger DY, Hirsch LJ, Bruner HJ, et al. Experience with the ketogenic diet in infants. *Pediatrics* (2001) 108(1):129–33. doi: 10.1542/peds.108.1.129

105. Brunengraber H. Potential of ketone body esters for parenteral and oral nutrition. *Nutrition* (1997) 13(3):233–5. doi: 10.1016/S0899-9007(96)00409-1
106. Clarke K, Tchabanenko K, Pawlosky R, Carter E, Todd King M, Musa-Veloso K, et al. Kinetics, safety and tolerability of (R)-3-hydroxybutyl (R)-3-hydroxybutyrate in healthy adult subjects. *Regul Toxicol Pharmacol* (2012a) 63(3):401–8. doi: 10.1016/j.yrtph.2012.04.008
107. Cahill GF. Starvation in man. *Clin Endocrinol Metab* (1976) 5(2):397–415. doi: 10.1016/S0300-595X(76)80028-X
108. Cahill GF. Fuel metabolism in starvation. *Annu Rev Nutr* (2006) 26:1–22. doi: 10.1146/annurev.nutr.26.061505.111258
109. McDonald TJW, Henry-Barron BJ, Felton EA, Gutierrez EG, Barnett J, Fisher R, et al. Improving compliance in adults with epilepsy on a modified Atkins diet: a randomized trial. *Seizure* (2018) 60:132–8. doi: 10.1016/j.seizure.2018.06.019
110. Clarke K, Tchabanenko K, Pawlosky R, Carter E, Knight NS, Murray AJ, et al. Oral 28-day and developmental toxicity studies of (R)-3-hydroxybutyl (R)-3-hydroxybutyrate. *Regul Toxicol Pharmacol* (2012b) 63(2):196–208. doi: 10.1016/j.yrtph.2012.04.001
111. Tate RL, Mehlman MA, Tobin RB. Metabolic fate of 1,3-butanediol in the rat: conversion to -hydroxybutyrate. *J Nutr* (1971) 101(12):1719–26. doi: 10.1093/jn/101.12.1719
112. Schönfeld P, Wojtczak L. Short- and medium-chain fatty acids in energy metabolism: the cellular perspective. *J Lipid Res* (2016) 57(6):943–54. doi: 10.1194/jlr.R067629
113. Henderson ST. Ketone bodies as a therapeutic for Alzheimer's disease. *Neurotherapeutics* (2008) 5(3):470–80. doi: 10.1016/j.nurt.2008.05.004
114. Chen L, Miao Z, Xu X. β-hydroxybutyrate alleviates depressive behaviors in mice possibly by increasing the histone3-lysine9-β-hydroxybutyrylation. *Biochem Biophys Res Commun* (2017) 490(2):117–22. doi: 10.1016/j.bbrc.2017.05.184
115. Yamanashi T, Iwata M, Kamiya N, Tsunetomi K, Kajitani N, Wada N, et al. Beta-hydroxybutyrate, an endogenic NLRP3 inflammasome inhibitor, attenuates stress-induced behavioral and inflammatory responses. *Sci Rep* (2017) 7(1):7677. doi: 10.1038/s41598-017-08055-1
116. Yang J, Chen T, Sun L, Zhao Z, Qi X, Zhou K, et al. Potential metabolite markers of schizophrenia. *Mol Psychiatry* (2013) 18(1):67–78. doi: 10.1038/mp.2011.131
117. Huang YC, Lin PY, Lee Y, Hung CF, Hsu ST, Wu CC, et al. Serum levels of β-hydroxybutyrate and pyruvate, metabolic changes and cognitive function in patients with schizophrenia during antipsychotic treatment: a preliminary study. *Neuropsychiatr Dis Treat* (2018) 14:799–808. doi: 10.2147/NDT.S157055
118. Setoyama D, Kato TA, Hashimoto R, Kunugi H, Hattori K, Hayakawa K, et al. Plasma metabolites predict severity of depression and suicidal ideation in psychiatric patients—a multicenter pilot analysis. *PLoS One* (2016) 11(12):e0165267. doi: 10.1371/journal.pone.0165267
119. Simeone TA, Simeone KA, Rho JM. Ketone bodies as anti-seizure agents. *Neurochem Res* (2017) 42:2011–8. doi: 10.1007/s11064-017-2253-5
120. Phelps JR, Siemers SV, El-Mallakh RS. The ketogenic diet for type II bipolar disorder. *Neurocase* (2013) 19(5):423–6. doi: 10.1080/13554794.2012.690421
121. Kraeuter AK, Loxton H, Lima BC, Rudd D, Sarnyai Z. Ketogenic diet reverses behavioral abnormalities in an acute NMDA receptor hypofunction model of schizophrenia. *Schizophr Res* (2015) 169(1–3):491–3. doi: 10.1016/j.schres.2015.10.041
122. Murphy P, Likhodii S, Nylen K, Burnham WM. The antidepressant properties of the ketogenic diet. *Biol Psychiatry* (2004) 56(12):981–3. doi: 10.1016/j.biopsych.2004.09.019
123. Ruskin DN, Fortin JA, Bisnauth SN, Masino SA. Ketogenic diets improve behaviors associated with autism spectrum disorder in a sex-specific manner in the EL mouse. *Physiol Behav* (2017a) 168:138–45. doi: 10.1016/j.physbeh.2016.10.023
124. Murphy P, Burnham WM. The ketogenic diet causes a reversible decrease in activity level in Long-Evans rats. *Exp Neurol* (2006) 201(1):84–9. doi: 10.1016/j.expneurol.2006.03.024
125. Packer RM, Law TH, Davies E, Zanghi B, Pan Y, Volk HA. Effects of a ketogenic diet on ADHD-like behavior in dogs with idiopathic epilepsy. *Epilepsy Behav* (2016) 55:62–8. doi: 10.1016/j.yebeh.2015.11.014
126. Sato K, Kashiwaya Y, Keon CA, Tsuchiya N, King MT, Radda GK, et al. Insulin, ketone bodies, and mitochondrial energy transduction. *FASEB J* (1995) 9(8):651–8. doi: 10.1096/fasebj.9.8.7768357
127. Juge N, Gray JA, Omote H, Miyaji T, Inoue T, Hara C, et al. Metabolic control of vesicular glutamate transport and release. *Neuron* (2010) 68:99–112. doi: 10.1016/j.neuron.2010.09.002
128. Won YJ, Lu VB, Puhl HL, 3rd, Ikeda SR. β-Hydroxybutyrate modulates N-type calcium channels in rat sympathetic neurons by acting as an agonist for the G-protein-coupled receptor FFA3. *J Neurosci* (2013) 33(49):19314–25. doi: 10.1523/JNEUROSCI.3102-13.2013
129. Lund TM, Ploug KB, Iversen A, Jensen AA, Jansen-Olesen I. The metabolic impact of β-hydroxybutyrate on neurotransmission: reduced glycolysis mediates changes in calcium responses and KATP channel receptor sensitivity. *J Neurochem* (2015) 132(5):520–31. doi: 10.1111/jnc.12975
130. Sharma AK, Rani E, Waheed A, Rajput SK. Pharmacoresistant epilepsy: a current update on non-conventional pharmacological and non-pharmacological interventions. *J. Epilepsy Res* (2015) 5:1–8. doi: 10.14581/jer.15001
131. Otani K, Yamatodani A, Wada H, Mimaki T, Yabuuchi H. Effect of ketogenic diet on the convulsive threshold and brain amino acid and monoamine levels in young mice. *No To Hattatsu* (1984) 16(3):196–204. doi: 10.11251/ojjscn1969.16.196
132. Dahlin M, Månsson JE, Åmark P. CSF levels of dopamine and serotonin, but not norepinephrine, metabolites are influenced by the ketogenic diet in children with epilepsy. *Epilepsy Res* (2012) 99(1–2):132–8. doi: 10.1016/j.eplepsyres.2011.11.003
133. Haas HL, Greene RW. Adenosine enhances afterhyperpolarization and accommodation in hippocampal pyramidal cells. *Pflugers Arch* (1984) 402:244–7. doi: 10.1007/BF00585506
134. Kovács Z, Kékesi KA, Juhász G, Dobolyi A. The antiepileptic potential of nucleosides. *Curr Med Chem* (2014) 21:788–821. doi: 10.2174/13816128196 66131119154505
135. Poulsen SA, Quinn RJ. Adenosine receptors: new opportunities for future drugs. *Bioorg Med Chem* (1998) 6(6):619–41. doi: 10.1016/S0968-0896(98)00038-8
136. Van der Putten C, Zuiderwijk-Sick EA, van Straalen L, de Geus ED, Boven LA, Kondova I, et al. Differential expression of adenosine A3 receptors controls adenosine A2A receptor-mediated inhibition of TLR responses in microglia. *J Immunol* (2009) 182(12):7603–12. doi: 10.4049/jimmunol.0803383
137. Almeida CG, de Mendonça A, Cunha RA, Ribeiro JA. Adenosine promotes neuronal recovery from reactive oxygen species induced lesion in rat hippocampal slices. *Neurosci Lett* (2003) 339(2):127–30. doi: 10.1016/S0304-3940(02)01478-7
138. Hu S, Dong H, Zhang H, Wang S, Hou L, Chen S, et al. Noninvasive limb remote ischemic preconditioning contributes neuroprotective effects *via* activation of adenosine A1 receptor and redox status after transient focal cerebral ischemia in rats. *Brain Res* (2012) 1459:81–90. doi: 10.1016/j.brainres.2012.04.017
139. Elamin M, Ruskin DN, Masino SA, Sacchetti P. Ketone-based metabolic therapy: is increased NAD+ a primary mechanism? *Front Mol Neurosci* (2017) 10:377. doi: 10.3389/fnmol.2017.00377
140. Maalouf M, Sullivan PG, Davis L, Kim DY, Rho JM. Ketones inhibit mitochondrial production of reactive oxygen species production following glutamate excitotoxicity by increasing NADH oxidation. *Neuroscience* (2007) 145(1):256–64. doi: 10.1016/j.neuroscience.2006.11.065
141. Fu SP, Wang JF, Xue WJ, Liu HM, Liu BR, Zeng YL, et al. Anti-inflammatory effects of BHBA in both *in vivo* and *in vitro* Parkinson's disease models are mediated by GPR109A-dependent mechanisms. *J Neuroinflammation* (2015) 12:9. doi: 10.1186/s12974-014-0230-3
142. Graff EC, Fang H, Wanders D, Judd RL. Anti-inflammatory effects of the hydroxycarboxylic acid receptor 2. *Metabolism* (2016) 65(2):102–13. doi: 10.1016/j.metabol.2015.10.001
143. Yang X, Cheng B. Neuroprotective and anti-inflammatory activities of ketogenic diet on MPTP-induced neurotoxicity. *J Mol Neurosci* (2010) 42(2):145–53. doi: 10.1007/s12031-010-9336-y
144. Levy M, Thaiss CA, Elinav E. Taming the inflammasome. *Nat Med* (2015) 21(3):213–5. doi: 10.1038/nm.3808

145. Patel MN, Carroll RG, Galván-Peña S, Mills EL, Olden R, Triantafilou M, et al. Inflammasome priming in sterile inflammatory disease. *Trends Mol Med* (2017a) 23(2):165–80. doi: 10.1016/j.molmed.2016.12.007
146. Bae HR, Kim DH, Park MH, Lee B, Kim MJ, Lee EK, et al. β-Hydroxybutyrate suppresses inflammasome formation by ameliorating endoplasmic reticulum stress *via* AMPK activation. *Oncotarget* (2016) 7(41):66444–54. doi: 10.18632/oncotarget.12119
147. Emerit J, Edeas M, Bricaire F. Neurodegenerative diseases and oxidative stress. *Biomed Pharmacother* (2004) 58(1):39–46. doi: 10.1016/j.biopha.2003.11.004
148. Kashiwaya Y, Pawlosky R, Markis W, King MT, Bergman C, Srivastava S, et al. A ketone ester diet increases brain malonyl-CoA and Uncoupling proteins 4 and 5 while decreasing food intake in the normal Wistar Rat. *J Biol Chem* (2010) 285(34):25950–6. doi: 10.1074/jbc.M110.138198
149. Xiao XQ, Zhao Y, Chen GQ. The effect of 3-hydroxybutyrate and its derivatives on the growth of glial cells. *Biomaterials* (2007) 28(25):3608–16. doi: 10.1016/j.biomaterials.2007.04.046
150. Kim DY, Simeone KA, Simeone TA, Pandya JD, Wilke JC, Ahn Y, et al. Ketone bodies mediate antiseizure effects through mitochondrial permeability transition. *Ann Neurol* (2015) 78(1):77–87. doi: 10.1002/ana.24424
151. Li X. Using the conditioned fear stress (CFS) animal model to understand the neurobiological mechanisms and pharmacological treatment of anxiety. *Shanghai Arch Psychiatry* (2012) 24(5):241–9. doi: 10.3969/j.issn.1002-0829.2012.05.001
152. Nagy J, Zámbó K, Decsi L. Anti-anxiety action of diazepam after intra-amygdaloid application in the rat. *Neuropharmacology* (1979) 18(6):573–6. doi: 10.1016/0028-3908(79)90104-7
153. Tang HH, McNally GP, Richardson R. The effects of FG7142 on two types of forgetting in 18-day-old rats. *Behav Neurosci* (2007) 121(6):1421–5. doi: 10.1037/0735-7044.121.6.1421
154. Lee H, Kim JJ. Amygdalar NMDA receptors are critical for new fear learning in previously fear-conditioned rats. *J Neurosci* (1998) 18(20):8444–54. doi: 10.1523/JNEUROSCI.18-20-08444.1998
155. Nishikawa H, Inoue T, Masui T, Izumi T, Koyama T. Effects of cytochrome P450 (CYP) 3A4 inhibitors on the anxiolytic action of tandospirone in rat contextual conditioned fear. *Prog Neuropsychopharmacol Biol Psychiatry* (2007) 31(4):926–31. doi: 10.1016/j.pnpbp.2007.02.010
156. Helmstetter FJ, Bellgowan PS. Effects of muscimol applied to the basolateral amygdala on acquisition and expression of contextual fear conditioning in rats. *Behav Neurosci* (1994) 108(5):1005–9. doi: 10.1037/0735-7044.108.5.1005
157. Diamond DM, Zoladz PR. Dysfunctional or hyperfunctional? The amygdala in posttraumatic stress disorder is the bull in the evolutionary China shop. *J Neurosci Res* (2016) 94(6):437–44. doi: 10.1002/jnr.23684
158. LeDoux JE, Pine DS. Using neuroscience to help understand fear and anxiety: a two-system framework. *Am J Psychiatry* (2016) 173(11):1083–93. doi: 10.1176/appi.ajp.2016.16030353
159. Zoladz PR, Diamond DM. Current status on behavioral and biological markers of PTSD: a search for clarity in a conflicting literature. *Neurosci Biobehav Rev* (2013) 37(5):860–95. doi: 10.1016/j.neubiorev.2013.03.024
160. Etkin A, Prater KE, Schatzberg AF, Menon V, Greicius MD. Disrupted amygdalar subregion functional connectivity and evidence of a compensatory network in generalized anxiety disorder. *Arch Gen Psychiatry* (2009) 66(12):1361–72. doi: 10.1001/archgenpsychiatry.2009.104
161. Teicher MH, Samson JA, Anderson CM, Ohashi K. The effects of childhood maltreatment on brain structure, function and connectivity. *Nat Rev Neurosci* (2016) 17(10):652–66. doi: 10.1038/nrn.2016.111
162. Thomaes K, Dorrepaal E, Draijer N, de Ruiter MB, van Balkom AJ, Smit JH, et al. Reduced anterior cingulate and orbitofrontal volumes in child abuse-related complex PTSD. *J Clin Psychiatry* (2010) 71(12):1636–44. doi: 10.4088/JCP.08m04754blu
163. Woon FL, Sood S, Hedges DW. Hippocampal volume deficits associated with exposure to psychological trauma and posttraumatic stress disorder in adults: a meta-analysis. *Prog Neuropsychopharmacol Biol Psychiatry* (2010) 34(7):1181–8. doi: 10.1016/j.pnpbp.2010.06.016
164. Miller AH, Raison CL. The role of inflammation in depression: from evolutionary imperative to modern treatment target. *Nat Rev Immunol* (2016) 16(1):22–34. doi: 10.1038/nri.2015.5
165. Einat H, Yuan P, Manji HK. Increased anxiety-like behaviors and mitochondrial dysfunction in mice with targeted mutation of the Bcl-2 gene: further support for the involvement of mitochondrial function in anxiety disorders. *Behav Brain Res* (2005) (2):172–80. doi: 10.1016/j.bbr.2005.06.012
166. Schiavone S, Trabace L. Pharmacological targeting of redox regulation systems as new therapeutic approach for psychiatric disorders: a literature overview. *Pharmacol Res* (2016) 107:195–204. doi: 10.1016/j.phrs.2016.03.019
167. Kahn RS, Sommer IE. The neurobiology and treatment of first-episode schizophrenia. *Mol Psychiatry* (2015) 20(1):84–97. doi: 10.1038/mp.2014.66
168. McCullumsmith RE, Clinton SM, Meador-Woodruff JH. Schizophrenia as a disorder of neuroplasticity. *Int Rev Neurobiol* (2004) 59:19–45. doi: 10.1016/S0074-7742(04)59002-5
169. Yoon JH, Maddock RJ, Rokem A, Silver MA, Minzenberg MJ, Ragland JD, et al. GABA concentration is reduced in visual cortex in schizophrenia and correlates with orientation-specific surround suppression. *J Neurosci* (2010) 30(10):3777–81. doi: 10.1523/JNEUROSCI.6158-09.2010
170. Wassef A, Baker J, Kochan LD. GABA and schizophrenia: a review of basic science and clinical studies. *J Clin Psychopharmacol* (2003) 23(6):601–40. doi: 10.1097/01.jcp.0000095349.32154.a5
171. Haijma SV, Van Haren N, Cahn W, Koolschijn PC, Hulshoff Pol HE, Kahn RS. Brain volumes in schizophrenia: a meta-analysis in over 18 000 subjects. *Schizophr Bull* (2013) 39(5):1129–38. doi: 10.1093/schbul/sbs118
172. Shenton ME, Dickey CC, Frumin M, McCarley RW. A review of MRI findings in schizophrenia. *Schizophr Res* (2001) 49(1–2):1–52. doi: 10.1016/S0920-9964(01)00163-3
173. Thompson PM, Vidal C, Giedd JN, Gochman P, Blumenthal J, Nicolson R, et al. Mapping adolescent brain change reveals dynamic wave of accelerated gray matter loss in very early-onset schizophrenia. *Proc Natl Acad Sci U S A* (2001) 98(20):11650–5. doi: 10.1073/pnas.201243998
174. Schnieder TP, Dwork AJ. Searching for neuropathology: gliosis in schizophrenia. *Biol Psychiatry* (2011) 69(2):134–9. doi: 10.1016/j.biopsych.2010.08.027
175. Catts VS, Catts SV, McGrath JJ, Féron F, McLean D, Coulson EJ, et al. Apoptosis and schizophrenia: a pilot study based on dermal fibroblast cell lines. *Schizophr Res* (2006) 84(1):20–8. doi: 10.1016/j.schres.2006.03.016
176. Ben-Shachar D, Laifenfeld D. Mitochondria, synaptic plasticity, and schizophrenia. *Int Rev Neurobiol* (2004) 59:273–96. doi: 10.1016/S0074-7742(04)59011-6
177. Holper L, Ben-Shachar D, Mann JJ. Multivariate meta-analyses of mitochondrial complex I and IV in major depressive disorder, bipolar disorder, schizophrenia, Alzheimer disease, and Parkinson disease. *Neuropsychopharmacology* (2019) 44:837–49. doi: 10.1038/s41386-018-0090-0
178. Kim YK, Na KS. Neuroprotection in schizophrenia and its therapeutic implications. *Psychiatry Investig* (2017) 14(4):383–91. doi: 10.4306/pi.2017.14.4.383
179. Miller BJ, Buckley P, Seabolt W, Mellor A, Kirkpatrick B. Meta-analysis of cytokine alterations in schizophrenia: clinical status and antipsychotic effects. *Biol Psychiatry* (2011) 70(7):663–71. doi: 10.1016/j.biopsych.2011.04.013
180. Yegin A, Ay N, Aydin O, Yargici N, Eren E, Yilmaz N. Increased oxidant stress and inflammation in patients with chronic schizophrenia. *Intl J Clin Med* (2012) 3(5):368–76. doi: 10.4236/ijcm.2012.35070
181. Rajkowska G, Miguel-Hidalgo JJ, Wei J, Dilley G, Pittman SD, Meltzer HY, et al. Morphometric evidence for neuronal and glial prefrontal cell pathology in major depression. *Biol Psychiatry* (1999) 45(9):1085–98. doi: 10.1016/S0006-3223(99)00041-4
182. Schmaal L, Veltman DJ, van Erp TG, Sämann PG, Frodl T, Jahanshad N, et al. Subcortical brain alterations in major depressive disorder: findings from the ENIGMA Major Depressive Disorder working group. *Mol Psychiatry* (2016) 21(6):806–12. doi: 10.1038/mp.2015.69
183. Schmaal L, Hibar DP, Sämann PG, Hall GB, Baune BT, Jahanshad N, et al. Cortical abnormalities in adults and adolescents with major depression based on brain scans from 20 cohorts worldwide in the ENIGMA Major Depressive Disorder Working Group. *Mol Psychiatry* (2017) (6):900–9. doi: 10.1038/mp.2016.60
184. Hamilton JP, Etkin A, Furman DJ, Lemus MG, Johnson RF, Gotlib IH. Functional neuroimaging of major depressive disorder: a meta-analysis and new integration of base line activation and neural response data. *Am J Psychiatry* (2012) 169(7):693–703. doi: 10.1176/appi.ajp.2012.11071105

185. Mayberg HS. Positron emission tomography imaging in depression: a neural systems perspective. *Neuroimaging Clin N Am* (2003) 13(4):805–15. doi: 10.1016/S1052-5149(03)00104-7
186. Satterthwaite TD, Kable JW, Vandekar L, Katchmar N, Bassett DS, Baldassano CF, et al. Common and dissociable dysfunction of the reward system in bipolar and unipolar depression. *Neuropsychopharmacology* (2015) 40(9):2258–68. doi: 10.1038/npp.2015.75
187. Feer H. The catecholamine hypothesis of depressions: further arguments. *Compr Psychiatry* (1967) 8(1):1–6. doi: 10.1016/S0010-440X(67)80008-7
188. Müller N, Schwarz MJ. The immune-mediated alteration of serotonin and glutamate: towards an integrated view of depression. *Mol Psychiatry* (2007) 12(11):988–1000. doi: 10.1038/sj.mp.4002006
189. Krystal JH, Sanacora G, Blumberg H, Anand A, Charney DS, Marek G, et al. Glutamate and GABA systems as targets for novel antidepressant and mood-stabilizing treatments. *Mol Psychiatry* (2002) 7 (Suppl 1):S71–80. doi: 10.1038/sj.mp.4001021
190. Petty F. GABA and mood disorders: a brief review and hypothesis. *J Affect Disord* (1995) 34(4):275–81. doi: 10.1016/0165-0327(95)00025-I
191. Su WJ, Zhang Y, Chen Y, Gong H, Lian YJ, Peng W, et al. NLRP3 gene knockout blocks NF-κB and MAPK signaling pathway in CUMS-induced depression mouse model. *Behav Brain Res* (2017) 322(Pt A):1–8. doi: 10.1016/j.bbr.2017.01.018
192. Zhu W, Cao FS, Feng J, Chen HW, Wan JR, Lu Q, et al. NLRP3 inflammasome activation contributes to long-term behavioral alterations in mice injected with lipopolysaccharide. *Neuroscience* (2017) 343:77–84. doi: 10.1016/j.neuroscience.2016.11.037
193. Alcocer-Gómez E, de Miguel M, Casas-Barquero N, Núñez-Vasco J, Sánchez-Alcazar JA, Fernández-Rodríguez A, et al. NLRP3 inflammasome is activated in mononuclear blood cells from patients with major depressive disorder. *Brain Behav Immun* (2014) 36:111–7. doi: 10.1016/j.bbi.2013.10.017
194. Kaufmann FN, Costa AP, Ghisleni G, Diaz AP, Rodrigues ALS, Peluffo H, et al. NLRP3 inflammasome-driven pathways in depression: clinical and preclinical findings. *Brain Behav Immun* (2017) 64:367–83. doi: 10.1016/j.bbi.2017.03.002
195. Stetler C, Miller GE. Depression and hypothalamic–pituitary–adrenal activation: a quantitative summary of four decades of research. *Psychosom Med* (2011) (2):114–26. doi: 10.1097/PSY.0b013e31820ad12b
196. Brown GM, McIntyre RS, Rosenblat J, Hardeland R. Depressive disorders: processes leading to neurogeneration and potential novel treatments. *Prog Neuropsychopharmacol Biol Psychiatry* (2018b) 80(Pt C):189–204. doi: 10.1016/j.pnpbp.2017.04.023
197. Hardingham GE, Fukunaga Y, Bading H. Extrasynaptic NMDARs oppose synaptic NMDARs by triggering CREB shut-off and cell death pathways. *Nat Neurosci* (2002) (5):405–14. doi: 10.1038/nn835
198. Zhu CB, Lindler KM, Owens AW, Daws LC, Blakely RD, Hewlett WA. Interleukin-1 receptor activation by systemic lipopolysaccharide induces behavioral despair linked to MAPK regulation of CNS serotonin transporters. *Neuropsychopharmacology* (2010) 35(13):2510–20. doi: 10.1038/npp.2010.116
199. Capuron L, Pagnoni G, Drake DF, Woolwine BJ, Spivey JR, Crowe RJ, et al. Dopaminergic mechanisms of reduced basal ganglia responses to hedonic reward during interferon alfa administration. *Arch Gen Psychiatry* (2012) 69(10):1044–53. doi: 10.1001/archgenpsychiatry.2011.2094
200. Goodwin FK, Jamison KR. *Manic-depressive illness: bipolar disorders and recurrent depression*. New York: Oxford University Press (2007), ISBN: 978-0-19-513579-4.
201. Kurita M, Nishino S, Numata Y, Okubo Y, Sato T. The noradrenaline metabolite MHPG is a candidate biomarker between the depressive, remission, and manic states in bipolar disorder I: two long-term naturalistic case reports. *Neuropsychiatr Dis Treat* (2015) 11:353–8. doi: 10.2147/NDT.S74550
202. Yatham LN, Kennedy SH, Parikh SV, Schaffer A, Bond DJ, Frey BN, et al. Canadian Network for Mood and Anxiety Treatments (CANMAT) and International Society for Bipolar Disorders (ISBD) 2018 guidelines for the management of patients with bipolar disorder. *Bipolar Disord* (2018) 20(2):97–170. doi: 10.1111/bdi.12609
203. Berk M, Kapczinski F, Andreazza AC, Dean OM, Giorlando F, Maes M, et al. Pathways underlying neuroprogression in bipolar disorder: focus on inflammation, oxidative stress and neurotrophic factors. *Neurosci Biobehav Rev* (2011) 35(3):804–17. doi: 10.1016/j.neubiorev.2010.10.001
204. Mertens J, Wang QW, Kim Y, Yu DX, Pham S, Yang B, et al. Differential responses to lithium in hyperexcitable neurons from patients with bipolar disorder. *Nature* (2015) 527(7576):95–9. doi: 10.1038/nature15526
205. Blumberg HP, Kaufman J, Martin A, Whiteman R, Zhang JH, Gore JC, et al. Amygdala and hippocampal volumes in adolescents and adults with bipolar disorder. *Arch Gen Psychiatry* (2003) 60(12):1201–8. doi: 10.1001/archpsyc.60.12.1201
206. Cao B, Passos IC, Mwangi B, Bauer IE, Zunta-Soares GB, Kapczinski F, et al. Hippocampal volume and verbal memory performance in late-stage bipolar disorder. *J Psychiatr Res* (2016) 73:102–7. doi: 10.1016/j.jpsychires.2015.12.012
207. Hibar DP, Westlye LT, Doan NT, Jahanshad N, Cheung JW, Ching CRK, et al. Cortical abnormalities in bipolar disorder: an MRI analysis of 6503 individuals from the ENIGMA Bipolar Disorder Working Group. *Mol Psychiatry* (2018) 23(4):932–42. doi: 10.1038/mp.2017.73
208. Rao JS, Harry GJ, Rapoport SI, Kim HW. Increased excitotoxicity and neuroinflammatory markers in postmortem frontal cortex from bipolar disorder patients. *Mol Psychiatry* (2010) 15(4):384–92. doi: 10.1038/mp.2009.47
209. Lange N, Travers BG, Bigler ED, Prigge MB, Froehlich AL, Nielsen JA, et al. Longitudinal volumetric brain changes in autism spectrum disorder ages 6-35 years. *Autism Res.* (2015) 8(1):82–93. doi: 10.1002/aur.1427
210. Paul LK, Corsello C, Kennedy DP, Adolphs R. Agenesis of the corpus callosum and autism: a comprehensive comparison. *Brain* (2014) 137(Pt 6):1813–29. doi: 10.1093/brain/awu070
211. Tyszka JM, Kennedy DP, Paul LK, Adolphs R. Largely typical patterns of resting-state functional connectivity in high-functioning adults with autism. *Cereb Cortex* (2014) 24(7):1894–905. doi: 10.1093/cercor/bht040
212. Zielinski BA, Prigge MB, Nielsen JA, Froehlich AL, Abildskov TJ, Anderson JS, et al. Longitudinal changes in cortical thickness in autism and typical development. *Brain* (2014) 137(Pt 6):1799–812. doi: 10.1093/brain/awu083
213. Bear MF, Huber KM, Warren ST. The mGluR theory of fragile X mental retardation. *Trends Neurosci* (2004) 27(7):370–7. doi: 10.1016/j.tins.2004.04.009
214. Erickson CA, Mullett JE, McDougle CJ. Open-label memantine in fragile X syndrome. *J Autism Dev Disord* (2009) 39(12):1629–35. doi: 10.1007/s10803-009-0807-3
215. Green J, Garg S. Annual Research Review: the state of autism intervention science: progress, target psychological and biological mechanisms and future prospects. *J Child Psychol Psychiatry* (2018) 59(4):424–43. doi: 10.1111/jcpp.12892
216. Lemonnier E, Villeneuve N, Sonie S, Serret S, Rosier A, Roue M, et al. Effects of bumetanide on neurobehavioral function in children and adolescents with autism spectrum disorders. *Transl Psychiatry* (2017) 7(3):e1056. doi: 10.1038/tp.2017.10
217. Chandana SR, Behen ME, Juhász C, Muzik O, Rothermel RD, Mangner TJ, et al. Significance of abnormalities in developmental trajectory and asymmetry of cortical serotonin synthesis in autism. *Int J Dev Neurosci* (2005) 23(2–3):171–82. doi: 10.1016/j.ijdevneu.2004.08.002
218. Cheffer A, Castillo ARG, Corrêa-Velloso J, Gonçalves MCB, Naaldijk Y, Nascimento IC, et al. Purinergic system in psychiatric diseases. *Mol Psychiatry* (2018) 23(1):94–106. doi: 10.1038/mp.2017.188
219. Masino SA, Kawamura M, Jr., Plotkin LM, Svedova J, DiMario FJ Jr, Eigsti IM. The relationship between the neuromodulator adenosine and behavioral symptoms of autism. *Neurosci Lett* (2011) 500(1):1–5. doi: 10.1016/j.neulet.2011.06.007
220. Masino SA, Kawamura M. Jr, Cote JL, Williams RB, Ruskin DN. Adenosine and autism: a spectrum of opportunities. *Neuropharmacology* (2013) 68:116–21. doi: 10.1016/j.neuropharm.2012.08.013
221. Rodriguez JI, Kern JK. Evidence of microglial activation in autism and its possible role in brain underconnectivity. *Neuron Glia Biol* (2011) 7(2–4):205–13. doi: 10.1017/S1740925X12000142
222. Hughes HK, Mills Ko E, Rose D, Ashwood P. Immune dysfunction and autoimmunity as pathological mechanisms in autism spectrum disorders. *Front Cell Neurosci* (2018) 12:405. doi: 10.3389/fncel.2018.00405

223. Vargas DL, Nascimbene C, Krishnan C, Zimmerman AW, Pardo CA. Neuroglial activation and neuroinflammation in the brain of patients with autism. *Ann Neurol* (2005) 57(1):67–81. doi: 10.1002/ana.20315
224. Zimmerman AW, Jyonouchi H, Comi AM, Connors SL, Milstien S, Varsou A, et al. Cerebrospinal fluid and serum markers of inflammation in autism. *Pediatr Neurol* (2005) 33(3):195–201. doi: 10.1016/j.pediatrneurol.2005.03.014
225. Filipek PA, Juranek J, Smith M, Mays LZ, Ramos ER, Bocian M, et al. Mitochondrial dysfunction in autistic patients with 15q inverted duplication. *Ann Neurol* (2003) 53(6):801–4. doi: 10.1002/ana.10596
226. Frye RE, Rossignol DA. Treatments for biomedical abnormalities associated with autism spectrum disorder. *Front Pediatr* (2014) 2:66. doi: 10.3389/fped.2014.00066
227. Rossignol DA, Frye RE. Evidence linking oxidative stress, mitochondrial dysfunction, and inflammation in the brain of individuals with autism. *Front Physiol* (2014) 5:150. doi: 10.3389/fphys.2014.00150
228. Cortese S, Kelly C, Chabernaud C, Proal E, Di Martino A, Milham MP, et al. Toward systems neuroscience of ADHD: a meta-analysis of 55 fMRI studies. *Am J Psychiatry* (2012) 169(10):1038–55. doi: 10.1176/appi.ajp.2012.11101521
229. Greven CU, Bralten J, Mennes M, O'Dwyer L, van Hulzen KJ, Rommelse N, et al. Developmentally stable whole-brain volume reductions and developmentally sensitive caudate and putamen volume alterations in those with attention-deficit/hyperactivity disorder and their unaffected siblings. *JAMA Psychiatry* (2015) 72(5):490–9. doi: 10.1001/jamapsychiatry.2014.3162
230. Courvoisie H, Hooper SR, Fine C, Kwock L, Castillo M. Neurometabolic functioning and neuropsychological correlates in children with ADHD-H: preliminary findings. *J Neuropsychiatry Clin Neurosci* (2004) 16(1):63–9. doi: 10.1176/appi.neuropsych.16.1.63
231. Edden RA, Crocetti D, Zhu H, Gilbert DL, Mostofsky SH. Reduced GABA concentration in attention-deficit/hyperactivity disorder. *Arch Gen Psychiatry* (2012) 69(7):750–3. doi: 10.1001/archgenpsychiatry.2011.2280
232. Briars L, Todd T. A review of pharmacological management of attention-deficit/hyperactivity disorder. *J Pediatr Pharmacol Ther* (2016) 21(3):192–206. doi: 10.5863/1551-6776-21.3.192
233. Gizer IR, Ficks C, Waldman ID. Candidate gene studies of ADHD: a meta-analytic review. *Hum Genet* (2009) 126(1):51–90. doi: 10.1007/s00439-009-0694-x
234. Oades RD, Slusarek M, Velling S, Bondy B. Serotonin platelet-transporter measures in childhood attention-deficit/hyperactivity disorder (ADHD): clinical versus experimental measures of impulsivity. *World J Biol Psychiatry* (2002) 3(2):96–100. doi: 10.3109/15622970209150607
235. Sowinski H, Karpawich PP. Management of a hyperactive teen and cardiac safety. *Pediatr Clin North Am* (2014) 61(1):81–90. doi: 10.1016/j.pcl.2013.09.021
236. Leffa DT, Bellaver B, de Oliveira C, de Macedo IC, de Freitas JS, Grevet EH, et al. Increased oxidative parameters and decreased cytokine levels in an animal model of attention-deficit/hyperactivity disorder. *Neurochem Res* (2017) 42(11):3084–92. doi: 10.1007/s11064-017-2341-6

15

Psychiatric and Cognitive Aspects of Phenylketonuria: The Limitations of Diet and Promise of New Treatments

*Killian Ashe[1], Wendy Kelso[1], Sarah Farrand[1], Julie Panetta[2], Tim Fazio[2,3], Gerard De Jong[2,3] and Mark Walterfang[1,4,5]**

[1] Neuropsychiatry Unit, Royal Melbourne Hospital, Melbourne, VIC, Australia, [2] Statewide Adult Metabolic Service, Royal Melbourne Hospital, Melbourne, VIC, Australia, [3] Melbourne Medical School, University of Melbourne, Melbourne, VIC, Australia, [4] Melbourne Neuropsychiatry Centre, University of Melbourne and North-Western Mental Health, Melbourne, VIC, Australia, [5] Florey Institute of Neuroscience and Mental Health, University of Melbourne, Melbourne, VIC, Australia

Correspondence:
Mark Walterfang
mark.walterfang@mh.org.au

Phenylketonuria (PKU) is a recessive disorder of phenylalanine metabolism due to mutations in the gene for phenylalanine hydroxylase (PAH). Reduced PAH activity results in significant hyperphenylalaninemia, which leads to alterations in cerebral myelin and protein synthesis, as well as reduced levels of serotonin, dopamine, and noradrenaline in the brain. When untreated, brain development is grossly disrupted and significant intellectual impairment and behavioral disturbance occur. The advent of neonatal heel prick screening has allowed for diagnosis at birth, and the institution of a phenylalanine restricted diet. Dietary treatment, particularly when maintained across neurodevelopment and well into adulthood, has resulted in markedly improved outcomes at a cognitive and psychiatric level for individuals with PKU. However, few individuals can maintain full dietary control lifelong, and even with good control, an elevated risk remains of—in particular—mood, anxiety, and attentional disorders across the lifespan. Increasingly, dietary recommendations focus on maintaining continuous dietary treatment lifelong to optimize psychiatric and cognitive outcomes, although the effect of long-term protein restricted diets on brain function remains unknown. While psychiatric illness is very common in adult PKU populations, very little data exist to guide clinicians on optimal treatment. The advent of new treatments that do not require restrictive dietary management, such as the enzyme therapy Pegvaliase, holds the promise of allowing patients a relatively normal diet alongside optimized mental health and cognitive functioning.

Keywords: phenylketonuria, psychiatric, anxiety, depression, cognitive function

INTRODUCTION

Phenylketonuria (PKU; OMIM 261600 and 261630) is a rare autosomal recessive and inborn error of metabolism (1). Caused by one of almost 1,000 gene variants (2), it is characterized by a variable deficiency in the activity of the phenylalanine hydroxylase (PAH) enzyme necessary for the conversion of the amino acid phenylalanine (Phe) to tyrosine (Tyr). The resultant accumulation of Phe throughout the body due to reduced PAH activity leads to significant neurodevelopmental sequelae including intellectual disability, growth retardation, and seizures (1), and is the most common biochemical cause of intellectual impairment (3). In addition, there are a range of neuropsychiatric and cognitive changes that can be associated with PKU at varying levels of hyperphenylalaninemia.

Phenylalanine is an essential amino acid, present in most natural proteinaceous foods, and is metabolized in the liver by the PAH system. The hydroxylation of Phe to Tyr requires tetrahydrobiopterin (BH4), iron, and molecular oxygen as co-factors (1). Defects in either PAH or the production or recycling of BH4 may result in hyperphenylalaninemia. The disorder was first discovered in 1934 by Følling who identified elevated Phe metabolites (phenylketones) in the urine of two intellectually disabled siblings, thus giving the disorder its name (4); the defect in PAH was isolated in 1953 (5), and a Phe-restricted diet was also shown to improve intellectual outcomes (6). In 1962, the Guthrie method to detect elevated Phe levels in dried blood spots was developed, which facilitated newborn screening of the disorder, facilitating early diagnosis and dietary management of PKU (7), and thus the prevention of many hundreds of thousands of cases of intellectual disability. The "Guthrie Test," conducted by neonatal heel prick, was implemented widely across North America and Europe in the 1960s (7). It identifies affected infants at birth and has a 99.2% sensitivity and 99.9% specificity for those with classical and mild PKU (8), and has been demonstrated to have a favorable benefit–cost ratio (9).

Two Australian studies reported the incidence of PKU to be 1 in 11,226 (10) and 1 in 8,900, mirroring the figures found in other Caucasian populations (3). The reported incidence of PKU ranges from 1 per 13,500 to 1 per 19,000 newborns in the United States, and does vary by ethnic group, with incidence being higher in Caucasians and Native Americans and lower in Hispanics, Blacks, and Asians (11).

Depending on the genotype and severity of the enzyme defect, various forms of PKU with different clinical outcomes have been described (12). These can be classified on the basis of blood Phe levels at diagnosis and dietary Phe tolerance. The natural history of untreated PKU consists of progressive irreversible neurological impairment during infancy and childhood. The most common outcome is severe intellectual disability often associated with a "mousy" odor, eczema, and reduced hair, skin, and iris pigmentation. There is often growth retardation, microcephaly, and neurological signs including tremor and epilepsy. All untreated patients have behavioral problems including hyperactivity, stereotypy, and anxiety. The severity of the clinical phenotype directly correlates with blood phenylalanine levels that reflect the degree of enzymatic deficiency (1).

Until recently, a strict low-Phe diet, the use of medical foods consisting of Phe-free protein substitutes, and supplementation containing large neutral amino acids (LNAAs) such as Tyr were the only therapies available (13). Foods high in Phe, such as eggs, meat, poultry, fish, bread, and pasta, are largely eliminated. Dietary treatment has been shown to be very effective in the prevention of impaired cognitive development, but still has its shortcomings. Specific deficiencies of calcium, zinc, selenium, iron, and vitamin B12 were reported with the early formulas, as was growth delay (14).This diet was initially discontinued after 6 years of age, when the majority of significant neurodevelopment was thought to be complete ("early-treated" patients); this age was later increased to 12 years of age; however, these discontinuation points often varied between jurisdictions. Later epochs of treatment recommendations suggested cessation at early adulthood, with only a return to diet being necessitated during pregnancy. However, over time, it has been increasingly recognized that ongoing adherence to diet is associated with better cognitive and psychosocial outcomes throughout adulthood ("continuously treated" patients), as increasingly hyperphenylalaninemia has been recognized to not just impact upon neurodevelopment, but dynamic functioning within the adult brain (15). Current guidelines indicate that individuals with PKU should aim to maintain lifelong Phe levels between 120 and 360 µmol/L in the US, or up to 600 µmol/L in Europe, even though this is still up to a fivefold increase over Phe levels in non-PKU individuals (16, 17).

When treatment is instituted from birth, PKU patients are likely to have a normal intellectual quotient (IQ), but it is now apparent that there is often an IQ gap when compared to their non-PKU siblings, and these patients may have deficits in certain neuropsychological functioning, particularly executive function (18). They may also demonstrate elevated rates of neuropsychiatric illness, increasingly being recognized, which contribute to significant impairments in psychosocial functioning and quality of life in adults with treated PKU. This review aims to discuss the range of neuropsychiatric and cognitive manifestations associated with PKU and their management.

Pathophysiology of PKU

Deficient PAH activity results in two key pathological states: hyperphenylalaninemia and hypotyrosinemia (19). High Phe competes with tyrosine, tryptophan, and other LNAAs at the L-type amino acid carrier (LAT1) at the blood–brain barrier (BBB), resulting in decreased concentrations of dopamine and serotonin in the brain (20). The transport of Phe across the BBB has been found to be highly variable, translating to heterogeneous clinical outcomes across individuals even when "on-diet" or with similar plasma Phe levels (11, 20).

There are multiple possible downstream effects of hyperphenylalaninemia, for which the evidence and hypotheses are drawn from human and animal studies. These are summarized in broad categories below, with respect to neuropsychiatric and cognitive profiles. The mechanisms by which these effects occur are summarized in **Figure 1**.

Neurotransmission and Protein Synthesis

Hyperphenylalaninemia causes dysfunction in neurotransmission and cerebral protein synthesis, *via* relative hypotyrosinemia, impaired transport of large amino acids into the brain, and impairment of other enzymatic systems. Not only is the biosynthesis of tyrosine reduced due to PAH deficiency, but also in a state of hyperphenylalaninemia, there is competitive binding at LAT1 carrier, resulting in Phe preferentially crossing the blood–brain barrier and a relative lack of other LNAAs including tryptophan and tyrosine, the building blocks of serotonin and dopamine (21). The low bioavailability of these LNAAs then has downstream effects on cerebral protein synthesis in evidence drawn from the PKU mouse model (21). Evidence from mice and human models also suggests that hyperPhe impairs the function of the tyrosine and tryptophan hydroxylase systems (22–24), as well as 3-hydroxy-3-methylglutaryl-coenzyme A reductase

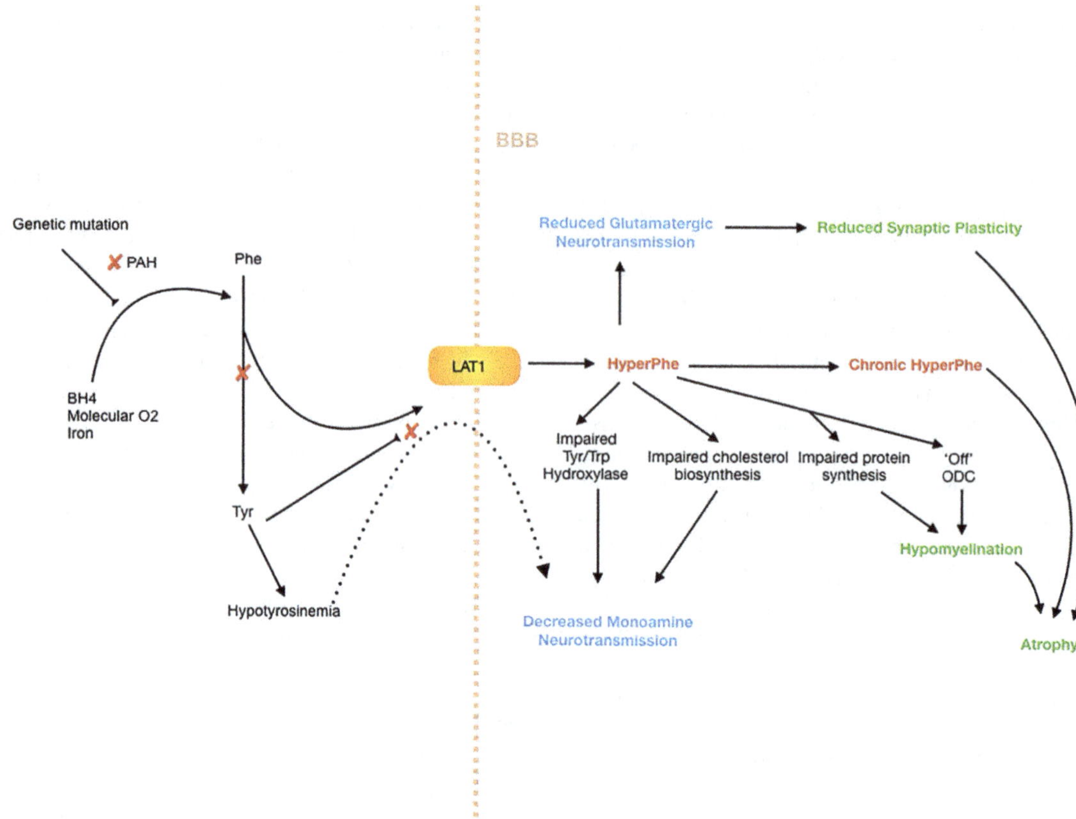

FIGURE 1 | Neuropathophysiology of PKU. Decreased PAH activity results in hyperphenylalaninemia as well as hypotyrosinemia. The high Phe levels further restrict transport of tyrosine across the blood–brain barrier, as well as impairing tyrosine and tryptophan hydroxylase systems, as well as cholesterol synthesis, creating a hypomonoaminergic state in the brain, predominantly in frontal and limbic circuits where these neurotransmitters predominate. There is also reduced glutamatergic neurotransmission, which results in reduced synaptic plasticity, and in turn atrophy. Myelination is critically affected by high Phe levels, which impair protein synthesis, as well as switch oligodendrocytes to an "off" or non-myelinating state.

and thus impairing cholesterol biosynthesis (21), all of which effects a reduction in neurotransmitter production.

Glutamate is the most abundant neurotransmitter and plays an important role in synaptic plasticity, learning, memory, and modulation of function within the limbic system (25). In the PKU mouse model, hyperPhe was found to reduce glutamate transmission resulting in compensatory changes in the expression of the glutamate receptor (26). This occurred *via* competitive binding at the NMDA receptor, reduction in release of neurotransmitters, and competition for binding to sites on other receptors (such as AMPA and kainate glutamatergic receptors) (27). Importantly these findings were reversible, suggesting a degree of reversibility of neuropsychiatric symptoms seen in PKU. Glutamate has also been increasingly recognized for its role in stress-related conditions, including anxiety and depression. While acute stress can transiently increase glutamate output and transmission, chronic stress is associated with similar findings to those seen in the hyperPhe state, with reduced synaptic plasticity and attenuated glutamatergic neurotransmission (28).

Synaptic and Dendritic Changes

Animal studies have greatly informed the field about the microstructural effects of hyperPhe. Treating newborn rodents with high levels of Phe during early life results in malformed dendritic trees (29, 30) and reduced neocortical synaptic density (31), possibly through the altered expression of cytoskeletal proteins (32). Studies of hippocampal cultures in the PAH^{enu2} mouse model treated with phenylalanine show a reduction in density of synapses, and length of dendrites (33), with synaptic morphological alterations (34). At least some of these morphological changes in the mouse model appear to be remediable by a specific nutrient combination, suggesting that attenuating synaptic deficits may be one potential mechanism of dietary intervention in PKU (30, 35).

Dysmyelination

A number of studies have demonstrated abnormal myelination in PKU patients (36, 37). Bauman and Kemper undertook histoanatomic assessment of three brains in untreated, intellectually disabled adult PKU patients and found that there was pallor of myelin staining, particularly in areas that undergo significant postnatal myelination, as compared with those areas that undergo myelination shortly before or after birth, which were comparable to age matched controls (38). Later-myelinating areas include the axonal connections to the prefrontal cortex and other frontal and parietal regions, as well as cortico-hippocampal relay circuits, which undergo myelination in adolescence (39, 40). Elevations in Phe resultsin the non-competitive inhibition of HMG-CoA reductase, which impairs the production of cholesterol, one of the major lipids in the myelin membrane (41), and the reduction of LNAAs available for myelin-related proteins may compromise myelin synthesis further (42, 43).

These late-myelinating regions may be more vulnerable to suboptimal environmental conditions. Areas that undergo myelination later in development have smaller axons and fewer lamellae, and originate from oligodendrocytes that myelinate many more axons than those that undergo early myelination (44). In a review of the relationship of late-myelinating regions and neurodegeneration, Bartzokis postulated that this resulted in three broad sequelae—that these regions would have greater surface area exposed to the extracellular environment and thus greater vulnerability to a toxic (i.e., HyperPhe) environment, higher myelin density, and a greater impact when there is breakdown of these areas due to the thinner myelin sheaths (44). This model, while applied by Bartzokis to primary neurodegenerative disorders, has relevance to all neuropsychiatric disorders, and in combination with the specific areas involved in late myelination, gives reasonable account as to the high rates of psychiatric and cognitive symptoms seen in PKU.

Supporting this are data from both animal and human studies. In normal rats, chronic hyperPhe resulted in impaired myelination and axonal maturation (45). In the PAH^{enu2} mouse model, when exposed to higher levels of Phe, myelin-rich areas had the lowest rates of protein synthesis (46), and to further this, Dyer and colleagues found that when oligodendrocytes were exposed to high Phe levels, they adopt a "non-myelinating" phenotype, effectively switching off myelination (47). There is a strong relationship between dopamine signaling and myelination, in addition to axonal maturation. Myelination itself facilitates axonal maturation through triggering heavy phosphorylation of neurofilaments, cytoskeleton rearrangement, and axonal swelling beneath the compact myelin lamellae (48). These myelin/axonal interactions may up-regulate the production of enzymes involved in dopamine biosynthesis pathway such as tyrosine hydroxylase (TH), or the phosphorylation of TH, which thus up-regulates dopamine synthesis. Thus, the hypodopaminergic state seen in PKU results not just from reduced precursor penetration into the CNS, but also indirectly through impaired myelination. Supporting this, when PKU mice are treated with a low Phe diet, myelination increases in concert with central DA levels, supporting the strong relationship between these two measures. In humans, this would support the findings that white matter abnormalities on MRI are most significantly related to recent Phe levels (at the time of MRI and in the 12 months prior) and appear to be somewhat reversible (49–51). Additionally, neuroimaging in humans suggests that in addition to hypomyelination in developing axonal tracts, intramyelinic edema may also contribute to the altered T2-weighted signal that is frequently seen in the posterior white matter in PKU patients (52), and changes in posterior white matter on imaging correlate well with serum Phe levels (53).

It is important to note that in Mastrangelo et al.'s retrospective longitudinal long-term study on the outcome of white matter abnormalities in early treated phenylketonuric patients (54), there was no significant association found between cognitive outcome and alterations in white matter structure. However, significant interindividual variability was found, and incongruity was often seen between biochemical control and the trajectory of white matter alterations. About 30% of the variability of white matter alterations remains unexplained by the known quantifiable variables of the disease.

PSYCHIATRIC DISORDERS

Children, adolescents, and adults with PKU can display disturbed emotional and behavioral functioning with evidence of a heterogeneous range of phenotypes, as summarized in **Table 1**. However, review of the literature continues to demonstrate that the prevalence and severity of problems correlate strongly with the degree and timing of exposure to elevations in blood Phe levels (55). Neuropsychiatric symptoms are likely to be driven by multiple mechanisms, through which hyperPhe impacts brain function, including disruption of amino acid transport across the blood–brain barrier, myelin abnormalities, and reductions in neurotransmitters, as described previously (43).

Untreated PKU patients have long been known to present with significant neuropsychiatric disturbance, dating back to Følling's initial descriptions of the disease in 1934, where a spectrum of presentations was noted, ranging from shy and anxious, irritable, agitated and with anger outbursts, through to grossly disturbed, psychotic, and catatonic (56). Further mid-twentieth century literature correlated untreated PKU status with severe behavioral disturbance, largely autistic and psychotic spectrum illnesses, frequently with marked levels of agitation and aggression (57). Literature from that time indicates that this group was particularly challenging to manage in institutions for the intellectually disabled; these patients often display aggression, self-mutilation, impulsivity, and even psychosis (58). In 10 previously undiagnosed and 1 previously diagnosed but untreated individuals, Mazur et al. identified the most frequent behaviors as aggression, affective symptoms including euphoria/elation, as well as agitation and aberrant motor symptoms, but also noted the marked heterogeneity of presentations—including anxiety, delusions and hallucinations, and dysphoria/depression (59).

However with the advent of dietary treatment of PKU, the degree of cognitive and neuropsychiatric impairment markedly

TABLE 1 | Neuropsychiatric symptoms as a function of treatment Initiation.

Untreated	Early-treated children and adolescents	Early-treated adults
Psychotic symptoms	Attentional problems	Depressed mood
Autistic behaviors	School problems	Social isolation/withdrawal
Hyperactivity	Less achievement motivation	Generalized anxiety
Aggression	Low self-esteem	Phobias
Anxiety	Decreased social competence	Social maturity deficits
Depressed mood	Decreased autonomy	Decreased positive emotions
Impaired social skills associated with profound intellectual disability		Low self-esteem
		Lack of autonomy

reduced in the PKU patient group, with most individuals more assimilated in mainstream educational and vocational settings (60). Given that with strict dietary control, Phe levels in treated patients are usually elevated significantly over Phe levels in non-PKU individuals, it is not unexpected that even with continuous clinical management, psychosocial and/or neuropsychiatric impairments have been observed in clinically treated cohorts (61). Burton et al. demonstrated that >50% of adults with PKU screened positive for the presence of clinically significant psychiatric symptoms, the most common being depression and anxiety (62).

Depression

Rates of depression are significantly higher among adults with PKU than the general population (63). Depression is reported by up to half of adult patients in survey data (64, 65). A meta-analysis of reported neuropsychiatric complications demonstrated that overall point prevalence rates of depression were 18% in the population with PKU, further subdivided into 12% in the early-treated group, versus 35% in the late-treated (18). This is corroborated in Bilder's 2017 retrospective cohort study, showing that rates of depression are markedly higher in the overall adult PKU cohort compared to the general population cohort—and this was demonstrated in significantly higher rates of depression in all age groups over the age of 20 years (66). This study of 3,715 individuals with PKU demonstrated depression in 19.5%, which was comparable with depression in a population with diabetes mellitus (21.1%), and exceeding that seen in the in the general population (11.8%).

The underpinning pathophysiology of depression in PKU is likely to be multifaceted. A number of biological processes underpin the development of complex mental illness such as depression, including neurochemical, neurohumoral, and neuroinflammatory processes (67), which are also mediated by psychosocial factors including dietary adherence (68). However, given the key involvement of dopamine, norepinephrine, and serotonin in regulating cognition, emotion, and mood, and the marked elevation of rates of depression in PKU, it is likely that depressive symptoms are strongly associated with hyperPhe-driven low central monoaminergic transmission. This is supported by one study showing that short-term elevations in Phe do result in acutely lowered mood (69). Monoaminergic networks that project to frontal cortical and cortico-limbic regions play an important role in the modulation of mood, and dysfunction in these networks is implicated in the pathophysiology of depression (70, 71). Similarly, antidepressant medications likely act, at least in part if not indirectly, by restoring impaired monoaminergic transmission in these regions (72, 73), particularly through neuroplastic change driven by changes in gene expression and synaptic plasticity (74). Antidepressants may also act by increasing neurogenesis in the dentate gyrus of the hippocampus (75), in addition to other sites, such as the amygdala (76). Adult hippocampal neurogenesis may mediate antidepressant effects *via* its influence on the HPA axis (77).

Unfortunately, the role of antidepressants in the treatment of PKU-associated depression has never been formally studied, so it is not clear if efficacy rates of treatment are comparable to those seen in non-PKU individuals (68), although symptomatic patients may benefit from antidepressant treatment.

Anxiety

Rates of anxiety disorders are also significantly higher in the overall adult PKU population (15.6%) compared to the general population (9.2%), as evidenced in Bilder's recent retrospective cohort study (66), and heterogeneity in presentations of anxiety and depression can be largely explained by blood Phe level and PKU treatment (early vs. late/untreated) (18). Anxiety, alongside depression, is one of the most frequently self-reported symptoms in both adult and pediatric PKU patients (15, 64).

A range of anxiety disorders, including generalized anxiety, panic disorder, specific phobias, and obsessive-compulsive disorder, have been associated with low serotonin in the brain (73). Anxiety has been associated with a number of alterations in the serotonergic system including polymorphisms in the serotonin transporter gene (SERT) (78) and also the gene for the CNS-form of tryptophan hydroxylase (TPH2) (79). Given this, it is unsurprising that hyperphenylalaninemia in PKU, and the consequent reduction of central serotonin levels, has been associated with an increased prevalence of anxiety disorders (80). As dietary recommendations in PKU were introduced and, over time, shifted toward a more sustained restriction of Phe intake across the developmental lifespan, symptoms reported by patients also shifted in favor of internalizing symptoms (80). Non-treated children continued to prominently display externalizing symptoms of aggression and agitation in addition to mental retardation, as compared with early-treated children described as exhibiting anxiety, phobias, obsessionality, low self-esteem, and withdrawal (81, 82). Additionally, anxiety measures have been found to correlate with elevations, and significant variability over time, of blood Phe (83). Patients who maintain Phe-restricted diets into adolescence appear less likely to develop an anxiety disorder (15), and those that do have an anxiety disorder are less likely to experience symptoms when they return to dietary treatment (84). Serum Phe levels in PKU have also been shown to correlate to platelet serotonin levels (85), although peripheral are not necessarily a correlate for central serotonin levels (86). An alternate hypothesis for elevated rates of anxiety is that the burden of strict follow-up and dietary treatment constitutes a psychological stressor for children and their families; one study found that patients who adhered to the dietary recommendations during their first decade were more likely to be diagnosed with a psychiatric disorder compared to those patients with poor metabolic control (80); most other studies, however, do suggest that hyperPhe is associated with significant anxiety. For the majority of patients, a reduction in Phe levels often results in a significant attenuation of anxiety symptoms. For a subgroup of patients, particularly those who are unable to effectively lower Phe levels, treatment with serotonergic antidepressants—particularly selective serotonin reuptake inhibitors (SSRIs)—may be beneficial, although data in PKU patients are lacking.

Psychosis

Psychotic disorders including schizophrenia and bipolar affective disorder, while not the most common neuropsychiatric manifestation of PKU, still occur at higher rates than the general population (66). Early studies of PKU families identified a twice expected rate of psychosis in PKU (87), which has been replicated in more recent retrospective cohort studies (66). Early studies exploring the relationship between Phe, Tyr, and Trp with schizophrenia had mixed results, likely owing to low study numbers and methodological issues. More recent studies in the last 5–10 years have consistently shown a more compelling relationship. Genetic association studies have suggested an association between schizophrenia and PAH polymorphisms, though the functional impact of these genetic changes is not well understood (88, 89). In 2014, Okusaga and colleagues measured plasma Phe in 950 patients with schizophrenia compared with 1,000 controls, and found increased Phe and increased Phe/Tyr ratios, suggesting aberrant PAH function in schizophrenia hypothesized to be as a result of neuroinflammation (90). A small sample of medicated chronic schizophrenic patients was also found to have decreased Phe kinetics as measured by a Phe breath test, as compared to controls, further supporting the role of phenylalanine imbalance in schizophrenia (91). There is significant overlap in the pathophysiology of PKU and schizophrenia, accounting for the increased rates of psychosis seen in this PKU, as well as providing novel avenues for enquiry for the understanding and treatment of schizophrenia.

Attention Deficit Hyperactivity Disorder

Attention deficit hyperactivity disorder (ADHD) occurs in approximately 3–5% of the population (92). This disorder is characterized by developmentally inappropriate levels of impulsivity, hyperactivity, and/or inattention (93). ADHD is currently categorized into three subtypes with varying rates of prevalence: ADHD-inattentive subtype (approximately 25–30%), the ADHD-hyperactive/impulsive subtype (< 5%), and an ADHD-combined subtype (65–70%) (94). Both PKU and ADHD are highly heritable conditions, though ADHD occurs at approximately twice the rate in those with PKU compared with the general population (66).

Antshel and Waisbren studied 46 children with early- and continuously-treated classical PKU, 15 maternal PKU (mPKU) offspring, and 18 typically developing controls. They demonstrated that both the PKU and mPKU groups had higher ADHD prevalence rates compared to controls (95).

Of note, the inattentive type far exceeded the hyperactive impulsive variant, with the authors postulating that the developmental timing of exposure to elevated levels of Phe may affect the expression of ADHD symptoms. Prenatal exposure is associated with greatly increased hyperactive/impulsive symptoms, whereas exposure at any time affects attention regulation. There is a demonstrated dose-dependent relationship between Phe levels and ADHD symptoms; a greater number of ADHD symptoms were associated with a higher level of Phe exposure (95). Arnold et al.'s study in 2004 mirrored these findings (96).

In examining stimulant use in a group of 38 young people with early- and continuously treated classical PKU (as compared with age-matched type 1 diabetic controls), 50% of youths with PKU reportedly had significant inattentive symptoms, with 26% prescribed a stimulant medication (96). Stimulant use in the diabetic control group was 6.5% comparatively, and population studies suggest the rate of medication use in general ADHD populations is 2–8% (97). Importantly, while the mean Phe levels over 12 months for the PKU sample were significantly associated with inattentive symptoms, medication was reported efficacious in all PKU subjects, without a significant lowering of Phe levels (96).

The link between ADHD and PKU can be at least partially explained by a hypodopaminergic hypothesis (98, 99). In ADHD and PKU affected individuals, this hypodopaminergic state is particularly prominent in the prefrontal cortex and striatum, which rely heavily on optimal neurochemical functioning in order to perform critical roles in attention and behavior (100).

Diamond and colleagues conducted executive function testing in children with PKU longitudinally over 4 years and found that with Phe levels three to five times normal (despite early dietary restriction), they were impaired on tests of working memory and inhibition that were dependent on the functioning of the dorsolateral prefrontal cortex (101). These findings were most correlated to the current Phe level, suggesting that mesocortical system dysfunction underpinned by Phe/Tyr imbalance and subsequently reduced dopamine dysfunction was the underlying issue (101). Projections to prefrontal areas are thought to be more vulnerable to this hypodopaminergic state owing to their higher turnover of dopamine (102). A number of studies have linked dopamine to the neurobiology of ADHD, including those showing a link with dopamine system genes (103), overexpression of the dopamine transporter (104), and the pharmacological basis for effective treatments (105).

Given the particular sensitivity of the prefrontal cortex to low levels of dopamine, it is not surprising that this area is disproportionally affected by the sequelae of even mild elevations of Phe (102), and this provides a likely mechanism for the increased rates of ADHD in PKU. There are limited studies of the link between the two disorders, despite the link in neurobiological mechanisms.

The PKU ASCEND study was conducted to evaluate the therapeutic effects of sapropterin versus placebo on ADHD and executive functioning in PKU patients, and undertaken in individuals who had a demonstrated therapeutic blood Phe response to sapropterin therapy. Burton et al. conducted a randomized control trial including 206 children and adults with PKU (mean age = 20 years), of whom 118 responded to sapropterin therapy (106). There were 38 individuals that had sapropterin responsive PKU and ADHD symptoms at baseline. Primary endpoints were changed on ADHD Rating Scale (ADHD RS—child parental report and ADHD-ASRS—adult self-report versions), the Clinical Global Impression of Improvement (CGI-I), the Clinical Global Impression of Severity (CGI-S), and the Behavioural Rating Inventory of Executive Function (BRIEF). Sapropterin therapy was found to reduce inattentive ADHD symptoms in the first 4 weeks of treatment, and throughout the 26 weeks of treatment, these improvements were maintained. There were no changes noted between groups on the hyperactivity and impulsivity measures from the ADHD RS/ASRS. One third of the 118 individuals were found to have ADHD inattentive symptoms, similar to the findings of Antshel et al. (95).

COGNITION IN PKU

Cognitive Functioning in Early Treated Children With PKU

The historical literature on neurocognitive outcomes in children with early treated PKU is vast, and a number of meta-analyses have been conducted to try and overcome some of the methodological challenges, including small sample sizes, heterogeneous samples, small effect sizes, and large variability in outcomes. Mild to moderate deficits have been reported in a range of domains, including general intelligence (107, 108), attention (109–112), processing speed (112–114), working memory (115, 116), new learning and memory (112), motor skills and co-ordination (117), and executive functioning (112). Aspects of executive functioning are particularly sensitive to high Phe levels, and deficits have been reported in a variety of executive subdomains, including inhibitory control (101, 114), conceptual reasoning (118), planning (118–120), mental flexibility (114), and organizational strategy (115). Academic achievement differences have also been observed in some studies (112). White matter pathology in PKU is diffuse, and as a consequence, multiple pathways may be compromised, causing a broad array of neuropsychological difficulties in the PKU population (121).

DeRoche and Welsh (122) conducted a meta-analysis looking at 25 years of neurocognitive outcomes in children and adolescents with PKU, spanning from 1980 to 2004 including 33 studies (122). Effect sizes for intelligence (in comparison to unrelated controls) was small to moderate (0.20 to 0.42) with no significant heterogeneity among outcomes. The effect sizes for executive functioning (and its component processes) were in the "moderate to large" range including working memory (0.59), planning (0.51), inhibition (0.78), and flexibility (1.15). Significant heterogeneity among effect sizes was noted, though all domains of executive functioning were found to be significant ($p < 0.001$). DeRoche and Welsh concluded that individuals with early and continuous treatment will likely have IQ scores in the average range, albeit possibly lower than genetically related controls. However, they may experience significant impairments in executive functioning, including flexibility of thinking, inhibition, working memory, and planning (122).

As early treated children and adolescents with PKU commonly demonstrate executive difficulties on neuropsychological examination, it is important for parents, teachers, and the individuals themselves to be mindful of potential challenges in academic and social situations. As children progress through their schooling, they face many novel and challenging situations, demanding of executive skills and goal-directed behavior. Self-regulation and cognitive control are related to successful school achievement and social adjustment (123). Therefore, individuals with PKU may require additional educational support and counselling to help compensate for executive difficulties (122).

Cognitive Effects of Phe Variability in Children With PKU

Relatively few studies have examined the neuropsychological outcomes in mild hyperphenylalaninemia, in part due to a lack of consensus regarding the definition of mHPA (61). However as blood Phe concentrations can increase with age, children should be monitored during the first year of life at a minimum (124, 125). The evidence regarding cognitive outcomes in children with blood Phe levels just under 600μmol/L is inconsistent, with small sample sizes and methodological flaws (126, 127). A number of studies have focused solely on IQ assessment, rather than a comprehensive review of cognitive abilities, including executive functioning. The existing literature indicates that children with mHPA generally do not have intellectual impairment, but usually perform between those of individuals with phenylketonuria and those of comparison groups on broader neuropsychological measures (126, 127). However there is evidence that even modest elevations in Phe can affect selected cognitive functions, including attention, working memory and executive functioning (61, 126, 127). The complete European guidelines for PKU diagnosis and treatment err on the side of caution and recommend that children with blood Phe levels between 360μmol/L and 600μmol/L should be treated during the first 12 years of life to optimize cognitive functioning (17).

Cognitive Functioning in Early Treated Adults with PKU

There has been considerable research into the cognitive functioning of children with PKU but less so in adult populations (128, 129). For the majority of adults that commenced treatment shortly after birth, individuals generally fall within the normal range of general cognitive ability, have professional and educational achievements similar to their non-PKU siblings, and are able to live independent and productive lives (17, 128). However, there are some individuals that continue to demonstrate neuropsychological, social, and behavioral difficulties throughout their adult lives. These challenges can impact on education and training, employment, relationships, emotional wellbeing, and quality of life (1, 130, 131).

Palermo et al., (132) undertook comprehensive neuropsychological assessment on 37 early treated adults with PKU (AwPKU) with good dietary control (average 432 μmol/L childhood and <850 μmol/L in adulthood) and 30 controls (132). They found that only 5.4% of the PKU participants showed severe impairment (> 2 SD below the mean); however, a much greater number showed an abnormal cognitive profile in terms of proportion of impaired measures (46%). Overall, a quarter of the sample showed clear cognitive impairment in terms of average performance and cognitive profile, whereas 38% performed as well as controls with z scores always within 0.5 of the mean across all assessed domains.

When comparing AwPKU and controls, the largest difference (Cohen's D) was found for planning and switching (Tower of Hanoi, Wisconsin Card Sorting Test, Semantic Fluency), verbal reasoning (WASI Similarities and Vocabulary), short-term memory (Digit Span and Non-Word Repetition), and sustained attention (Rapid Visual Information Processing). Visuo-motor coordination (Grooved Pegboard and Digit Symbol) was reduced in comparison to controls but was thought to reflect general cognitive slowing rather than a specific difficulty with motor coordination or peripheral motor speed. Reading speed was slower than controls but was accurate. Spelling was intact, as was picture naming. Memory and learning were preserved [Rey Auditory Verbal Learning Test (RAVLT), Paired Associate Learning (PAL)].

Hofman et al. (129) reviewed 22 peer-reviewed publications, reporting on the outcomes of 16 studies of cognition in early treated PKU (129). Across studies, the most consistent findings were deficits in motor skills, working memory, and vigilance. However, impairments in other cognitive domains were less consistently observed. The relationship between Phe levels and cognition across the lifespan was variable, with no definitive linear pattern of association found. This was thought to reflect a number of core challenges in studying cognition in PKU. These included high heterogeneity in the nature of study samples, resulting in large variability in phenylalanine levels, as well as wide variation in the type and sensitivity of neuropsychological measures used to assess cognitive functioning. Study samples were often small, with cohorts exhibiting different levels of disease severity, age ranges, and socioeconomic status. No standard PKU core neuropsychological battery had been uniformly used. Hofman et al. concluded that the long-term cognitive outcome of continuous early management of PKU remained unclear.

Weglage et al. (133) conducted a longitudinal neuropsychological and neurological study of 57 early-treated classical PKU adults aged between 19 and 41 years and 46 controls over a 5-year period (133). PKU participants and controls were assessed on IQ, attention, and information-processing abilities. Magnetic resonance imaging (MRI) of the brain was performed in all patients. Neuropsychological assessments and MRI were repeated at a 5-year follow-up. In the 5-year interval, there was no change in processing speed or attentional measures. At both assessment times, IQ scores were significantly lower in PKU individuals as compared to controls. Older adult patients (> 32 years) showed poorer attention and information processing at both timepoints compared to young adult patients (aged <32 years) and controls. Intellectual quotients, attention, and information processing showed no correlation to imaging results; however, they were significantly correlated to blood phenylalanine (Phe) levels throughout childhood and adolescence. Phe levels had also been higher in the adolescent years of older adult patients, suggestive of an early relaxation of diet recommended when the older patients were adolescents. Weglage's results indicated a benefit of dietary control during adolescence in PKU (133).

Cognitive Outcomes in Late Treatment or Untreated PKU

Untreated PKU is characterized by motor deficits, intellectual disability, microcephaly, autism, seizures, developmental problems, behavioral issues, and a range of psychiatric symptoms (17). Failure to implement treatment in the neonatal period causes substantial lifelong disability through the toxic effects of excess Phe exposure to the brain, in particular to myelin and dendritic projections during critical postnatal periods of neuronal development (18). Brain MRI and histopathology of individuals with late- or never-treated PKU demonstrate diffuse cortical atrophy, hypomyelination, white matter vacuolization, and astrocytic gliosis (47, 134).

Gonzalez et al. (135) conducted a retrospective study of 121 PKU individuals (mean age = 16, range 1 month to 46 years) diagnosed and treated from 1985 to 2010 (135). The aim was to investigate the relationship between neurological complications and behavioral problems, age at diagnosis and dietary control among a follow-up group (135). Of these, 76% were diagnosed through neonatal screening. There were 12.4% with mild PKU, 19% moderate PKU, and 68.6% classic PKU. Eighty-eight percent of patients were treated with a protein-restricted diet, and the remainder with BH4. Almost all (97.7%) of the early-diagnosed patients had normal IQ, while 46.3% of late diagnosed patients had intellectual disability, 28.5% were borderline, and 25% had normal IQ.

In early-diagnosed patients, there was a significantly negative correlation between IQ and the index of dietary control during the first 6 years of life and that of the immediately preceding year. The proportion of patients with late diagnosis and neurological and behavioral problems was significantly higher than that of those diagnosed early. In addition, the proportion of early-diagnosed patients with behavioral and neurological problems who had good, intermediate, or poor dietary control during the first 6 years of life (and the immediate-past year) also differed significantly (135).

The severe cognitive impairments seen in untreated PKU can be partially reversed with dietary treatment in many individuals, and the prompt initiation of treatment following newborn metabolic screening remains essential for the prevention of disability and optimal neurodevelopment.

Intelligence in PKU

PKU results, in untreated patients, a profound intellectual disability and more subtle cognitive deficits in individuals who were treated early and continuously. The assessment of intellectual functioning in PKU has been an important target outcome variable since the implementation of neonatal PKU screening programs in the 1960s (108, 136). Research on intellectual functioning in individuals with PKU has played a significant role in guiding treatment recommendations and mproving outcomes (136).

Brumm and Grant (136) conducted a literature review examining the relationship between intellectual outcome and treatment parameters including initiation of treatment, duration of treatment, and blood phenylalanine (Phe) levels from infancy through adulthood. While current PKU treatment practices have eliminated severe neurological and cognitive impairment, evidence suggests that intellectual functioning, although typically within the average range when PKU is treated early and continuously, may not be maximized under the current definition of well-controlled PKU, which is based on blood Phe levels (136).

Two prior meta-analyses examining blood Phe concentrations and intellectual functioning in pediatric populations found a strong inverse relationship between historical blood Phe measurements and IQ (137, 138). Future research assessing intellectual and neurocognitive outcome in PKU should enhance the development of new treatment strategies.

Executive Functioning in PKU

Executive function is an umbrella term that refers to cognitive processes that are necessary for purposeful, future orientated behavior. Metaphorically speaking, the executive functions are the brain's chief executive officer. These processes are necessary to plan and complete tasks in spite of potential distracting or irrelevant information (139).

Executive functions include cognitive processes such as regulation of attention, inhibition of inappropriate responses, coordination of information in working memory, and cognitive flexibility. Higher-order executive functions require the simultaneous use of multiple basic executive functions and include planning, reasoning, and problem-solving (140).

Reviews of executive functions have found that the most consistent phenylalanine-related impairments have been observed in working memory, sustained attention, and inhibitory control (65, 129, 141). There have been several investigations to try and establish a theoretical model of executive functioning deficit in individuals with PKU, which has resulted in detailed analysis of various aspects of executive functioning (142). Part of the difficulty in the assessment of executive functioning in PKU populations has been the lack of consistent use of valid and sensitive tools that are suitable for both children and adults (141). Another challenge has been that many traditional "executive functioning" tasks do not solely measure one specific cognitive process. As an example, an executive test such as Trails B indexes both speed and mental switching (143).

Traditional tasks that have been used to assess executive functioning in PKU are the Wisconsin Card Sorting Test (WCST) and Brixton Spatial Anticipation Test (rule detection), Tower of London and Tower of Hanoi (planning and problem solving), Rey Complex Figure Test (visuo-spatial organization), Trails A and B and the Contingency Naming Test (mental flexibility and switching), the Controlled Oral Word Association Test/Verbal Fluency (verbal generativity and planned searching), and the Go-No Go Task, Stroop Test, and Haylings Sentence Completion Test (Inhibitory Control) (113, 122, 129, 142). Computerized test batteries have also been used to assess executive skills in PKU populations, including the Amsterdam Neuropsychological Test and the Cambridge Neuropsychological Test Automated Battery (CANTAB) (65, 69, 141). Studies have demonstrated significant variability in their findings, in part due to the methodological challenges in conducting research in rare and diverse PKU populations. In the future, it will be important for a consistent and sensitive core neuropsychological battery to be implemented across international PKU centers, to try and standardize consensus regarding cognitive treatment outcomes (17, 129).

Cognition in Offspring of Mothers With PKU

High Phe blood levels during pregnancy have a known teratogenic effect on the developing fetus, resulting in growth retardation, microcephaly, intellectual disability, and birth defects (144). There have been several studies that have assessed the cognitive outcomes of children born to mothers with PKU (144-146). A summary of the literature suggests that children who are born to mothers with PKU who have attained metabolic control before or very early in pregnancy seem to have a normal developmental trajectory. However, a delay in attainment of maternal metabolic control is associated with declines in offspring developmental outcome, including lower IQ and higher rates of externalizing behavioral difficulties (145).

Waisbren and Azen (145) conducted a prospective longitudinal study that assessed cognitive and behavioral outcomes in treated (mPKU) offspring (145). Two hundred and twenty-eight children who were born to mothers with treated PKU or untreated mild hyperphenylalaninemia were compared with 70 control subjects at 7 years of age. They found that the offspring cognitive outcome negatively correlated with the number of gestational weeks that elapsed until maternal metabolic control was achieved ($r = -0.61$). There was an increased risk of low IQ in PKU offspring if the mother came from a lower SES background and was also unable to provide a stimulating early home environment (145). The postnatal environment also significantly affected outcome. Interventions to improve dietary compliance before and throughout pregnancy may reduce the risks associated with mPKU (17).

Social Cognition and PKU

Social cognition is a domain of cognition involving all mental processes that underlie social interactions, and encompasses the ability to perceive, interpret, and then respond appropriately to social cues. Some basic social cognitive skills include face and emotion recognition and theory-of-mind (the capacity to attribute and understand feelings, thoughts, and intentions to/of others) (147). While there has been comprehensive investigation into the role of executive functions in PKU, there has only been one study to date that has assessed social-cognitive abilities (148). Deficits in social cognitive abilities are consistently reported in individuals with executive dysfunction, because of shared underlying neurobiology and neuroanatomy (149–151). In other disorders affecting the CNS, impairments in executive function have been correlated with deficits in communication skills and social relationships (152). High Phe levels may in some cases result in irritability, impacting on adaptive social skills.

(148) investigated whether early treated PKU patients have specific Phe-related problems with respect to social-cognitive functioning and social skills (148). Ninety-five PKU patients (mean age 21.6 ± 10.2 years) and 95 healthy controls (mean age 19.6 ± 8.7 years) were compared on performance of computerized and paper-and-pencil tasks measuring social-cognitive abilities and on parent and self-reported social skills. Early treated AwPKU performed worse than controls on all four tasks included; however, when age was controlled for, impairments were only observed on two tasks. In addition, comparisons were made between patients using tetrahydrobiopterin (BH4, $n = 30$) and patients who were not. PKU patients demonstrated poorer social cognition and had poorer social skills than controls, regardless of general cognitive abilities. The quality of patients' social cognition was inversely related to recent Phe levels, and to levels between 8 and 12 years, for PKU adolescents. The quality of social skills was also inversely related to lifetime phenylalanine levels in adult patients, and more specifically to Phe levels up to 12 years of age. No differences with respect to social outcome measures were observed between the BH4 and non-BH4 groups. Jahja and colleagues concluded that PKU patients have difficulties with social cognition and social

skills that appear to be strongly related to Phe levels. Impairments in functioning seem to be more evident among adolescents and adults with PKU, with high Phe levels during childhood and early adolescence (presumably during critical periods of development of frontal circuits subserving social cognitive functioning) seem to be of greater influence than current and recent Phe levels in PKU individuals (148).

Neuropsychological Mechanisms in PKU

While there has been no consensus agreement about the exact mechanism/s for cognitive changes in PKU, the general belief has been that the deficits are related to individuals' Phe levels at several stages throughout life (153). These include concurrent Phe levels, lifetime Phe levels, variation in Phe levels, and altered Phe/Tyrosine ratio. Two theories have been postulated regarding the mechanism of action of the disrupted Phe metabolism in individuals with PKU. The first theory suggests that because Phe competes with other LNAAs (tryptophan and tyrosine) for transport across the blood–brain barrier, high levels of Phe saturate the LNAA transporters. This leads to PKU individuals presenting with lower brain concentrations of other LNAA and important neurotransmitters such as dopamine, norepinephrine, and serotonin (153), which are known to be important in cognitive functioning (154). The second theory suggests that high brain Phe concentrations cause neurotoxicity. This interferes with cerebral protein synthesis, increases myelin turnover, and inhibits neurotransmitter synthesis (43).

One of the primary cognitive changes that is consistently seen in the AwPKU literature is a reduction in speed of processing. This is reflective of cognitive slowing, rather than a peripheral reduction in motor speed (132). Information processing speed relies on the speed with which action potentials are able to travel along the long myelinated axons. If myelination of these axons was damaged or incomplete, there would be a reduction in processing speed. Previous studies have found that slowing occurs at a cognitive level, consistent with the apparently toxic effects of hyperPhe on oligodendrocytes (132, 155, 156), but not on the peripheral nervous system's Schwann cells (157).

Neuropsychological Assessment Recommendations

There is currently no consensus regarding a standardized PKU neuropsychological battery for children or adults. The European guidelines suggest that neuropsychological assessment should occur on an "as needed" basis in childhood, with routine evaluations at 12 and 18 years of age. This correlates with changes in treatment targets for blood Phe and life changes including school transitions, living situation, and transfer to adult clinics and brain development (see **Table 2**).

When conducting a neuropsychological assessment in individuals with PKU, it is important for clinicians to conduct a comprehensive examination encompassing all cognitive domains. If time is limited, the domains most likely to be susceptible to high Phe levels are attention, working memory, motor control, complex speed of processing, and executive functioning (17, 129, 141). Intellectual functioning as a stand-alone outcome measure has been found to be less sensitive than the above-mentioned cognitive abilities (141). While memory retention is often sound, attentional difficulties can affect registration and encoding of new information and should be assessed.

A thorough clinical history should be obtained prior to an assessment being conducted, to help guide test selection, with a particular focus on cognitive strengths and weaknesses, social cognition, psychiatric symptoms, psychosocial adjustment, quality of life, and behavioral difficulties (17, 158). As there is emerging evidence that social cognition skills (facial and emotional recognition and theory of mind) and emotional and behavioral regulation are affected in individuals with PKU, it is important to consider assessment of these domains as part of a comprehensive neuropsychological examination (148). A brief psychiatric history should also be obtained, as conditions such as depression and anxiety can negatively impact on cognitive test performance, particularly on measures of attention and speed. Mood and anxiety symptoms can be treated, which may lead to an improvement in cognitive functioning. By conducting a comprehensive neuropsychological examination, cognitive, psychological, and social cognition interventions can be individually tailored to best assist individuals with PKU to achieve their highest potential and enhance quality of life.

TABLE 2 | Neuropsychological assessment recommendations.

Neuropsychological assessments should be conducted at 12 and 18 years in all patients
If any of the stated risk factors applies, perform (additional) neuropsychological assessment: • Non-optimal metabolic control; <50% of the Phe levels are out of target range over a period of 6–12 months (depending on age <12 or >12 years) • Problems at school or work • Concerns of parents/caregivers/family/teachers • Concern of PKU patient • Concern of metabolic team
Cognitive Domains for Inclusion
Estimation of intelligence
Academic achievement
Immediate, divided, and sustained attention
Speed of processing
Visuo-spatial functioning
Verbal new learning and memory
Expressive and receptive language
Motor speed and coordination
Executive functions: • Working memory • Inhibitory control/self-monitoring • Planning and organization • Cognitive flexibility/shifting • Verbal fluency
Social cognition
Psychiatric screening
Psychosocial adjustment/quality of life
Behavioral rating scales

Table 2 *is adapted and expanded from Statement #24, European Guidelines for Diagnosis and Treatment of PKU (17).*

CASE VIGNETTES

Case 1

Ms T was a 43-year-old single woman who was not diagnosed with PKU until after 12 months of age and only started dietary treatment at 18 months of age. Prior to this period, she had significant irritability, childhood anxiety, delayed milestones, and failure to thrive and progress (**Figure 2**). She continued dietary treatment until the age of 9, at which time the family was told to stop dietary management. Ms T's IQ was in the intellectually disabled range (<70). She did not resume diet until 30 years of age. She presented with attentional deficits, hyperactivity, and social cognition issues throughout childhood, and then developed a psychotic illness in her late teens. This remained largely treatment refractory, and during periods of poor dietary control (Phe >1500), she suffered from poor frustration tolerance and impulse control, anxiety, and worsened chronic hallucinations. When dietary control was good (Phe 400–600), psychotic symptoms were significantly attenuated, anxiety was minimal, and impulse control returned to normal.

Case 2

Mr C was a 47-year-old married engineer and father of two, who was diagnosed at birth on bloodspot screening. His dietary control was "strict" until age 13, "relaxed" until age 17, then ceased dietary control altogether. At times of increased protein intake, he noted increased mood lability, irritability, and anxiety, with inattention and a sense of "cloudy" thinking; this occurred with Phe levels at 1,200–1,400. His anxiety was generalized, with occasional panic episodes and periods of low mood with mild neurovegetative disturbance. With improved dietary control (Phe < 700) he noted that his mood lifted, anxiety levels reduced, and sleep improved significantly. After 12 months of dietary control, anxiety levels had improved markedly, and his mood was persistently euthymic.

Mr C underwent comprehensive neuropsychological assessment prior to commencing a low Phe diet (baseline) and after 12 months of good dietary control. At baseline, Mr C was estimated to be of "Average–High Average" intelligence. He performed in keeping with these estimates on all tasks, with the exception of verbal new learning and memory, where he was in the *Borderline Impaired* range. Mr C reported that he found it challenging to attend to the verbal information being presented.

After 18 months on diet, Mr C demonstrated statistically significant improvements in the domains of processing speed (from 34 percentile at baseline to 77 percentile on-diet) and new learning and memory (from 7 percentile at baseline to 50 percentile on diet). A number of executive functioning measures also improved, although the improvements were mild and not statistically significant. He reported being able to think more clearly and quickly, with improved concentration.

Case 3

Ms N was a 36 year-old married lady who was diagnosed at birth on bloodspot screening. She adhered to a low Phe diet for the first 7 years of her life then ceased dietary control. She recommenced on diet at age 35 due to symptomatic PKU affecting her cognitive functioning and mental health. Ms N had a long history of mental health difficulties starting in childhood. She had difficulties regulating her mood and had episodes of depression. She had her first panic attack in her mid-teens, along with generalized anxiety symptoms and infrequent self-harming behaviors. She had been under psychiatric care since her teenage years and had several psychiatric admissions. She had worked in a variety of semi-skilled roles in a part-time capacity, but had found it difficult to maintain employment due to fluctuating mental health. She saw a psychologist on a regular basis and had been on pharmacological treatment with SSRIs since her early 30s, with some improvement. She reported significant cognitive limitations, including difficulties with attention and concentration, memory, planning, and organization

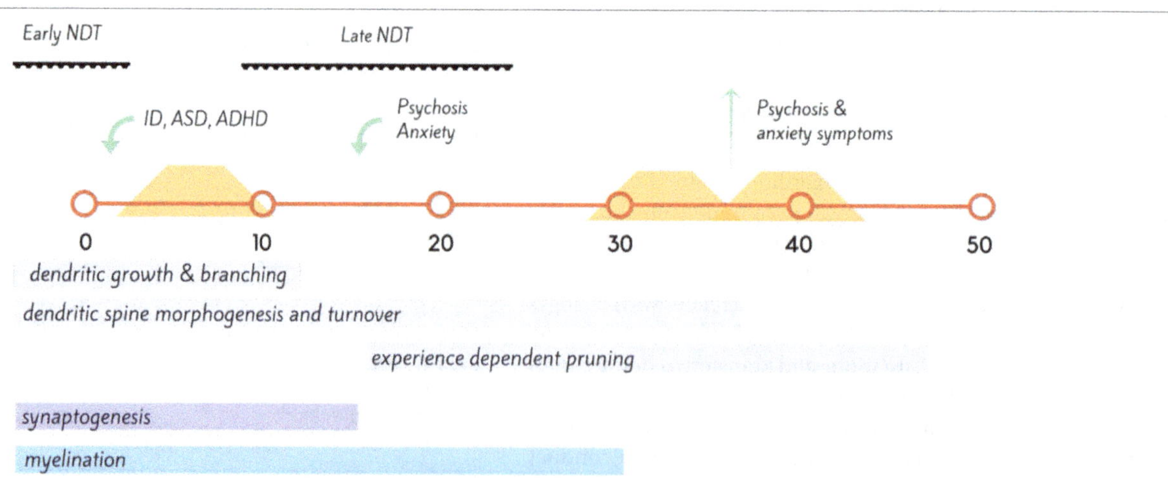

FIGURE 2 | Timeline (in years) of proposed neural development, onset of neuropsychiatric disorder (green) and dietary coverage (orange) for Case Vignette 1. This case highlights the importance of neuronal development across the lifespan, with insult during the early neurodevelopmental (NDT) stages resulting in intellectual disability (ID), autism spectrum disorder (ASD), and attention deficit hyperactivity disorder (ADHD); while insult during the later stages of neurodevelopment, during adolescence with disruption of synaptic pruning leading to disorders such as bipolar disorder and in this instance, schizophrenia (159, 160).

and slowed mental processing. These difficulties had affected her ability to maintain productive employment, leading to feelings of inferiority and low self-esteem. Baseline neuropsychological assessment prior to resuming a low Phe diet revealed that Ms N was of average intelligence. However, she demonstrated moderate impairments on tasks of divided attention and psychomotor speed and severe impairments on task of planning, organization, and self-monitoring. After 12 months of good dietary control (reducing Phe from ~700 to <300), Ms N had made statistically significant improvements on tasks of psychomotor speed (from 9 percentile at baseline to 63 percentile on diet), planning and organization (from <0.1 percentile at baseline to 77 percentile on diet), divided attention (from 9 percentile at baseline to 50 percentile on diet), and self-monitoring (from 1 percentile on diet to 37 percentile on diet). She also showed a significant regression in white matter lesions (**Figure 3**). Her depression and anxiety symptoms also improved; however, they did not fully resolve and she benefitted from the introduction of escitalopram, initially at 20 mg but ultimately required a dose escalation to 40 mg.

Treatment Considerations: Current and Future

Though rare, PKU is an important cause of preventable neurodevelopmental disability that requires lifelong commitment to Phe restriction. The literature supports treatment being initiated as early as possible, even before 10 days, in order to minimize neurological damage. Every 4-week delay in starting treatment has been shown to cause a decline of IQ score by approximately 4 points (1).

There is consensus in the literature that patients with untreated blood Phe concentrations > 600 μmol/L should be treated, and that patients with untreated blood Phe levels < 360 μmol/L should remain untreated, as this is not considered to be indicative of disease (138). What is less clear is treatment in the group of patients with PKU whose levels are in the 360 and 600 μmol/L range. The most reliable literature suggests they should be treated during the first 12 years of age to prevent cognitive function impairment in PKU (161). Because of the consequences of elevated blood Phe levels, guidelines from the American College of Medical Genetics and Genomics (ACMG) recommend lifelong treatment of PKU, with the primary goal of therapy to lower blood Phe to the range of 120 to 360 μmol/L (16).

Dietary treatment is comprised of three aspects: natural protein restriction, Phe-free- L-amino acid supplements, and low protein food (17). Though central to the treatment, dietary modification remains very challenging for patients and their families, due to cost and impact on quality of life, and despite optimal dietary treatment, outcomes remain suboptimal, hence the ongoing exploration into alternate treatments.

A patient's Phe tolerance will vary over their lifetime, depending on many factors such as the stage of growth and development and net protein catabolism-synthesis ration, target Phe levels, severity of illness, energy intake, compliance with diet and supplementation, as well as use of adjunctive treatments such as BH4 (162, 163). Striking a balance between adequate protein intake and maintaining acceptable Phe levels needs to be individualized to each patient (17).

Amino Acid Supplementation

Phe is an essential amino acid for protein synthesis both in childhood and adulthood and is gained through dietary protein intake (164). Traditional treatment of PKU has been to restrict overall dietary protein intake (165). However, as the understanding of PKU neuropathophysiology has unfolded, it has become clear that just keeping Phe levels low does not constitute optimal treatment.

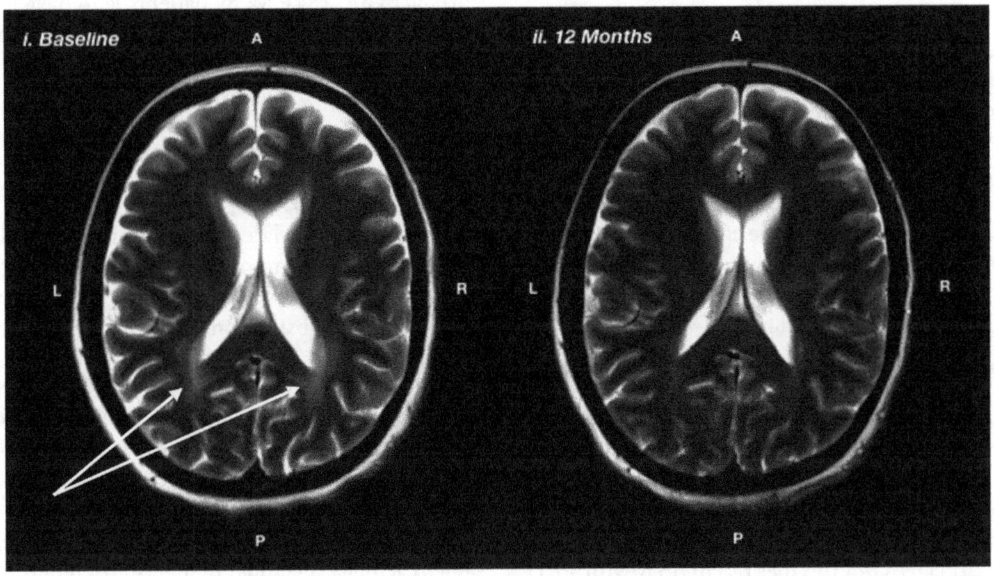

FIGURE 3 | T2-weighted magnetic resonance imaging showing i) baseline: prior to the recommencing diet, and ii) 12 months after recommencing diet, showing reduction in white matter hyperintensity, particularly in the posterior regions, as indicated by the white arrows.

A mainstay of dietary treatment is supplementation with Phe-free L-amino acid supplements. The 2017 van Wegberg et al. European Guidelines on Phenylketonuria Diagnosis and Treatment state that supplementation should be evenly administered throughout the day in at least three equal portions to minimize losses of L-amino acids due to oxidation, and to help minimize fluctuations in blood Phe concentrations over a 24-h period (17, 166).

Oral supplementation with LNAAs has been proven to be helpful in reducing brain Phe concentrations *via* competitive binding at LAT1, which improves neuropsychological functioning (167, 168). LNAA supplementation either alone or in combination with a low-Phe diet has been shown to improve health outcome for individuals unable to follow the low-Phe diet. However, long-term outcome studies assessing efficacy and safety of LNAA supplementation are needed (169).

Promising developments include van Vliet et al.'s studies on mice showing that LNAA supplementation without dietary phenylalanine restriction improves brain biochemistry through all three hypothesized biochemical mechanisms: namely, the normalization of brain phenylalanine, non-phenylalanine LNAA, and the concentration of monoaminergic neurotransmitters. They demonstrated that utilizing LNAAs with a strong affinity for the LNAA transporter type 1, such as Leu and Ile, is most efficacious in reducing Brain Phe concentrations. Additionally, Tyr and Trp in conjunction serve to optimally ameliorate brain monoaminergic neurotransmitter concentrations (170). They also compared several LNAA supplements with a very phenylalanine-restricted diet on measures of brain monoamine and amino acid concentrations in adult C57Bl/6 Pah-enu2 mice, and the results indicated that the supplementation of the eight LNAAs was as effective as the highly Phe-restricted diet in restoring CNS monoamines, even while brain and plasma phenylalanine concentrations remained highly elevated (171).

Advances in Dietary Supplementation

Dietary modification has continued to evolve to ensure that foods are affordable, palatable, and supplemented with micronutrients otherwise lacking in a low-Phe diet. One such advancement is the utility of glycomacropeptide (GMP), an intact protein source derived from cheese whey that improves Phe utilization and protein retention (172). Compliance has been shown to be improved with GMP as compared with traditional amino acid foods due to greater acceptability and fewer gastrointestinal side effects (173).

Other supplementation changes include improved caloric content, addition of taurine and other micronutrients, and addition of long-chain polyunsaturated fats (LCPUFAs) (171).

Long-Chain Polyunsaturated Fatty Acids

LCPUFAs have been found to be decreased in systematic review and meta-analysis of studies in PKU, likely secondary to dietary restriction and possibly metabolic changes, though the latter is only partially understood (174, 175). The addition of omega-3 docosahexaenoic acid (DHA) to the diet of children with PKU has been shown to increase central nervous system processing speed (as measured by visual evoked potentials) as well as motor and coordination skills, suggesting DHA is an essential part of the treatment of PKU (176).

Tetrahydropterin as Enzyme Enhancement Therapy for PKU

Tetrahydropterin acts as a molecular chaperone in PKU patients and promotes correct folding and stability of the PAH enzyme, thus acting as a critical co-factor in a normal PAH system (177). A subset of patients with PKU benefit from adjunctive treatment with pharmacological doses of tetrahydropterin (BH4) or sapropterin hydrochloride (178). Robust evidence from two systematic reviews demonstrates that BH4 is effective in reducing blood Phe concentrations and in increasing the Phe "tolerance" in BH4-responsive PKU patients (179, 180). Long-term treatment with sapropterin of such responsive patients with PKU also appears to improve Phe tolerance and may allow patients to discontinue highly restrictive diets (181).

However, not all patients benefit, and those with Phe levels > 360 μmol/L need to be tested for responsiveness. This requires multiple levels to be taken pre and post the initiation of BH4, and a decrease in blood Phe of 30% or more from baseline indicates response to sapropterin therapy (130). Patients with high residual activity of the PAH enzyme have a greater probability of BH4 response, but a minority of patients with classical PKU have been shown to benefit from BH4 treatment (182, 183). Understandably, BH4 responsive patients have been shown to have a higher natural protein tolerance (182, 183).

There is ongoing research required to establish if other molecules in addition to tetrahydrobiopterin may act as chaperones to assist in the folding of PAH; however, there are some promising studies including one by Pey et al, which performed a high-throughput ligand screening of over 1,000 pharmacological agents, identifying four compounds that enhanced the stability of PAH activity (184). Many patients who have little or no residual PAH activity do not respond to BH4. Studies have identified various figures from 20% to 50% of patients responding in the studies to combination sapropterin and dietary Phe restriction (185, 186).

Enzyme Therapy

Pegvaliase, PEGylated recombinant *Anabaena variabilis* phenylalanine ammonia lyase (PAL), converts Phe to transcinnamic acid and ammonia, and is now FDA-approved as an enzyme substitution therapy to lower blood Phe in adults with PKU (187). As per Thomas et al., Pegvaliase has now been investigated in a single Phase 1 clinical trial, four Phase 2 clinical trials, and two Phase 3 clinical trials, PRISM-1 and PRISM-2, the results of which are now reported (188–190). These studies have evaluated over 350 adults with PKU being treated with Pegvaliase.

The PRISM clinical program exemplified that with a manageable self-administration program, patients with PKU were able to achieve sustained reductions in blood Phe concentration, that were associated with sustained improvements in associated neuropsychiatric symptoms (188). Evidence from Vockley et al. is demonstrating that long-term treatment with Pegvaliase showed consistent and clinically meaningful improvements across all inattention and mood outcomes evaluated (191), representing an exciting new treatment pathway (192).

Individual Variation and Compliance

Interestingly, studies indicate that while there are patients with PKU suffering from all the sequelae of non-treatment, or poor adherence to treatment, so too there is likely a subset of patients who are over-restricting their protein consumption. Blood levels of Phe do not necessarily fluctuate with small changes in dietary intake (162, 193). For those with either late diagnosis or no previous treatment, there is a growing body of evidence that introduction of the low Phe diet and adjunctive treatments will benefit patients and can reverse some of the IQ loss in reported cases, particularly in the younger age group 4 to 6 years old (194). Concerningly, there are high rates of attrition from services, with some services reporting that a majority of adults with PKU were lost to follow-up and, without the support of specialist services, are likely to have suboptimal metabolic control (195, 196).

The Role of Sleep

Accumulating evidence increasingly indicates that improving quality of sleep is an important target for intervention in optimizing the cognitive and psychiatric state of those with PKU. Bruinenberg et al. explored the link between PKU and sleep disturbance in men and mice in their 2017 study and asserted that PKU patients demonstrated more sleep disorders, a reduced sleep quality, an increased latency to fall asleep, and more sleepiness during the day. Additionally they identified an increased fragmentation and a shift in diurnality, in PKU mice (197). Previously, results of the study by DeGiorgis et al. had shown a consistent delay in the maturation of trace-alternant and spindle scores in children with PKU (198). Surendran et al. identified that qualifying and addressing sleep disturbance may mitigate cognitive and psychiatric sequelae of PKU in the mouse model (199, 200).

CONCLUSIONS

Elevated rates of psychiatric illness and cognitive impairment occur in PKU, and their nature and prevalence vary in accordance with the severity of the deficit in PAH function, the degree of dietary treatment, and—perhaps most crucially—the timing of attempts to attenuate the hyperPhe that defines the illness. The differing epochs of treatment availability and recommendations—from untreated patients, through varying duration of "early-treated" patients, through to more recent moves to ensure that "continuously treated" patients are treated lifelong—have resulted in vast differences in cognitive and psychiatric outcomes. Increasingly it is recognized that lifelong treatment offers not just the best dietary "coverage" of crucial developmental periods, but has significant implications for functional outcome and quality of life.

Although some of the effects of hyperPhe on monoaminergic function and myelination appear reversible, persistent and prolonged hyperPhe across key neurodevelopmental periods appears to cause permanent alterations to the trajectory of brain development. When this occurs across early periods of neurodevelopment, gross intellectual and behavioral changes occur.

While the emerging data show consistent elevations in rates of these disorders, very little data exist on treatment of psychiatric illness, in particular in the setting of PKU. For some off-diet patients, a return to diet may afford significant improvement in common psychiatric symptoms. It is not known, however, how likely diet alone is to effect a full remission in psychiatric illness; nor is evidence available to guide clinicians on the use of commonly utilized treatments for these disorders—such as antidepressants in mood and anxiety disorders, and stimulants in attentional disorders. Further evaluation of specific agents in these patient populations is warranted.

The broad range of neuropsychological difficulties seen in children, adolescents and adults with PKU reflects the population's heterogeneity in overall functioning. Early treated individuals with PKU that maintain a strict low Phe diet throughout life are more likely to fulfil their academic potential, without compromise to intellectual functioning. The accumulating body of literature suggests that "diet for life" also negates the likelihood of attention, processing speed, and executive deficits in early treated adults with PKU. As a significant number of PKU individuals with cognitive inefficiencies have co-morbid mood and anxiety symptoms, future research should consider looking at the contribution of depression and anxiety on the neuropsychological profile in PKU. It is possible that enhanced psychological and pharmacological treatment of psychiatric symptoms may alleviate subtle cognitive deficits, particularly in the areas of complex attention and speed of information processing. Further research is required to look at the relationship between social cognition, psychological adjustment, and quality of life with optimal illness control.

The evidence available suggests that dietary adherence attenuates, but does not completely eliminate, the elevated risk for psychiatric illness and cognitive impairment in PKU. This may be in part because reductions in Phe down to the levels seen in non-PKU individuals are very difficult to achieve by diet alone; furthermore, the degree of protein restriction required may have other downstream effects on brain structure and function that are not yet clearly understood. It is, however, important to also acknowledge that the need to adhere to a restrictive diet, have separate "PKU foods" and supplementation, is a stressor in itself. For both pediatric and adult patients, this need for diet can be stigmatizing and socially limiting and affect a patient's self-concept significantly. This, along with diet adherence itself, is onerous and often difficult to maintain. Treatment modalities, such as pegvaliase, that do not involve significant dietary restriction may allow PKU patients to have the best of both worlds: a relatively normal diet, free of restriction and stigma, alongside stable mental health and optimal cognitive functioning.

AUTHOR CONTRIBUTIONS

MW conceived and provided the methodological framework for the review and completed the manuscript. KA, SF, and WK contributed to manuscript design and writing. JP, TF, and GJ contributed to the manuscript.

FUNDING

BioMarin Pharmaceutical Inc provided support to cover the cost of open-access publication, but were not involved in the development or review of this manuscript at any stage.

REFERENCES

1. Blau N, van Spronsen FJ, Levy HL. Phenylketonuria. *Lancet* (2010) 376(9750):1417–27. doi: 10.1016/S0140-6736(10)60961-0
2. Blau N. Genetics of phenylketonuria: then and now. *Hum Mutat* (2016) 37(6):508–15. doi: 10.1002/humu.22980
3. Scriver C, Kaufman S. Hyperphenylalaninemia: phenylalanine hydroxylase deficiency. In: *the metabolic and molecular bases of inherited disease*. McGraw-Hill Inc (2001). p. 1667–724.
4. Følling A. Uber Ausscheidung von Phenylbrenztraubensaure in den Harn als Stoffwechselanomalie in Vebindung mit Imbezzillitat. *Hoppe-Seyler's Z Physiol Chem* (1934) 227:169–76. doi: 10.1515/bchm2.1934.227.1-4.169
5. Jervis GA. Phenylpyruvic oligophrenia deficiency of phenylalanine-oxidizing system. *Proc Soc Exp Biol Med* (1953) 82(3):514–5.
6. Bickel H, Gerrard J, Hickmans EM. Influence of phenylalanine intake on phenylketonuria. *Lancet* (1953) 265(6790):812–3. doi: 10.1016/S0140-6736(53)90473-5
7. Guthrie R, Susi A. A simple phenylalanine method for detecting phenylketonuria in large populations of newborn infants. *Pediatrics* (1963) 32(3):338–43.
8. Hanley WB, Demshar H, Preston MA, Borczyk A, Schoonheyt WE, Clarke JTR, et al. Newborn phenylketonuria (PKU) Guthrie (BIA) screening and early hospital discharge. *Early Hum Dev* (1997) 47(1):87–96. doi: 10.1016/S0378-3782(96)01846-4
9. Dhondt JL, Farriaux JP, Sailly JC, Lebrun T. Economic evaluation of cost-benefit ratio of neonatal screening procedure for phenylketonuria and hypothyroidism. *J Inherit Metab Dis* (1991) 14:633–9. doi: 10.1007/BF01797933
10. Boneh A, Francis DE, Humphrey M, Upton HJ, Peters HL. Three-year audit of the hyperphenylalaninaemia/phenylketonuria spectrum in Victoria. *J Paediatr Child Health* (2006) 42(9):496–8. doi: 10.1111/j.1440-1754.2006.00909.x
11. Weglage J, Wiedermann D, Denecke J, Feldmann R, Koch H-G, Ullrich K, et al. Individual blood–brain barrier phenylalanine transport determines clinical outcome in phenylketonuria. *Ann Neurol* (2001) 50(4):463–7. doi: 10.1002/ana.1226
12. Blau N, Hennermann JB, Langenbeck U, Lichter-Konecki U. Diagnosis, classification, and genetics of phenylketonuria and tetrahydrobiopterin (BH4) deficiencies. *Mol Genet Metab* (2011) 104 Suppl:S2–9. doi: 10.1016/j.ymgme.2011.08.017
13. Walterfang M, Bonnot O, Mocellin R, Velakoulis D. The neuropsychiatry of inborn errors of metabolism. *J Inherit Metab Dis* (2013) 36(4):687–702. doi: 10.1007/s10545-013-9618-y
14. Dobbelaere D, Michaud L, Debrabander A, Vanderbecken S, Gottrand F, Turck D, et al. Evaluation of nutritional status and pathophysiology of growth retardation in patients with phenylketonuria. *J Inherit Metab Dis.* (2003) 26:1–11. doi: 10.1023/A:1024063726046
15. Koch R, Burton B, Hoganson G, Peterson R, Rhead W, Rouse B, et al. phenylketonuria in adulthood: a collaborative study. *J Inherit Metab Dis* (2002) 25(5):333–46. doi: 10.1023/A:1020158631102
16. Vockley J, Andersson HC, Antshel KM, Braverman NE, Burton BK, Frazier DM, et al. Phenylalanine hydroxylase deficiency: diagnosis and management guideline. *Genet Med* (2014) 16(2):188–200. doi: 10.1038/gim.2013.157
17. van Wegberg AMJ, MacDonald A, Ahring K, Belanger-Quintana A, Blau N, Bosch AM, et al. The complete European guidelines on phenylketonuria: diagnosis and treatment. *Orphanet J Rare Dis* (2017) 12(1):162. doi: 10.1186/s13023-017-0685-2
18. Bilder DA, Noel JK, Baker ER, Irish W, Chen Y, Merilainen MJ, et al. Systematic review and meta-analysis of neuropsychiatric symptoms and executive functioning in adults with phenylketonuria. *Dev Neuropsychol* (2016) 41(4):245–60. doi: 10.1080/87565641.2016.1243109
19. Hanley WB, Lee AW, Hanley AJG, Lehotay DC, Austin VJ, Schoonheyt WE, et al. "Hypotyrosinemia" in phenylketonuria. *Mol Genet Metab* (2000) 69(4):286–94. doi: 10.1006/mgme.2000.2985
20. Pietz J, Kreis R, Rupp A, Mayatepek E, Rating D, Boesch C, et al. Large neutral amino acids block phenylalanine transport into brain tissue in patients with phenylketonuria. *J Clin Invest* (1999) 103(8):1169–78. doi: 10.1172/JCI5017
21. González MJ, Gassió R, Artuch R, Campistol J. Impaired neurotransmission in early-treated phenylketonuria patients. *Semin Pediatr Neurol* (2016) 23(4):332–40. doi: 10.1016/j.spen.2016.11.007
22. van Spronsen FJ, Hoeksma M, Reijngoud D-J. Brain dysfunction in phenylketonuria: is phenylalanine toxicity the only possible cause? *J Inherit Metab Dis* (2009) 32(1):46. doi: 10.1007/s10545-008-0946-2
23. Pascucci T, Andolina D, Ventura R, Puglisi-Allegra S, Cabib S. Reduced availability of brain amines during critical phases of postnatal development in a genetic mouse model of cognitive delay. *Brain Res* (2008) 1217:232–8. doi: 10.1016/j.brainres.2008.04.006
24. Puglisi-Allegra S, Cabib S, Pascucci T, Ventura R, Cali F, Romano V. Dramatic brain aminergic deficit in a genetic mouse model of phenylketonuria. *Neuroreport* (2000) 11(6):1361–4. doi: 10.1097/00001756-200004270-00042
25. Price DL, Brady ST, Siegel GJ, Albers RW. *Basic neurochemistry: principles of molecular, cellular, and medical neurobiology*. Amsterdam: Elsevier Ltd (2012).
26. Nardecchia F, Orlando R, Iacovelli L, Colamartino M, Fiori E, Leuzzi V, et al. Targeting mGlu5 metabotropic glutamate receptors in the treatment of cognitive dysfunction in a mouse model of phenylketonuria. *Front Neurosci* (2018) 12:154. doi: 10.3389/fnins.2018.00154
27. Martynyuk AE, Glushakov AV, Sumners C, Laipis PJ, Dennis DM, Seubert CN. Impaired glutamatergic synaptic transmission in the PKU brain. *Mol Genet Metab* (2005) 86(SUPPL):S34–42. doi: 10.1016/j.ymgme.2005.06.014
28. Popoli M, Yan Z, McEwen BS, Sanacora G. The stressed synapse: the impact of stress and glucocorticoids on glutamate transmission. *Nat Rev Neurosci* (2011) 13:22. doi: 10.1038/nrn3138
29. Cordero ME, Trejo M, Colombo M, Aranda V. Histological maturation of the neocortex in phenylketonuric rats. *Early Hum Dev* (1983) 8(2):157–73. doi: 10.1016/0378-3782(83)90072-5
30. Andolina D, Conversi D, Cabib S, Trabalza A, Ventura R, Puglisi-Allegra S, et al. 5-Hydroxytryptophan during critical postnatal period improves cognitive performances and promotes dendritic spine maturation in genetic mouse model of phenylketonuria. *Int J Neuropsychopharmacol* (2011) 14(4):479–89. doi: 10.1017/S1461145710001288
31. Horster F, Schwab MA, Sauer SW, Pietz J, Hoffmann GF, Okun JG, et al. Phenylalanine reduces synaptic density in mixed cortical cultures from mice. *Pediatr Res* (2006) 59(4 Pt 1):544–8. doi: 10.1203/01.pdr.0000203091.45988.8d
32. de Freitas MS, de Mattos-Dutra A, Schroder N, Wannmacher CM, Pessoa-Pureur R. Effect of hyperphenylalaninemia chemically induced on *in vitro* incorporation of 32P into cytoskeletal proteins from cerebral

cortex of developing rats. *Exp Neurol* (1997) 143(2):188–95. doi: 10.1006/exnr.1996.6351

33. Schlegel G, Scholz R, Ullrich K, Santer R, Rune GM. Phenylketonuria: direct and indirect effects of phenylalanine. *Exp Neurol* (2016) 281:28–36. doi: 10.1016/j.expneurol.2016.04.013
34. Liang L, Gu X, Lu L, Li D, Zhang X. Phenylketonuria-related synaptic changes in a BTBR-Pah(enu2) mouse model. *Neuroreport* (2011) 22(12):617–22. doi: 10.1097/WNR.0b013e3283495acc
35. Bruinenberg VM, van Vliet D, Attali A, de Wilde MC, Kuhn M, van Spronsen FJ, et al. A specific nutrient combination attenuates the reduced expression of PSD-95 in the proximal dendrites of hippocampal cell body layers in a mouse model of phenylketonuria. *Nutrients* (2016) 8(4):185. doi: 10.3390/nu8040185
36. Shah SN, Peterson NA, McKean CM. Lipid composition of human cerebral white matter and myelin in phenylketonuria. *J Neurochem* (1972) 19(10):2369–76. doi: 10.1111/j.1471-4159.1972.tb01291.x
37. Malamud N. Neuropathology of phenylketonuria. *J Neuropathol Exp Neurol* (1966) 25(2):254–68. doi: 10.1097/00005072-196604000-00006
38. Bauman ML, Kemper TL. Morphologic and histoanatomic observations of the brain in untreated human phenylketonuria. *Acta Neuropathol* (1982) 58:55–63. doi: 10.1007/BF00692698
39. Paus T. Mapping brain maturation and cognitive development during adolescence. *Trends Cogn Sci* (2005) 9(2):60–8. doi: 10.1016/j.tics.2004.12.008
40. Fuster JM. Frontal lobe and cognitive development. *J Neurocytol* (2002) 31(3):373–85.
41. Shefer S, Tint GS, Jean-Guillaume D, Daikhin E, Kendler A, Nguyen LB, et al. Is there a relationship between 3-hydroxy-3-methylglutaryl coenzyme a reductase activity and forebrain pathology in the PKU mouse? *J Neurosci Res* (2000) 61(5):549–63. doi: 10.1002/1097-4547(20000901)61:5<549::AID-JNR10>3.0.CO;2-0
42. Hoeksma M, Reijngoud DJ, Pruim J, de Valk HW, Paans AM, van Spronsen FJ. Phenylketonuria: high plasma phenylalanine decreases cerebral protein synthesis. *Mol Genet Metab* (2009) 96(4):177–82. doi: 10.1016/j.ymgme.2008.12.019
43. Surtees R, Blau N. The neurochemistry of phenylketonuria. *Eur J Pediatr* (2000) 159 Suppl 2:S109–13. doi: 10.1007/PL00014370
44. Bartzokis G. Quadratic trajectories of brain myelin content: unifying construct for neuropsychiatric disorders. *Neurobiol Aging* (2004) 25(1):49–62. doi: 10.1016/j.neurobiolaging.2003.08.001
45. Reynolds R, Burri R, Herschkowitz N. Retarded development of neurons and oligodendroglia in rat forebrain produced by hyperphenylalaninemia results in permanent deficits in myelin despite long recovery periods. *Exp Neurol* (1993) 124(2):357–67. doi: 10.1006/exnr.1993.1206
46. Smith CB, Kang J. Cerebral protein synthesis in a genetic mouse model of phenylketonuria. *Proc Natl Acad Sci USA* (2000) 97(20):11014–9. doi: 10.1073/pnas.97.20.11014
47. Dyer CA, Kendler A, Philibotte T, Gardiner P, Cruz J, Levy HL. Evidence for central nervous system glial cell plasticity in phenylketonuria. *J Neuropathol Exp Neurol* (1996) 55(7):795–814. doi: 10.1097/00005072-199607000-00005
48. Sanchez I, Hassinger L, Paskevich PA, Shine HD, Nixon RA. Oligodendroglia regulate the regional expansion of axon caliber and local accumulation of neurofilaments during development independently of myelin formation. *J Neurosci* (1996) 16(16):5095–105. doi: 10.1523/JNEUROSCI.16-16-05095.1996
49. Thompson AJ, Youl BD, Kendall B, Lees AJ, Smith I, Brenton D, et al. Neurological deterioration in young adults with phenylketonuria. *Lancet* (1990) 336(8715):602–5. doi: 10.1016/0140-6736(90)93401-A
50. Cleary MA, Walter JH, Wraith JE, Alani SM, Whittle D, Jenkins JPR, et al. Magnetic resonance imaging of the brain in phenylketonuria. *Lancet* (1994) 344(8915):87–90. doi: 10.1016/S0140-6736(94)91281-5
51. Leuzzi V, Trasimeni G, Gualdi GF, Antonozzi I. Biochemical, clinical and neuroradiological (MRI) correlations in late-detected PKU patients. *J Inherit Metab Dis* (1995) 18(5):624–34. doi: 10.1007/BF02436009
52. Leuzzi V, Tosetti M, Montanaro D, Carducci C, Artiola C, Carducci C, et al. The pathogenesis of the white matter abnormalities in phenylketonuria. A multimodal 3.0 tesla MRI and magnetic resonance spectroscopy (1H MRS) study. *J Inherit Metab Dis* (2007) 30(2):209–16. doi: 10.1007/s10545-006-0399-4
53. Kono K, Okano Y, Nakayama K, Hase Y, Minamikawa S, Ozawa N, et al. Diffusion-weighted MR imaging in patients with phenylketonuria: relationship between serum phenylalanine levels and ADC values in cerebral white matter. *Radiology* (2005) 236(2):630–6. doi: 10.1148/radiol.2362040611
54. Mastrangelo M, Chiarotti F, Berillo L, Caputi C, Carducci C, Di Biasi C, et al. The outcome of white matter abnormalities in early treated phenylketonuric patients: a retrospective longitudinal long-term study. *Mol Genet Metab* (2015) 116(3):171–7. doi: 10.1016/j.ymgme.2015.08.005
55. Bilder DA, Burton BK, Coon H, Leviton L, Ashworth J, Lundy BD, et al. Psychiatric symptoms in adults with phenylketonuria. *Mol Genet Metab* (2013) 108(3):155–60. doi: 10.1016/j.ymgme.2012.12.006
56. Folling A. [Phenylketonuria]. *Tidsskr Nor Laegeforen* (1967) 87(5):451–4.
57. Nagler B, Wood J. Progress Report on PKU1965. 386-91 p.
58. Penrose LS. *The biology of mental defect.* 3d rev. and reset ed. London: Sidgwick and Jackson (1963). xxiv, 374 p.
59. Mazur A, Jarochowicz S, Ołtarzewski M, Sykut-Cegielska J, Gradowska W, Januszek-Trzciąkowska A, et al. An investigation of the neurological and neuropsychiatric disturbances in adults with undiagnosed and/or untreated phenylketonuria in Poland. *J Appl Res Intellect Disabil* (2011) 24(5):482–8. doi: 10.1111/j.1468-3148.2011.00628.x
60. Bone A, Kuehl AK, Angelino AF. A neuropsychiatric perspective of phenylketonuria I: overview of phenylketonuria and its neuropsychiatric sequelae. *Psychosomatics* (2012) 53(6):517–23. doi: 10.1016/j.psym.2012.04.010
61. Gassio R, Artuch R, Vilaseca MA, Fuste E, Boix C, Sans A, et al. Cognitive functions in classic phenylketonuria and mild hyperphenylalaninaemia: experience in a paediatric population. *Dev Med Child Neurol* (2005) 47(7):443–8. doi: 10.1017/S0012162205000861
62. Burton BK, Leviton L, Vespa H, Coon H, Longo N, Lundy BD, et al. A diversified approach for PKU treatment: routine screening yields high incidence of psychiatric distress in phenylketonuria clinics. *Mol Genet Metab* (2013) 108(1):8–12. doi: 10.1016/j.ymgme.2012.11.003
63. Pietz J, Fatkenheuer B, Burgard P, Armbruster M, Esser G, Schmidt H. Psychiatric disorders in adult patients with early-treated phenylketonuria. *Pediatrics* (1997) 99(3):345–50. doi: 10.1542/peds.99.3.345
64. Ford S, O'Driscoll M, MacDonald A. Living with Phenylketonuria: lessons from the PKU community. *Mol Genet Metab Rep* (2018) 17:57–63. doi: 10.1016/j.ymgmr.2018.10.002
65. Jahja R, Huijbregts SCJ, de Sonneville LMJ, van der Meere JJ, Legemaat AM, Bosch AM, et al. Cognitive profile and mental health in adult phenylketonuria: a PKU-COBESO study. *Neuropsychology* (2017) 31(4):437–47. doi: 10.1037/neu0000358
66. Bilder DA, Kobori JA, Cohen-Pfeffer JL, Johnson EM, Jurecki ER, Grant ML. Neuropsychiatric comorbidities in adults with phenylketonuria: a retrospective cohort study. *Mol Genet Metab* (2017) 121(1):1–8. doi: 10.1016/j.ymgme.2017.03.002
67. Hasler G. Pathophysiology of depression: do we have any solid evidence of interest to clinicians? *World Psychiatry* (2010) 9(3):155–61. doi: 10.1002/j.2051-5545.2010.tb00298.x
68. Brumm VL, Bilder D, Waisbren SE. Psychiatric symptoms and disorders in phenylketonuria. *Mol Genet Metab* (2010) 99 Suppl 1:S59–63. doi: 10.1016/j.ymgme.2009.10.182
69. ten Hoedt AE, de Sonneville LM, Francois B, ter Horst NM, Janssen MC, Rubio-Gozalbo ME, et al. High phenylalanine levels directly affect mood and sustained attention in adults with phenylketonuria: a randomised, double-blind, placebo-controlled, crossover trial. *J Inherit Metab Dis* (2011) 34(1):165–71. doi: 10.1007/s10545-010-9253-9
70. Leonard BE. The role of noradrenaline in depression: a review. *J Psychopharmacol* (1997) 11(4 Suppl):S39–47.
71. Maes M, Meltzer H. The serotonin hypothesis of major depression. In: Bloom F, Kupfer D, editors. *Psychopharmacology: The Fourth Generation.* Raven Press (1995).
72. Morilak DA, Frazer A. Antidepressants and brain monoaminergic systems: a dimensional approach to understanding their behavioural effects in depression and anxiety disorders. *Int J Neuropsychopharmacol* (2004) 7(2):193–218. doi: 10.1017/S1461145704004080
73. Ressler KJ, Nemeroff CB. Role of serotonergic and noradrenergic systems in the pathophysiology of depression and anxiety disorders. *Depress Anxiety* (2000) 12 Suppl 1:2–19. doi: 10.1002/1520-6394(2000)12:1+<2::AID-DA2>3.3.CO;2-W

74. Racagni G, Popoli M. Cellular and molecular mechanisms in the long-term action of antidepressants. *Dialogues Clin Neurosci* (2008) 10(4):385–400.
75. Eliwa H, Belzung C, Surget A. Adult hippocampal neurogenesis: is it the alpha and omega of antidepressant action? *Biochem Pharmacol* (2017) 141:86–99. doi: 10.1016/j.bcp.2017.08.005
76. Jhaveri DJ, Tedoldi A, Hunt S, Sullivan R, Watts NR, Power JM, et al. Evidence for newly generated interneurons in the basolateral amygdala of adult mice. *Mol Psychiatry* (2018) 23(3):521–32. doi: 10.1038/mp.2017.134
77. Mahar I, Bambico FR, Mechawar N, Nobrega JN. Stress, serotonin, and hippocampal neurogenesis in relation to depression and antidepressant effects. *Neurosci Biobehav Rev* (2014) 38:173–92. doi: 10.1016/j.neubiorev.2013.11.009
78. Homberg JR, Lesch KP. Looking on the bright side of serotonin transporter gene variation. *Biol Psychiatry* (2011) 69(6):513–9. doi: 10.1016/j.biopsych.2010.09.024
79. Waider J, Araragi N, Gutknecht L, Lesch KP. Tryptophan hydroxylase-2 (TPH2) in disorders of cognitive control and emotion regulation: a perspective. *Psychoneuroendocrinology* (2011) 36(3):393–405. doi: 10.1016/j.psyneuen.2010.12.012
80. Manti F, Nardecchia F, Chiarotti F, Carducci C, Carducci C, Leuzzi V. Psychiatric disorders in adolescent and young adult patients with phenylketonuria. *Mol Genet Metab* (2016) 117(1):12–8. doi: 10.1016/j.ymgme.2015.11.006
81. Smith I, Beasley MG, Wolff OH, Ades AE. Behavior disturbance in 8-year-old children with early treated phenylketonuria. Report from the MRC/DHSS phenylketonuria register. *J Pediatr* (1988) 112(3):403–8. doi: 10.1016/S0022-3476(88)80320-2
82. Smith I, Knowles J. Behaviour in early treated phenylketonuria: a systematic review. *Eur J Pediatr* (2000) 159 Suppl 2:S89–93. doi: 10.1007/PL00014392
83. Didycz B, Bik-Multanowski M. Blood phenylalanine instability strongly correlates with anxiety in phenylketonuria. *Mol Genet Metab Rep* (2018) 14:80–2. doi: 10.1016/j.ymgmr.2017.12.003
84. Waisbren SE, Levy HL. Agoraphobia in phenylketonuria. *J Inherit Metab Dis* (1991) 14(5):755–64. doi: 10.1007/BF01799946
85. Ormazabal A, Vilaseca MA, Perez-Duenas B, Lambruschini N, Gomez L, Campistol J, et al. Platelet serotonin concentrations in PKU patients under dietary control and tetrahydrobiopterin treatment. *J Inherit Metab Dis* (2005) 28(6):863–70. doi: 10.1007/s10545-005-0153-3
86. Mann JJ, McBride PA, Brown RP, Linnoila M, Leon AC, DeMeo M, et al. Relationship between central and peripheral serotonin indexes in depressed and suicidal psychiatric inpatients. *Arch Gen Psychiatry* (1992) 49(6):442–6. doi: 10.1001/archpsyc.1992.01820060022003
87. Munro TA. Phenylketonuria: data on forty-seven British families. *Ann Eugen* (1947) 14(1):60–88. doi: 10.1111/j.1469-1809.1947.tb02379.x
88. Talkowski ME, McClain L, Allen T, Bradford LD, Calkins M, Edwards N, et al. Convergent patterns of association between phenylalanine hydroxylase variants and schizophrenia in four independent samples. *Am J Med Genet B Neuropsychiatr Genet* (2009) 150B(4):560–9. doi: 10.1002/ajmg.b.30862
89. Richardson MA, Read LL, Clelland JD, Chao HM, Reilly MA, Romstad A, et al. Phenylalanine hydroxylase gene in psychiatric patients: screening and functional assay of mutations. *Biol Psychiatry* (2003) 53(6):543–53. doi: 10.1016/S0006-3223(02)01528-7
90. Okusaga O, Muravitskaja O, Fuchs D, Ashraf A, Hinman S, Giegling I, et al. Elevated levels of plasma phenylalanine in schizophrenia: a guanosine triphosphate cyclohydrolase-1 metabolic pathway abnormality? *PLoS One* (2014) 9(1):e85945–e. doi: 10.1371/journal.pone.0085945
91. Teraishi T, Ozeki Y, Hori H, Sasayama D, Chiba S, Yamamoto N, et al. 13C-phenylalanine breath test detects altered phenylalanine kinetics in schizophrenia patients. *Transl Psychiatry* (2012) 2:e119. doi: 10.1038/tp.2012.48
92. Polanczyk G, de Lima MS, Horta BL, Biederman J, Rohde LA. The Worldwide Prevalence of ADHD: a Systematic Review and Metaregression Analysis. *Am J Psychiatry* (2007) 164(6):942–8. doi: 10.1176/ajp.2007.164.6.942
93. Epstein JN, Loren REA. Changes in the Definition of ADHD in DSM-5: subtle but Important. *Neuropsychiatry* (2013) 3(5):455–8. doi: 10.2217/npy.13.59
94. American Psychiatric Association. *Diagnostic and statistical manual of mental disorders: DSM-5*. 5th Edition. Arlington, VA: American Psychiatric Association (2013).
95. Antshel KM, Waisbren SE. Developmental timing of exposure to elevated levels of phenylalanine is associated with ADHD symptom expression. *J Abnorm Child Psychol* (2003) 31(6):565–74.
96. Arnold GL, Vladutiu CJ, Orlowski CC, Blakely EM, DeLuca J. Prevalence of stimulant use for attentional dysfunction in children with phenylketonuria. *J Inherit Metab Dis* (2004) 27(2):137–43. doi: 10.1023/B:BOLI.0000028725.37345.62
97. Rowland AS, Lesesne CA, Abramowitz AJ. The epidemiology of attention-deficit/hyperactivity disorder (ADHD): a public health view. *Ment Retard Dev Disabil Res Rev* (2002) 8(3):162–70. doi: 10.1002/mrdd.10036
98. Faraone SV, Perlis RH, Doyle AE, Smoller JW, Goralnick JJ, Holmgren MA, et al. Molecular Genetics of Attention-Deficit/Hyperactivity Disorder. *Biol Psychiatry* (2005) 57(11):1313–23. doi: 10.1016/j.biopsych.2004.11.024
99. Antshel KM. ADHD, learning, and academic performance in phenylketonuria. *Mol Genet Metab* (2010) 99:S52–S8. doi: 10.1016/j.ymgme.2009.09.013
100. Arnsten AF. Fundamentals of attention-deficit/hyperactivity disorder: circuits and pathways. *J Clin Psychiatry* (2006) 67 Suppl 8:7–12.
101. Diamond A, Prevor MB, Callender G, Druin DP. Prefrontal Cortex Cognitive Deficits in Children Treated Early and Continuously for PKU. *Monogr Soc Res Child Dev* (1997) 62(4):i–206. doi: 10.2307/1166208
102. Tam SY, Elsworth JD, Bradberry CW, Roth RH. Mesocortical dopamine neurons: high basal firing frequency predicts tyrosine dependence of dopamine synthesis. *J Neural Transm Gen Sect* (1990) 81(2):97–110. doi: 10.1007/BF01245830
103. Li D, Sham PC, Owen MJ, He L. Meta-analysis shows significant association between dopamine system genes and attention deficit hyperactivity disorder (ADHD). *Hum Mol Genet* (2006) 15(14):2276–84. doi: 10.1093/hmg/ddl152
104. Dougherty DD, Bonab AA, Spencer TJ, Rauch SL, Madras BK, Fischman AJ. Dopamine transporter density in patients with attention deficit hyperactivity disorder. *Lancet* (1999) 354(9196):2132–3. doi: 10.1016/S0140-6736(99)04030-1
105. Levy F. The Dopamine Theory of Attention Deficit Hyperactivity Disorder (ADHD). *Aust N Z J Psychiatry* (1991) 25(2):277–83. doi: 10.3109/00048679109077746
106. Burton B, Grant M, Feigenbaum A, Singh R, Hendren R, Siriwardena K, et al. A randomized, placebo-controlled, double-blind study of sapropterin to treat ADHD symptoms and executive function impairment in children and adults with sapropterin-responsive phenylketonuria. *Mol Genet Metab* (2015) 114(3):415–24. doi: 10.1016/j.ymgme.2014.11.011
107. Griffiths PV, Demellweek C, Fay N, Robinson PH, Davidson DC. Wechsler subscale IQ and subtest profile in early treated phenylketonuria. *Arch Dis Child* (2000) 82(3):209–15. doi: 10.1136/adc.82.3.209
108. Burgard P. Development of intelligence in early treated phenylketonuria. *Eur J Pediatr* (2000) 159 Suppl 2:S74–9. doi: 10.1007/PL00014388
109. Huijbregts SC, de Sonneville LM, Licht R, van Spronsen FJ, Verkerk PH, Sergeant JA. Sustained attention and inhibition of cognitive interference in treated phenylketonuria: associations with concurrent and lifetime phenylalanine concentrations. *Neuropsychologia* (2002) 40(1):7–15. doi: 10.1016/S0028-3932(01)00078-1
110. Schmidt E, Burgard P, Rupp A. Effects of concurrent phenylalanine levels on sustained attention and calculation speed in patients treated early for phenylketonuria. *Eur J Pediatr* (1996) 155 Suppl 1:S82–6. doi: 10.1007/PL00014258
111. Weglage J, Pietsch M, Funders B, Koch HG, Ullrich K. Deficits in selective and sustained attention processes in early treated children with phenylketonuria–result of impaired frontal lobe functions? *Eur J Pediatr* (1996) 155(3):200–4. doi: 10.1007/BF01953938
112. Anderson PJ, Wood SJ, Francis DE, Coleman L, Anderson V, Boneh A. Are neuropsychological impairments in children with early-treated phenylketonuria (PKU) related to white matter abnormalities or elevated phenylalanine levels? *Dev Neuropsychol* (2007) 32(2):645–68. doi: 10.1080/87565640701375963

113. Channon S, Mockler C, Lee P. Executive functioning and speed of processing in phenylketonuria. *Neuropsychology* (2005) 19(5):679–86. doi: 10.1037/0894-4105.19.5.679
114. Huijbregts S, de Sonneville L, Licht R, Sergeant J, van Spronsen F. Inhibition of prepotent responding and attentional flexibility in treated phenylketonuria. *Dev Neuropsychol* (2002) 22(2):481–99. doi: 10.1207/S15326942DN2202_4
115. White DA, Nortz MJ, Mandernach T, Huntington K, Steiner RD. Deficits in memory strategy use related to prefrontal dysfunction during early development: evidence from children with phenylketonuria. *Neuropsychology* (2001) 15(2):221–9. doi: 10.1037//0894-4105.15.2.221
116. Huijbregts SC, de Sonneville LM, van Spronsen FJ, Licht R, Sergeant JA. The neuropsychological profile of early and continuously treated phenylketonuria: orienting, vigilance, and maintenance versus manipulation-functions of working memory. *Neurosci Biobehav Rev* (2002) 26(6):697–712. doi: 10.1016/S0149-7634(02)00040-4
117. Huijbregts SC, De Sonneville LM, Van Spronsen FJ, Berends IE, Licht R, Verkerk PH, et al. Motor function under lower and higher controlled processing demands in early and continuously treated phenylketonuria. *Neuropsychology* (2003) 17(3):369–79. doi: 10.1037/0894-4105.17.3.369
118. Leuzzi V, Pansini M, Sechi E, Chiarotti F, Carducci C, Levi G, et al. Executive function impairment in early-treated PKU subjects with normal mental development. *J Inherit Metab Dis* (2004) 27(2):115–25. doi: 10.1023/B:BOLI.0000028781.94251.1f
119. Welsh MC, Pennington BF, Ozonoff S, Rouse B, McCabe ER. Neuropsychology of early-treated phenylketonuria: specific executive function deficits. *Child Dev* (1990) 61(6):1697–713. doi: 10.1111/j.1467-8624.1990.tb03560.x
120. Cappelletti S, Cotugno G, Goffredo BM, Nicolo R, Bernabei SM, Caviglia S, et al. Cognitive findings and behavior in children and adolescents with phenylketonuria. *J Dev Behav Pediatr* (2013) 34(6):392–8. doi: 10.1097/DBP.0b013e31829a79ef
121. Anderson PJ, Leuzzi V. White matter pathology in phenylketonuria. *Mol Genet Metab* (2010) 99 Suppl 1:S3–9. doi: 10.1016/j.ymgme.2009.10.005
122. DeRoche K, Welsh M. Twenty-five years of research on neurocognitive outcomes in early-treated phenylketonuria: intelligence and executive function. *Dev Neuropsychol* (2008) 33(4):474–504. doi: 10.1080/87565640802101482
123. Blair C. School readiness. Integrating cognition and emotion in a neurobiological conceptualization of children's functioning at school entry. *Am Psychol* (2002) 57(2):111–27. doi: 10.1037//0003-066X.57.2.111
124. Schulze A, Mayatepek E, Hoffmann GF. Evaluation of 6-year application of the enzymatic colorimetric phenylalanine assay in the setting of neonatal screening for phenylketonuria. *Clin Chim Acta* (2002) 317(1-2):27–37. doi: 10.1016/S0009-8981(01)00736-7
125. Berlin CM, Levy HL, Hanley WB. Delayed increase in blood phenylalanine concentration in phenylketonuric children initially classified as mild hyperphenylalaninemia. *Screening* (1995) 4:35–9. doi: 10.1016/0925-6164(95)00105-U
126. Campistol J, Gassio R, Artuch R, Vilaseca MA. Unit PKUF-u. Neurocognitive function in mild hyperphenylalaninemia. *Dev Med Child Neurol* (2011) 53(5):405–8. doi: 10.1111/j.1469-8749.2010.03869.x
127. van Spronsen FJ. Mild hyperphenylalaninemia: to treat or not to treat. *J Inherit Metab Dis* (2011) 34(3):651–6. doi: 10.1007/s10545-011-9283-y
128. Burlina AP, Lachmann RH, Manara R, Cazzorla C, Celato A, van Spronsen FJ, et al. The neurological and psychological phenotype of adult patients with early-treated phenylketonuria: a systematic review. *J Inherit Metab Dis* (2019) 42(2):209–19. doi: 10.1002/jimd.12065
129. Hofman DL, Champ CL, Lawton CL, Henderson M, Dye L. A systematic review of cognitive functioning in early treated adults with phenylketonuria. *Orphanet J Rare Dis* (2018) 13(1):150. doi: 10.1186/s13023-018-0893-4
130. Blau N, Belanger-Quintana A, Demirkol M, Feillet F, Giovannini M, MacDonald A, et al. Management of phenylketonuria in Europe: survey results from 19 countries. *Mol Genet Metab* (2010) 99(2):109–15. doi: 10.1016/j.ymgme.2009.09.005
131. Enns GM, Koch R, Brumm V, Blakely E, Suter R, Jurecki E. Suboptimal outcomes in patients with PKU treated early with diet alone: revisiting the evidence. *Mol Genet Metab* (2010) 101(2-3):99–109. doi: 10.1016/j.ymgme.2010.05.017
132. Palermo L, Geberhiwot T, MacDonald A, Limback E, Hall SK, Romani C. Cognitive outcomes in early-treated adults with phenylketonuria (PKU): a comprehensive picture across domains. *Neuropsychology* (2017) 31(3):255–67. doi: 10.1037/neu0000337
133. Weglage J, Fromm J, van Teeffelen-Heithoff A, Moller HE, Koletzko B, Marquardt T, et al. Neurocognitive functioning in adults with phenylketonuria: results of a long term study. *Mol Genet Metab* (2013) 110 Suppl:S44–8. doi: 10.1016/j.ymgme.2013.08.013
134. Huttenlocher PR. The neuropathology of phenylketonuria: human and animal studies. *Eur J Pediatr* (2000) 159 Suppl 2:S102–6. doi: 10.1007/PL00014371
135. Gonzalez MJ, Gutierrez AP, Gassio R, Fuste ME, Vilaseca MA, Campistol J. Neurological complications and behavioral problems in patients with phenylketonuria in a follow-up unit. *Mol Genet Metab* (2011) 104 Suppl:S73–9. doi: 10.1016/j.ymgme.2011.07.015
136. Brumm VL, Grant ML. The role of intelligence in phenylketonuria: a review of research and management. *Mol Genet Metab* (2010) 99 Suppl 1:S18–21. doi: 10.1016/j.ymgme.2009.10.015
137. Lindegren ML, Krishnaswami S, Fonnesbeck C, Reimschisel T, Fisher J, Jackson K et al. *Adjuvant Treatment for Phenylketonuria (PKU).* Rockville (MD): AHRQ Comparative Effectiveness Reviews (2012).
138. Waisbren SE, Noel K, Fahrbach K, Cella C, Frame D, Dorenbaum A, et al. Phenylalanine blood levels and clinical outcomes in phenylketonuria: a systematic literature review and meta-analysis. *Mol Genet Metab* (2007) 92(1-2):63–70. doi: 10.1016/j.ymgme.2007.05.006
139. Diamond A. Executive functions. *Annu Rev Psychol* (2013) 64:135–68. doi: 10.1146/annurev-psych-113011-143750
140. Welsh MC. Developmental and clinical variations in executive functions. In: *Developmental variations in learning: Applications to social, executive function, language, and reading skills.* Lawrence Erlbaum Associates Publishers (2002). p. 139–85.
141. van Spronsen FJ, Huijbregts SC, Bosch AM, Leuzzi V. Cognitive, neurophysiological, neurological and psychosocial outcomes in early-treated PKU-patients: a start toward standardized outcome measurement across development. *Mol Genet Metab* (2011) 104 Suppl:S45–51. doi: 10.1016/j.ymgme.2011.09.036
142. Christ SE, Huijbregts SC, de Sonneville LM, White DA. Executive function in early-treated phenylketonuria: profile and underlying mechanisms. *Mol Genet Metab* (2010) 99 Suppl 1:S22–32. doi: 10.1016/j.ymgme.2009.10.007
143. Salthouse TA. What cognitive abilities are involved in trail-making performance? *Intelligence* (2011) 39(4):222–32. doi: 10.1016/j.intell.2011.03.001
144. Koch R, Hanley W, Levy H, Matalon K, Matalon R, Rouse B, et al. The Maternal Phenylketonuria International Study: 1984-2002. *Pediatrics* (2003) 112(6 Pt 2):1523–9.
145. Waisbren SE, Azen C. Cognitive and behavioral development in maternal phenylketonuria offspring. *Pediatrics* (2003) 112(6 Pt 2):1544–7.
146. Guttler F, Lou H, Andresen J, Kok K, Mikkelsen I, Nielsen KB, et al. Cognitive development in offspring of untreated and preconceptionally treated maternal phenylketonuria. *J Inherit Metab Dis* (1990) 13(4):665–71. doi: 10.1007/BF01799522
147. Hughes C, Leekam S. What are the Links Between Theory of Mind and Social Relations? Review, Reflections and New Directions for Studies of Typical and Atypical Development. *Soc Dev* (2004) 13(4):590–619. doi: 10.1111/j.1467-9507.2004.00285.x
148. Jahja R, van Spronsen FJ, de Sonneville LMJ, van der Meere JJ, Bosch AM, Hollak CEM, et al. Social-cognitive functioning and social skills in patients with early treated phenylketonuria: a PKU-COBESO study. *J Inherit Metab Dis* (2016) 39(3):355–62. doi: 10.1007/s10545-016-9918-0
149. Arnsten AF, Rubia K. Neurobiological circuits regulating attention, cognitive control, motivation, and emotion: disruptions in neurodevelopmental psychiatric disorders. *J Am Acad Child Adolesc Psychiatry* (2012) 51(4):356–67. doi: 10.1016/j.jaac.2012.01.008
150. Heinz AJ, Beck A, Meyer-Lindenberg A, Sterzer P, Heinz A. Cognitive and neurobiological mechanisms of alcohol-related aggression. *Nat Rev Neurosci* (2011) 12(7):400–13. doi: 10.1038/nrn3042
151. Murphy FC, Smith KA, Cowen PJ, Robbins TW, Sahakian BJ. The effects of tryptophan depletion on cognitive and affective processing in healthy

volunteers. *Psychopharmacology* (2002) 163(1):42–53. doi: 10.1007/s00213-002-1128-9

152. Beauchamp MH, Anderson V. SOCIAL: an integrative framework for the development of social skills. *Psychol Bull* (2010) 136(1):39–64. doi: 10.1037/a0017768
153. Burlina AB, Bonafe L, Ferrari V, Suppiej A, Zacchello F, Burlina AP. Measurement of neurotransmitter metabolites in the cerebrospinal fluid of phenylketonuric patients under dietary treatment. *J Inherit Metab Dis* (2000) 23(4):313–6. doi: 10.1023/A:1005694122277
154. Antenor-Dorsey JA, Hershey T, Rutlin J, Shimony JS, McKinstry RC, Grange DK, et al. White matter integrity and executive abilities in individuals with phenylketonuria. *Mol Genet Metab* (2013) 109(2):125–31. doi: 10.1016/j.ymgme.2013.03.020
155. Moyle JJ, Fox AM, Arthur M, Bynevelt M, Burnett JR. Meta-analysis of neuropsychological symptoms of adolescents and adults with PKU. *Neuropsychol Rev* (2007) 17(2):91–101. doi: 10.1007/s11065-007-9021-2
156. Moller HE, Weglage J, Bick U, Wiedermann D, Feldmann R, Ullrich K. Brain imaging and proton magnetic resonance spectroscopy in patients with phenylketonuria. *Pediatrics* (2003) 112(6 Pt 2):1580–3.
157. Joseph B, Dyer CA. Relationship between myelin production and dopamine synthesis in the PKU mouse brain. *J Neurochem* (2003) 86(3):615–26. doi: 10.1046/j.1471-4159.2003.01887.x
158. Bodin D, Beetar JT, Yeates KO, Boyer K, Colvin AN, Mangeot S. A survey of parent satisfaction with pediatric neuropsychological evaluations. *Clin Neuropsychol* (2007) 21(6):884–98. doi: 10.1080/13854040600888784
159. Tau GZ, Peterson BS. Normal development of brain circuits. *Neuropsychopharmacology* (2009) 35:147. doi: 10.1038/npp.2009.115
160. Forrest MP, Parnell E, Penzes P. Dendritic structural plasticity and neuropsychiatric disease. *Nat Rev Neurosci* (2018) 19:215. doi: 10.1038/nrn.2018.16
161. Fonnesbeck CJ, McPheeters ML, Krishnaswami S, Lindegren ML, Reimschisel T. Estimating the probability of IQ impairment from blood phenylalanine for phenylketonuria patients: a hierarchical meta-analysis. *J Inherit Metab Dis* (2013) 36(5):757–66. doi: 10.1007/s10545-012-9564-0
162. MacLeod EL, Gleason ST, van Calcar SC, Ney DM. Reassessment of phenylalanine tolerance in adults with phenylketonuria is needed as body mass changes. *Mol Genet Metab* (2009) 98(4):331–7. doi: 10.1016/j.ymgme.2009.07.016
163. Rohde C, Mutze U, Weigel JF, Ceglarek U, Thiery J, Kiess W, et al. Unrestricted consumption of fruits and vegetables in phenylketonuria: no major impact on metabolic control. *Eur J Clin Nutr* (2012) 66(5):633–8. doi: 10.1038/ejcn.2011.205
164. Macleod EL, Ney DM. Nutritional management of phenylketonuria. *Ann Nestle Eng* (2010) 68(2):58–69. doi: 10.1159/000312813
165. Haberle J, Boddaert N, Burlina A, Chakrapani A, Dixon M, Huemer M, et al. Suggested guidelines for the diagnosis and management of urea cycle disorders. *Orphanet J Rare Dis* (2012) 7:32. doi: 10.1186/1750-1172-7-32
166. MacDonald A, Rylance G, Hall SK, Asplin D, Booth IW. Factors affecting the variation in plasma phenylalanine in patients with phenylketonuria on diet. *Arch Dis Child* (1996) 74(5):412–7. doi: 10.1136/adc.74.5.412
167. Schindeler S, Ghosh-Jerath S, Thompson S, Rocca A, Joy P, Kemp A, et al. The effects of large neutral amino acid supplements in PKU: an MRS and neuropsychological study. *Mol Genet Metab* (2007) 91(1):48–54. doi: 10.1016/j.ymgme.2007.02.002
168. Matalon R, Michals-Matalon K, Bhatia G, Grechanina E, Novikov P, McDonald JD, et al. Large neutral amino acids in the treatment of phenylketonuria (PKU). *J Inherit Metab Dis* (2006) 29(6):732–8. doi: 10.1007/s10545-006-0395-8
169. Strisciuglio P, Concolino D. New Strategies for the Treatment of Phenylketonuria (PKU). *Metabolites* (2014) 4(4):1007–17. doi: 10.3390/metabo4041007
170. van Vliet D, Bruinenberg VM, Mazzola PN, van Faassen MH, de Blaauw P, Pascucci T, et al. Therapeutic brain modulation with targeted large neutral amino acid supplements in the Pah-enu2 phenylketonuria mouse model. *Am J Clin Nutr* (2016) 104(5):1292–300. doi: 10.3945/ajcn.116.135996
171. van Vliet D, van der Goot E, Bruinenberg VM, van Faassen M, de Blaauw P, Kema IP, et al. Large neutral amino acid supplementation as an alternative to the phenylalanine-restricted diet in adults with phenylketonuria: evidence from adult Pah-enu2 mice. *J Nutr Biochem* (2018) 53:20–7. doi: 10.1016/j.jnutbio.2017.09.020
172. Cabana MD, Kiyoshi-Teo H. The broader picture on guideline adherence. *JPEN J Parenter Enteral Nutr* (2010) 34(6):593–4. doi: 10.1177/0148607110375698
173. Ney DM, Stroup BM, Clayton MK, Murali SG, Rice GM, Rohr F, et al. Glycomacropeptide for nutritional management of phenylketonuria: a randomized, controlled, crossover trial. *Am J Clin Nutr* (2016) 104(2):334–45. doi: 10.3945/ajcn.116.135293
174. Lohner S, Fekete K, Decsi T. Lower n-3 long-chain polyunsaturated fatty acid values in patients with phenylketonuria: a systematic review and meta-analysis. *Nutr Res (New York, NY)* (2013) 33(7):513–20. doi: 10.1016/j.nutres.2013.05.003
175. Drzymala-Czyz S, Kaluzny L, Krzyzanowska-Jankowska P, Walkowiak D, Mozrzymas R, Walkowiak J. Deficiency of long-chain polyunsaturated fatty acids in phenylketonuria: a cross-sectional study. *Acta Biochim Pol* (2018) 65(2):303–8. doi: 10.18388/abp.2018_2565
176. Koletzko B, Beblo S, Demmelmair H, Hanebutt FL. Omega-3 LC-PUFA supply and neurological outcomes in children with phenylketonuria (PKU). *J Pediatr Gastroenterol Nutr* (2009) 48 Suppl 1:S2–7. doi: 10.1097/MPG.0b013e3181977399
177. Pey AL, Stricher F, Serrano L, Martinez A. Predicted effects of missense mutations on native-state stability account for phenotypic outcome in phenylketonuria, a paradigm of misfolding diseases. *Am J Hum Genet* (2007) 81(5):1006–24. doi: 10.1086/521879
178. Cerone R, Andria G, Giovannini M, Leuzzi V, Riva E, Burlina A. Testing for tetrahydrobiopterin responsiveness in patients with hyperphenylalaninemia due to phenylalanine hydroxylase deficiency. *Adv Ther* (2013) 30(3):212–28. doi: 10.1007/s12325-013-0011-x
179. Lindegren ML, Krishnaswami S, Reimschisel T, Fonnesbeck C, Sathe NA. McPheeters ML. A Systematic Review of BH4 (Sapropterin) for the Adjuvant Treatment of Phenylketonuria. *JIMD Rep* (2013) 8:109–19. doi: 10.1007/8904_2012_168
180. Somaraju UR, Merrin M. Sapropterin dihydrochloride for phenylketonuria. *Cochrane Database Syst Rev* (2015) (3), CD008005. doi: 10.1002/14651858.CD008005.pub4
181. Trefz FK, Burton BK, Longo N, Casanova MM, Gruskin DJ, Dorenbaum A, et al. Efficacy of sapropterin dihydrochloride in increasing phenylalanine tolerance in children with phenylketonuria: a phase III, randomized, double-blind, placebo-controlled study. *J Pediatr* (2009) 154(5):700–7. doi: 10.1016/j.jpeds.2008.11.040
182. Burlina A, Blau N. Effect of BH(4) supplementation on phenylalanine tolerance. *J Inherit Metab Dis* (2009) 32(1):40–5. doi: 10.1007/s10545-008-0947-1
183. Keil S, Anjema K, van Spronsen FJ, Lambruschini N, Burlina A, Belanger-Quintana A, et al. Long-term follow-up and outcome of phenylketonuria patients on sapropterin: a retrospective study. *Pediatrics* (2013) 131(6):e1881–8. doi: 10.1542/peds.2012-3291
184. Pey AL, Ying M, Cremades N, Velazquez-Campoy A, Scherer T, Thony B, et al. Identification of pharmacological chaperones as potential therapeutic agents to treat phenylketonuria. *J Clin Invest* (2008) 118(8):2858–67. doi: 10.1172/JCI34355
185. Burton BK, Grange DK, Milanowski A, Vockley G, Feillet F, Crombez EA, et al. The response of patients with phenylketonuria and elevated serum phenylalanine to treatment with oral sapropterin dihydrochloride (6R-tetrahydrobiopterin): a phase II, multicentre, open-label, screening study. *J Inherit Metab Dis* (2007) 30(5):700–7. doi: 10.1007/s10545-007-0605-z
186. Levy HL, Milanowski A, Chakrapani A, Cleary M, Lee P, Trefz FK, et al. Efficacy of sapropterin dihydrochloride (tetrahydrobiopterin, 6R-BH4) for reduction of phenylalanine concentration in patients with phenylketonuria: a phase III randomised placebo-controlled study. *Lancet* (2007) 370(9586):504–10. doi: 10.1016/S0140-6736(07)61234-3
187. Bell SM, Wendt DJ, Zhang Y, Taylor TW, Long S, Tsuruda L, et al. Formulation and PEGylation optimization of the therapeutic PEGylated phenylalanine ammonia lyase for the treatment of phenylketonuria. *PLoS One* (2017) 12(3):e0173269. doi: 10.1371/journal.pone.0173269

188. Thomas J, Levy H, Amato S, Vockley J, Zori R, Dimmock D, et al. Pegvaliase for the treatment of phenylketonuria: results of a long-term phase 3 clinical trial program (PRISM). *Mol Genet Metab* (2018) 124(1):27–38. doi: 10.1016/j.ymgme.2018.03.006
189. Longo N, Harding CO, Burton BK, Grange DK, Vockley J, Wasserstein M, et al. Single-dose, subcutaneous recombinant phenylalanine ammonia lyase conjugated with polyethylene glycol in adult patients with phenylketonuria: an open-label, multicentre, phase 1 dose-escalation trial. *Lancet* (2014) 384(9937):37–44. doi: 10.1016/S0140-6736(13)61841-3
190. Zori R, Thomas JA, Shur N, Rizzo WB, Decker C, Rosen O, et al. Induction, titration, and maintenance dosing regimen in a phase 2 study of pegvaliase for control of blood phenylalanine in adults with phenylketonuria. *Mol Genet Metab* (2018). 125(3):217–227. doi: 10.1016/j.ymgme.2018.06.010
191. Harding CO, Amato RS, Stuy M, Longo N, Burton BK, Posner J, et al. Pegvaliase for the treatment of phenylketonuria: a pivotal, double-blind randomized discontinuation Phase 3 clinical trial. *Mol Genet Metab* (2018) 124(1):20–6. doi: 10.1016/j.ymgme.2018.03.003
192. Pascucci T, Rossi L, Colamartino M, Gabucci C, Carducci C, Valzania A, et al. A new therapy prevents intellectual disability in mouse with phenylketonuria. *Mol Genet Metab* (2018) 124(1):39–49. doi: 10.1016/j.ymgme.2018.03.009
193. van Rijn M, Hoeksma M, Sauer PJ, Modderman P, Reijngoud DJ, van Spronsen FJ. Adult patients with well-controlled phenylketonuria tolerate incidental additional intake of phenylalanine. *Ann Nutr Metab* (2011) 58(2):94–100. doi: 10.1159/000324924
194. Grosse SD. Late-treated phenylketonuria and partial reversibility of intellectual impairment. *Child Dev* (2010) 81(1):200–11. doi: 10.1111/j.1467-8624.2009.01389.x
195. MacDonald A, Gokmen-Ozel H, van Rijn M, Burgard P. The reality of dietary compliance in the management of phenylketonuria. *J Inherit Metab Dis* (2010) 33(6):665–70. doi: 10.1007/s10545-010-9073-y
196. Berry SA, Brown C, Grant M, Greene CL, Jurecki E, Koch J, et al. Newborn screening 50 years later: access issues faced by adults with PKU. *Genet Med* (2013) 15(8):591–9. doi: 10.1038/gim.2013.10
197. Bruinenberg VM, Gordijn MCM, MacDonald A, van Spronsen FJ, Van der Zee EA. Sleep disturbances in phenylketonuria: an explorative study in men and mice. *Front Neurol* (2017) 8:167. doi: 10.3389/fneur.2017.00167
198. De Giorgis GF, Nonnis E, Crocioni F, Gregori P, Rosini MP, Leuzzi V, et al. Evolution of daytime quiet sleep components in early treated phenylketonuric infants. *Brain Dev* (1996) 18(3):201–6. doi: 10.1016/0387-7604(96)00005-8
199. Surendran S, Campbell GA, Tyring SK, Matalon K, McDonald JD, Matalon R. High levels of orexin A in the brain of the mouse model for phenylketonuria: possible role of orexin A in hyperactivity seen in children with PKU. *Neurochem Res* (2003) 28(12):1891–4. doi: 10.1023/A:1026184127689
200. Surendran S, Rady PL, Szucs S, Michals-Matalon K, Tyring SK, Matalon R. High level of orexin A observed in the phenylketonuria mouse brain is due to the abnormal expression of prepro-orexin. *Biochem Biophys Res Commun* (2004) 317(2):522–6. doi: 10.1016/j.bbrc.2004.03.079

Permissions

All chapters in this book were first published by Frontiers; hereby published with permission under the Creative Commons Attribution License or equivalent. Every chapter published in this book has been scrutinized by our experts. Their significance has been extensively debated. The topics covered herein carry significant findings which will fuel the growth of the discipline. They may even be implemented as practical applications or may be referred to as a beginning point for another development.

The contributors of this book come from diverse backgrounds, making this book a truly international effort. This book will bring forth new frontiers with its revolutionizing research information and detailed analysis of the nascent developments around the world.

We would like to thank all the contributing authors for lending their expertise to make the book truly unique. They have played a crucial role in the development of this book. Without their invaluable contributions this book wouldn't have been possible. They have made vital efforts to compile up to date information on the varied aspects of this subject to make this book a valuable addition to the collection of many professionals and students.

This book was conceptualized with the vision of imparting up-to-date information and advanced data in this field. To ensure the same, a matchless editorial board was set up. Every individual on the board went through rigorous rounds of assessment to prove their worth. After which they invested a large part of their time researching and compiling the most relevant data for our readers.

The editorial board has been involved in producing this book since its inception. They have spent rigorous hours researching and exploring the diverse topics which have resulted in the successful publishing of this book. They have passed on their knowledge of decades through this book. To expedite this challenging task, the publisher supported the team at every step. A small team of assistant editors was also appointed to further simplify the editing procedure and attain best results for the readers.

Apart from the editorial board, the designing team has also invested a significant amount of their time in understanding the subject and creating the most relevant covers. They scrutinized every image to scout for the most suitable representation of the subject and create an appropriate cover for the book.

The publishing team has been an ardent support to the editorial, designing and production team. Their endless efforts to recruit the best for this project, has resulted in the accomplishment of this book. They are a veteran in the field of academics and their pool of knowledge is as vast as their experience in printing. Their expertise and guidance has proved useful at every step. Their uncompromising quality standards have made this book an exceptional effort. Their encouragement from time to time has been an inspiration for everyone.

The publisher and the editorial board hope that this book will prove to be a valuable piece of knowledge for researchers, students, practitioners and scholars across the globe.

List of Contributors

Adriana Lori
Department of Psychiatry and Behavioral Sciences, Emory University School of Medicine, Atlanta, GA, United States

Stephanie A. Maddox
Neurobiology of Fear Laboratory, Division of Depression and Anxiety Disorders, McLean Hospital, Belmont, MA, United States
Department of Psychiatry, Harvard Medical School, Boston, MA, United States

Sumeet Sharma
Department of Psychiatry and Behavioral Sciences, Emory University School of Medicine, Atlanta, GA, United States
Neurobiology of Fear Laboratory, Division of Depression and Anxiety Disorders, McLean Hospital, Belmont, MA, United States

Raül Andero
Institut de Neurociènces, Universitat Autònoma de Barcelona, Bellaterra, Spain CIBERSAM, Corporació Sanitaria Parc Taulí, Sabadell, Spain
Department of Psychobiology and Methodology in Health Sciences, Universitat Autònoma de Barcelona, Bellaterra, Spain

Kerry J. Ressler
Department of Psychiatry and Behavioral Sciences, Emory University School of Medicine, Atlanta, GA, United States
Neurobiology of Fear Laboratory, Division of Depression and Anxiety Disorders, McLean Hospital, Belmont, MA, United States
Department of Psychiatry, Harvard Medical School, Boston, MA, United States

Alicia K. Smith
Department of Psychiatry and Behavioral Sciences, Emory University School of Medicine, Atlanta, GA, United States
Department of Gynecology and Obstetrics, Emory University School of Medicine, Atlanta, GA, United States

Harumi Jyonouchi
Department of Pediatrics, Saint Peter's University Hospital, New Brunswick, NJ, United States
Robert Wood Johnson Medical School-Rutgers, New Brunswick, NJ, United States

Lee Geng
Department of Pediatrics, Saint Peter's University Hospital, New Brunswick, NJ, United States

Shannon Rose and Sirish C. Bennuri
Arkansas Children's Research Institute, Little Rock, AR, United States
Department of Pediatrics, University of Arkansas of Medical Sciences, Little Rock, AR, United States

Richard E. Frye
Department of Child Health, University of Arizona College of Medicine-Phoenix, Phoenix, AZ, United States
Barrow Neurological Institute at Phoenix Children's Hospital, Phoenix, AZ, United States

Melanie M. Ashton
IMPACT Strategic Research Centre, School of Medicine, Barwon Health, Deakin University, Geelong, VIC, Australia
Florey Institute for Neuroscience and Mental Health, University of Melbourne, Parkville, VIC, Australia
Professorial Unit, The Melbourne Clinic, Department of Psychiatry, University of Melbourne, Richmond, VIC, Australia

Olivia M. Dean
IMPACT Strategic Research Centre, School of Medicine, Barwon Health, Deakin University, Geelong, VIC, Australia
Florey Institute for Neuroscience and Mental Health, University of Melbourne, Parkville, VIC, Australia
Department of Psychiatry, Royal Melbourne Hospital, University of Melbourne, Parkville, VIC, Australia

Adam J. Walker and Wolfgang Marx
IMPACT Strategic Research Centre, School of Medicine, Barwon Health, Deakin University, Geelong, VIC, Australia

Chiara C. Bortolasci and Ken Walder
Centre for Molecular and Medical Research, School of Medicine, Deakin University, Geelong, VIC, Australia

Chee H. Ng
Professorial Unit, The Melbourne Clinic, Department of Psychiatry, University of Melbourne, Richmond, VIC, Australia

Malcolm Hopwood
Professorial Psychiatry Unit, Albert Road Clinic, University of Melbourne, Melbourne, VIC, Australia

Brian H. Harvey and Marisa Möller
Centre of Excellence for Pharmaceutical Sciences, School of Pharmacy (Pharmacology), North West University, Potchefstroom, South Africa

John J. McGrath
Queensland Centre for Mental Health Research, The Park Centre for Mental Health, Wacol, QLD, Australia
Queensland Brain Institute, University of Queensland, St. Lucia, QLD, Australia
National Centre for Register-Based Research, Aarhus University, Aarhus, Denmark

Alyna Turner
IMPACT Strategic Research Centre, School of Medicine, Barwon Health, Deakin University, Geelong, VIC, Australia
Department of Psychiatry, Royal Melbourne Hospital, University of Melbourne, Parkville, VIC, Australia

Seetal Dodd
IMPACT Strategic Research Centre, School of Medicine, Barwon Health, Deakin University, Geelong, VIC, Australia
Department of Psychiatry, Royal Melbourne Hospital, University of Melbourne, Parkville, VIC, Australia
Centre of Youth Mental Health, University of Melbourne, Parkville, VIC, Australia

James G. Scott
Queensland Centre for Mental Health Research, The Park Centre for Mental Health, Wacol, QLD, Australia
Faculty of Medicine, The University of Queensland, Herston, QLD, Australia
Metro North Mental Health, Royal Brisbane and Women's Hospital, Brisbane, QLD, Australia

Jon-Paul Khoo
IMPACT Strategic Research Centre, School of Medicine, Barwon Health, Deakin University, Geelong, VIC, Australia
Faculty of Medicine, The University of Queensland, Herston, QLD, Australia

Jerome Sarris
Professorial Unit, The Melbourne Clinic, Department of Psychiatry, University of Melbourne, Richmond, VIC, Australia
NICM Health Research Institute, Western Sydney University, Westmead, NSW, Australia

Jean Bastin
Sorbonne Paris Cité, Faculté des Sciences Fondamentales et Biomédicales, Université Paris Descartes, Paris, France
INSERM, UMR-S 1124, Toxicologie, Pharmacologie et Signalisation Cellulaire, Paris, France

Rita Barone
Child Neurology and Psychiatry, Department of Clinical and Experimental Medicine, University of Catania, Catania, Italy
Referral Centre for Inherited Metabolic Disorders, Department of Clinical and Experimental Medicine, University of Catania, Catania, Italy

Michael Berk
IMPACT Strategic Research Centre, School of Medicine, Barwon Health, Deakin University, Geelong, VIC, Australia
Florey Institute for Neuroscience and Mental Health, University of Melbourne, Parkville, VIC, Australia
Department of Psychiatry, Royal Melbourne Hospital, University of Melbourne, Parkville, VIC, Australia
Centre of Youth Mental Health, University of Melbourne, Parkville, VIC, Australia
Orygen Youth Health Research Centre, Parkville, VIC, Australia

Samuel F. Yanuck
Program on Integrative Medicine, Department of Physical Medicine and Rehabilitation, University of North Carolina School of Medicine, Chapel Hill, NC, United States

Salvatore Alaimo, Alfredo Pulvirenti and Alfredo Ferro
Bioinformatics Unit, Department of Clinical and Experimental Medicine, University of Catania, Catania, Italy

Marianna Messina
Referral Centre for Inherited Metabolic Disorders, Department of Clinical and Experimental Medicine, University of Catania, Catania, Italy

Richard E. Frye
University of Arizona College of Medicine, Phoenix, AZ, United States
Phoenix Children's Hospital, Phoenix, AZ, United States

Renata Rizzo
Child Neurology and Psychiatry, Department of Clinical and Experimental Medicine, University of Catania, Catania, Italy

Rickinder Sethi
Department of Psychiatry, Western University, London, ON, Canada

Nieves Gómez-Coronado
Unidad de Gestión Clinica Salud Mental, Hospital Universitario Virgen del Rocio, Sevilla, Spain

Adam J. Walker and Bruno Agustini
IMPACT Strategic Research Centre, Deakin University, Geelong, VIC, Australia

Oliver D'Arcy Robertson
IMPACT Strategic Research Centre, Deakin University, Geelong, VIC, Australia
University Hospital Geelong, Barwon Health, Geelong, VIC, Australia

Michael Berk
IMPACT Strategic Research Centre, Deakin University, Geelong, VIC, Australia
University Hospital Geelong, Barwon Health, Geelong, VIC, Australia
Department of Psychiatry, The University of Melbourne, Parkville, VIC, Australia
Orygen, The National Centre of Excellence in Youth Mental Health, Parkville, VIC, Australia
Department of Psychiatry, Florey Institute of Neuroscience and Mental Health, Parkville, VIC, Australia

Seetal Dodd
IMPACT Strategic Research Centre, Deakin University, Geelong, VIC, Australia
University Hospital Geelong, Barwon Health, Geelong, VIC, Australia
Department of Psychiatry, The University of Melbourne, Parkville, VIC, Australia
Orygen, The National Centre of Excellence in Youth Mental Health, Parkville, VIC, Australia

Lucija Tudor, Marcela Konjevod, Matea Nikolac Perkovic, Dubravka Svob Strac, Gordana Nedic Erjavec and Nela Pivac
Laboratory for Molecular Neuropsychiatry, Division of Molecular Medicine, Rudjer Boskovic Institute, Zagreb, Croatia

Suzana Uzun and Oliver Kozumplik
Department of Biological Psychiatry and Psychogeriatry, University Psychiatric Hospital Vrapce, Zagreb, Croatia
Faculty of Medicine, Josip Juraj Strossmayer University of Osijek, Osijek, Croatia

Marina Sagud
School of Medicine, University of Zagreb, Zagreb, Croatia
Department of Psychiatry, University Hospital Centre Zagreb, Zagreb, Croatia

Zrnka Kovacic Petrovic
Department of Biological Psychiatry and Psychogeriatry, University Psychiatric Hospital Vrapce, Zagreb, Croatia
Department of Psychopharmacology, Croatian Institute for Brain Research, School of Medicine, University of Zagreb, Zagreb, Croatia

Sirish C. Bennuri and Shannon Rose
Arkansas Children's Research Institute and Department of Pediatrics, University of Arkansas for Medical Sciences, Little Rock, AR, United States

Richard E. Frye
Barrow Neurologic Institute at Phoenix Children's Hospital, Phoenix, AZ, United States
Department of Child Health, University of Arizona College of Medicine—Phoenix, Phoenix, AZ, United States

Seyed A. Safavynia
Department of Anesthesiology, Weill Cornell Medical College, New York, United States

Peter A. Goldstein
Department of Anesthesiology, Weill Cornell Medical College, New York, United States
Department of Medicine, Weill Cornell Medical College, New York, United States
Neuroscience Graduate Program, Weill Cornell Medical College, New York, United States

Ane Gretesdatter Rogne and Sigrun Hope
Department for Neurohabilitation, Oslo University Hospital and University of Oslo, Oslo, Norway

Shibani Dhir, Maya Tarasenko and Eleonora Napoli
Department of Molecular Biosciences, School of Veterinary Medicine, University of California, Davis, Davis, CA, United States

Cecilia Giulivi
Department of Molecular Biosciences, School of Veterinary Medicine, University of California, Davis, Davis, CA, United States
Medical Investigations of Neurodevelopmental Disorders (MIND) Institute, University of California, Davis, Davis, CA, United States

Sina Hafizi
Department of Psychiatry, Rady Faculty of Health Sciences, Max Rady College of Medicine, University of Manitoba, Winnipeg, MB, Canada

Dina Tabatabaei
School of Medicine, Tehran University of Medical Sciences, Tehran, Iran

Meng-Chuan Lai
Centre for Addiction and Mental Health and The Hospital for Sick Children, Department of Psychiatry, University of Toronto, Toronto, ON, Canada
Autism Research Centre, Department of Psychiatry, University of Cambridge, Cambridge, United Kingdom
Department of Psychiatry, National Taiwan University Hospital and College of Medicine, Taipei, Taiwan

Bjørnar Hassel
Department for Neurohabilitation, Oslo University Hospital and University of Oslo, Oslo, Norway
Norwegian Defence Research Establishment (FFI), Kjeller, Norway

Terry Harville
Department of Pathology, University of Arkansas for Medical Sciences, Little Rock, AR, United States
Department of Internal Medicine, University of Arkansas for Medical Sciences, Little Rock, AR, United States

Bobbie Rhodes-Clark
Department of Pathology, University of Arkansas for Medical Sciences, Little Rock, AR, United States

Sirish C. Bennuri, Marie Tippett, Shannon Rose and Stephen Kahler
Department of Pediatrics, College of Medicine, University of Arkansas for Medical Sciences, Little Rock, AR, United States
Arkansas Children's Research Institute, Little Rock, AR, United States

Leanna Delhey
School of Public Health, University of Arkansas for Medical Sciences, Little Rock, AR, United States
Arkansas Children's Research Institute, Little Rock, AR, United States

Rebecca Wynne
National Center for Toxicological Research, Jefferson, AR, United States

Richard E. Frye
Barrow Neurological Institute at Phoenix Children's Hospital, Phoenix, AZ, United States
Department of Child Health, University of Arizona College of Medicine, Phoenix, AZ, United States

Zsolt Kovács
Savaria Department of Biology, ELTE Eötvös Loránd University, Savaria University Centre, Szombathely, Hungary

Dominic P. D'Agostino
Department of Molecular Pharmacology and Physiology, Laboratory of Metabolic Medicine, Morsani College of Medicine, University of South Florida, Tampa, FL, United States
Institute for Human and Machine Cognition, Ocala, FL, United States

Killian Ashe, Wendy Kelso and Sarah Farrand
Neuropsychiatry Unit, Royal Melbourne Hospital, Melbourne, VIC, Australia

David Diamond
Department of Molecular Pharmacology and Physiology, Laboratory of Metabolic Medicine, Morsani College of Medicine, University of South Florida, Tampa, FL, United States
Department of Psychology, Hyperbaric Neuroscience Research Laboratory, University of South Florida, Tampa, FL, United States

Mark S. Kindy
Department of Pharmaceutical Sciences, College of Pharmacy, University of South Florida, Tampa, FL, United States
James A. Haley VA Medical Center, Tampa, FL, United States
Shriners Hospital for Children, Tampa, FL, United States

Christopher Rogers
Department of Molecular Pharmacology and Physiology, Laboratory of Metabolic Medicine, Morsani College of Medicine, University of South Florida, Tampa, FL, United States

Csilla Ari
Department of Psychology, Hyperbaric Neuroscience Research Laboratory, University of South Florida, Tampa, FL, United States

John Slattery
BioRosa Technologies Inc, San Francisco, CA, United States

Julie Panetta
Statewide Adult Metabolic Service, Royal Melbourne Hospital, Melbourne, VIC, Australia

Tim Fazio and Gerard De Jong
Statewide Adult Metabolic Service, Royal Melbourne Hospital, Melbourne, VIC, Australia
Melbourne Medical School, University of Melbourne, Melbourne, VIC, Australia

Mark Walterfang
Neuropsychiatry Unit, Royal Melbourne Hospital, Melbourne, VIC, Australia
Melbourne Neuropsychiatry Centre, University of Melbourne and North-Western Mental Health, Melbourne, VIC, Australia
Florey Institute of Neuroscience and Mental Health, University of Melbourne, Melbourne, VIC, Australia

Index

N

O

P

Q

R

S

T

W